# Nursing and Health Interventions

# Nursing and Health Interventions

## Design, Evaluation, and Implementation

### SECOND EDITION

## Souraya Sidani

Ryerson University
Toronto, ON, Canada

## Carrie Jo Braden

University of Texas Health Science Center
San Antonio, TX, USA

**WILEY** Blackwell

*Registered Offices*
John Wiley & Sons, Inc., 111 River Street, Hoboken, NJ 07030, USA
John Wiley & Sons Ltd, The Atrium, Southern Gate, Chichester, West Sussex, PO19 8SQ, UK

*Editorial Office*
9600 Garsington Road, Oxford, OX4 2DQ, UK

For details of our global editorial offices, customer services, and more information about Wiley products visit us at www.wiley.com.

Wiley also publishes its books in a variety of electronic formats and by print-on-demand. Some content that appears in standard print versions of this book may not be available in other formats.

*Library of Congress Cataloging-in-Publication Data*

Names: Sidani, Souraya, author. | Braden, Carrie Jo, 1944– author.
Title: Nursing and health interventions : design, evaluation and
    implementation / Souraya Sidani, Carrie Jo Braden.
Other titles: Design, evaluation, and translation of nursing interventions
Description: Second edition. | Hoboken, NJ : Wiley-Blackwell, 2021. |
    Preceded by Design, evaluation, and translation of nursing interventions
    / Souraya Sidani, Carrie Jo Braden. 2011. | Includes bibliographical
    references and index.
Identifiers: LCCN 2021013467 (print) | LCCN 2021013468 (ebook) | ISBN
    9781119610120 (paperback) | ISBN 9781119610137 (adobe pdf) | ISBN
    9781119610090 (epub)
Subjects: MESH: Nursing Care | Evaluation Studies as Topic | Nursing
    Research | Research Design | Translational Medical Research
Classification: LCC RT81.5 (print) | LCC RT81.5 (ebook) | NLM WY 100.1 |
    DDC 610.73072–dc23
LC record available at https://lccn.loc.gov/2021013467
LC ebook record available at https://lccn.loc.gov/2021013468

Cover Design: Wiley
Cover Image: © Alexkich/iStock/Getty Images

Set in 10.5/13pt STIXTwoText by SPi Global, Pondicherry, India
Printed and bound by CPI Group (UK) Ltd, Croydon, CR0 4YY

C9781119610120_020421

# Contents

# Preface

Interventions constitute the essence of nursing and health care. To be successful in promoting health and well-being, health interventions have to be carefully designed, delivered, and evaluated, before they are implemented in practice.

Over the past decades, advances in intervention research generated a range of designs, methods, and procedures for developing, providing, and determining the effectiveness of health interventions. The advances were motivated by cumulating evidence pointing to limitations in traditional approaches to intervention research, by the widening recognition of the value of client-centered care, and by the increasing demand for interventions that are acceptable and adaptable to practice and for evidence that is relevant and meaningful in informing treatment decisions in practice. Practice-relevant evidence indicates: what clients, presenting with which personal and health characteristics, benefit, to what extent, from what health intervention, provided in what mode or format and what dose, in what context, as well as how health interventions work in producing the beneficial outcomes that are of importance to clients.

Advances in intervention research have been described in a multitude of sources spanning different disciplines and professions, and often using different terminology. This book is intended to serve as a helpful "one-stop" resource for researchers and health professionals planning to engage in intervention research. The book is divided into five sections. The first section provides an overview of the conditions that instigated the advances, and of the systematic process for designing and evaluating health interventions. The second section presents approaches for developing new interventions that culminate in the generation of the intervention theory. The central role of the theory in guiding the planning and conduct of intervention delivery and evaluation is clarified. The third section details approaches and methods for delivering the intervention with fidelity and flexibility. The fourth section describes traditional and alternative research designs, methods, and procedures for evaluating the interventions' acceptance, feasibility, process, and outcomes. The fifth section provides an overview of initiatives aimed at implementing evidence-based interventions in practice.

The content of the book covers conceptual, empirical, and practical knowledge needed for the optimal design, delivery, evaluation, and implementation of health interventions. The conceptual knowledge clarifies the rationale or the "why" of the approaches and methods for designing and evaluating interventions; it explains the principles and logic underlying them and discusses their strengths and limitations. Empirical knowledge supports the utility of the approaches and methods by providing evidence on their strengths and limitations. The conceptual and empirical knowledge are combined to justify methodological decisions in intervention research. Practical knowledge describes the "what" and "how" of the approaches and methods; it provides guidance for applying them.

The goal is to support students, researchers, and health professionals in making appropriate decisions in:

1. Selecting the optimal approaches and methods for designing, delivering, evaluating, and implementing health interventions.
2. Generating evidence that informs treatment decisions in practice.
3. Promoting the adoption, adaptation, and implementation of intervention in practice, which ultimately lead to the provision of high-quality, client-centered, healthcare.

# Acknowledgments

The authors gratefully acknowledge the informal feedback from colleagues, the constant challenge of students, and the instrumental support of staff (at the Health Intervention Research Center), which contributed to the refinement of our thinking and continuous expansion and evaluation of their conceptual and methodological knowledge.

This work could not be accomplished without the love, encouragement, and unlimited support of their family (in particular Cara Ager and Leila Sidani) and mentors.

This work was partially supported by the Canada Research Chairs Program.

# INTRODUCTION

# CHAPTER 1

# Introduction to Intervention Research

Clients experience health problems and seek assistance from health professionals to address these problems. Health professionals are responsible for providing high-quality healthcare that successfully manages the clients' problems and promotes their well-being. Specifically, health professionals are expected to engage with clients in making treatment-related decisions; provide the selected treatment or intervention; monitor clients' responses to treatment, that is, changes in the experience of the health problems; and adapt the intervention, as needed, to clients' responses. Thus, interventions constitute the central elements of healthcare, and their careful selection and appropriate delivery form the basis of high-quality care. Sound decision-making demands that health professionals: are aware of available interventions addressing the health problem with which clients present and of evidence regarding the benefits or effectiveness and the risks or discomfort associated with alternative interventions; inquire about clients' values and preferences; and collaboratively choose the intervention that is beneficial yet consistent with clients' values and preferences. Intervention research is concerned with generating evidence on the benefits and risks of health interventions, to inform treatment decision-making in practice.

What constitutes empirical evidence that is useful in informing treatment decisions in practice is evolving. With the adoption of evidence-based practice in the early 1990s, evidence from randomized controlled or clinical trials (RCTs), also known as experimental designs, was admitted as the most reliable or robust evidence of health interventions' benefits; the RCT is believed to have features that enhance the validity of inferences regarding the causal impact of interventions on outcomes (Holm et al., 2017). Consequently, evidence synthesized across RCTs was relied on to generate guidelines that inform decision-making in practice.

In the past decades, experiences with evidence-based practice revealed limitations of this approach to healthcare (Horwitz et al., 2017). These limitations, along with increasing societal value and demand for person-centeredness, are contributing to shifts in perspectives on what constitutes high-quality healthcare and what methods and strategies are appropriate for the design, delivery, and evaluation of interventions.

In this chapter, the treatment decision-making steps and the information needed to guide decision-making in practice are briefly reviewed. Limitations of evidence

*Nursing and Health Interventions: Design, Evaluation, and Implementation*, Second Edition.
Souraya Sidani and Carrie Jo Braden.
© 2021 John Wiley & Sons Ltd. Published 2021 by John Wiley & Sons Ltd.

derived from RCTs in informing decision-making in practice are highlighted and related to disregarding the principles of client-centeredness and the complexity of the real world. Advances in research methodology that account for complexity are introduced. The overall process for designing, delivering, and evaluating interventions, and implementing them in practice, is briefly described.

## 1.1   TREATMENT DECISION-MAKING

Health professionals (i.e. practitioners, clinicians, therapists) include nurses, physicians, psychologists, dietitians, health educators, and allied health therapists such as respiratory, physical, occupational, and speech-language therapists. They work independently and collaboratively to provide high-quality healthcare to individuals, families, and communities (hereafter collectively referred to as clients) in a range of settings such as primary, home, acute, rehabilitation, and long-term care.

Provision of high-quality healthcare aims to: promote health; prevent and manage health problems; prevent complications; and maintain or improve well-being. Currently, person-, patient-, or client-centered care is viewed as the cornerstone of high-quality care (Van Belle et al., 2019), and client participation in treatment decisions and in health management as the pillar of client-centered care (Britten et al., 2017). Client participation is enacted in shared decision-making. Shared decision-making is an interactive process that involves collaboration between clients and health professionals, focused on making treatment decisions (Stacey & Légaré, 2015). The application of shared decision-making in practice involves several steps (Coutu et al., 2015; Elwyn et al., 2014; Muscat et al., 2015; Shay & Lafata, 2014):

1. Health professionals conduct a comprehensive and thorough assessment of clients' condition. The assessment covers all domains of health, including biophysiological, physical, cognitive, emotional, behavioral, sociocultural, and spiritual domains, as well as the clients' personal account of the health problem and its impact on their life.

2. Health professionals critically analyze the findings of the assessment and, together with the clients, formulate the clients' health needs, that is, the potential (i.e. at risk) and actual health problems with which clients present and requiring remediation; in addition health professionals work with clients to prioritize their problems. An in-depth and lucid understanding of the clients' health problems is necessary for selecting the remediation interventions.

3. Health professionals appraise alternative interventions; discuss with the clients the benefits and risks of the interventions; elicit clients' preferences for interventions; and collaboratively select the most appropriate, effective, and safe ones.

4. Health professionals deliver the selected interventions for, on behalf, or with clients.

5. Health professionals and clients monitor clients' status on a regular basis to determine the extent to which the interventions were successful in addressing clients' health problems. If unsuccessful, health professionals and clients investigate factors that may influence the effectiveness of the interventions and should be accounted for in adapting the same interventions or providing alternative ones.

The application of decision-making in practice requires a sound theoretical and empirical knowledge base of the health problem and the interventions. This implies that health professionals have access to:

1. A conceptualization of the health problem with which clients present. The conceptualization clarifies the nature of the problem; specifies its indicators; presents a comprehensive list of its determinants experienced in different domains of health and at different levels (e.g. interpersonal, environmental); and delineates the relationships between the health problem and other co-occurring problems, which are likely to be observed with the increasing prevalence of multiple chronic conditions, particularly among older adults (Golfam et al., 2015). The conceptualization helps health professionals understand the clients' health problem and overall condition, which, in turn, guides the search for relevant interventions.

2. A conceptualization of alternative (if available) interventions addressing the same health problems. The conceptualization describes the components and activities comprising each intervention, and explains its mechanism of action (i.e. why and how the interventions work in addressing the health problem). This conceptualization is important for understanding the interventions and for adapting them to the clients' context or life circumstances (Levinton, 2017). Health professionals find it difficult to apply interventions they do not understand (Kazdin, 2007).

3. Empirical evidence that indicates the extent to which each alternative intervention is effective and safe in addressing the health problem, as well as its relative effectiveness (i.e. compared to other interventions).

Empirical evidence on the effectiveness of interventions has been regarded as a credible source to inform health professionals' practice and to guide decision-making. It forms the foundation of evidence-based practice.

## 1.2   EVIDENCE-BASED PRACTICE

Evidence-informed or evidence-based practice refers to "the conscientious, explicit, and judicious use of current, best evidence in making decisions about the care of individual patients" (Sackett et al., 1997, p. 2). Proponents of evidence-based practice believe that interventions, evaluated in the context of research studies and found effective and safe, can be delivered in the same and consistent manner to produce the same effects in clients presenting with the same health problem, under the conditions of day-to-day practice. They advocate the development of guidelines to inform practice. Guidelines consist of systematically developed statements about recommendations for interventions that have demonstrated effectiveness and can be used to address a health problem, and procedures for monitoring the intervention's outcomes. The guidelines are disseminated to health professionals who are expected to implement the recommended interventions (Fernandez et al., 2015).

Proponents of evidence-based practice developed a hierarchy of research designs that are most appropriate for generating evidence on the effectiveness of interventions. They place high value on evidence derived from primary or meta-analytic studies that used the RCT design to investigate the effects of interventions. The RCT is deemed the most reliable, even the "gold standard" for intervention evaluation research because its features are believed to minimize potential biases. Controlling for biases is required for demonstrating the causal effects of the intervention on outcomes (Hansen & Tjørnhøj-Thomsen, 2016; Holm et al., 2017).

To date, experiences with evidence-based practice have been less than optimal. It is estimated that up to 55% of clients receive interventions recommended in guidelines for acute, chronic, and preventive healthcare, and if provided, wide variations in implementing the evidence-based interventions were observed (Greenhalgh et al., 2014; Harris et al., 2017). Several factors related to the characteristics of the healthcare system, organization, health professionals, clients, and the interventions affect the implementation of evidence-based interventions and guidelines in daily practice (Lau et al., 2016). Evidence suggests that health professionals do not depend on research as a source of information to guide practice. Rather, they rely on other sources, primarily clinical knowledge either gained personally or shared by colleagues, as well as client experience (Spenceley et al., 2008).

Recently, concerns have been raised about the applicability of evidence, derived from primary and meta-analytic studies using the RCT design, in informing practice (Ioannidis, 2016). Overall, the concerns stem from limitations of the RCT design in generating evidence that is relevant to the practice context (Braithwaite et al., 2018; Reeve et al., 2016). The limitations are related to the features of the RCT (i.e. careful selection of participants, random assignment, standardized delivery of treatment) that enable the focus on the direct causal effects of an intervention on outcomes and the control of potential sources of bias. As such, the RCT features ignore the complexity of the real world, the individuality of clients' experiences of the health problem and life circumstances as well as responses to treatment, and clients' participation in treatment decisions.

Careful selection of participants confines the RCT sample to a select subgroup of the target client population (e.g. clients with no comorbid conditions), which limits the applicability of the findings to other subgroups of clients seen in practice (Greenhalgh et al., 2014). Random assignment of participants to treatment groups does not reflect the treatment decision-making process followed in practice. Therefore, random assignment is not well received by clients participating in the RCT (thereafter referred to as participants) and has been found to affect enrollment in the trial, attrition and nonadherence to treatment, which weaken the validity of inferences regarding the effectiveness of an intervention (see Chapter 14). Standardized delivery of interventions is not responsive to clients' individual experiences, life circumstances, and preferences. Standardization also is difficult to transport into practice due to the complex and inter-related influence of factors pertaining to clients, health professionals, and context (Chu & Leino, 2017; Leask et al., 2019). The focus on the average direct causal effects of the intervention ignores individual variability in clients' responses to treatment (i.e. level of improvement in outcomes observed following treatment completion) and the mechanism through which the treatment produces its benefits; yet, health professionals need to understand what client subgroups respond favorably to the intervention and how the intervention produces its benefits for making appropriate treatment decisions (Horwitz et al., 2017; Lipsitz & Markowitz, 2013; Van Belle et al., 2016).

The limitations extend to meta-analytic studies or systematic reviews of RCT findings, which form the basis for recommendations stated in guidelines. Attempts at synthesizing RCT-derived evidence face challenges associated with limited replication (e.g. Pereira & Ioannidis, 2011). Limited replication is manifested in conflicting and, therefore, inconclusive evidence of the intervention's effectiveness (Hesselink et al., 2014). Accordingly, the guidelines' recommendations are usually stated in general terms that simply identify the interventions that can be used in addressing a health problem (Edwards et al., 2007). In addition, reports of primary and meta-analytic studies as well as guidelines provide a brief description of the interventions. Insufficient description of the interventions constrains their replication and proper implementation in research and practice (Bach-Mortensen et al., 2018; Levinton, 2017). For instance, Glasziou et al. (2010) found that health professionals were able to replicate the interventions evaluated in half of 80 studies published in the journal of Evidence-Based Medicine. Furthermore, the guidelines do not offer instructions on how to adapt the design and delivery of interventions in a way that preserves their active ingredients yet is responsive to the characteristics, preferences, and life circumstances of clients and to the resources available in local practice contexts (Bach-Mortensen et al., 2018; Westfall et al., 2009).

Accordingly, the evidence generated in primary and meta-analytic studies using the RCT design is of limited utility in informing practice. It does not address the questions that health professionals ask when making treatment decisions (Bonell et al., 2018; Levinton, 2017). The questions include:

- Who (i.e. clients with what sociodemographic and health or clinical profiles) most benefit (i.e. demonstrate improvement in outcomes) from an intervention, delivered in what mode and at what dose?
- What are the intervention's active ingredients (operationalized in what specific components) responsible for its benefits?
- What risks or discomforts are associated with the intervention?
- How and why does the intervention work to produce its benefits? Or, what is the mechanism of action responsible for the intervention's effectiveness in addressing the health problem?
- What resources are needed to deliver the intervention?
- What contextual factors influence the delivery of the intervention by health professionals, its uptake and enactment by clients, and its effectiveness?
- To what extent and how can the intervention be tailored to the individual clients' characteristics or preferences, and/or adapted to the local practice context?
- What alternative interventions are available to address the health problem, and what are their relative benefits (effectiveness) and risks (safety)?

Intervention research needs to be reoriented toward developing well-conceptualized yet practice-relevant interventions, and generating the evidence that addresses these questions. The goal is to consolidate the theoretical and empirical knowledge that informs practice, and ultimately improves the quality of healthcare and the health of clients. To be useful in informing practice, intervention research should embrace a realist, pragmatic perspective in reflecting the characteristics of practice: client-centeredness and complexity. This can be achieved through client engagement and use of a range of relevant research designs and methods.

## 1.3  CLIENT-CENTERED CARE

The less-than-optimal experiences with evidence-based practice, the limited applicability of RCT-derived evidence to practice, in combination with clients' demand for an approach to healthcare that reflects their individuality, values, and preference, have led to the resurgence of client-centered care as the "core" of high-quality healthcare (Beck et al., 2010; de Boer et al., 2013; Sidani & Fox, 2014; Van Belle et al., 2019; Vijn et al., 2018).

Client-centeredness is an approach to healthcare familiar to health professionals. Professionals are instructed, socialized, and expected to deliver client-centered care. Client-centered care is applied at different levels. At the individual level, it involves the application of tailored and adaptive interventions addressing the presenting health problem or aiming to change health behaviors (Hekler et al., 2018) and personalized or precision medicine (Bothwell et al., 2016). At the group level, client-centeredness is illustrated by family-centered care or the provision of health interventions that are adapted to the demands and preferences of particular communities such as ethno-cultural communities (Barrera et al., 2013; Netto et al., 2010). At the healthcare organization level, client-centeredness involves the adaptation of evidence-based interventions and practice guidelines to the local context (Harrison et al., 2010; Powell et al., 2017) and at the system level, it is reflected in patient engagement (McNeil et al., 2016).

In general, the application of client-centered care involves: (1) a comprehensive and thorough assessment of the clients' condition to identify their health problems, beliefs, values and preferences; (2) collaboration and active participation of clients in prioritizing their problems, designing new or selecting available, evidence-based interventions, and implementing the selected interventions (as is done in shared decision-making); and (3) adaptation or tailoring of the intervention for consistency with clients' problems, beliefs, values, and preferences, as well as with their changing experiences of the health problem, and life circumstances, over time.

Cumulating evidence supports the benefits of client-centered care. At the individual level, client-centered care was found to improve clients' knowledge of their condition and treatment, experiences with healthcare, general health and well-being. It also enhanced adherence to treatment; self-efficacy in managing the health problem; and reduced health services use and cost (Barello et al., 2012; Fors et al., 2018; Hibbard & Greene, 2013; Ren et al., 2019; Vijn et al., 2018). Similarly, tailored interventions were reported to be more effective than non-tailored ones (Hawkins et al., 2008; Richards et al., 2007). At the community level, providing culturally tailored interventions was associated with increased client satisfaction but not with improvement in health outcomes (Renzoto et al., 2013). At the healthcare organization and system level, client-centered care contributed to the development of new and improved services (Mockford et al., 2012).

The provision of client-centered care, the cornerstone of high-quality healthcare (Van Belle et al., 2019), requires the availability of interventions with demonstrated appropriateness, acceptability, effectiveness, safety, and efficiency. Appropriate interventions are logical, reasonable, and sound treatments that address a specific health problem. This implies that the nature of the interventions, reflected in its active ingredients, is consistent with the nature of the health problem.

Acceptable interventions are desirable by clients expected to receive the interventions. Desirable interventions are perceived as consistent with the clients' beliefs about the health problem and its treatment, suitable to their lifestyle, safe and convenient to apply in their daily life (Sidani et al., 2018). Related to acceptability is the notion of cultural relevance of interventions; it refers to the congruence of the interventions' components, mode and dose of delivery, with the beliefs, values, and norms held by particular groups or ethno-cultural communities (Barrera et al., 2013). Effective interventions produce the best health outcomes by activating the anticipated mechanism of action (Dalkin et al., 2015); that is, they induce changes in clients' cognition, skills, or behaviors that mediate improvements in the experience of the health problem, health, and well-being. Safe interventions are associated with no or minimal risks or discomfort (Bonell et al., 2015). Efficient interventions are optimized in terms of content, delivery, and resources required for their implementation, to maximize health outcomes; that is, they yield the highest impact (i.e. large improvement in the outcomes in a large proportion of the population) within a reasonably short time period (i.e. speed of recovery) (Benedikt et al., 2016; Morin et al., 2014).

New approaches are needed to design and evaluate health interventions in ways that inform the application of client-centeredness in practice. Approaches for designing (1) appropriate health interventions rely on generating a comprehensive understanding of the health problem (see Chapter 3) and identification of the intervention's active ingredients (see Chapter 4), which are integrated into the intervention theory (see Chapter 5); (2) acceptable interventions involve the engagement of clients in the design of interventions, the development of tailored or adaptive interventions (see Chapter 4), and the assessment of clients' perceived acceptability of interventions (see Chapter 11). Approaches for evaluating the effectiveness, safety, and efficiency of health interventions entail the recognition of the complexity of the real world (see Section 1.4) and use of a range of research designs and methods to find answers to the practice-related questions listed in Section 1.2. The goal of intervention research is to generate evidence that is grounded in and useful to practice (Westfall et al., 2009), which is characterized as client-centered.

## 1.4  COMPLEXITY OF THE REAL WORLD

The complexity of the real world is a fact. Clients live in a complex environment where multiple factors contribute to their health and their capacity to promote healthy living. They may experience one or more health problems associated with a range of determinants. These complex health problems require complex interventions for successful remediation. Several health professionals are involved in the delivery of complex intervention, in a context that is characterized by factors, operating at different levels and contributing to the success (or failure) of the intervention implementation and effectiveness. The complexity of the real world should be accounted for, and not ignored as is the case in the RCT design, when developing and evaluating health interventions in order to generate evidence of relevance to practice.

Accounting for complexity demands acknowledgement of multi-causality in the design and evaluation of health interventions, as well as of the individuality of clients. This can be achieved with the development of theory of the health problem (see Chapter 3), multicomponent interventions (see Chapter 4), theory of change (see Chapter 4 and 5), as well as examining the influence of contextual factors on the implementation of the intervention (see Chapter 13) and individual variability in clients' responses to interventions.

### 1.4.1  Theory of the Health Problem

In practice, many clients present with one or more health problems and a range of life circumstances (or context). The experience of each problem may be associated with multiple determinants or causes, occurring in different domains of health (e.g. physical, psychological) and at different levels (e.g. intrapersonal, interpersonal, environmental) (Diez-Roux, 2011). The problems and their determinants are often inter-related, forming a "web of causation" (Golfam et al., 2015), also called multi-causality. Understanding these inter-relations is essential for designing and evaluating health interventions; this can be achieved with the development of the theory of the health problem to be targeted by an intervention. The theory of the health problem is a means for integrating the determinants of the health problem and delineating the complex inter-relationships among them (Fleury & Sidani, 2018). The theory of the health problem points to aspects of the problem amenable to change, which informs the design of interventions. Interventions based on a clear understanding of the health problem were found to be most successful (e.g. Glanz & Bishop, 2010; Prestwich et al., 2014). The theory is also useful in guiding practice; it delineates aspects of the health problem that should be assessed, thereby ensuring a comprehensive and thorough assessment and understanding of the clients' condition, as advocated in client-centered care.

### 1.4.2   Development of Multicomponent Interventions

Complex health problems require complex solutions. Complex interventions consist of multiple components (Medical Research Council, 2019). Each component involves a set of inter-related activities, performed by clients and health professionals that have the common goal of managing a particular aspect (e.g. one determinant) of the health problem (Greenwood-Lee et al., 2016). Complex interventions can be delivered in a standardized way whereby all clients are given all components, or tailored to the individual clients' experience of the health problem. In the latter case, clients are provided one component or a subset of components that is or are most appropriate to address the most salient aspect of the health problem as clients experience it.

### 1.4.3   Development of the Theory of Change

Each component of a complex health intervention targets a particular aspect of the health problem, and, therefore, activates a unique mechanism of action. When a combination of components is delivered, the components may act interdependently in producing complex, multiple causal pathways that represent the mechanism of action responsible for the intervention's effects on the outcomes. The theory of change integrates these pathways (Mayne, 2015; Montague, 2019; Powell, 2019) to explain how the complex intervention, in its totality, works to bring about beneficial changes in the health problem and other outcomes (Bleijenberg et al., 2018).

The theory of change guides the plan and conduct of intervention evaluation studies. It identifies the interventions' processes, mediators, and outcomes to be investigated; gives direction for their measurement as well as the timing of their assessment; and assists in interpreting the findings. In practice, health professionals' awareness of the theory empowers engagement in an enlightened and judicious decision-making process.

### 1.4.4   Examination of Contextual Factors

Interventions, complex or not, are delivered in real-world context. The context includes the practice setting in which health professionals provide the interventions, and the environment in which clients apply the treatment recommendations. In either case, context is complex, characterized by variability on a multitude of factors, occurring at different levels (Chandler et al., 2016; Masterson-Algar et al., 2018) and at different points in time (Cambon et al., 2019). The factors are embedded within the physical, psycho-socio-cultural, economic, and political setting or environment, and encountered at the micro (e.g. individual, home), meso (e.g. workplace, organization), or macro (e.g. healthcare system) levels. Contextual factors influence the implementation and the effectiveness of interventions (Craig et al., 2018). It, therefore, is essential to account for context in the design and evaluation of interventions. This can be achieved by: (1) engaging various stakeholder groups (e.g. clients, health professionals, decision-makers) in the design and adaptation of interventions (Braithwaite et al., 2018; Greenwood-Lee et al., 2016)—the groups are knowledgeable of the local context and provide valuable feedback on what factors are operating in that context, how to address the factors, and how to modify the intervention to enhance its fit with the features and resources available at the local context; and (2) incorporating a process evaluation within an intervention evaluation study (see Chapter 13) aimed to monitor the implementation of the intervention, examine its mechanism of action, and exploring if and how contextual factors affect interventions' implementation and effectiveness (Moore et al., 2019). The findings of a process evaluation are critical for the validity of a study's conclusions; specifically, they point to factors that contributed, positively or negatively, to the interventions' effects.

### 1.4.5   Examination of Client Individuality

Individuality of clients adds to the complexity of real-world practice. In addition to their experience of co-occurring health problems, clients vary in their sociodemographic and health profiles, and most importantly differ in their beliefs about health in general and the presenting health problem such as possible causes of the problem. These beliefs influence clients' health behaviors and shape their preferences for treatment (De las Cuevas et al., 2018). Respecting their beliefs and accounting for their preferences are principles of client-centered care that are gaining wide interest in intervention research. This is evident in: (1) calls to determine the social acceptability, in addition to clinical effectiveness and economic efficiency, of interventions (Staniszewska et al., 2010), and to design tailored interventions that customize interventions to individual clients' characteristics and preferences (Radhakrishan, 2012); and (2) widening recognition of the utility of pragmatic and preference trials for evaluating interventions. Clients also differ in their response to interventions: some experience improvement in the health problem, whereas others show no change or even deterioration. The latter subgroups of clients may require modification of their treatment, also referred to as adaptive interventions. The modification or adaptation may include a range of possibilities such as intensifying the interventions (e.g. increasing its dose) or providing different ones (e.g. stepped-up care) based on their responses (Hekler et al., 2018). Advances in health technology are facilitating the design and delivery of adaptive interventions, and innovative research designs are proposed to evaluate them. Planned subgroup analysis can be applied to determine the profiles of clients who most benefit from the intervention.

### 1.5   CLIENT ENGAGEMENT IN INTERVENTION RESEARCH

The high value placed on client-centered care and the less-than-optimal implementation of evidence-based interventions by health professionals, and uptake and enactment by clients, served as the impetus for engaging clients in intervention research. Client engagement takes place in different stages and steps of research:

1. Identifying research priorities for funding agencies (e.g. Patient-Centered Outcomes Research Institute in the US), most pressing health needs of the general public, or services requiring improvement in a healthcare organization

or system: The James Lind Alliance has developed a systematic process for engaging clients (e.g. persons experiencing a health problem, health professionals) in identifying research priorities (Cowan, 2010; Manafò et al., 2018).

2. Setting the research questions to be addressed in a study: Clients join the research team as collaborators. They actively participate in stating the study aims, and may assist in preparing or reviewing the grant proposal prior to submission.

3. Designing new interventions, co-creating or co-producing the intervention protocol and materials (Hwakins et al., 2017; Kildea et al., 2019), selecting and adapting evidence-based interventions (Aarons et al., 2012; Sidani et al., 2017): This involves a systematic process in which clients serve as consultants or as participants in a research study aimed to adapt or co-create interventions.

4. Delineating the study protocol: As collaborators, clients have experiential knowledge that is useful in determining: the target populations' acceptance of randomization and of methods for data collection; effective sources and strategies for recruitment; convenient locations for delivering the interventions; and suitability (comprehension, readability, response burden) of measures to a range of participants.

5. Recruiting participants, facilitating data collection, and assisting in the interpretation and dissemination of findings: Clients serving as collaborators or participants in a study can assume these responsibilities.

Client engagement in intervention research may reduce research waste. Client involvement is expected to: (1) identify research questions relevant to research or evidence users including clients or the general public, health professionals, and decision-makers (Ioannidis, 2016; McLeod et al., 2014); (2) yield interventions that are optimally designed (Bleijenberg et al., 2018) and acceptable to users, which is likely to improve their uptake in practice; and (3) enhance participants' enrollment and retention, thereby reducing the resources, cost, and time needed to complete the study.

## 1.6   ADVANCES IN INTERVENTION RESEARCH METHODS

The increasing demand for addressing questions of relevance to practice (Chavez-MacGregor & Giordano, 2016; Concato et al., 2010) and mounting evidence dispelling misconceptions about the strengths of the RCT and the weaknesses of non-RCT or observation designs (Frieden, 2017) have brought to the forefront the importance of the research questions or aims in informing the selection of research designs and methods in intervention research (Skivington et al., 2018). Accordingly, researchers have a more inclusive range of research designs and methods to choose from. Designs considered appropriate for evaluating health interventions are presented in several publications (e.g. Medical Research Council guidance, 2019; Shadish et al., 2002; Sidani, 2015). The main categories of designs and methods are described in Chapters 14 and 15, respectively. The overall trend is toward embracing a pragmatic, realist approach to intervention evaluation research that is conducted within the context of practice and reflects the complexity of inter-relations among client, health professional and contextual factors, intervention implementation, and outcomes. Practical trials, preference trials, adaptive designs, and multiple or mixed-methods designs are relevant methodological innovations. The selection of a research design should be informed by the research questions, taking into consideration feasibility, ethical and safety issues (Lobo et al., 2017).

## 1.7  PROCESS FOR DESIGNING, EVALUATING, AND IMPLEMENTING INTERVENTIONS

The process for designing, evaluating, and implementing interventions is systematic and rigorous, yet flexible and iterative (Czajkowski et al., 2015; Medical Research Council, 2019). It involves phases that are logically sequenced. Although some may be conducted simultaneously, the results of each phase drive the work forward toward the next phase or backward toward earlier phases. For instance, feasibility and acceptability can be examined simultaneously rather than sequentially. Newly developed interventions found acceptable to the target population are moved to the next phase for evaluating their effectiveness, whereas interventions deemed unacceptable should be reconceptualized to optimize their design (i.e. moved back to the drawing board!). Each phase is carried out using research designs and methods that are most pertinent to address the respective research questions or achieve the stated aims, and to maintain the validity of findings. The phases are briefly mentioned in Table 1.1, with an emphasis on what they aim to achieve. The book is organized into sections that detail the research methods that can be used in designing, evaluating, and implementing interventions. Different methods are discussed, consistent with the recommendation for selecting those that are most appropriate to address the research questions and are feasible within the practice context.

**TABLE 1.1**  Phases of the process for designing, evaluating, and implementing interventions.

| Process | Phase | Aims |
|---|---|---|
| *Designing interventions* | Generating an understanding of health problem | 1. Clarify the health problem requiring remediation<br>    a. conceptual and operational definition<br>    b. determinants<br>    c. consequences<br>2. Develop a theory of the health problem<br>3. Identify aspects of the health problem that are amenable to change or remediation |
| | Developing intervention | 1. Conceptualize the intervention's active ingredients<br>2. Operationalize the intervention's active ingredients in specific and nonspecific components<br>3. Operationalize the components<br>    a. goals and activities<br>    b. mode of delivery<br>    c. dose<br>4. Delineate the intervention's mechanism of action<br>5. Develop the theory of change |
| | Developing intervention theory | 1. Integrate theory of the problem and theory of change<br>2. Identify contextual factors affecting intervention's delivery, mechanism of action, and effectiveness<br>3. Operationalize the intervention theory |

*(Continued)*

**TABLE 1.1**    (Continued)

| Process | Phase | Aims |
|---|---|---|
| *Delivering interventions* | Developing intervention protocol | 1. Describe in detail the content to be covered and activities to be performed by health professionals (or interventionists) and clients during intervention delivery |
| | Training health professionals or interventionists | 1. Select interventionists based on well-defined professional qualifications and personal characteristics<br>2. Provide training and support |
| | Monitoring fidelity | 1. Assess theoretical fidelity<br>2. Develop or select measures for assessing operational fidelity<br>3. Investigate operational fidelity throughout the intervention delivery period |
| *Evaluating interventions* | Examining perceptions of intervention | 1. Assess clients' perceptions of interventions before, during, and following delivery |
| | Examining feasibility of intervention and research methods | 1. Assess interventionists' perceptions of the intervention's feasibility<br>2. Assess clients' perceptions of the intervention's feasibility<br>3. Determine the acceptability and feasibility of the research methods for intervention evaluation<br>4. Revise the design of the intervention and the research methods as necessary |
| | Evaluating process | 1. Monitor the delivery of the intervention<br>2. Examine the intervention's mechanism of action<br>3. Explore contextual factors affecting the intervention's delivery, mechanism of action, and effectiveness<br>4. Revise the conceptualization, operationalization, and delivery of the intervention, based on process evaluation results |
| | Evaluating outcomes | 1. Determine the effectiveness of the intervention in producing the intended beneficial health outcomes<br>2. Explore the safety (risks or discomforts associated with the intervention) and unintended outcomes |
| *Implementing interventions* | Adapting evidence-based interventions | 1. Examine the acceptability and feasibility of the intervention to the local context<br>2. Explore modifications required to enhance the fit of the intervention to the local context<br>3. Assess barriers and facilitators of implementation in the local context<br>4. Select implementation techniques |
| | Implementing evidence-based interventions | 1. Support the implementation initiative |

# REFERENCES

Aarons, G.A., Green, A.E., Palinkas, L.A., et al. (2012) Dynamic adaptation process to implement an evidence-based child maltreatment intervention. *Implementation Science*, 7, 32–40.

Bach-Mortensen, A.M, Lange, B.C.L., & Montgomery, P. (2018) Barriers and facilitators to implementing evidence-based interventions among third sector organization: A systematic review. *Implementation Science*, 13, 103–121.

Barello S, Graffigna G, & Vegni E. (2012) Patient engagement as an emerging challenge for healthcare services: Mapping the literature. *Nursing Research and Practice*, 2012, 905–934.

Barrera, M., Castro, F.G., Strycker, L.A., et al. (2013) Cultural adaptations of behavioral health interventions: A Progress report. *Journal of Consulting and Clinical Psychology*, 81(2), 196–205.

Beck, C., McSweeney, J.C., Richards, K.C., et al. (2010) Challenges in tailored intervention research. *Nursing Outlook*, 58(2), 104–110.

Benedikt, C., Kelly, S.L., Wilson, D., & Wilson, D.P., on behalf of the Optima Consortium (2016) Allocative and implementation efficiency in HIV prevention and treatment for people who inject drugs. *International Journal of Drug Policy*, 38, 73–80.

Bleijenberg, N., de Man-van Ginkel, J.M., Trappenburg, J.C.A., et al. (2018) Increasing value and reducing waste by optimizing the development of complex interventions: Enriching the development phase of the Medical Research Council (MRC) framework. *International Journal of Nursing Studies*, 79, 86–93.

de Boer, D., Delnoij, D., & Rademakers, J. (2013) The importance of patient-centered care for various groups. *Patient Education and Counseling*, 90, 405–410.

Bonell, C., Jamal, F., Melendez-Torres, G.J., & Cummins, S. (2015) 'Dark logic': Theorizing the harmful consequences of public health interventions. *Journal of Epidemiology & Community Health*, 69, 95–98.

Bonell, C., Moore, G., Warren, E., & Moore, L. (2018) Are randomised controlled trials positivist? Reviewing the social science and philosophy literature to assess positivist tendencies of trials of social interventions in public health and health services. *Trials*, 19(1), 238–249.

Bothwell, L.E., Greene, J.A., Podolsky, S.H., et al. (2016) Assessing the gold standard—Lessons from the history of RCTs. *New England Journal of Medicine*, 374, 2175–2181.

Braithwaite, J, Churruca, K, Long, J.C., et al. (2018) When complexity science meets implementation science: A theoretical and empirical analysis of system change. *BMC Medicine*, 16, 63–76.

Britten N, Moore L, Lydahl D, et al. (2017) Elaboration of the Gothenburg model of person-centred care. *Health Expectations*, 20, 407–418.

Cambon, L., Terral, P., & Alla, F. (2019) From intervention to interventional system: towards greater theorization in population health intervention research. *BMC Public Health*, 19, 389–345.

Chandler, J., Rycroft-Malone, J., Hawkes, C., & Noyes, J. (2016) Application of simplified complexity theory concepts for healthcare social systems to explain the implementation of evidence into practice. *Journal of Advanced Nursing*, 72(2), 461–480.

Chavez-MacGregor, M. & Giordano, S.H. (2016) Randomized clinical trials and observational studies: Is there a battle? *Journal of Clinical Oncology*, 34, 772–773.

Chu, J. & Leino, A. (2017) Advancement in the maturing science of cultural adaptations of evidence-based interventions. *Journal of Consulting and Clinical Psychology*, 85(1), 45–57.

Concato, J., Peduzzi, P., Huang, G.D., et al. (2010) Comparative effectiveness research: What kind of studies do we need? *Journal of Investigative Medicine*, 58, 764–769.

Coutu, M.-F., Légaré, F., Stacey, D., et al. (2015) Occupational therapists' shared decision-making behaviors with patients having persistent pain in a work rehabilitation context: A cross-sectional study. *Patient Education & Counseling*, 98, 864–970.

Cowan, K. (2010) The James Lind Alliance: Tackling treatment uncertainties together. *The Journal of Ambulatory Care Management*, 33(3), 241–248.

Craig, P., Di Ruggiero, E., Frohlich, K.L., Mykhalovskiy, E., & White, M., on behalf of the Canadian Institutes of Health Research (CIHR)—National Institute for Health Research (NIHR). (2018). *Taking Account of Context in Population Health Intervention Research: Guidance for Producers, Users and Funders of Research*. NIHR Evaluation, Trials and Studies Coordinating Centre, Southampton.

Czajkowski, S.M., Powell, L.H., Adler N., et al. (2015) From ideas to efficacy: The ORBIT model for developing behavioral treatments for chronic diseases. *Health Psychology*, 34(10), 971–982.

Dalkin, S.M., Greenhalgh, J., Jones, D., et al. (2015) What's in a mechanism? Development of a key concept in realist evaluation. *Implementation Science*, 10, 49–55.

De las Cuevas, C., Motuca, M., Baptista, T., & de Leon, J. (2018) Skepticism and phamacophobia toward medication may negatively impact adherence to psychiatric medications: A comparison among outpatient samples recruited in Spain, Argentina, and Venezuela. *Patient Preference and Adherence*, 12, 301–310.

Diez-Roux, A.V. (2011). Complex system thinking and current impasses in health disparities research. *American Journal of Public Health*, 101(9), 1627–1634.

Edwards, N., Davies, B., Ploeg, J., Virani, T. & Skelly, J. (2007) Implementing nursing best practice guidelines: Impact on patient referrals. *BMC Nursing*, 6, 4–12.

Elwyn, G., Frosch, D., Thomson, R., et al. (2014) Shared decision making: A model for clinical practice. *Journal of General Internal Medicine*, 27(10), 1361–1367.

Fernandez, A., Sturmberg, J., Lukersmith, S., et al. (2015) Evidence-based medicine: Is it a bridge too far? *Health Research Policy and Systems*, 13, 66–74.

Fleury, J. & Sidani, S. (2018). Using theory to guide intervention studies. In: B.M. Melnyk & D. Morrison-Beedy (eds) *Intervention Research and Evidence-Based Quality Improvement Second Edition: Designing, Conducting, Analyzing, and Funding*. Springer, New York, NY

Fors, A., Blanck, E., Ali, L., et al. (2018) Effects of a person-centred telephone-support in patients with chronic obstructive pulmonary disease and/or chronic heart failure—A randomized controlled trial. *PLoS One*, 13(8), e0203031.

Frieden, T.R. (2017) Evidence for health decision making—Beyond randomized, controlled trials. *New England Journal of Medicine*, 377, 465–475.

Glanz, K. & Bishop, D.B. (2010) The role of behavioral science theory in development and implementation of public health interventions. *Annual Review of Public Health*, 31, 399–418.

Glasziou, P., Chalmers, I., Altman, D.G., et al. (2010) Taking healthcare interventions from trial to practice. *BMJ*, 341, c3852.

Golfam, M., Beall, R., Brehaut J., et al. (2015) Comparing alternative design options for chronic disease prevention interventions. *European Journal of Clinical Investigation*, 45, 87–99.

Greenhalgh, T., Howick, J., & MasKreg, N, for the Evidence Based Medicine Renaissance Group (2014) Evidence based medicine: A movement in crisis? *BMJ*, 348, g3725.

Greenwood-Lee, J., Hawe, P., Nettel-Aguirre, A., et al. (2016) Complex intervention modelling should capture the dynamics of adaptation. *BMC Medical Research Methodology*, 16, 51–57.

Hansen, H.P. & Tjørnhøj-Thomsen, T. (2016) Meeting the challenges of intervention research in health science: An argument for a multimethod research approach. *Patient*, 9, 193–200.

Harris, M., Lawn, S.J., Morello, A., et al. (2017) Practice change in chronic conditions care: An appraisal of theories. *BMC Health Services Research*, 17, 170–179.

Harrison, M., Legare, F., Graham, I., & Fervers, B. (2010) Adapting clinical practice guidelines to local context and assessing barriers to their use. *CMAJ*, 182 (2), 78–84.

Hawkins, R.P., Kreuter, M., Resnicow, K., et al. (2008) Understanding tailoring in communicating about health. *Health Education Research,* 23(3), 454–466.

Hawkins, J., Madden, K., Fletcher, A., et al. (2017) Development of a framework for the co-production and prototyping of public health interventions. *BMC Public Health*, 17, 689–699.

Hekler, E.B., Rivera, D.E., Martin, C.A., et al. (2018) Optimizing adaptive interventions: Tutorial on when and how to use control systems engineering to optimize adaptive mHealth intervention. *Journal of Medical Internet Reseach*, 20(6), e214.

Hesselink, G., Zegers, M., Vernooij-Dassen, M., et al. (2014) Improving patient discharge and reducing hospital readmissions by using intervention mapping. *BMC Health Services Research*, 14, 389–399.

Hibbard, J.H. & Greene, J. (2013) What the evidence shows about patient activation: Better health outcomes and care experiences. *Health Affairs*, 32(2), 207–214.

Holm, M., Alvariza, A., Fürst, C-J, et al. (2017) Recruiting participants in a randomized controlled trial testing an intervention in palliative cancer care—The perspectives of health care professionals. *European Journal of Oncology Nursing*, 31, 6–11.

Horwitz, R.I., Hayes-Conroy, A., Coricchio, R., & Singer, B.H. (2017) Fromm evidence based medicine to medicine based evidence. *The American Journal of Medicine*, 130, 1246–1250.

Ioannidis, J.P.A. (2016) Why most clinical research is not useful. *PLoS Medicine*, 13(6), e1002049.

Kazdin, A.E. (2007) Mediators and mechanisms of change in psychotherapy research. *The Annual Review of Clinical Psychology*, 3, 1–27.

Kildea, J., Battista, J., Cabral, B., et al. (2019) Design and development of a person-centered patient portal using participatory stakeholder co-design. *Journal of Medical Internet Research*, 21(2), e11371.

Lau, R., Stevenson, F., Ong, B.N., et al. (2016) Achieving change in primary care—causes of the evidence to practice gap: Systematic reviews of reviews. *Implementation Science*, 11, 40—50.

Leask, C.F., Sandlund, M., Skelton, D.A., et al. (2019) Framework, principles and recommendations for utilising participatory methodologies in the co-creation and evaluation of public health interventions. *Research Involvement and Engagement*, 5, 2–17.

Levinton, L.C. (2017) Generalizing about public health intervention: A mixed-methods approach to external validity. *Annual Review of Public Health*, 38, 371–391.

Lipsitz, J.D & Markowitz, J.C. (2013) Mechanisms of change in interpersonal therapy (IPT). *Clinical Psychology Review*, 33 (8), 1134–1147.

Lobo, M.A., Kagan, S.H., & Corrigan, J.D. (2017) Research design options for intervention studies. *Pediatric Physical Therapy*, 29(Suppl 3), S57–S63.

Manafò, E., Petermann, L., Vandall-Walker, V., et al. (2018) Patient and public engagement in priority setting: A systematic rapid review of the literature. *PLoS One*, 13(3), e0193579

Masterson-Algar, P., Burton, C.R., & Rycroft-Malone, J. (2018) The generation of consensus guidelines for carrying out process evaluations in rehabilitation research. *BMC Medical Research Methodology*, 18, 180–190.

Mayne, J. (2015). Useful theory of change models. *The Canadian Journal of Program Evaluation*, 30(2), 119–142.

McLeod, M., Michie, S., Roberts, I., et al. (2014) Biomedical research: Increasing value, reducing waste. *Lancet*, 383(9912), 101–104.

McNeil, H., Elliot, J., Huson, K., et al. (2016) Engaging older adults in healthcare research and planning: A realist synthesis. *Research Involvement and Engagement*, 2, 10–27.

Medical Research Council (2019) *Developing and Evaluating Complex Interventions.* Author. www.mrc.ac.uk/complexinterventionsguidance

Mockford, C., Staniszewska, S., Griffiths, F., & Herron-Marx, S. (2012) The impact of patient and public involvement in UK NHS health care: A systematic review. *International Journal of Quality in Health Care*, 24(1), 28–38.

Montague, S. (2019) Does your implementation fit your theory of change? *Canadian Journal of Program Evaluation/La Revue canadienne d'évaluation de programme*, 33(3), 316–335.

Moore, G.F., Evans, R., Hawkins, J., et al. (2019) From complex social interventions to interventions in complex social systems: Future directions and unresolved questions for intervention development and evaluation. *Evaluation*, 25(1), 23–45

Morin, C.M., Beaulier-Bonneau, S., Ivers, H., et al. (2014) Speed and trajectory of changes of insomnia symptoms during acute treatment with cognitive-behavioral therapy, singly and combined with medication. *Sleep Medicine*, 15(6), 701–707.

Muscat, D.M., Morony, S., Shepherd, H.L., et al. (2015) Development and field testing of a consumer shared decision-making program for adults with low literacy. *Patient Education and Counseling*, 98, 1180–1188.

Netto, G., Bohpal, R., Leberle, N., et al. (2010) How can health promotion interventions be adapted for minority ethnic communities? Five principles for guiding the development of behavioural interventions. *Health Promotion International*, 25(2), 248–257.

Pereira, T.V. & Ioannidis, J.P. (2011) Statistically significant meta-analyses of clinical trials have modest credibility and inflated effects. *Journal of Clinical Epidemiology*, 64, 1060–1069.

Powell, S. (2019) Theories of change: Making value-explicit. *Journal of MultiDisciplinary Evaluation*, 15(32), 37–52.

Powell, B.J., Beidas, R.S., Lewis, C.C., et al. (2017) Methods to improve the selection and tailoring of implementation strategies. *Journal of Behavioral Health Services and Research*, 44(2), 177–194.

Prestwich, A., Sniehotta, F. F., Whittington, C., et al. (2014) Does theory influence the effectiveness of health behavior interventions? Meta-analysis. *Health Psychology*, 33(5), 465–474.

Radhakrishan, K. (2012) The efficacy of tailored interventions for self-management outcomes of type 2 diabetes, hypertension or heart disease: A systematic review. *Journal of Advanced Nursing*, 68(3), 496–510.

Reeve, J., Cooper, L., Harrington, S., et al. (2016) Developing, delivering and evaluating primary mental health care: The co-production of a new complex intervention. *BMC Health Services Research*, 16, 470–483.

Ren, J., Li, Q., Zhang, T., et al. (2019) Perceptions of engagement in health care among patients with tuberculosis: A qualitative study. *Patient Preference and Adherence*, 13, 107–117.

Renzoto, A.M.W., Romios, P., Crock, C., & Sφnderlund, A.L. (2013). The effectiveness of cultural competence program in ethnic minority patient-centered health care—A systematic review of the literature. *International Journal of Quality in Health Care*, 25(3), 261–269.

Richards, K.C., Enderlin, C.A., Beck, C., et al. (2007) Tailored biobehavioral interventions: A literature review and synthesis. *Research and Theory for Nursing Practice: An international Journal*, 21(4), 271–282.

Sackett, D.L., Richardson, W.S., Rosenberg, W.M., & Haynes, R.B. (1997) *Evidence-Based Medicine: How to Practice and Teach EBM*. Churchill Livingstone, New York.

Shadish, W.R., Cook, T.D., & Campbell, D.T. (2002) *Experimental and Quasi-Experimental Design for Generalized Causal Inference*. Houghton-Mifflin, Boston, MA.

Shay, L.A. & Lafata, J.E. (2014). Understanding patient perceptions of shared decision making. *Patient Education & Counseling*, 96, 295–301.

Sidani, S. (2015) *Health Intervention Research: Advances in Research Design and Methods*. Sage, London, UK.

Sidani, S. & Fox, M. (2014) Patient-centered care: A clarification of its active ingredients. *Journal of Interprofessional Care*, 28(2), 134–141.

Sidani, S., Fox, M., & Esptein, D.R. (2017) Contribution of treatment acceptability to acceptance of randomization: An exploration. *Journal of Evaluation in Clinical Practice*, 23(1), 14–20.

Sidani, S., Epstein, D.R., Miranda, J., & Fox, M. (2018) Psychometric properties of the treatment perception and preferences scale. *Clinical Nursing Research*, 27(6), 743–761.

Skivington, K., Matthews, L., Simpson, P.C., & Moore, L. (2018) Developing and evaluating complex interventions: Updating Medical Research Council guidance to take account of new methodological and theoretical approaches. *The Lancet*, 392(2), S2.

Spenceley, S.M., O'Leary, K.A., Chizawsky, L.L.K., et al. (2008) Sources of information used by nurses to inform practice. An integrative review. *International Journal of Nursing Studies*, 45, 954–970.

Stacey, D. & Légaré, F. (2015). Engaging patients using an interprofessional approach to shared decision making. *Canadian Oncology Nursing Journal/Revue canadienne de soins infirmiers en oncologie*, 25(4), 455–461.

Staniszewska, S., Crowe, S., Badenoch, D., et al. (2010) The PRIME project: Developing a patient evidence-base. *Health Expectations*, 13, 312–322.

Van Belle, S., Wong, G., Westrop, G. et al. (2016) Can "realist" randomised controlled trials be genuinely realist? *BMC Trials*, 17, 313

Van Belle, E., Giesen, J., Conroy, T. et al. (2019) Exploring person-centred fundamental nursing care in hospital wards: A multi-site ethnography. *Journal of Clinical Nursing*, 29(11–12), 1933–1944.

Vijn, T.W., Wollersheim, H., Faber, M.J., et al. (2018) Building a patient-centered and interprofessional training program with patients, students and care professional: Study protocol of a participatory design and evaluation study. *BMC Health Services Research*, 13, 387–398.

Westfall, J.M., Mold, J., & Fagnan, L. (2009. Practice-based research—"Blue highways" on the NIH roadmap. *JAMA*, 297(4), 403–406.

CHAPTER 2

# Overview of Interventions

For health interventions to be appropriate, acceptable, effective, safe, and efficient, they should be carefully designed. Designing interventions rests on an awareness of what constitutes interventions. This chapter presents a definition of interventions that distinguishes it from related terms (e.g. strategies, programs). The interventions' elements (goals and components) and characteristics (mode, structure, dose) are clarified and described. The elements and characteristics are taken into account when developing, operationalizing, delivering, evaluating, and implementing interventions.

## 2.1 DEFINITION OF INTERVENTIONS

In the health-related literature, different terms are used to reflect health professionals' practices or services they provide to clients: strategies, interventions, treatments, techniques, therapies, complex or multicomponent interventions, and programs. These terms are not necessarily interchangeable. There is a distinction between strategies; interventions (including treatments, techniques, therapies); and programs (including complex or multicomponent interventions).

### 2.1.1 Strategies

A strategy refers to a general conceptual approach to address a health problem. It is derived from and consistent with the conceptualization of the health problem requiring remediation. A strategy is used to frame the overall design of an intervention. For instance, conceptualizing chronic insomnia from a cognitive perspective only (Harvey et al., 2007) highlights the need for a cognitive approach for intervention. The cognitive approach focuses on information processing (e.g. beliefs about factors contributing to and consequences of insomnia). In contrast, viewing chronic insomnia as a behavioral problem (e.g. Bootzin & Epstein, 2011) indicates the need for a behavioral approach for intervention. The behavioral approach focuses on sleep-related behaviors and habits. As such, a strategy offers general principles to guide the selection and/or design of interventions that are commensurate with the overarching conceptualization of the health problem.

*Nursing and Health Interventions: Design, Evaluation, and Implementation*, Second Edition.
Souraya Sidani and Carrie Jo Braden.
© 2021 John Wiley & Sons Ltd. Published 2021 by John Wiley & Sons Ltd.

## 2.1.2  Interventions

The terms "intervention," "treatment," and "therapy" are interchangeable. Although widely used in written (e.g. books, published research reports) and verbal (e.g. case conference, end of shift report in the practice setting) communications, only a few formal definitions of interventions have been located in recent literature (Table 2.1). A thorough examination of these definitions points to two key attributes that define interventions. The first attribute is that interventions are essentially activities. They involve the application of specific techniques by the health professional delivering interventions and the clients receiving interventions. The second attribute is rationality. Rationality means that interventions are given in response to an actual or potential health problem, and directed toward attainment of desired goals. Accordingly, interventions are sets of activities performed by health professionals and clients, independently or collaboratively, to address problems experienced by clients and to achieve beneficial outcomes.

Interventions are more specific than strategies. Strategies provide general principles informing the generation of new or the selection of available evidence-based techniques. For instance, a behavioral conceptualization of chronic insomnia provided guidance for developing the stimulus control therapy. The stimulus control therapy consists of specific recommendations for sleep behaviors (known to perpetuate

**TABLE 2.1**  Formal definitions of interventions.

| Field | Definition | Reference |
|---|---|---|
| Nursing | Deliberate cognitive, physical, or verbal activities performed with, or on behalf of, individuals and their families, that are directed toward accomplishing particular therapeutic objectives relative to individuals' health and well-being | Grove et al. (2015) |
| | Actions, treatments, or technologies, that are physical, psychological, social in nature, with predicted outcomes | Forbes (2009) |
| Public health | Planned actions to prevent or reduce a particular health problem or the determinants of the problem | Wight et al. (2015) |
| | An act performed for, with, or on behalf of a person or population with the purpose to assess, improve, promote, or modify health, functioning, or health conditions | Cambon et al. (2019) |
| Behavior health | Coordinated sets of activities or techniques introduced at a given time and place to change the behavior of individuals, communities, or populations through a hypothesized or known mechanism | Araújo-Soares et al. (2018) |
| Social/ implementation science | Events within systems, aimed to disrupt the functioning of complex systems through changing relationships, displacing entrenched practice, and redistributing and transforming resources | Moore et al. (2019) |
| | Attempts to disrupt mechanisms which perpetuate and sustain a problem in a given time and place | Moore and Evans (2017) |
| Program evaluation | Specific activities undertaken to make a positive difference in outcomes | Mayne (2015) |

insomnia) to do or avoid, and specific techniques to assist clients in carrying out these recommendations. The techniques include providing information on the association between sleep behaviors and insomnia, prompting identification of barriers and possible solutions, and encouraging self-monitoring of sleep behaviors and parameters. These three specific techniques are described as replicable behavior change techniques designed to alter behaviors (Abraham & Michie, 2008; Carey et al., 2018).

### 2.1.3   Programs

Programs, complex interventions, and multicomponent interventions consist of multiple interventions that have been grouped into a package. The package is often designed to address: (1) a health problem that is conceptualized from different perspectives and experienced in different domains of health (e.g. cognitive and behavioral, as is the case with chronic insomnia); (2) a health problem that is attributable to a range of determinants occurring in different domains of health (e.g. physical, psychological, social) and at different levels (e.g. individual, community, healthcare system); or (3) co-occurring and inter-related health problems (e.g. comorbidity or multi-morbidity that is, the presence of multiple acute and chronic conditions among older adults). Examples of programs are provided in Table 2.2.

## 2.2   INTERVENTION ELEMENTS

Interventions are described in terms of the goals they are set to achieve and the components comprising them.

### 2.2.1   Intervention Goals

Interventions are designed to attain one or more goals related to a particular health problem. An intervention goal is a statement of what exactly the intervention is expected to achieve relative to the health problem it targets. Some interventions aim to modify the determinants or causes of the health problem and, hence, to prevent its occurrence. For example, changing a nonambulatory client's position in bed every two hours aims to prevent pressure ulcer, and instructing clients with asthma to avoid irritants such as dust and smoke is directed at preventing dyspnea. Other interventions are designed to manage the health problem, to reduce its burden, and/or to mitigate its negative consequences. For instance, taking a medication is useful in self-managing muscle pain whereas listening to music is helpful in reducing the emotional reactions to pain such as anxiety (i.e. its burden); both interventions relieve pain and minimize its contribution to limited physical functioning (i.e. its negative consequences). Other interventions are directed at promoting engagement in health-related behaviors such as physical activity and smoking cessation and consequently, enhancing general health and well-being.

### 2.2.2   Intervention Components

Interventions are comprised of one or more components. A component is a set of activities or techniques that are directed toward addressing a common goal. For example, the multicomponent intervention for insomnia described in Table 2.2 consists of four components, each addressing one goal: (1) sleep education and hygiene

**TABLE 2.2** Examples of programs or multicomponent interventions.

| Health problem | Chronic insomnia | Stroke and multi-morbidity | Promotion of physical health |
|---|---|---|---|
| Program/intervention name | Multicomponent intervention | Hospital-to-home transitional care intervention | For health, I move in my neighborhood! |
| Description | 1. Sleep education and hygiene<br>  • Discussion of factors that contribute to insomnia<br>  • Presentation of behavioral and environmental recommendations to promote a good night's sleep<br>2. Stimulus control therapy<br>  • Discussion of instructions for sleep-related behaviors<br>  • Application of recommendations in daily life<br>3. Sleep restriction therapy<br>  • Identification of sleep needs<br>  • Working out a sleep–wake schedule<br>  • Application of schedule in daily life<br>4. Behavior change support<br>  • Identification of barriers and strategies to overcome barriers to the application of recommendations in daily life<br>  • Self-monitoring of sleep behaviors and sleep parameters | 1. Person-centered care<br>  • Comprehensive health assessment<br>  • Medication review and reconciliation<br>  • Self-management education and support<br>  • Provision of caregiver support<br>2. Care coordination/system navigation<br>  • In-person (inter-professional case conferences) and electronic (web-based application) communication among health professionals<br>  • Timely referral to appropriate health professionals and community resources | 1. Improved offering and accessibility to physical activity<br>  • Provision of new activities (e.g. walking, yoga) in schools<br>2. Communication about physical activity (i.e. information about benefits of physical activity)<br>  • Distribution of flyers or brochures<br>  • Physical activity instructor's visits to different structures (e.g. schools, community centers) and availability for consultation<br>  • Sports festival<br>3. Environmental changes<br>  • Orientation pathways (i.e. information on distance and duration of walk to different services)<br>  • Provision of additional sports devices at community centers<br>4. Urban redevelopment<br>  • Road work (e.g. bike path, widening sidewalk)<br>  • Redevelopment of green areas<br>5. "Shape and Health Challenge" program<br>  • Physical and sports activities program |
| Reference | Adapted from Sidani et al. (2019) | Adapted from Markle-Reid et al. (2019) | Adapted from Buscail et al. (2016) |

aims to help clients understand the factors that perpetuate insomnia, and the general behavioral and environmental recommendations to promote a good night's sleep; (2) stimulus control therapy focuses on reassociating the bed with sleep; (3) sleep restriction therapy aims to consolidate sleep; and (4) behavior change support is set to facilitate clients' initiation, engagement, and adherence to all treatment recommendations in their daily life context.

There are two categories of intervention components: specific and nonspecific. Specific components are unique and essential in distinguishing the intervention. They represent the "active ingredients," which are theoretically hypothesized to bring about the intended changes in the health problem and to produce related beneficial outcomes (Carey et al., 2018; Kühne et al., 2015; Michie et al., 2009). The nonspecific components are techniques used to enable, support, reinforce, or facilitate the implementation of the intervention's specific components (Sidani et al., 2020). Nonspecific components are usually not unique to a particular intervention and, therefore, are not expected to contribute significantly to the intended beneficial outcomes (Araújo-Soares et al., 2018). Recent evidence, however, suggests that nonspecific components, in combination with the way the intervention is delivered, may enhance or undermine its effectiveness (Dombrowski et al., 2016). For example, sleep education and hygiene, stimulus control therapy and sleep restriction therapy are specific components of the multicomponent intervention for insomnia. The behavior change support is a nonspecific component because it is generic and can be integrated in other health behavior change interventions.

## 2.3    CHARACTERISTICS OF INTERVENTIONS

Interventions are characterized by their elements (i.e. goals and components), which define them conceptually, and the way in which the interventions and their components are delivered. This encompasses features through which interventions' content is conveyed (Dombrowski et al., 2016) and specific components and activities are implemented. The features include mode of delivery, structure, and dose.

### 2.3.1    Mode of Delivery

The mode of intervention delivery is described in terms of medium and format.

*Medium* is the means through which the intervention and its components and respective activities are carried out. Medium is defined by the intersection of person-dependency and method. For the former, medium can be classified as person-dependent and person-independent (Beall et al., 2014; Cutrona et al., 2010). In the person-dependent medium, individuals, including health professionals and/or laypersons, offer the intervention to clients, whereas these individuals are not directly involved in the intervention delivery in person-independent medium. There are two methods of delivery: verbal/oral and written.

*Format* refers to the specific technique used within the verbal and written method for providing the intervention. Examples of specific media illustrating the intersectionality of person-dependency, method, and format are presented in Table 2.3.

Different *modes* can be used to deliver different components of an intervention and more than one mode can be used to deliver each component. For instance, the sleep education and hygiene component of the multicomponent intervention for insomnia can be provided via the combination of: (1) formal presentation of pertinent

**TABLE 2.3**   Examples of specific media for providing interventions.

| Method | Person-dependent | Person-independent |
| --- | --- | --- |
| Verbal | 1. Face-to-face format<br>  • Large group presentation<br>  • Small (6–10 persons) group meetings/sessions<br>  • Individual meetings/contacts<br>2. Distance format<br>  • Telephone calls<br>  • Videoconferencing<br>  • Digital media contacts | • Recorded (audio/video) presentations<br>• Automated telephone calls<br>• Message disseminated via media (radio, television, mobile telephones-text messaging) |
| Written | • Slide presentation | • Posters located in public places<br>• Information distributed via diverse modes (e.g. regular mail, electronic mail, mobile telephones)<br>• Information available via digital media (World Wide Web, mobile applications, portable media players) |

content by a health professional to a small group of persons with insomnia, complemented by a slide presentation; (2) involvement of persons in a group discussion to clarify the information; and (3) a booklet summarizing the key points that serves as a reference for persons carrying out the sleep hygiene recommendations.

## 2.3.2   Structure

Structure has to do with the approach and sequence for providing the intervention components. Approach represents the manner in which the intervention is given. It can be standardized or tailored/adaptive.

The *standardized* approach consists of giving the same intervention components, in the same mode, to all clients, regardless of the relevance of the intervention's components, activities, and mode of delivery to the characteristics and preferences of clients. The *tailored* approach involves customizing or individualizing the intervention to the characteristics and preferences of clients (Mannion & Exworthy, 2017). It is conceivable to provide some components and respective activities in a standardized approach and others in a tailored approach. In the example of the multicomponent intervention for chronic insomnia, the instructions of the stimulus control therapy are applicable to all clients and, thus, relayed in a standardized approach; however, setting a regular sleep–wake schedule, which is the specific component of sleep restriction therapy, is informed by clients' sleep needs and negotiated to suit individual clients' life circumstances.

The components comprising the intervention can be provided simultaneously or sequentially. *Simultaneous* provision implies that the components and respective activities are presented, discussed, and carried out all together at one point in time. For instance, Sidani et al. (2019) designed the multicomponent intervention for chronic insomnia in a way whereby the information and recommendations of the sleep education and hygiene, stimulus control therapy, and sleep restriction therapy were conveyed to clients in the first intervention session; clients were instructed to apply all recommendations associated with these three components simultaneously.

*Sequential* provision means that the intervention components are given progressively, that is, one component is introduced at a time. This is illustrated with how Holmqvist et al. (2014) designed and delivered the cognitive behavioral therapy for insomnia: Clients were exposed to the therapy's components in the following sequence: (1) psychoeducation about sleep and models or factors contributing to insomnia; (2) relaxation training; (3) concepts of stimulus control therapy and sleep restriction therapy; (4) cognitive therapy; (5) information on sleep hygiene and stimulus control; and (6) mindfulness meditation.

### 2.3.3  Dose

Dose (also called intensity) refers to the level at which the intervention as-a-whole (i.e. including all its components) is delivered in order to effectively address the health problem and produce beneficial changes in other outcomes. Similar to the dose of medications, the dose of health interventions is operationalized in four aspects: purity, amount, frequency, and duration.

*Purity* reflects the concentration of the active ingredients of the intervention; it can be quantified as the ratio of specific to nonspecific elements constituting the intervention. Amount, frequency, and duration reflect exposure to the intervention. Specifically, *amount* refers to the quantity with which the intervention is given. Quantity is represented by the number of contacts (e.g. individual or group sessions, home visits) planned with the health professional or laypersons responsible for delivering the intervention; or the number of modules (e.g. sections in a paper or electronic booklet) to be completed by clients. Quantity also quantifies the time it takes to complete each contact (e.g. length of a group session) or module (e.g. length of time to read the information presented in each section of the booklet).

*Frequency* is the number of times the contacts are given or the modules are self-completed, over a specified period of time such as a week or month. *Duration* is the total length of time during which the intervention is given. Amount, frequency, and duration are commonly reported to specify the dose of health interventions (Beall et al., 2014). For instance, the dose of the multicomponent intervention for insomnia can be specified as: four group sessions of 60 minutes each and two individual telephone contacts of 20 minutes each, for a total of six contacts (amount). The six contacts are given once a week (frequency), over a six-week period (duration).

### REFERENCES

Abraham, C. & Michie, S. (2008) A taxonomy of behavior change techniques used in interventions. *Health Psychology*, 27(3), 379–387.

Araújo-Soares, V., Hankonen, N., Presseau, J., et al. (2018) Developing behavior change interventions for self-management in chronic illness. *European Psychologist*, 24(1), 7–25.

Beall, R.F., Baskerville, N., Golfam, M., et al. (2014) Modes of delivery in prevention intervention studies: A rapid review. *European Journal of Clinical Investigation*, 44(7), 688–696.

Bootzin, R.R. & Epstein, D.R. (2011) Understanding and treating insomnia. *Annual Review of Clinical Psychology*, 7, 435–458.

Buscail, C., Menai, M., Salanave, B., et al. (2016) Promoting physical activity in a low-income neighborhood of the Paris suburb of Saint-Denis: Effects of a community-based intervention to increase physical activity. *BMC Public Health*, 16, 667–675.

Cambon, L., Terral, P., & Alla, F. (2019) From intervention to interventional system: Towards greater theorization in population health intervention research. *BMC Public Health*, 19, 389–345.

Carey, R.N., Connell, L.E., Johnston, M., et al. (2018) Behavior change techniques and their mechanisms of action: A synthesis of links described in published intervention literature. *Annals of Behavioral Medicine*, 53(8), 693–707.

Cutrona, S., Choudhry, N., Fisher, M., et al. (2010) Modes of delivery for interventions to improve cardiovascular medication adherence: Review. *American Journal of Managed Care*, 16(12), 929–942.

Dombrowski, S.U., O'Carroll, R.E., & Williams, B. (2016) Form of delivery as a key "active ingredient" in behavior change interventions. *British Journal of Health Psychology*, 21, 733–740.

Forbes, A. (2009) Clinical intervention research in nursing. *International Journal of Nursing Studies*, 46(4), 557–568.

Grove, S.K., Gray, J.R., & Burns, N. (2015) *Understanding Nursing Research: Building an Evidence-Based Practice* (6th Ed). Elsevier, St. Louis, Missouri.

Harvey, A.G., Sharpley, A.L., Ree, M.J., et al. (2007) An open trial of cognitive therapy for chronic insomnia. *Behavior Research and Therapy*, 45(10), 2491–2501.

Holmqvist, M., Vincent, N., & Walsh, K. (2014) Web- vs telehealth-based delivery of cognitive behavioral therapy for insomnia: A randomized controlled trial. *Sleep Medicine*, 15, 187–195.

Kühne, F., Ehmcke, R., Härter, M., et al. (2015) Conceptual decomposition of complex health care interventions for evidence synthesis: A literature review. *Journal of Evaluation in Clinical Practice*, 21, 817–823.

Mannion, R. & Exworthy, M. (2017) (Re) making the proscrustean bed? Standardization and customization as competing logics in healthcare. *International Journal of Health Policy and Management*, 6(6), 301–304.

Markle-Reid, M., Valaitis, R., Bartholomew, A., et al. (2019) Feasibility and preliminary effects of an integrated hospital-to-home transition care intervention for older adults with stroke and multimorbidity : A study protocol. *Journal of Comorbidity*, 9, 1–22.

Mayne, J. (2015) Useful theory of change models. *The Canadian Journal of Program Evaluation*, 30(2), 119–142.

Michie, S., Fixsen, D., Grimshaw, J.M., & Eccles, M.P. (2009) Editorial. Specifying and reporting complex behavior change interventions: The need for a scientific method. *Implementation Science*, 4, 40–45.

Moore, G.F. & Evans, R.E. (2017) What theory, for whom and in which context? Reflections on the application of theory in the development and evaluation of complex population health intervention. *SSM—Population Health*, 3, 132–135.

Moore, G.F., Evans, R.E., Hawkins, J., et al. (2019) From complex social interventions to interventions in complex social systems: Future directions and unresolved questions for intervention development and evaluation. *Evaluation*, 25(1), 23–45.

Sidani, S., Epstein, D.R., & Fox, M. (2019) Comparing the effects of single and multiple component therapies for insomnia on sleep outcomes. *Worldviews on Evidence-Based Nursing*, 16(3), 195–203.

Sidani, S., El-Masri, M., & Fox, M.T. (2020) Guidance for the reporting of an interventions theory. *Research and Theory for Nursing Practice*, 34(1), 35–48.

Wight, D., Wimbush, E., Jepson, R., & Doi, L. (2015) Six steps in quality intervention development (6SQuID). *Journal of Epidemiology and Community Health*, 70, 520–525.

# DEVELOPING INTERVENTIONS

CHAPTER 3

# Understanding Health Problems

Poorly designed interventions can waste resources (Moore et al., 2019): Despite the effort expanded by health professionals and clients in carrying them out, the interventions are not useful in preventing, managing, or resolving the health problem. Therefore, it is essential to carefully design health interventions in order to improve their success in addressing the health problem.

The process for designing or developing health interventions is systematic and rigorous. It involves critical analysis and thorough application of relevant approaches and methods to gain a lucid understanding of the health problem requiring remediation, which is represented in the theory of the problem (Chapter 3). This understanding informs the specification of the intervention's elements, which is represented in the implementation theory, and the delineation of the mechanism underlying the intervention's effects on the outcomes, which is reflected in the theory of change (Chapter 4). The process culminates in the generation of the intervention theory (Chapter 5) that guides the delivery and evaluation of the intervention.

The development of a thorough and comprehensive understanding of the health problem requiring remediation is foundational for designing interventions (Bleijenberg et al., 2018; Wight et al., 2016). The understanding entails clarification of what the problem is, how it is experienced, by what population and in what context (Aráujo-Soares et al., 2018). Different approaches and methods can be utilized to gain an understanding of the problem; using a combination of approaches and methods is recommended to iteratively delineate the theory of the problem that is well grounded in pertinent theory, supported by evidence, and reflective of the target client population's experience and context.

In this chapter, the importance of understanding the health problem, captured in the theory of the problem, is explained. The elements of the theory are identified and illustrated with examples. The theoretical, empirical, and experiential approaches, and their respective methods, for developing the theory of the problem are discussed.

*Nursing and Health Interventions: Design, Evaluation, and Implementation*, Second Edition.
Souraya Sidani and Carrie Jo Braden.
© 2021 John Wiley & Sons Ltd. Published 2021 by John Wiley & Sons Ltd.

## 3.1   IMPORTANCE OF UNDERSTANDING HEALTH PROBLEMS

The terms health problem, diagnosis, and need are often used (in different health-related discipline or professions) interchangeably to reflect a situation requiring a solution. Clients (individuals, families, communities) experience a range of health problems and seek health professionals' assistance in selecting and applying appropriate interventions to address the problems. Health problems are the triggers for designing interventions since remedying the problem requires understanding it first (Kok et al., 2016). Poor conceptualization of the problem could result in the design of inappropriate and potentially ineffective intervention, that is, type III error (Renger, 2011). Accordingly, understanding the health problem requiring remediation provides directions for: specifying the goals of the intervention; identifying its active ingredients that are expected to successfully address the problem; and delineating contextual factors that should be considered in operationalizing and providing an intervention. Interventions designed in a way that is responsive to the target client populations' experience of the health problem and context are likely to be acceptable, efficient, and effective (Huntink et al., 2014; Yardley et al., 2015). For instance, Glanz and Bishop (2010) stated that the most successful public health interventions are based on an understanding of health behaviors and the contexts in which they occur. The understanding is best represented in the theory of the problem.

## 3.2   THEORY OF THE PROBLEM

The theory of the problem is also called logic model of the problem (Dalager et al., 2019). It presents a systematic articulation of the health problem requiring remediation. Health problems are experienced in different domains of health, in different ways, by different clients presenting with different personal and health profiles. The problems are brought about, caused, or influenced by a range of factors operating at different levels, in different contexts. This heterogeneity or variation in experience demands a clarification of the health problem as encountered in the clients' circumstances or contexts (Butner et al., 2015; Leask et al., 2019). The theory of the problem is a middle range theory that provides a comprehensive conceptualization of the health problem requiring remediation. The theory defines the problem, identifies influential factors, and explains the relationships among them, that is, how the factors contribute to the problem. The theory can also specify possible consequences if the problem is not addressed.

### 3.2.1   Definition of the Health Problem

The theory identifies the health problem (i.e. what it is called such as insomnia), defines it at the conceptual and operational levels. The conceptual definition describes the nature of the problem, whereas the operational definition delimits its attributes.

#### 3.2.1.1   Conceptual Definition

The nature of the health problem characterizes what it is about. It is described in terms of its categorization as actual or potential, and by the domain of health in which it is experienced.

## Categorization of Health Problems

An actual problem is an existing situation with which clients present that requires intervention. It reflects an alteration in health, or a dysfunction, and/or an undesirable behavior that clients actually experience or exhibit, respectively at a particular point in time. Examples of actual health problems include symptoms such as pain and fatigue; difficulty performing activities of daily living; less-than-optimal adherence to treatment recommendations; an epidemic or spread of infectious disease in the community; and caregiving burden.

A potential problem refers to a discrepancy between a current situation (i.e. the way things are) and an ideal situation (i.e. the way things ought to be). It reflects an inadequacy in the type or level of current functioning, and/or an inadequacy in the type or level of healthcare services, that increases the probability of resulting in an actual problem. Potential problems are illustrated by: engagement in undesirable health behaviors such as smoking that increases the risk of lung cancer; the need for information, support, or additional services to promote engagement in physical activity; or shortage in the number of nurse practitioners with expertise in geriatrics care to provide comprehensive care to the growing aging population and prevent admission to acute care hospitals.

The categorization of health problems determines the overall goal of the intervention and the timing within the trajectory of the health problem experience for its delivery. For actual health problems, interventions are designed to manage them, that is, to improve the problems' experience, treat or resolve them, or assist clients to manage them successfully. The interventions are provided after the occurrence of the actual problem. For potential health problems, interventions are geared to prevent them, that is, reduce the chances of their occurrence. The interventions are offered before the occurrence of the problems.

## Domains of Health Problems

The nature of the health problem also reflects the domain of health in which it is experienced. Actual or potential problems exhibit as alterations in any or combination of health domains: biological (e.g. bone fracture, muscle injury); physiological (e.g. high blood pressure or glucose levels); physical (e.g. difficulty walking); cognitive (e.g. difficulty remembering things); psychological/emotional (e.g. stress); behavioral (e.g. substance abuse); social (e.g. lack of social support network); cultural (e.g. proscribed practices); and spiritual (e.g. lost meaning in life).

The conceptualization of the problem as experienced in a particular or combination of health domains informs the general strategy underlying the intervention. The strategy should be consistent with the nature of the problem. For instance, conceptualizing insomnia as a cognitive problem (e.g. Harvey et al., 2017), or a behavioral problem (e.g. Bootzin & Epstein, 2011), or a combined cognitive and behavioral problem (e.g. Schwartz & Carney, 2012) suggests the need for a cognitive, behavioral, or cognitive-behavioral approach, respectively, for its management. Interventions focusing only on education are not consistent with these conceptualizations of insomnia and, therefore, are likely to be ineffective in resolving this health problem.

### 3.2.1.2 Operational Definition

The attributes of the health problem are the indicators of its presence and distinguish it from other problems. The attributes are described in terms of the type and level of indicators that define the problem, as well as the severity and duration with which the problem is experienced.

*Type and Level of Indicators*

Indicators reflect how the problem is manifested. They are the particular alterations or changes in structure or function that point to the presence of the problem. The indicators may be objectively observed (i.e. signs) or subjectively reported (i.e. symptoms). For example, difficulty initiating sleep (i.e. falling asleep) and maintaining sleep (i.e. staying asleep) are two indicators of insomnia. It is important to note that the experience of the indicators may vary within and across client populations. The variation may be associated with different client characteristics such as age, gender, and culture. For example, the indicators of insomnia vary with age: Middle-aged persons frequently report experiencing difficulty falling asleep, whereas older persons frequently report difficulty staying asleep (Sidani et al., 2018a).

The identification of the indicators can be supplemented by the specification of the level at which they are experienced in order to operationally define the health problem. Level of experiencing the indicators is reflected in a range of values or cutoff scores that should be observed or reported to indicate the presence of the problem. For example, difficulty falling asleep and/or staying asleep may be experienced by anyone, under a wide range of circumstances (e.g. clients may not sleep well a few days before surgery). To indicate the presence of insomnia, these sleep difficulties or disturbances should occur for 30 minutes or more per night, over at least three nights per week.

*Severity and Duration of the Health Problem*

Severity refers to the intensity with which the health problem is experienced. It has to do with "how badly," serious and/or distressing the problem is. The level of severity can be objectively assessed (e.g. level of dependence in performance of activities of daily living, or number of cigarettes smoked) or subjectively rated for its distress or burden by clients, using relevant measures and rating scales. For example, the Insomnia Severity Index assesses clients' perception of how distressing their sleep problem is, and how much it interferes with daytime functioning; the total score quantifies the level of insomnia severity (Morin et al., 2011).

Duration refers to the time period over which the health problem is experienced. It determines the acuity or chronicity of the problem, which may be associated with different sets of contributing factors. For example, the experience of the sleep difficulties as described previously, over at least three months, indicates the presence of chronic insomnia, which is primarily associated with sleep-related behaviors; acute insomnia is experienced as a result of life events.

Generating a list of indicators, describing each indicator accurately, and specifying the severity and duration of the health problem's experience are important. A critical analysis of the indicators points to those that are amenable to change and for which interventions or components of an intervention can be designed to directly address them and, hence, contribute to the management or resolution of the problem. For example, dyspnea is manifested by rapid short breathing, suggesting that clients can be instructed to perform deep breathing exercises to control this specific indicator of dyspnea. The severity and duration of the health problem's experience inform the identification of factors that contribute to the problem.

### 3.2.1.3    Factors Contributing to the Problem

Generating a comprehensive understanding of the health problem requires the identification of influential factors and the delineation of their inter-relationships with the problem.

## Identification of Factors

Causative factors, risk factors, or determinants of the health problem are circumstances, events, conditions, or capabilities that contribute to its experience. It is now well recognized that multiple factors, taking place at different levels, conduce to the occurrence (e.g. Aráujo-Soares et al., 2018; Golfam et al., 2015) or maintenance (e.g. Glanz & Bishop, 2010) of a particular problem. The factors exhibit in any domain of health and life, at the intrapersonal, interpersonal, social, and environmental levels (Bartholomew et al., 2016). Intrapersonal factors include biological characteristics (e.g. sex and age) and physiological, physical, behavioral, psychological, and cognitive conditions. Interpersonal factors entail challenges in the relationships between individual clients and others in their immediate environment (e.g. home, work) and the availability or accessibility of resources and support. Social factors relate to beliefs, values, and norms commonly held by a group or community. Environmental factors represent features of the physical, socioeconomic, and political setting or context in which clients reside (Craig et al., 2018).

In addition to identifying the types and levels at which the factors occur, it may be useful to (1) categorize them into factors that contribute to the development or to the maintenance of the health problem (Butner et al., 2015; Glanz & Bishop, 2010); (2) determine if and how they are inter-related and (3) if they vary across populations and time. Overall, the factors can be categorized into predisposing, precipitating, and perpetuating factors as was done for factors contributing to insomnia.

1. *Predisposing* factors are usually innate characteristics that increase clients' susceptibility or tendency to experience the problem. This category of factors is illustrated with sex and age, which have been found to increase clients' vulnerability to experience insomnia.
2. *Precipitating* (also called enabling) factors are conditions or events that bring about or trigger the problem. This category of factors is illustrated with the onset of illness or stress-related events that disrupt sleep.
3. *Perpetuating* (also called reinforcing) factors serve to maintain the problem. In the case of insomnia, perpetuating factors represent sleep habits or behaviors that clients engage in an attempt to deal with poor sleep but are ineffective.

## Delineation of Inter-relationships

In the real world, the determinants are interconnected, forming a web of factors contributing to the experience of the health problem. The determinants can co-occur simultaneously or sequentially, and interact with each other to produce the health problem. For instance, older persons are prone to arousability (i.e. light sleep), which may be exacerbated if they reside in a noisy neighborhood (simultaneous); they start drinking alcohol (sequential) thinking that it would help them sleep better; alcohol causes light sleep thereby further contributing to awakenings at night, and intensifies the effects of medications such as sleeping pills and other antidepressants (interaction). The specific determinants or combination of factors contributing to the health problem could vary across client populations or within the same population over time. For example, young and middle-aged adults (compared to older adults) report difficulty falling asleep, which they attribute to stress related to daily life and work; the level at which they experience this sleep difficulty fluctuates over time as a result of changes in life and work events and clients' use of effective strategies to promote sleep (e.g. engagement in relaxation).

The identification and the specification of the inter-relationships among determinants are essential for understanding why and how the health problem is generated and maintained. A critical analysis of the inter-relationships (described in Chapter 4) assists in determining the factors that are and are not amenable to change (Aráujo-Soares et al., 2018; Bartholomew et al., 2016; Fernandez et al., 2019; Lippe & Ziegelman, 2008). Factors that are malleable and have the greatest scope for change are targeted by the intervention (Wight et al., 2016); they inform the specification of its active ingredients. Factors that cannot be modified (e.g. personal and contextual characteristics) are considered as potential moderators, indicating the need for tailoring of the intervention (Fleury & Sidani, 2018).

### 3.2.2  Consequences of the Problem

Consequences of the health problem represent complications that may arise if the problem is not effectively addressed. Complications are changes in condition resulting from the problem and interfering with clients' general functioning, health and well-being. Examples of consequences associated with insomnia include: physical and mental fatigue that limit physical and psychosocial functioning, which in turn, contributes to accidents. The experience of consequences may be the reason for which clients seek healthcare. As such, interventions are designed to address the health problem with the ultimate goal of preventing or minimizing the severity of its consequences.

### 3.2.3  Illustrative Example

Once developed, the theory or logic model of the health problem is presented textually to detail the conceptual and operational definitions of the problem; identify and describe its determinants and consequences; and explain the proposed direct and indirect (mediated and/or moderated) relationships among them. The theory is also summarized in a table and its main propositions illustrated in a figure. Table 3.1 and Figure 3.1 illustrate the theory of insomnia.

## 3.3  APPROACHES FOR GENERATING THEORY OF THE HEALTH PROBLEM

Different approaches can be utilized, independently or in combination, to gain an understanding of the health problem and generate a theory of the problem. The approaches include theoretical, empirical, and experiential. They reflect different logic and methods of reasoning: deductive (top-down), inductive (bottom-up), retroductive (backtracking process of logical inference going beyond an existing theory and empirical observations), and abductive (alternative explanation process). The approaches can be used independently. With the emphasis on evidence-based practice, the empirical approach was considered the most robust. With the recent emphasis on client engagement in the design of health services and in research, and the widening recognition of the role of context in health and healthcare, the experiential approach has been increasingly advocated. Since each approach has its

**TABLE 3.1**   Summary of the theory of insomnia.

| | | |
|---|---|---|
| Conceptual definition | Nature | Insomnia is conceptualized as a learned behavior<br>Insomnia refers to self-reported disturbed sleep in the presence of adequate opportunity and circumstances for sleep<br>Insomnia is actually experienced by clients across the life span |
| Operational definition | Defining indicators | Types:<br>Insomnia is manifested in any or a combination of difficulty initiating or maintain sleep<br><br>Levels:<br>Sleep difficulties reported at ≥30 minutes per night, reported on ≥3 nights per week |
| | Severity | Insomnia Severity Index total score:<br>≤7 = no clinically significant insomnia<br>8–14 = subthreshold insomnia<br>15–21 = clinical insomnia of moderate severity<br>22–28 = clinically severe insomnia |
| | Duration | Acute insomnia: indicators experienced at the specified level, periodically for <3 months<br>Chronic insomnia: indicators experienced at the specified level for ≥3 months |
| Contributing factors | Determinants | Precipitating factors: onset of illness, stress, life or work-related events that disrupt sleep<br><br>Perpetuating factors: cognitions (unrealistic beliefs about sleep, insomnia and its consequences); general behaviors (physical inactivity, smoking); sleep habits or behaviors (irregular sleep schedules, engaging in activities in bed); and engagement in behaviors (extended time in bed) that fuel or maintain insomnia |
| | Moderators | Predisposing factors: innate characteristics (age, sex, familial or genetic tendency) that increase vulnerability to poor sleep |
| | Environment | Features (light, noise, temperature) in the sleep environment that interfere with good sleep |
| Consequences | | Physical and mental daytime fatigue; reduced engagement in physical and psychosocial functions; home, work, or traffic accidents; development of physical (e.g. hypertension) and psychological (e.g. depression) health conditions |

strengths and limitations, the use of a combination of approaches is recommended (e.g. Aráujo-Soares et al., 2018; Bartholomew et al., 2016; Bleijenberg et al., 2018) to develop a comprehensive understanding of the health problem as experienced by the target client population in the respective context. The approaches and methods for applying them are discussed next.

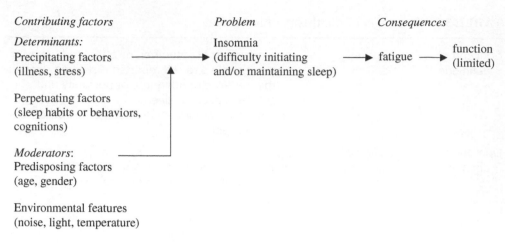

**FIGURE 3.1** Representation of theory of insomnia.

## 3.3.1   Theoretical Approach

### 3.3.1.1   Overview

The theoretical approach relies on relevant theories to develop an understanding of the health problem requiring intervention. Middle range theories are most useful because they describe the health problem and explain its associations with determinants, within a particular context (Moore & Evans, 2017).

### *Elements of Theory*

Theories consist of a group of statements, based on careful reasoning and/or evidence that present a systematic and logical view of the health problem. The statements are logically organized to identify, define, and describe the problem and its determinants, and to explain the direct and indirect relationships among the determinants and the problem. The explanations clarify conceptually why and how the relationships come about, that is, what goes on that connects each determinant to the problem. For example, the following pathway explains the association between age and insomnia: As individuals age, they spend more time in light, than deep, stages of sleep; they are prone to arousability resulting in frequent awakenings during the night, manifested in difficulty maintaining sleep.

### *Types of Relationships*

A *direct relationship* reflects an immediate linkage between a determinant and the problem, where the problem flows straightforwardly from or is a function of the determinant. For example, there is a direct association between caffeine and nicotine intake close to bedtime and insomnia; caffeine and nicotine are stimulants that interfere with sleep.

An *indirect relationship* can take either of two forms: mediated or moderated. The relationship between a determinant and the health problem is considered *mediated* when another factor intervenes between the two, whereby the determinant influences the mediator (also called intervening factor), which in turn affects the health problem (MacKinnon & Fairchild, 2009). For example, cognitions are erroneous beliefs, resulting from worry or rumination about sleep-related issues such as inability to get eight hours of sleep and the negative impact of insomnia on daytime functions. These cognitions increase arousal and drive engagement in sleep behaviors in an attempt to alleviate arousal; however, these behaviors may be ineffective and the repeated experience of arousal in bed results in conditional arousal (i.e. associating the bed with wakefulness), which contributes to insomnia (Schwartz & Carney, 2012). The relationship between a determinant and the health problem is characterized as *moderated* when it is affected by another factor (also called moderator). The moderator is the condition (e.g. personal or environmental feature) under which the relationship exists, that is, the presence, strength or magnitude, and/or direction of the relationship between the determinant and the health problem vary according to the value of the moderator (Fleury & Sidani, 2018). For instance, gender could moderate the association between arousal and insomnia; women may experience life stress (because of multiple roles' demands) and worry, which is likely to strengthen the relationship between arousal and insomnia if not well managed.

### Examples of Theory

A wide range of middle range theories are available and have been used to generate an understanding of health problems. Theories that have commonly informed the understanding of the occurrence of health behaviors (e.g. physical inactivity, diet, medication adherence) include the health beliefs model, the transtheoretical model, social cognitive theory, social ecological model, and theory of planned behavior (Beall et al., 2014; Durks et al.m 2017; Fassier et al., 2019; Glanz & Bishop, 2010; Lamort-Bouché et al., 2018). Other theories include self-determination theory and self-regulation theory (e.g. Muellmann et al., 2019). Cognitive theories have been used to understand some psychological health problems such as depression (Vittengl et al., 2014) and insomnia (Harvey et al., 2007). Kwasnicka et al. (2016) reviewed theories that explain how behaviors are maintained.

### Selection of Theory

Different middle range theories propose different conceptualizations of the same health problem. The theories identify different sets of determinants, operating at different levels and/or related to the health problem through different pathways or mechanisms. Selection of a theory or theories should take into consideration the complexity of the real world (i.e. multiple factors, at different levels, contribute to the health problem). Attending to complexity demands the careful review, appraisal, and, if necessary, integration of different theories (or elements of theories) to explain the health problem as experienced by the target client population within the respective context (Bleijenberg et al., 2018; Moore & Evans, 2017). For example, conceptualizing insomnia from a behavioral perspective alone may not be adequate, as it is recognized that behaviors are shaped by cognitions (i.e. beliefs), attitudes, personal sense of control, sociocultural norms, and physical environment (Dohnke et al., 2018). Therefore, the selection of middle range theories to generate the theory of the health problem should be carefully done.

### 3.3.1.2 Methods

To be useful in understanding the health problem, middle range theories need to be relevant to the problem of interest. This necessitates a clarification of the problem, identification of available theories, and critical analysis of the theories' description of the problem and propositions regarding its determinants.

*Step 1 – Clarification of the Problem*
Clarification of the health problem entails an initial delineation of its nature. This is done by addressing the questions: What is the problem exactly about? Is it an actual or potential problem? How is the problem manifested? In what domain of health is it experienced, in what way, by whom, in what context, at what time? Is the concern about the occurrence or the maintenance of the problem? Answers to these questions generate a clear definition of the problem and specification of its attributes, experienced by a particular client population, in a particular context. For example health behaviors are described relative to target, action, context, time, and actors (Aráujo-Soares et al., 2018). The clarification of the problem guides the search for relevant theories; it provides key terms and sets limits (e.g. client population, context) for conducting the search.

*Step 2 – Identification of Theories*
Two general methods can be used to identify relevant theories that explain the health problem as defined in Step 1. The first method relies on *consultation* with scholars and/or health professionals who have expert theoretical and/or clinical knowledge of the health problem. They may have developed, adapted, or been aware of relevant theories. The second method consists of a *literature search*. The search covers a wide range of sources including: theoretical or conceptual papers that focus on the presentation of the theory or its adaptation to a particular client population or context; textbooks or chapters that describe the health problem from a theoretical or clinical perspective; and grey literature such as professional organizations' websites providing access to white papers or conference presentations about the problem and relevant theories. The search may be extended to empirical papers reporting on studies that tested the theories in different client populations and contexts. Literature sources are selected if they offer a clear description of the theory, which contains a definition of the health problem, identification of its determinants, and propositions explaining the relationships (direct and indirect) between the determinants and the problem.

*Step 3 – Analysis of Theories*
The analysis of theories consists of the following:

1. The analysis begins by extracting from the selected sources, information on the following elements of each theory identified as relevant to the health problem: name of the theory; conceptual definition of the problem; operational definition of the problem; and possible variations in its indicators across client populations, subgroups comprising a population, and contexts; specification of determinants at different levels; definition of each determinant; delineation of the relationships (direct, indirect) among determinants and the health problem; conceptual explanation of the proposed relationships; and if available, empirical evidence supporting the proposed relationships.

2. The information pertaining to each theory is synthesized across all sources in order to generate a full and accurate description of the theory and its elements. The description is entered into a matrix illustrated in Table 3.2, in preparation for the analysis.

3. The analysis is done for each theory to determine its logical coherence (i.e. consistency between conceptual and operational definitions, logical explanation of the proposed relationships), usefulness in generating a comprehensive and in-depth understanding of the health problem (e.g. comprehensive list of determinants at different levels), and applicability to the context of the target client population (Mayne, 2017; The Improved Clinical Effectiveness through Behavioral Research Group, 2006).

**TABLE 3.2**   Matrix for analysis of theories.

| Element of theory | Theory 1 | Theory 2 |
| --- | --- | --- |
| Name | | |
| Conceptual definition of health problem | | |
| Operational definition of health problem<br>a. Defining indicators<br>b. Variations in indicators | | |
| Determinants<br>a. List of determinants at each level<br>b. Definition of determinants<br>c. Direct determinants<br>d. Indirect determinants:<br>  • Mediators<br>  • Moderators | | |
| Conceptual explanation of<br>a. Direct relationships<br>b. Mediated relationships<br>c. Moderated relationships | | |
| Empirically supported relationships | | |

4. The analysis is also done across theories. This analysis consists of comparing and contrasting, qualitatively, the different elements of the theories, as well as their logical coherence, usefulness, and applicability. The results indicate whether (1) a particular theory is most appropriate, logical and consistent with the initial clarification of the problem experienced by the client population within the context of interest; this theory is selected as the theory of the health problem; (2) elements of different theories are complementary or provide supplementary information about the problem and its determinants; these elements are integrated into the theory of the health problem to present a complete and clear understanding of the problem and its determinants; or (3) a theory or integrated elements is(are) useful in understanding the problem but its(their) applicability to the target client population and context cannot be confirmed; in this case, other approaches (e.g. empirical, experiential) could be used to generate the theory of the problem.

The information gained from this analysis assists in formulating the theory or logic model of the health problem. Specifically, the initial definition of the problem is refined as needed. A comprehensive list of determinants is generated and their direct and indirect relationships with the problem are delineated and explained, and where available, supported by empirical evidence.

### 3.3.1.3   Strengths

The theoretical approach to generate an understanding of the health problem is advantageous. Theories provide a generalizable conceptualization of the problem and its determinants (Foy et al., 2007). By transcending individual cases, middle range theories describe clearly the nature of the problem and identify its determinants or "root causes" (Davidoff et al., 2015). They provide explicit, logical explanations of why and how the determinants affect the problem directly or indirectly.

Thus, theories prevent the danger of (1) mislabeling and vaguely defining health problems, (2) missing or omitting important determinants; and (3) misinterpreting associations (specifically bivariate ones that link the problem to one determinant) between the determinants and the problem, all of which have the potential to mislead the design of interventions. Middle range theories do not only explain the pathways linking the determinants to the problem, but also point to the context under which the problem is experienced and maintained, and the pathway is induced. Variations in the pathway across clients and contexts highlight the need to adapt or tailor the design of interventions. Briefly, theories are powerful tools to understand the health problem and to make informed decisions when designing interventions (e.g. Aráujo-Soares et al., 2018; Bleijenberg et al., 2018; Medical Research Council, 2019).

### 3.3.1.4    Limitations

The theoretical approach has some limitations in gaining a comprehensive understanding of the health problem. The reliance on one single middle range theory constrains the perspective on the nature and determinants of the problem to those identified in the theory. Therefore, additional factors (in particular contextual or environmental) that may contribute to the problem could be missed; this limits the capacity to account for all possible determinants pertinent to complex problems experienced by particular client populations in particular contexts. For many health-related problems there is a limited, if any, number of relevant middle range theories that provide an adequate understanding of the problem and all its determinants. Further, of the available middle range theories, a few have been subjected to extensive empirical test across the range of client populations and contexts, and for those tested (e.g. transtheoretical model), the results are often mixed.

Middle range theories may have limited utility if they are not supported empirically. The theoretical approach can be complemented with the empirical approach to gain a comprehensive and accurate understanding of the health problem as actually experienced in the target client population and context.

### 3.3.2    Empirical Approach

The empirical approach relies on systematically generated evidence to gain an understanding of the health problem. The evidence is obtained through these methods: a review of pertinent literature, conduct of primary studies, and/or analysis of available data.

### 3.3.2.1    Literature Review

*Overview*

Literature reviews are essential to analyze and synthesize available empirical evidence on the health problem. The literature encompasses primary quantitative and qualitative studies that investigated the problem, as well as reviews that synthesized the evidence on the experience of the problem (i.e. its indicators) and its association with determinants.

*Review of Quantitative Studies*

Quantitative studies to include in the review are the ones that aimed to describe the health problem and/or to examine its relationships, direct or indirect, with its determinants and consequences within particular client populations and settings. The studies may use different research designs.

Results of *descriptive cross-sectional* studies indicate the prevalence of the problem in different client populations and clarify the nature of the problem, its indicators, and level of severity as reported by clients presenting with diverse sociodemographic, cultural, and health or clinical characteristics, at one point in time. Differences in the health problem experience across client populations or subgroups of the same target population have implications for the design of interventions, whereby different components are selected or their delivery is adapted or tailored to variations in the clients' experience of the problem.

Results of *descriptive longitudinal* studies indicate changes in the experience, indicators, and severity levels of the health problem over time. Awareness of changes in the problem experience over time is informative as it guides the selection of the timing, within the health problem trajectory, for delivering the intervention; of the optimal dose at which the intervention is given which may incorporate "booster" sessions to prevent relapse; and the organization or sequence with which the intervention components are offered.

Results of *correlational cross-sectional* studies support the existence, direction, and magnitude or size of the associations between the health problem, and its determinants. They shed light on the nature of the relationships (i.e. whether direct or indirect) between the problem and determinants. Findings of *correlational longitudinal* studies provide evidence of the sustainability or changes in the existence, direction, or magnitude of these relationships over time; they have the potential to identify the temporal sequence linking determinants to the problem, which is required to support naturally occurring causal linkages. For example, cross-sectional evidence has long supported the existence of a positive correlation between insomnia and depression; but it was not clear which of these two problems caused the other. Recent longitudinal evidence suggests that insomnia predicts depression and that interventions addressing insomnia could contribute to improvement in depression and not the other way as implied in cross-sectional evidence (e.g. Fernandez-Mendoza et al., 2015).

### Review of Qualitative Studies

Qualitative studies to include in the review are those that focused on exploring the experience of the health problem from the clients' perspective. Clients are well known to hold implicit theories of the health problem; these theories reflect their personal construction of the problem and explanation of contributing factors (Armstrong & Dregan, 2014). Qualitative studies using different approaches (e.g. phenomenology, grounded theory) are selected if they aim to describe clients' experience of the problem (e.g. indicators, impact on daily life); elucidate factors that contributed to the problem; or generate a theory or a model summarizing and explaining the intricate relationships among the determinants and the problem. Results of qualitative studies highlight the unique way in which the health problem is experienced by particular subgroups of the client population. They also assist in clarifying the pathway linking the determinants with the problem and in providing conceptual explanations of these associations.

### Review of Reviews

Many types of literature reviews are useful in developing a comprehensive understanding of the health problem. These are well described by Snilstveit et al. (2012), Paré et al. (2015), and Hong et al. (2017). Of interest to the generation of an understanding of the health problem are reviews that synthesize theoretical or conceptual knowledge and quantitative and qualitative empirical evidence related to the problem experience and its associations with determinants.

*Theoretical or conceptual reviews* are exemplified with concept analysis (Hupcey & Penrod, 2005) and framework synthesis (Carroll et al., 2013). Essentially, these consist of reviewing theoretical, empirical, and sometimes grey literature, for the purposes of: clarifying the attributes of the health problem; defining it at the theoretical and operational levels and distinguishing it from related concepts or problems; and identifying its determinants.

*Quantitative reviews* include systematic reviews, meta-analyses, and umbrella reviews that focus on the relationships among determinants and the health problems. The reviews apply a systematic process for searching the literature; identifying and selecting studies that meet the pre-specified criteria; appraising the study quality; and extracting data on the existence, direction, and magnitude of the associations between the determinants and the problem. However, they differ in the method for synthesizing the evidence. Systematic reviews use vote count or content analysis to integrate evidence on the associations. Meta-analyses use statistical techniques to estimate the direction and magnitude of the association reported in each study; to determine the extent of variability in the estimates across studies. When the variability is minimal, the estimates are synthesized to indicate the average level of associations between the problem and its determinants. Where there is high variability, statistical tests are used to identify conceptual and/or methodological factors that account for the observed variability in the estimates. Recently, umbrella reviews (also called reviews of reviews, meta-reviews or meta-evaluation/meta-epidemiology; Gough et al., 2012) have been conducted to compare, contrast, reconcile, and/or explain differences in the results of systematic reviews and meta-analyses (Paré et al., 2015). Findings of systematic reviews, meta-analyses, and umbrella reviews indicate: the extent to which the associations between the determinants and the health problem exist within particular client populations and contexts, or are replicated across populations and settings; the expected direction and magnitude (or size) of the associations; and the factors that moderate the associations.

### Qualitative Reviews

Meta-syntheses entail methods for integrating findings of qualitative studies (Edwards & Kaimal, 2016) that investigated the health problem. Examples of methods include meta-ethnography and thematic synthesis that consist of searching the literature, identifying and selecting relevant studies, extracting and coding the findings of each study, then comparing and contrasting the codes to generate themes (Sandelowski & Barraso, 2007; Snilstveit et al., 2012). The themes can provide a list of determinants and explanation of the inter-relationships among the determinants and the problem, embedded within or across contexts.

### Mixed Reviews

Mixed reviews are increasingly performed to understand the health problem. They consist of integrating evidence synthesized from quantitative and qualitative studies. Mixed reviews are justified with the increasing complexity of the inter-relationships among determinants (occurring at different levels) and health problems (experienced in different domains), and the acknowledgement of the unique and complementary contribution of quantitative and qualitative research methods (Edwards & Kaimal, 2016;

Fleming, 2010; Hong et al., 2017). Mixed method reviews (e.g. critical interpretive synthesis) follow the same steps for searching the literature; identifying, selecting, and appraising quantitative and qualitative studies; and extracting data on the experience of the health problem and its determinants from each study. In some mixed-method reviews, the synthesis is conducted separately for the quantitative (e.g. through vote counting, estimating effect size) and the qualitative (e.g. coding, generating themes) findings; then, the synthesized quantitative and qualitative evidence is compared and contrasted to identify convergence and divergence. In other mixed-method reviews, the quantitative and qualitative data are integrated (i.e. brought together) during the analysis and synthesis stages of the review.

The integration of the quantitative and qualitative evidence can be done by aggregation or configuration. Aggregation is used when quantitative and qualitative findings address the same association between a determinant and the health problem, and the purpose is to examine convergence (i.e. whether the findings confirm each other). The aggregation may be accomplished at the data or study level. Data-based aggregation involves the transformation of one type of data into another (e.g. quanticizing qualitative codes/themes) and analyzing the transformed data using the same analytic method (e.g. descriptive statistics). Study-based aggregation consists of juxtaposing the findings of quantitative and qualitative studies, using grids, tables or matrices, where the interface between the two types of findings occurs in the cells; the latter evidence is compared and contrasted to identify convergence (Fleming, 2010; Hong et al., 2017). Aggregation by configuration entails the arrangement of diverse findings into a coherent form or model. The quantitative and qualitative findings are carefully examined and analyzed to determine if they complement, extend, explain each other (e.g. why and how a determinant contribute to the health problem), or reflect variability in the problem experience and in the association of the determinant with the problem in different contexts (Sandelowski et al., 2012).

All types of literature review are useful for understanding the health problem. The mixed-method reviews are most promising in generating a comprehensive list of factors contributing to the problem, delineating direct and indirect relationships that are context-dependent, and providing explanation of why and how the determinants contribute to the health problem.

## Methods

The process for conducting literature reviews is systematic. It has been extensively described in different sources (e.g. Heyvaert et al., 2016) as comprised of several steps. The steps are briefly reviewed with a particular emphasis on understanding the health problem.

1. *Clarifying the health problem:* This first step involves delineating the nature of the health problem and specifying the context (i.e. characteristics of the client population and context) of interest. This step is important for specifying the key words to be used in searching the literature and the criteria for selecting literature sources. The goal is to enhance relevance of the literature to the problem and context of interest.

2. *Specifying the key words:* The key words are the terms used to refer to the health problem. They include the specific words (e.g. insomnia) and its synonyms (e.g. sleep problem, disorder, difficulty) frequently appearing in the scientific literature and mentioned in lay conversation or documents. Consultation

with librarians is very helpful in finalizing the list of key words. The key words are used independently or in combination with other key words representing the target client population (e.g. older adults), context (e.g. primary care), and determinants of the problem (e.g. stress) if the determinants are known (e.g. derived from pertinent middle range theories); alternatively, the terms "factors," "determinants," "causes," "predictors," or similar ones are used in the initial search; and additional terms reflecting the specific factors identified through the review of the initial literature sources are used to refocus the search.

3. *Conducting the search:* The search for literature relevant to the experience and determinants of the health problem is carried out using multiple bibliographic databases pertaining to health literature in general or to specific health-related disciplines (e.g. CINAHL, MEDLINE, PSYCHINFO), for comprehensiveness. The search may yield a large number of studies whose abstracts should be reviewed to determine their relevance. Setting reasonable limits to the search (e.g. language of publication and time period) enhances the relevance of the literature to the most recent conceptualization of the problem; further, the limits may render the review more focused and manageable.

4. *Specifying the selection criteria:* The criteria ensure the relevance of the literature sources to be selected. As mentioned previously, theoretical or conceptual and empirical sources can be included in the review if they address any aspect of the health problem (e.g. presentation of its conceptual definition, description of its indicators, and examination of its determinants). Quantitative and qualitative studies utilizing a range of research designs are sought, regardless of their quality. Quality is defined in terms of appropriately preventing or addressing biases that threaten validity of findings. Quality of the studies can be assessed with available tools and taken into account during the data analysis and synthesis steps.

5. *Identifying and selecting sources*: Having a list of the preset selection criteria and clearly specified definitions and indicators of these criteria facilitates the review of the sources. The selection is done in two stages. First, the abstract of the identified source is read and its content evaluated for relevance (i.e. meet all criteria). Second, copies of relevant sources are obtained for full review and, if considered to meet all preset criteria, are selected for inclusion in the literature review.

6. *Extracting data:* Selected sources are carefully reviewed to extract methodological (e.g. type of design, sample size, study quality) and substantive (e.g. conceptual and operational definitions of the problem and determinants investigated, target population, main findings related to the experience of the problem and its association with determinants). The data extracted are incorporated in a database in preparation for synthesis of quantitative, qualitative, or both types of findings.

7. *Synthesizing data:* Different strategies and techniques can be used to synthesize descriptive and correlational (representing the reported associations between determinants and the health problem) quantitative and qualitative findings, and to integrate quantitative and qualitative evidence (for detail, refer to Hong et al., 2017). The selection of a particular technique is informed by the type of data extracted, the number of studies included in the review, and the availability of resources needed to apply the technique.

**TABLE 3.3**  Narrative review of literature on determinants of insomnia.

| Category of predictors | Results | Sources |
|---|---|---|
| *Predisposing factors* | Age: Older adults are prone to sleep disturbances (explanation: due to fragmented sleep or comorbid medical conditions)<br><br>Gender: Women of all age groups have a higher prevalence of sleep problems than men | Kao et al. (2008), López-Torres Hidalgo et al. (2012), Paparrigopoulos et al. (2010), Rybarczyk et al. (2013), Singareddy et al. (2012), Zhang et al. (2012) |
| *Precipitating factors* | Comorbidity: Having one or more chronic diseases (e.g. cancer, angina, multiple sclerosis); symptoms (e.g. pain); and sleep disorders (e.g. restless leg syndrome), increases the odds of experiencing sleep problems | Dragiotti et al. (2018), Fernandez-Mendoza et al. (2012), Gindin et al. (2014), López-Torres Hidalgo et al. (2012), Rybarczyk et al. (2013) |
| | Psychological conditions: depressive symptomatology and perceived distress | Gindin et al. (2014), Isaia et al. (2011), Paparrigopoulos et al. (2010), Pillai et al. (2014), Vgontzas et al. (2012). |
| | Social conditions: marital status, level of education and socioeconomic status | Gellis et al. (2005), López-Torres Hidalgo et al. (2012), Moscou-Jackson et al. (2016) |
| *Perpetuating factors* | Health behaviors: smoking, alcohol consumption, and limited engagement in physical activity | Colagiuri et al. (2011), Endeshaw and Yoo (2010), Fernandez-Mendoza et al. (2012), Paparrigopoulos et al. (2010) |
| *Factors identified by persons with insomnia* | Worry, illness/discomfort<br><br>Note: varied by age such as worry more frequently reported in early working life and illness by older adults | Armstrong and Dregan (2014) |

The results of the literature review point to similarities or variations, across client populations, settings, and time occasions, in the experience of the health problem relative to its indicators and level of severity. They also identify the range of possible determinants and those most significant. They delineate the nature (direct or indirect); direction (positive or negative); and size (small, moderate, large) of the relationships among determinants and the health problem experience. The findings, particularly those synthesized from qualitative studies and from theoretical sources, provide probable explanations (why and how) of the relationships. Table 3.3 illustrates the results of a narrative review of the literature on the determinants of insomnia.

*Strengths*

The advantages of literature reviews rest on grounding the understanding of the health problem on actual data obtained by multiple researchers, from different client populations under different contexts, using different designs and methods. Results that are consistent across populations, contexts, and research methods enhance the accuracy of the conceptualization of the problem. Comprehensive lists of indicators and determinants of the problem are generated, reflecting different but complementary perspectives. These comprehensive lists reduce the likelihood of omitting a potentially significant indicator or determinant. The range of the severity level with which the problem is experienced by different client populations and in different contexts is identified. Factors contributing to different levels of problem severity may be revealed. Discrepancies in findings point to variability in the problem experience. This empirical knowledge of the health problem is useful in directing the development of interventions and in identifying the need for tailoring the intervention to the characteristics of different client populations and contexts.

### Limitations

The limitations of literature reviews relate to the (often limited) availability of well-planned and executed studies that investigated the health problem. Where available, there is the potential for publication bias (Chan et al., 2014), non-replication of findings, or having mixed or inconclusive findings, all of which weaken the confidence in the validity or accuracy of the generated knowledge, and hence its utility in informing the design of interventions (Ioannidis et al., 2014: Van Assen et al., 2015).

### 3.3.2.2   Conduct of Primary Studies

### Overview

The decision to conduct a primary study to understand the health problem is made when: (1) there is a small number of studies that investigated the problem, thereby limiting the knowledge of the problem experience and its determinants; (2) the quality of available studies is appraised as low, which may be related to a range of conceptual and methodological concerns, such as unclear definition of the health problem, omission of theoretically important determinants, and use of measures with questionable reliability and validity; and (3) available studies have not investigated the health problem in the client population and context of interest, raising questions about the relevance and applicability of available evidence to the target population and context.

The primary studies can be prospective quantitative, qualitative, or mixed (quantitative and qualitative, concurrent, or sequential) method. Mixed-method studies are promising in generating a comprehensive, in-depth understanding of the problem as experienced by the target population in the particular context of interest.

### Methods

The process for planning and conducting primary studies is well described in basic and advanced research textbooks, and is not reviewed here. However, some key considerations are briefly mentioned.

- The main focus of the study is on the health problem and its determinants, as experienced by the target client population in the context of interest.
- The study is designed to address the specific gap in knowledge about the problem as *experienced by the target client population and the context of interest*. Quantitative, cross-sectional or longitudinal studies aim to: (1) describe the experience of the problem (e.g. frequency of occurrence, severity, most common indicators) and its determinants and consequences at one point in time, or changes in the problem experience and determinants over time;

(2) examine factors that operate at different levels and contribute most significantly to the problem as experienced by the target client population and the context of interest; or (3) test the theory of the problem derived from relevant middle range theories or empirical evidence. Qualitative studies can be designed to: (1) generate inductively the conceptualization of the health problem held by the target client population, or (2) elicit clients' perceptions of the determinants and consequences, as well explanations of the inter-relationships among determinants, problem, and consequences. The gaps in knowledge to address dictate the general research approach to utilize.

- The specific research design and methods (e.g. online survey, face-to-face unstructured interviews) are selected for their consistency and appropriateness in addressing the study aims. The choice of methods should take into account the size of the accessible client population and anticipated response rate (e.g. low response rates have been reported for some populations like immigrant older adults); logistics of client recruitment in the context of interest (e.g. it may be hard to reach community-dwelling substance users); the preference or comfort of the client population with specific research methods (e.g. ability to access a computer, and skills enabling completion of online surveys); availability of validated instruments that measure the problem, determinants and consequences; and ability to access human and material resources required to conduct the study within a reasonable time frame.

- The data collection procedures are carefully planned and executed in order to minimize the potential for response burden and introduction of biases (such as acquiescence, social desirability) that threaten the validity of findings.

- The data analysis is done rigorously, using appropriate analytic techniques that allow the determination of factors that most significantly contribute to the problem experience, the delineation of the inter-relationships (direct and indirect) among the determinants and the problem, and the elucidation of the clients' explanations of these inter-relationships.

### Strengths

Conducting primary studies is advantageous in generating an understanding of the health problem. Large-scale quantitative studies that use validated measures of the problem and determinants provide opportunities to identify the most influential determinants and to delineate their direct and indirect influence on the problem, as experienced by the client population and in the context of interest. The use of psychometrically sound measures enhances construct validity. Qualitative studies have the advantage of capturing the target client population's views of the problem and explanations of how factors occurring at different levels inter-relate or interact in influencing the problem. The integration of quantitative and qualitative findings in mixed-method studies is effective in enhancing the validity and applicability of the knowledge of the problem to the client population and context of interest.

### Limitations

The conduct of primary studies is resource intensive and time consuming. It is often limited by potential biases associated with the inadequacy of the accrued sample size, restricted representation of all subgroups comprising the target client population, and the quality of the obtained data (e.g. missing data that reduce statistical power to detect significant relationships among determinants and problem; and non-normal response distribution that constrains the use of powerful statistical tests). Analysis of available data is a means to overcome some of these limitations

### 3.3.2.3    Analysis of Available Data

*Overview*

Large volumes of health and social data are collected by national and international groups of researchers, as well as healthcare, governmental, and nongovernmental agencies. These data are obtained through regularly scheduled surveys of the general population (e.g. Canadian Longitudinal Study on Aging, involving collection of data on a wide range of health indices from 30 000 persons, every five years; Healthy Aging and Retirement in Europe as mentioned by Hoffman et al., 2018); or routine assessment of health indices for clients using healthcare services, that is done in practice and compiled in administrative or claims data (e.g. Ammendolia et al., 2016). Electronic copies of these data are available for analysis aimed to describe the health problem and its associations with relevant determinants in the target client population and context. For instance, Sidani and Guruge (unpublished report) analyzed the first wave of data obtained by the Canadian Longitudinal Study on Aging to determine differences in the experience of insomnia between Canadian-born and immigrant older adults. Preliminary findings showed variability in the experience and the determinants of insomnia. Canadian-born older adults reported experiencing difficulty initiating sleep more frequently than immigrants, which was associated with having pain or discomfort and with lower level of education.

*Methods*

After determining the availability of a data set, the process for accessing the electronic copy starts. The process varies with the requirements of the agencies that own the data. For instance, there is a website for the Canadian Longitudinal Study on Aging that provides general information about the study, the specific variables measured (e.g. demographic, cognitive, sleep problems), and the process for acquiring a copy of the data of interest. This process consists of completing a request form that is approved by the research team, and of signing a confidentiality form. Once the data file is obtained, it should be carefully reviewed to get a clear understanding of the variables and their measurement, which has implications for planning the data analysis. The analysis follows the conventional steps of: (1) conducting descriptive statistics to examine the distribution of the data and the extent of missing data for each variable; (2) handling missing data with the most appropriate method (e.g. McKnight et al., 2007); (3) computing total scale scores for variables measured by multi-item scales; and (4) performing relevant correlational analyses to investigate the direct associations between the health problem and each determinant (e.g. bivariate correlation) or a set of determinants (e.g. regression analysis); the indirect relationships among the determinants and the problem (e.g. structural equation modeling); and/or the moderating effect of a factor (e.g. multigroup analysis).

*Strengths*

Analysis of available data has the advantages of: enhanced generalizability of the findings because the data were obtained from large, representative samples; ability to conduct the analysis on the client population and/or context of interest without losing statistical power; low reactivity (e.g. low social desirability) of the data collected routinely in practice (Baur, 2019); and opportunity to examine the contribution of a wide range of determinants.

*Limitations*

The drawbacks of this approach are attributable to the quality of the data. For instance, single items are often used to measure the concepts potentially threatening construct validity. The procedure for data collection may not be standardized or applied consistently across data collectors, which has the potential for incomplete or missing information and for introducing biases (Baur, 2019).

In summary, the empirical approach is an effective and efficient (if data are already collected) way of generating an understanding of the health problem. Literature reviews and analysis of available data are more efficient, whereas the conduct of primary studies is resource and time intensive. However, the available evidence may not be relevant and applicable to the specific client population and context of interest. The experiential approach is useful in this case (Baker et al., 2018).

### 3.3.3   Experiential Approach

#### 3.3.3.1   Overview

The experiential approach relies on input from the target client population to elicit the implicit theory or construction of the health problem requiring intervention. Exploring the target client population's perspective on how the problem is experienced in daily life and on the most important factors contributing to the problem is critical for designing interventions that are relevant, appropriate, and potentially effective in addressing the problem as actually experienced (Clark, 2015; Huntink et al., 2014; Leask et al., 2019; O'Brien et al., 2016; Wight et al., 2016; Yardley et al., 2015). The experiential approach is consistent with the principles of public or client engagement in research and in co-designing services, and with the collaborative participatory approach to research (Greenlagh et al., 2016). The highlight of this approach is that researchers work closely with members of the target client population to uncover the population's view of the health problem.

The experiential approach entails holding meetings with members of the target client population to formulate the population's perception of the health problem, its indicators, determinants, and consequences. Although the meetings can be scheduled with individual members (based on their comfort and preference), holding group sessions offers more advantages (Hawkins et al., 2017; O'Brien et al., 2016). Through group discussion, the members have the opportunity to exchange ideas; respond to each other's comments; question, clarify, elaborate, and explain points; and reach agreement that captures collective, in-depth, and comprehensive knowledge of the health problem (Sidani et al., 2017). Further, the group interaction promotes open and honest discussion of the problem, and prevents members from giving socially desirable and potentially misleading information. This, in turn, increases the likelihood of gaining collective knowledge of the problem that transcends individual idiosyncrasies and accurately captures the target population's perspective (Vogt et al., 2004). Participants in the group sessions are selected to represent a broad range of those who experience the problem, thereby ensuring that a variety of viewpoints are accounted for when describing the target client population's perspective. The number of participants in each group session should not exceed 12, to enable active and meaningful participation by all members. Multiple sessions may be held to accommodate participants representing different subgroups of the population (defined in terms of sociodemographic and health characteristics).

The group discussion should be carefully planned and executed in order to capture the target client population's conceptualization or construction of the health problem. Two procedures have been used to attain this goal, and are briefly reviewed here, as applied to gaining an understanding of the problem: concept mapping (Trochim, 1989; O'Brien et al., 2016; Vijn et al., 2018) and the first step of the integrated cultural adaptation strategy (Sidani et al., 2017).

### 3.3.3.2 Concept Mapping

*Overview*

Concept mapping is a structured process aimed at articulating thoughts or ideas related to complex phenomena or situations, and the relationships among them (Trochim, 1989). It results in a process map that delineates the inter-relationships among the health problem and determinants, as perceived by a client population in a particular setting (Ball et al., 2017; Hesselink et al., 2014).

*Methods*

The concept mapping process integrates a mix of quantitative and qualitative methods for data collection and analysis. It consists of the following steps described by Trochim and colleagues (Burke et al., 2005; Trochim & Kane, 2005).

*Step 1 – Preparation.* In this planning step, decisions are made on the selection of participants (as mentioned previously) and the focal questions to guide the group discussion. These questions focus on eliciting participants' experience of the problem; view of its indicators and determinants; input on the relative importance of the determinants; and pathways linking the determinants and the problem. Additional questions are generated to prompt for clarification of ideas or words (e.g. What do you mean?), for delineation of pathways (e.g. Can you explain how these factors are related? Which occurred first and brought/led to the other?), and for reaching agreement on points of discussion (e.g. Does this reflect your thoughts?).

*Step 2 – Generation of statements.* In this step, selected participants are invited to attend a group session. The group moderator poses the questions prepared in Step 1, requests participants to generate statements that reflect their ideas or thoughts related to how they experience the problem with a special attention to its indicators (e.g. what changes in their condition are considered as indicative of the presence of the problem); what factors contribute to the occurrence, severity, or maintenance of the problem (e.g. What happened that led to the problem or what brought this problem?); and what are the consequences of the problem (e.g. How did the problem affect you?). The moderator and an assistant record the participants' responses on resources (e.g. projected computer screen, board, flipchart) visible to all group members. The responses are recorded verbatim in the form of statements as expressed by the participants. Once all statements are documented, the moderator engages the group in a review of the statements to identify duplicates, to recognize irrelevant ones, and to confirm a final list of statements about the presenting problem. The investigators review the transcript of the group session to verify that the generated list of statements accurately and comprehensively reflects the discussion. When several group sessions are held, the investigators consolidate the statements obtained in each session into a final list that consists of an exhaustive nonoverlapping account of all ideas or thoughts about the problem expressed by participants.

*Step 3 – Structuring of statements.* The goal of this step is to gain an understanding of the inter-relationships among the ideas or thoughts generated in Step 2 that depict the target population's conceptualization of the problem. This is accomplished by having participants sort the statements into piles and rate the importance of statements in reflecting the problem. The sorting exercise is done individually by each participant. Each statement is printed on a card. Each participant is given the cards for all statements and instructed to put the cards into piles where each pile contains statements representing similar ideas, as perceived by the individual. No specific directions are given to do the sorting; rather, participants are given the freedom to arrange the statements in a way that is meaningful to them. However, they are requested to place each statement into one pile only, and not to put all statements into one pile. There is no restriction on the number of piles that can be generated. The data obtained with the sorting exercise are entered into a database for analysis. The database consists of a similarity matrix. The rows and columns of the matrix represent the statements, and the data in the cells represent the number of participants who place the pair of statements into the same pile. The similarity matrix is then subjected to multivariate analysis using multidimensional scaling technique and hierarchical cluster analysis. The analysis produces a map that locates nonoverlapping clusters of statements reflecting similar ideas (Trochim & Kane, 2005). In addition to sorting, the participants are asked to rate each statement in terms of its importance or relevance to the problem, on a five-point rating scale. These data are also entered in a database and analyzed descriptively. The Concept System software can integrate the importance rating with the sorting data to indicate clusters of statements with varying levels of importance (Burke et al., 2005). The map is presented to the participants for discussion.

*Step 4 – Representation.* The aim of this step is to choose a final set of clusters that best captures the target population's conceptualization of the problem. To this end, the same or another group of participants representative of the target population are invited to a session that proceeds as follows:

1. Read the statements generated in Step 2 to familiarize the participants with the ideas or thoughts about the problem.
2. Show the map of clusters and explain that it illustrates the groupings of statements obtained with quantitative data analysis performed in Step 3.
3. Review the statements grouped into each cluster and elicit the participants' feedback about the cluster. Specifically, their agreement is sought on the extent to which statements organized in a cluster reflect a common idea. The participants are given the freedom to challenge the presented clusters and to regroup the statements into clusters that are meaningful to them.
4. Review all clusters located on the map to determine the total number of clusters that reflect conceptually distinct ideas about the problem.
5. Review the statements within and across clusters that were rated most important to identify the ideas of relevance to the problem.

If more than one session is held, then the investigators reconcile the results and integrate them into one comprehensive set of clusters, which is discussed with the participants in the next step of concept mapping.

*Step 5 – Interpretation.* This step focuses on labeling the clusters and exploring the pathways delineating the relationships among the clusters, as conceived by members of the target population. Again, the members are invited to a session and requested, as a whole group or as small groups of four to five, to carefully review the statements organized into a cluster in Step 4; to discuss the ideas captured in the statements; to identify the common theme underlying the ideas; and to come up with a label (i.e. short phrase or word) that best describes the theme. The labeling may be based on statements, within a cluster, rated as most important in Step 4. Once all themes are labeled, the moderator engages the group in a cognitive exercise to identify themes that reflect determinants, indicators, and consequences of the problem, and to diagram relationships among them. Specifically, participants are asked to indicate (1) what each labeled cluster or theme represents: a determinant of the problem, that is, something that takes place before and leads to the problem; an indicator of the problem, that is, a change in functioning or condition that indicates the presence of the problem; or a consequence of the problem, that is, the impact of the problem on well-being or quality of life; and (2) which determinants are related to each other and to the problem and in what way. This exercise results in a concept map that includes concepts emerging from the labeled clusters and linking lines that delineate which concepts are related and in what way (illustrated with arrows linking related concepts), and a set of phrases that describe the proposed linkages among concepts.

The concept map guides the development of the theory of the problem and subsequently the design of interventions. Burke et al.'s (2005) work illustrates the application of concept mapping to explore women's perception of residential neighborhood factors that contribute to the experience of partner violence.

### Strengths

Concept mapping is a useful method for clarifying and accurately reflecting the target client population's conceptualization of the health problem. The integration of quantitative and qualitative methods for data collection and analysis allows exploration of complex problems and enhances the credibility of the results. Obtaining data from individual participants and from the group increases the richness of, and the likelihood of reaching collective agreement on, the resulting conceptualization.

### Limitations

The implementation of concept mapping is challenging. It is resource and labor intensive. The conduct of the group sessions requires availability of: suitable location for holding the meetings; well-trained and experienced group moderators; skilled research assistants for entering and analyzing data; appropriate software for analyzing the data; materials for documenting the statements and for sorting and rating them; and equipment/technology for visually presenting the clusters/map to the group. In addition, the group sessions are long (about three to four hours) and involve intensive cognitive work; the statement sorting exercise is burdensome (Burke et al., 2005).

### 3.3.3.3    Step 1 of the Integrated Cultural Adaptation Strategy

#### Overview

The integrated strategy was initially proposed as a systematic process for the cultural adaptation of evidence-based interventions (Sidani et al., 2017). It also has been applied to adapt interventions to the needs and contexts of different client populations including post-acute patients in rural areas (Fox et al., 2019) and elder abuse (Guruge et al., 2019).

*Methods*

The first step of the strategy focuses on eliciting the target population's conceptualization of the health problem. It uses a mix of quantitative and qualitative methods to obtain relevant data in group sessions.

Prior to the group session, the researchers generate a list of indicators and determinants of the health problem, from a review of pertinent theories, empirical studies, and practice sources (e.g. consultation with health professionals). The researchers prepare a brief description, in lay terms, of each indicator and determinant. The descriptions are incorporated in a questionnaire to assess their relevance and/or importance to the target client population. The questionnaire contains the following for each indicator and determinant: its name (e.g. difficulty falling asleep), its description (e.g. it takes 30 minutes or more to fall asleep), and a rating scale (e.g. numeric rating scale anchored with *not at all*—0 and *very much*—10) to determine its relevance (i.e. extent to which it is experienced by members of the target population) and importance in contributing to the experience of the health problem. In addition, researchers prepare a set of open-ended questions to engage the group in a discussion to elaborate on the population's perspective on the problem and identify other relevant indicators and determinants of the problem.

During the group session, the researchers:

1. Explain the purpose of the session, which is to get an understanding of the client population's view and experience of the health problem.
2. Give an overview of the health problem by describing what it is.
3. Distribute the questionnaire and provide instructions on how to rate the indicators and determinants; that is, their relevance and importance to the population.
4. For each indicator and determinant, read its name and description; clarify any misunderstanding; and invite participants to complete the rating, individually, by selecting the most appropriate response option.
5. Once all indicators and determinants are rated, engage participants in a discussion to further elaborate on the conceptualization of the problem. Guiding questions include: (1) Which indicators are commonly reported when people experience the health problem? Are there other indicators? Which indicators are most important and could be managed to help resolve the problem? (2) Which determinants significantly contribute to or cause the health problem? How do these determinants lead or cause the problem? Are there other determinants? Which determinants should be addressed to help resolve the problem? Which should be given priority? What makes them important? (3) Are the indicators and determinants important for all people or are some more or less important for particular groups of people (e.g. men/women, young/older)?

After all group sessions are completed, the quantitative ratings are analyzed descriptively to determine the most relevant and important indicators and determinants (indicated by high means and low variances). The transcripts of the qualitative comments are content analyzed. A matrix is used to integrate quantitative and qualitative findings and identify the most relevant indicator of the health problem, the most important determinants, how the determinants contribute to the problem, and possible differences across subgroups of the target population. The application of this method is illustrated in Sidani et al. (2018b) who found that Chinese Canadians experience insomnia as difficulty initiating sleep, which they attribute to high levels of stress.

### Strengths

The first step of the integrative strategy for cultural adaptation of interventions has the same advantages as concept mapping. However, its application is less cognitively burdensome.

### Limitations

Integration of the quantitative and qualitative data may be challenging.

#### 3.3.3.4   Strengths and Limitations

The experiential approach is a useful means for accessing the implicit theory or conceptualization of the health problem held by client populations, in contexts not represented or investigated in previous studies, as is often the case with marginalized groups or ethno-cultural communities (Buffel, 2018). However, this approach has some limitations related to the selection of the target population members and the size of the participating group. These limitations may lead to unrepresentative sample, yielding potentially biased results that may not be applicable to all subgroups of the target population.

### 3.3.4   Combined Approach for Understanding the Problem

#### 3.3.4.1   Overview

Each of the theoretical, empirical, and experiential approach is useful in gaining insights about the health problem. However, each approach has limitations. Combining the three approaches is recommended to overcome the limitations, and is applied in the first step of the intervention mapping process. Intervention mapping is a process for designing behavioral interventions (Bartholomew et al., 2016), which is described in more detail in Chapter 4. The first step in intervention mapping focuses on the analysis of the problem to clearly specify the individual and contextual determinants of the problem. This is accomplished by applying the three approaches concurrently or sequentially, and integrating the theoretical, empirical, and experiential information to generate the theory or logic model of the problem.

#### 3.3.4.2   Methods

As described by Bartholomew et al. (2016) and Kok et al. (2016), and implemented by numerous researchers, the first step of intervention mapping involves:

- Identification of the health problem or behavior in need of remediation, that is, clarification of what needs to be changed and for whom.
- Search for theoretical and empirical evidence to gain an understanding of the problem or behavior and its determinants. Determinants are reasons or causes of the problem or (non)engagement in the behavior, commonly occurring at the individual client (e.g. cognitions, emotions, beliefs) or context (e.g. social norms) levels. Different types of reviews have been conducted such as rapid

reviews (e.g. Baker et al., 2018), systematic reviews (e.g. Brendryen et al., 2013), scoping reviews (e.g. Dalager et al., 2019), and narrative reviews (e.g. Athilingam et al., 2018; Beck et al., 2018; Besharati et al., 2017).

- Integration of theoretical and empirical evidence into a comprehensive list of factors contributing to the problem or behavior.
- Engagement of stakeholder groups (e.g. clients, community leaders, health professionals) in events or activities aimed to explore the relevance of the determinants, identified from the literature, to the target client population and context. A range of activities have been used including: individual interviews with stakeholders (e.g. Baker et al., 2018; Beck et al., 2018), focus group discussions (e.g. Ammendolia et al., 2016; Besharati et al., 2017), roundtable meetings, workshops or nominal group techniques (e.g. Johnson et al., 2017; Meng et al., 2019), to review the determinants for their relevance and/or to prioritize the determinants that should be addressed when designing the intervention.
- Refinement of the theory or logic model of the problem so that it reflects the problem and its determinants, as experienced by the target client population.

### 3.3.4.3 Strengths

Combining the theoretical, empirical, and experiential approaches, as recommended in intervention mapping, provides complementary and supplementary information for developing the theory of the problem and for refining it to enhance its relevance and applicability to the target client population and context.

### 3.3.4.4 Limitations

The drawback of this combined approach is that it is time consuming and labor intensive.

Regardless of the approach used, the theory of the health problem forms the foundation for designing interventions, as explained in the next chapter.

## REFERENCES

Ammendolia, C., Côté, P., Cancelliere, C., et al. (2016) Healthy and productive workers: Using intervention mapping to design a workplace health promotion and wellness program to improve presenteeism. *BMC Public Health*, 16, 1190–1207.

Aráujo-Soares, V., Hankonen, N., Presseau, J., Rodrigues, A., & Sniehotta, F.F. (2018) Developing behavior change interventions for self-management in chronic illness. *European Psychologist*, 24(1), 7–25.

Armstrong, D. & Dregan, A (2014) A population-based investigation into the self-reported reasons for sleep problems. *PLoS One*, 9(7), e101368.

Athilingam, P., Clochesy, J.M., & Labrador, M.A. (2018) Intervention mapping approach in the design of an interactive mobile health application to improve self-care in heart failure. *Computers, Informatics, Nursing*, 36(2), 90–97.

Baker, P., Coole, C., Drummond, A., et al. (2018) Development of an occupational advice intervention for patients undergoing lower limb arthroplasty (the OPAL study). *Health Services Research*, 18, 504–511.

Ball, L., Ball, D., Leveritt, M., et al. (2017) Using logic models to enhance the methodological quality of primary health-care interventions: Guidance from an intervention to promote nutrition care by general practitioners and practice nurses. *Australian Journal of Primary Health*, 23, 53–60.

Bartholomew, L.K., Kok, G., & Markham, C.M. (2016) *Planning Health Promotion Programs: An Intervention Mapping Approach* (4th ed). John Wiley and Amp; Sons Inc, New York.

Baur, N. (2019). Linearity vs circularity? On some common misconceptions on the differences in the research process in qualitative and quantitative research. *Frontiers in Education*, 4, 53–67.

Beall, R.F., Baskerville, N., Golfam, M., Saeed, S., & Little, J. (2014) Modes of delivery in prevention intervention studies: A rapid review. *European Journal of Clinical Investigation*, 44(7), 688–696.

Beck, D., Been-Dahmen, J., Peeters, M., et al. (2018) A nurse-led self-management support intervention (ZENN) for kidney transplant recipients using intervention mapping: Protocol for a mixed-methods feasibility study. *JMIR Research Protocols*, 8(3), e11856

Besharati, F., Karimi-Shahanjarini, A., Hazavehei, S.M.M., et al. (2017) Development of a colorectal cancer screening intervention for Iranian adults: Appling intervention mapping. *Asian Pacific Journal of Cancer Prevention*, 18(8), 2193–2199.

Bleijenberg, N., de Man-van Ginkel, J.M., Trappenburg, J.C.A., et al. (2018) Increasing value and reducing waste by optimizing the development of complex interventions: Enriching the development phase of the Medical Research Council (MRC) framework. *International Journal of Nursing Studies*, 79, 86–93

Bootzin, R.R. & Epstein, D.R. (2011) Understanding and treating insomnia. *Annual Review of Clinical Psychology*, 7, 435–458.

Brendryen, H., Johansen, A., Nesvåg, S., Kok, G., & Duckert, F. (2013) Constructing a theory- and evidence-based treatment rationale for complex eHealth interventions: Development of an online alcohol intervention using an intervention mapping approach. *JMIR Research Protocols*, 2(1), e6.

Buffel, T. (2018) Social research and co-production with older people: Developing age-friendly communities. *Journal of Aging Studies*, 44, 52–60.

Burke, J.G., O'Campo, P., Peak, G.L., et al. (2005) An introduction to concept mapping as a participatory public health research method. *Qualitative Health Research*, 15, 1392–1410.

Butner, J.E., Gagnon, K.T., Geuss, M.N., Lessard, D.A., & Story, N. (2015) Utilizing typology to generate and test theories of change. *Psychological Methods*, 20(1), 1–25.

Carroll, C., Booth, A., Leaviss, J., & Rick, J. (2013) "Best fit" framework synthesis: Refining the method. *BMC Medical Research Methodology*, 13, 37–51.

Chan, A.-W., Song, F., Vickers, A., et al. (2014) Increasing value and reducing waste: Addressing inaccessible research. *Lancet*, 383(9913), 257–266.

Clark, M. (2015) Co-production in mental health care. *Mental Health Review Journal*, 20(4), .

Colagiuri, B., Christensen, S., Jensen, A.B., et al. (2011) Prevalence and predictors of sleep difficulty in a national cohort of women with primary breast cancer three to four months postsurgery. *Journal of Pain and Symptom Management*, 42(5), 710–720.

Craig, P., Di Ruggiero, E., Frohlich, K.L., Mykhalovskiy, E., & White, M., on behalf of the Canadian Institutes of Health Research (CIHR)—National Institute for Health Research (NIHR). (2018). *Taking account of context in population health intervention research: guidance for producers, users and funders of research*. NIHR Evaluation, Trials and Studies Coordinating Centre, Southampton.

Dalager, T., Højmark, A., Jensen, P.T., Søgaard, K. & Andersen, L.N. (2019) Using an intervention mapping approach to develop prevention and rehabilitation strategies for musculoskeletal pain among surgeons. *BMC Public Health*, 19, 320–332.

Davidoff, F., Dixon-Woods, M., Leviton, L., & Michie, S. (2015) Demystifying theory and its use in improvement. *BMJ Quality and Safety*, 24(3), 228–238.

Dohnke, B., Dewitt, T., & Steinhilber, A. (2018) A prototype-targeting intervention for the promotion of healthy eating in adolescents: Development and evaluation using intervention mapping. *Health Education*, 118(6), 450–469.

Dragiotti, E., Bernfort, L., Larsson, B., Gerdle, B. & Levin, L.A. (2018) Association of insomnia severity with well-being, quality of life and health care costs: A cross-sectional study in older adults with chronic pain (PainS65+). *European Journal of Pain*, 22, 414–425.

Durks, D., Fernandez-Llimos, F., Hossain, L.N., et al. (2017) Use of intervention mapping to enhance health care professional practice: A systematic review. *Health Education & Behavior*, 44(4), 524–535.

Edwards, J. & Kaimal, G. (2016) Using meta-synthesis to support application of qualitative methods findings in practice: A discussion of meta-ethnography, narrative synthesis, and critical interpretative synthesis. *The Arts in Psychotherapy*, 51, 30–35.

Endeshaw, Y.W. & Yoo, W. (2010) Association between social and physical activities and insomnia symptoms among community-dwelling older adults. *Journal of Aging and Health*, 28(6), 1073–1089.

Fassier, J.B., Sarnin, P., Rouat, S., et al. (2019) Interventions developed with the intervention mapping protocol in work disability prevention: A systematic review of the literature. *Journal of Occupational Rehabilitation*, 29, 11–24.

Fernandez, M.E., ten Hoor, G.A., van Lieshout, S., et al. (2019) Implementation mapping: Using intervention mapping to develop implementation strategies. *Frontiers in Public Health*, 7, 158.

Fernandez-Mendoza, J., Vgontzas, A.N., Bixler, E.O., et al. (2012) Clinical and polysomnographic predictors of the natural history of poor sleep in the general population. *Sleep*, 35(5), 689–697.

Fernandez-Mendoza, J., Shea, S., Vgontzas, A. N., et al. (2015) Insomnia and incident depression: Role of objective sleep duration and natural history. *Journal of Sleep Research*, 24(4), 390–398.

Fleming, K. (2010) Synthesis of quantitative and qualitative research: An example using critical interpretative synthesis. *Journal of Advanced Nursing*, 66(1), 201–217.

Fleury, J. & Sidani, S. (2018) Using theory to guide intervention studies. In: B.M. Melnyk & D. Morrison-Beedy (eds), *Intervention Research and Evidence-Based Quality Improvement Second Edition: Designing, Conducting, Analyzing, and Funding*. Springer, New York, NY.

Fox, M.T., Sidani, S., Butler, J.I., Skinner, M.W., & Alzghoul, M.M. (2019) Protocol of a multimethod descriptive study: Adapting hospital-to-home transitional care interventions to the rural healthcare context in Ontario, Canada. *BMJ Open*, 9, e028050.

Foy, R., Francis, J.J., Johnston, M., et al. (2007) The development of a theory-based intervention to promote appropriate disclosure of a diagnosis of dementia. *BMC Health Services Research*, 7, 207–215.

Gellis, L.A., Lichstein, K.L., Scarinci, I.C., et al. (2005) Socioeconomic status and insomnia. *Journal of Abnormal Psychology*, 114(1), 111–118.

Gindin, J., Shochat, T., Chetrit, A., et al., for the SHELTER project (2014) Insomnia in long-term care facilities: A comparison of seven European countries and Israel: The services and health for the elderly in long TERm care study. *Journal of the American Geriatric Society*, 62, 2033–2039

Glanz, K. & Bishop, D.B. (2010) The role of behavioral science theory in development and implementation of public health interventions. *Annual Review of Public Health*, 31, 399–418.

Golfam, M., Beall, R., Brehaut, J., et al. (2015) Comparing alternative design options for chronic disease prevention interventions. *European Journal of Clinical Investigation*, 45, 87–99.

Gough, D., Thomas, J., & Oliver, S. (2012) Clarifying differences between review designs and methods. *Systematic Reviews*, 1, 28–36.

Greenlagh, T., Jackson, C., Shaw, S., & Janamian, T. (2016) Achieving research impact through co-creation in community-based health services: Literature review and case study. *The Milbank Quarterly*, 94(2), 392–429.

Guruge, S., Sidani, S., Matsuoka, A., Man, G., & Pirner, D. (2019) Developing a comprehensive understanding of elder abuse prevention in immigrant communities: A comparative mixed methods study protocol. *BMJ Open*, 9, e022736.

Harvey, A.G., Sharpley, A.L., Ree, M.J., Stinson, K., & Clark, D.M. (2007) An open trial of cognitive therapy for chronic insomnia. *Behavior Research and Therapy*, 45(10), 2491–2501.

Harvey, A.G., Dong, L., Bélanger, L., & Morin, C.M. (2017) Mediators and treatment matching in behavior therapy, cognitive therapy and cognitive behavior therapy for chronic insomnia. *Journal of Consulting and Clinical Psychology*, 85(10), 975–987.

Hawkins, J., Madden, K., Fletcher, A., et al. (2017) Development of a framework for the co-production and prototyping of public health interventions. *BMC Public Health*, 17, 689–699.

Hesselink, G., Zegers, M., Vernooij-Dassen, M., et al., on behalf of the European HANDOVER Research Collaborative (2014) Improving patient discharge and reducing hospital readmissions by using intervention mapping. *BMC Health Services Research*, 14, 389–399.

Heyvaert, M., Hannes, K., & Onghena, P. (2016) *Using Mixed Methods Synthesis for Literature Reviews*. Volume 4 of Mixed Methods Research Series. Sage, Thousand Oaks.

Hoffman, R., Kröger, H., & Pakpohan, E. (2018) Pathways between socioeconomic status and health: Does health selection or social causation dominate in Europe? *Advances in Life Course Research*, 36, 23–36.

Hong, Q.N., Pluye, P., Bujold, M., & Wassef, M. (2017) Convergent and sequential synthesis designs: Implications for conducting and reporting systematic reviews of qualitative and quantitative evidence. *Systematic Reviews*, 6, 61–74.

Huntink, E., van Lieshout, J., Aakhus, E., et al. (2014) Stakeholders' contribution to tailored implementation programs: an observational study of group interview methods. *Implementation Science*, 9, 185–193.

Hupcey, J.E. & Penrod, J. (2005) Concept analysis: Examining the state of the science. *Research and Theory for Nursing Practice: An International Journal*, 19, 197–208.

Ioannidis, J. P.A., Greenland, S., Hlatky, M.A., et al. (2014) Increasing value and reducing waste in research design, conduct, and analysis. *The Lancet*, 383, 166–175.

Isaia, G., Corsinovi, L., Bo, M., et al. (2011) Insomnia among hospitalized elderly patients: Prevalence, clinical characteristics and risk factors. *Archives of Gerontology and Geriatrics*, 52, 133–137.

Johnson, K., Markham, C., Smith, R., & Tortolero, S.R. (2017) Be legendary—using intervention mapping and participatory strategies to develop a multi-component teen pregnancy prevention intervention for older teen males of color. *Journal of Applied Research on Children: Informing Policy for Children at Risk*, 8(1), Article 4.

Kao, C.-C., Huang, C.-J., Wang, M.-Y., & Tsai, P.-S. (2008) Insomnia: Prevalence and its impact on excessive daytime sleepiness and psychological well-being in the adult Taiwanese population. *Quality of Life Research*, 17, 1073–1080.

Kok, G., Gottlieb, N.H., Peters, G.-J.Y., et al. (2016) A taxonomy of behavior change methods: An intervention mapping approach. *Health Psychology Review*, 10, 297–312.

Kwasnicka, D., Dombrowski, S.U., White, M., & Sniehotta, F. (2016) Theoretical explanations for maintenance of behaviour change: A systematic review of behaviour theories. *Health Psychology Review*, 10(3), 277–296.

Lamort-Bouché, M., Sarnin, P., Kok, G., et al. (2018) Interventions developed with the intervention mapping protocol in the field of cancer: A systematic review. *Psycho-Oncology*, 27, 1138–1149.

Leask, C.F., Sandlund, M., Skelton, D.A., et al., on behalf of the Grand Stand, Safe Step and Teenage Girls on the Move Research Groups (2019) Framework, principles and recommendations for utilising participatory methodologies in the co-creation and evaluation of public health interventions. *Research Involvement and Engagement*, 5, 2–17.

Lippe, S. & Ziegelman, J.P. (2008) Theory-based health behavior change: Developing, testing, and applying theories for evidence-based interventions. *Applied Psychology. An International Review*, 57, 698–716.

López-Torres Hidalgo, J., Bravo, B.N., Martínez, I.P., et al. (2012) Understanding insomnia in older adults. *International Journal of Geriatric Psychiatry*, 27, 1086–1093.

MacKinnon, D.P. & Fairchild, A.J. (2009) Current directions in mediation analysis. *Current Directions in Psychological Science*, 18(1): 16–20.

Mayne, J. (2017) Theory of change analysis: Building robust theories of change. *The Canadian Journal of Program Evaluation*, 32(2), 155–173.

McKnight, P.E., McKnight, K.M., Sidani, S., & Figueredo, A.J. (2007) *Missing Data: A Gentle Introduction*. Guilford Publications, Inc., New York, NY

Medical Research Council (2019) *Developing and Evaluating Complex Interventions*. Author.

Meng, A., Borg, V., & Clausen, T. (2019) Enhancing the social capital in industrial workplaces: Developing workplace interventions using intervention mapping. *Evaluation and Program Planning*, 72, 227–236.

Moore, G.F. & Evans, R.E. (2017) What theory, for whom and in which context? Reflections on the application of theory in the development and evaluation of complex population health intervention. *SSM—Population Health*, 3, 132–135.

Moore, G.F., Evans, R., Hawkins, J., et al. (2019) From complex social interventions to interventions in complex social systems: Future directions and unresolved questions for intervention development and evaluation. *Evaluation*, 25(1), 23–45

Morin, C.M., Belleville, G., Bélanger, L., & Ivers, H. (2011) The insomnia severity index: Psychometric indicators to detect insomnia cases and evaluate treatment response. *Sleep*, 34(5), 601–608.

Moscou-Jackson, G., Allen, J., Kozachik, S., et al. (2016) Acute pain and depressive symptoms: Independent predictors of insomnia symptoms among adults with sickle cell disease. *Pain Management Nursing*, 17(1), 38–46.

Muellmann, S., Bucj, C., Voelcker-Rehage, C., et al. (2019) Effects of two web-based interventions promoting physical activity among older adults compared to a delayed intervention control group in northwestern Germany: Results of the PROMOTE community-based intervention trial. *Preventive Medicine Reports*, 15, 100958.

O'Brien, N., Heaven, B., Teal, G., et al. (2016) Integrating evidence from systematic reviews, qualitative research, and expert knowledge using co-design techniques to develop a web-based intervention for people in the retirement transition. *Journal of Medical Internet Research*, 18(8), e210.

Paparrigopoulos, T., Tzavara, C., Theleritis, C., et al. (2010) Insomnia and its correlates in a representative sample of the Greek population. *BMC Public Health*, 10, 531–537.

Paré, G., Trudel, M-C., Jaana, M., & Kitsiou, S. (2015) Synthesizing information systems knowledge: A typology of literature reviews. *Information & Management*, 52, 183–199.

Pillai, V., Roth, T., Mulins, H.M., & Drake, C.L. (2014) Moderators and mediators of the relationship between stress and insomnia: Stressor chronicity, cognitive intrusion, and coping. *Sleep*, 37(7), 1199–1208.

Renger, R. (2011) Constructing and verifying program theory using source documentation. *The Canadian Journal of Program Evaluation*, 25(1), 51–67.

Rybarczyk, B., Lund, H.G., Garroway, A.M., & Mack, L. (2013) Cognitive behavioral therapy for insomnia in older adults: Background, evidence, and overview of treatment protocol. *Clinical Gerontologist*, 36, 70–93.

Sandelowski, M. & Barraso, J. (2007) *Handbook for Synthesizing Qualitative Research*. Springer Publishing Company, New York.

Sandelowski, M., Voils, C.I., Leeman, J., & Crandell, J.L. (2012) Mapping the mixed-methods mixed research synthesis terrain. *Journal of Mixed Methods Research*, 6(4), 317–331.

Schwartz, D.R. & Carney, C.E. (2012) Mediators of cognitive-behavioral therapy for insomnia: A review of randomized controlled trials and secondary analysis studies. *Clinical Psychology Review*, 22, 664–675.

Sidani, S., Ibrahim, S., Lok, J., et al. (2017). An integrated strategy for the cultural adaptation of evidence-based interventions. *Health*, 9, 738–755.

Sidani, S., Ibrahim, S., Lok, J., et al. (2018a) Comparing the experience of and factors perpetuating chronic insomnia severity among young, middle-aged, and older adults. *Clinical Nursing Research*. Oct 15, 105477381880616. Doi: 10.1177/1054773818806164. [Epub ahead of print].

Sidani, S., Ibrahim, S., Lok, J., Fan, L., & Fox, M. (2018b) Implementing the integrated strategy for the cultural adaptation of evidence-based interventions: An illustration. *Canadian Journal of Nursing Research*, 50(4), 1–8.

Singareddy, R., Vgontzas, A.N., Fernandez-Mendoza, J., et al. (2012) Risk factors for incident chronic insomnia: A general population prospective study. *Sleep Medicine*, 13(4), 346–353.

Snilstveit, B., Oliver, S., & Vojtkova, M. (2012) Narrative approaches to systematic review and synthesis of evidence for international development policy and practice. *Journal of Development Effectiveness*, 4(3), 409–429.

The Improved Clinical Effectiveness through Behavioral Research Group (ICEBeRG) (2006) Designing theoretically-informed implementation interventions. *Implementation Science*, 1, 4–11.

Trochim, W.M.K. (1989) An introduction to concept mapping for planning and evaluation. *Evaluation and Program Planning*, 12, 1–16.

Trochim, W. & Kane, M. (2005) Concept mapping: An introduction to structured conceptualization in health care. *International Journal for Quality in Health Care*, 17, 187–191.

Van Assen, M.A.L.M., van Aert, R.C.M., & Wicherts, J.M. (2015) Meta-analysis using effect size distributions of only statistically significant studies. *Psychological Methods*, 20(3), 293–309.

Vgontzas, A.N., Fernandez-Mendoza, J., Bixter, E.O., Singareddy, R., & Shaffer, M.L. (2012) Persistent insomnia: The role of objective short sleep duration and mental health. *Sleep: Journal of Sleep and Sleep Disorders Research*, 35(1), 61–68.

Vijn, T.W., Wollersheim, H., Faber, M.J., Fluit, C.R.M.G., & Kremer, J.A.M. (2018) Building a patient-centered and interprofessional training program with patients, students and care professional: Study protocol of a participatory design and evaluation study. *BMC Health Services Research*, 13, 387–398.

Vittengl, J.R., Clark, L.A., Thase, M.E., & Jarrett, R.B. (2014) Are improvements in cognitive content and depressive symptoms correlates or mediators during acute-phase cognitive therapy for recurrent major depressive disorder? *International Journal of Cognitive Therapy*, 7(3), 255–271.

Vogt, D.S., King, D.W., & King, L.A. (2004) Focus groups in psychological assessment: Enhancing content validity by consulting members of the target population. *Psychological Assessment*, 16, 231–243.

Wight, D., Wimbush, E., Jepson, R., & Doi, L. (2016) Six steps in quality intervention development (6SQuID). *Journal of Epidemiology and Community Health*, 70, 520–525.

Yardley, L., Morrison, L., Bradbury, K., & Muller, I. (2015) The person-based approach to intervention development: Application to digital health-related behavior change interventions. *Journal of Medical Internet Research*, 17(1), e30.

Zhang, J., Lam, S.P., Li, S.X., et al. (2012) Long-term outcomes and predictors of chronic insomnia: A prospective study in Hong Kong Chinese adults. *Sleep Medicine*, 13, 544–462.

# CHAPTER 4

# Designing Interventions

Health interventions should be carefully designed or developed to enhance their potentials to successfully address health problems (Moore et al., 2019). This can be achieved by following a systematic process, in which the interventions are grounded in an understanding of the problem and designed to match the manner in which the problem is experienced by the target client population, in the context of interest (Beck et al., 2019; van Meijel et al., 2004). Results of systematic reviews indicate that interventions developed through a systematic and structured process such as intervention mapping are effective in addressing the respective health problem (e.g. Fassier et al., 2019; Garba & Gadanya, 2017; Lamort-Bouché et al., 2018).

In this chapter, the process for designing interventions is described and illustrated with an example. Approaches for delineating the intervention's active ingredients are discussed. The intervention design process results in the generation of the theory of implementation and the theory of change that clarifies the intervention components and mechanism of action, respectively.

## 4.1 PROCESS FOR INTERVENTION DESIGN

Intervention mapping (Bartholomew et al., 2016) is a systematic, well-structured process that is useful for designing interventions. Intervention mapping has been recently applied to design health interventions aimed at promoting performance of health behaviors including physical activity (e.g. Direito et al., 2018; Krops et al., 2018), engagement in screening tests (e.g. Besharati et al., 2017; Byrd et al., 2012), and self-management in chronic illness (e.g. Beck et al., 2019; Burrell et al., 2019). Intervention mapping has also been applied to design public health interventions (e.g. Abbey et al., 2017, Belansky et al., 2013) and implementation interventions that facilitate the adoption of clinical guidelines or evidence-based interventions in practice (e.g. Caminiti et al., 2017; Chambers et al., 2019), as well as to adapt evidence-based treatments to the local context (e.g. Koutoukidis et al., 2018; Perry et al., 2017).

Intervention mapping consists of a clearly described process for developing interventions that focus on changing health behaviors (Bartholomew et al., 2016; Kok et al., 2016). The process begins with an analysis of the health behavior to identify what needs to be changed, followed by the creation of matrices that combine change objectives with determinants of the health behavior, selection of theory-based intervention methods, translation of these methods into practical application, and integration of the practical applications into an organized program. In addition to theory, relevant evidence synthesized from the literature and input from stakeholder groups including clients, are integrated in the process. The application of the mapping process culminates in the design of interventions that are informed by theory and that match or are responsive to the target client population's experience of the health problem (Beck et al., 2019; Brendryen et al., 2013; Dalager et al., 2019).

The mapping process described next is adapted to enable the design of interventions addressing a range of health problems such as symptoms and cognitions, in addition to behaviors. The application of the steps comprising the process is illustrated with the design of an intervention for the management of insomnia.

*Step 1 – Clarify the Health Problem*
Clarification of the health problem is done by reviewing the theory or the logic model of the problem (detailed in Chapter 3). It is important to be familiar with the conceptual definition of the problem, as well as its indicators, level of severity, duration, determinants, and consequences, and to understand the direct and indirect relationships among the determinants and the problem experience. Special attention is given to the problem's indicators and determinants, and the explanations of the pathways linking the determinants to the problem. A lucid understanding of the problem is essential to guide the next steps of the intervention design process. The theory of the problem, exemplified for insomnia, is illustrated in Table 3.1. The theory summarizes the determinants, indicators, and consequences of insomnia.

*Step 2 – Analyze the Health Problem*
Analysis of the health problem is a foundational step in the process of designing interventions. The analysis consists of critically reviewing the theory of the problem (see Chapter 3) to determine "what about the problem needs to and can be changed" in order to prevent, manage, or resolve the problem. The analysis involves a critical and meticulous examination of: (1) the conceptual definition of the health problem, which highlights the nature of the problem and provides a general hint on its amenability to change; for example, a problem that is genetic in nature may be difficult, if not impossible, to change whereas unhealthy behaviors or cognitions are potentially modifiable; (2) the operational definition of the problem into attributes that are specified in respective indicators, which point to indicators that are potentially changeable; and (3) the determinants of the problem, which identify those potentially modifiable. The meticulous examination contributes to a judgment as to what can be actually changed (also referred to as aspects of the problem): the overall problem, some or all its indicators, or some or all its determinants (Araújo-Soares et al., 2018; Bello & Pillay, 2019; Besharati et al., 2017; Bleijenberg et al., 2018; Wight et al., 2016).

The judgment is based on logical thinking relative to the amenability of the problem, its indicators and determinants to change. The judgment is also informed and endorsed by the propositions of the middle range theory underpinning the conceptualization of the problem (selected if the theoretical approach is used to gain an understanding of the problem—see Chapter 3), the empirical evidence integrated to support the experience of the problem and its indicators and the association with its determinants (as is done if the empirical approach is used), and/or the explanations provided by stakeholder groups (as is done if the experiential approach is used).

The middle range theory of the problem provides statements about the conceptualization of the health problem and its associations with determinants. The theory also points to specific aspects of the problem that are malleable and have the greatest scope of change (Bleijenberg et al., 2018; Wight et al., 2016). These changeable aspects become the target of the intervention; that is, the intervention is designed to manage these aspects, with the ultimate goal of successfully addressing the health problem. For example, the social cognitive theory is frequently used to inform the conceptualization of health behaviors and the design of behavioral interventions (e.g. Durks et al., 2017; Lamort-Bouché et al., 2018). The social cognitive theory posits that (non)engagement in a behavior is influenced by: personal determinants such as cognitions (beliefs, attitudes, expected outcomes of the behavior); perceived behavioral control (self-efficacy); and social determinants such as norms and peer influence. The theory highlights cognitions and perceived behavioral control as determinants most malleable to change (e.g. Ball et al., 2017; Dalager et al., 2019; Direito et al., 2018).

The empirical evidence synthesizes the results of quantitative and/or qualitative studies pertaining to the experience if the health problem and its determinants. The evidence indicates aspects of the problem, in particular determinants, that could be potentially targeted by the intervention. Specifically, relevant evidence shows that the determinants (1) are consistently (across studies) and significantly associated with the experience of the problem; (2) are prioritized or considered important in contributing to the problem by the target client population; and (3) change over time, either normally or following treatment. Evidence of change confirms that the determinants are potentially modifiable. For example, incorrect beliefs and expectations about sleep have been found to perpetuate insomnia, and to be modified as a result of cognitive therapy (e.g. Eidelman et al., 2016; Morin et al., 2007).

In the absence of a middle range theory and empirical evidence on the health problem, the judgment is formed on the basis of systematic analysis of the problem and logical thinking; both are done either by the researchers alone or in collaboration with experts, including health professionals and clients. For example, the theory of insomnia presented in Chapter 3 is used here to illustrate the application of this analysis. As mentioned in Table 3.1, insomnia is conceptualized as a learned behavior. It is manifested as difficulty initiating and/or maintaining sleep (indicators), and influenced by predisposing, precipitating, and perpetuating factors (determinants). The analysis begins by questioning the extent to which insomnia, as a learned behavior, can be altered directly. Logically, this may be possible but not easy due to the complexity of the behavior. The conceptualization of insomnia as a learned behavior suggests that it can be "unlearned" and substituted with other behaviors that promote sleep. This perspective points to the need for behaviorally based interventions to manage this problem, but it does not indicate the specific behaviors to be changed. The analysis then moves to other aspects of insomnia to determine their amenability to change.

The analysis involves a review of the indicators and determinants of insomnia. There is no theoretical, empirical, or clinical/practical proposition that suggests that the indicators of insomnia (e.g. difficulty falling and/or staying asleep) can be directly manipulated or changed. However, a review and critical analysis of the three categories of determinants points to the following logic: (1) predisposing factors are innate characteristics of persons with insomnia and accordingly, they are not modifiable; (2) precipitating factors are often out the persons' control because they initiate or trigger poor sleep but dissipate once the persons start to experience insomnia; therefore they may not be changed at the time the persons start to experience insomnia and seek treatment; (3) perpetuating factors, representing behaviors and use of strategies or techniques that maintain insomnia are potentially modifiable—these behaviors can be unlearned and the strategies can be substituted with sleep-promoting ones.

The analysis results in the identification of what about the problem or aspects are modifiable. The identified aspects are defined at the conceptual and operational levels, based on the information presented in the theory of the problem, or relevant theoretical and empirical literature. These definitions are useful in specifying the desired changes in the next step.

*Step 3 – Identify Desired Changes*

In this step, desired changes are delineated for each aspect of the health problem identified as modifiable (Burrell et al., 2019). The changes represent alterations that should take place in the respective aspects of the problem and, subsequently, contribute to the prevention, management, or resolution of the problem. The changes are expected to occur at the level (e.g. intraindividual, environmental) at which the respective aspects of the problem are experienced. Two types of desired changes are specified. The first type, referred to as "change objectives" in the intervention mapping process described by Bartholomew et al. (2016), defines what clients need to do or alter to induce changes in the respective aspect of the problem (Beck et al., 2019); they reflect behaviors, activities, or actions in which clients engage to modify the aspect of the problem. The second type of desired changes, referred to as "performance objectives" in the intervention mapping process, defines the alterations in the aspects of the problem (Ball et al., 2017) that clients are expected to experience. Thus, desired changes reflect significant milestones, that is, changes in condition that clients experience and in behaviors in which clients engage, in the pathway to prevent, manage, or resolve the health problem (Brendryen et al., 2013; Czajkowski et al., 2015).

The desired changes are stated clearly, concisely, and in observable terms that accurately depict what is the specific alteration to be experienced and what is to be done, and who should make the change. The changes may be hypothesized to take place sequentially, whereby the occurrence of one leads to another, ultimately resulting in the prevention of or improvement in the experience of the health problem. The specification of the desired changes is critical (1) for designing interventions; the changes inform the delineation of the active ingredients (in step 4) and (2) for understanding the mechanism of action (represented in the sequence of desired changes) that explains how the intervention yields improvement in the health problem (Brendryen et al., 2013).

The identification of desired changes is illustrated in the example of insomnia. Of the factors that perpetuate insomnia and that are amenable to change, two health behaviors, physical inactivity and smoking, are reported to influence sleep. The following sequence of changes in condition is desired to help clients avoid these behaviors:

1. Heightened awareness of the general health-related behaviors that affect sleep.
2. Improved understanding of when, how, and why these behaviors interfere with sleep and contribute to insomnia
3. Increased knowledge of recommended techniques for handling these behaviors and, hence, mitigating their interference with sleep.
4. Enhanced self-confidence or self-efficacy in applying the recommended techniques.
5. Enhanced ability/skills in applying the recommended techniques.
6. Appropriate and consistent use of the recommended techniques.

*Step 4 – Delineate Intervention's Active Ingredients*

The active ingredients of a health intervention are the specific therapies or techniques (called "intervention methods" in the intervention mapping process) that are hypothesized to bring about the desired changes and, consequently, induce improvement in the health problem (Bleijenberg et al., 2018; Wight et al., 2016). The specific techniques encompass information that is relayed to clients and behaviors that clients engage in to address the problem. The techniques are delineated for each aspect of the problem identified as malleable, and relative to the respective desired changes. The techniques should be consistent with the aspect of the problem and capable of inducing the desired changes. The conceptual correspondence or match among the aspect of the problem, active ingredient or technique, and desired changes is essential to ensure the design of interventions with great potentials for being effective in addressing the health problem in the client population and context of interest (Dohnke et al., 2018; Mesters, et al., 2018).

The active ingredients or techniques can be identified from relevant theory, relevant empirical evidence, and/or consultation with experts or stakeholder groups, as explained in Section 4.2.

Delineation of the intervention's active ingredients is founded on logical reasoning. Logical reasoning is based on a thorough understanding of the nature of the aspect of the problem amenable to change and critical thinking of how it can be modified. The goal is to generate new or select available therapies or techniques that conceptually correspond with the nature of the problem or its aspects. This implies that the techniques should address the problem or its relevant aspects directly, effectively, and efficiently by triggering the respective desired changes.

In the example of insomnia, engagement in health behaviors (i.e. physical inactivity and smoking) perpetuates this sleep problem. To induce the desired changes identified for the behaviors in the step 3, it is logical to provide education (active ingredient 1) about the behaviors and how they interfere with sleep, and recommend techniques for handling them to produce desired changes 1–3, as well as to offer instrumental support (active ingredient 2) in applying the recommended techniques to induce desired changes 4–6.

*Step 5 – Operationalize the Active Ingredients*
In step 4, the intervention's active ingredients are delineated at the conceptual level; as such they are broadly defined (e.g. provide education about factors contributing to the health problem and offer support in changing these factors). While important, conceptually delineated active ingredients may not give specific instructions for how to deliver them; therefore, they should be diligently operationalized in a manner that maintains correspondence between their conceptual definition and delivery. This correspondence is necessary to enhance construct validity of the intervention (Sidani, 2015).

Operationalization of the intervention's active ingredients consists of:

1. *Specifying the components* that represent the active ingredients: This is accomplished by operationally defining each active ingredient in a component. The operationalization of each component involves detailing the content or information to be relayed to clients, the specific behaviors or activities in which clients engage, and the recommendations that clients are to apply in their daily life in order to attain the desired changes specified relative to the aspects of the problem amenable to change.

   In the example of insomnia, education and support were delineated as active ingredients for addressing the health behaviors that perpetuate insomnia. To operationalize these ingredients, one should ask the questions: education about what in particular and what type of support is useful for changing these two determinants of insomnia? The answers should be very specific detailing:

- The *content of education*: (1) inform clients of the health behaviors that perpetuate insomnia (what are the behaviors?)—for example, physical inactivity; (2) explain how the behaviors interfere with sleep (what is the pathway through which these behaviors lead to poor sleep and insomnia)—for example, physical inactivity influences circadian rhythm "synchronizers," daytime physical and mental health, arousal and body temperature around bedtime, and sleep architecture (Chennaoui et al., 2015; Irish et al., 2015); (3) describe, in detail, the recommended techniques for handling the behaviors—for example, develop a regular schedule of physical activity during the day, engage in physical activity in the later afternoon or early evening to help ward off feeling of early sleepiness or drowsiness, and avoid rigorous exercise immediately before bedtime.
- The *type of support*: (1) engage clients in an active discussion to select the physical activity they enjoy and afford performing, and to think through a plan or procedures to put in place to regularly perform the selected physical activity; (2) encourage clients to engage in the planned physical activity in daily life and monitor its impact on sleep; (3) review barriers and enablers, and generate or exchange ideas of what can be done to overcome barriers and reinforce enablers.

2. *Selecting the mode for delivering* the active ingredients: This consists of specifying the manner in which the active ingredients, as operationalized into respective components, are to be given to the client population in the context of interest. This exercise is referred to as practical applications in the intervention mapping process. Practical applications are concerned with the way the techniques are translated for practical use or delivery to fit the context of the client target population (Dohnke et al., 2018; Kok et al., 2016; Mesters et al., 2018). As described in Chapter 2, mode of delivery is characterized by different media and formats, some of which may be more appropriate for the operationalization of particular active ingredients than others. Therefore, the selection of delivery modes is based on an understanding of the active ingredients and of the range of media and formats.

   The mode of delivery is carefully selected to: (1) be consistent with the nature of the active ingredient, as operationalized in specific content, activities, and treatment recommendations; and (2) facilitate the delivery of the active ingredients in a way that is efficient yet maintains integrity of the active ingredient. Selection of the delivery mode is informed, where available, by evidence of the effectiveness of different media and formats, in different contexts, as well as evidence of their acceptability to the client population of interest and feasibility of use in the context of interest.

   In the example of insomnia, education, as an active ingredient, can be delivered in the written medium and in the format of an online module that covers the information on the health behaviors, the pathway through which they interfere with sleep, and the treatment recommendations. This mode of delivery (online module) is considered efficient, reaching a large proportion of adults with insomnia, with minimal human (e.g. therapist time) and material (e.g. costs of printing) resource expenses, and burden on clients who can assess and review the module at their convenience (i.e. reduced burden associated with time and cost of transportation). However, the online mode of delivery may not be accessible to some clients such as those with low reading and computer skills, vision problems, limited understanding of the language in which the module is written, and those who do not have access to a computer at home. Further, it may not be helpful to persons with low motivation and/or low self-confidence in the ability to carry out the treatment recommendations (Beall et al., 2014; Free et al., 2013; Murray, 2012). Lastly extant evidence, synthesized in systematic reviews, indicates that the effectiveness of online or web-based modes for delivering interventions in achieving the desired changes in a range of health problems is rather limited. Specifically, van Straten et al. (2018) found that the effects of self-help, web-based modes of providing cognitive behavioral therapy on insomnia severity and other sleep indicators, were smaller than those of person-dependent modes of delivery like group or individual sessions.

3. *Determining the optimal structure and intervention dose*: Once the active ingredients are operationalized into components and the most appropriate and effective mode of delivery is selected, the optimal structure and dose should be determined for delivering the intervention, comprised of all ingredients. The structure has to do with the approach and sequence for providing the intervention. The decision to use a standardized or tailored approach for giving the intervention is made based on a number of factors discussed in Section 4.5 related to the design of tailored interventions. The nature, complexity (i.e. type and number of components), sequence, and mode of delivery guide the specification of the optimal dose. If available, empirical evidence obtained in studies that compared the effectiveness of different dose levels for the same intervention is used to further justify the specified dose.

In the example of insomnia, two active ingredients, education and support, are delineated. It is logical to estimate that (1) education can be offered in one, 90-minute session; this session length provides ample time for the interventionist or therapist to present the detailed information at a pace suitable to clients who may vary in their ability or speed of grasping and processing the information, and for the clients to ask for clarification as needed; (2) support can be offered in four, 60-minute sessions; having four sessions provides clients the opportunity to apply the treatment recommendations in their daily life, and to reflect on their impact on sleep in the time interval between sessions, as well as to discuss ways or strategies to overcome barriers and reinforce enablers in subsequent sessions; thus, the plan is for four sessions (one for education and three for support). The selection of this dose is supported by empirical evidence showing that behavioral therapy delivered in four sessions is effective in managing insomnia (van Straten et al., 2018).

*Step 6 – Production of the Intervention Protocol and Materials*
After delineating all intervention components that operationalize the active ingredients, mode of delivery, and optimal structure and dose, it is important to develop the intervention protocol and produce relevant intervention materials (Ball et al., 2017; Byrd et al., 2012). The intervention protocol organizes the sequence for delivering the components, and within each component, the order for relaying the content and for engaging clients in the planned activities; it also describes the specific procedures to be followed, and the human and material resources required for delivering the intervention (see Chapter 7). The intervention materials refer to those used by the therapist in delivering the intervention (e.g. slide presentation) or provided to clients as a reference for application of the treatment recommendations in daily life (e.g. booklet).

## 4.2 APPROACHES FOR DELINEATING THE INTERVENTION'S ACTIVE INGREDIENTS

As introduced previously, there are three approaches for delineating the intervention's active ingredients: theoretical, empirical, and experiential. The approaches can be used independently or in combination. The selection of one or more approaches is contingent on the availability of pertinent theory and evidence that describe the health problem as experienced by and therapies or techniques that are acceptable to the client population and context of interest.

### 4.2.1 Theoretical Approach

#### 4.2.1.1 Overview

The theoretical approach is applied where a middle range theory of the problem is available and has guided the generation of the theory of the problem. This approach involves a meticulous review of the propositions of the middle range theory for delineating the intervention's active ingredients. The propositions of the theory point to aspects of the problem that are amenable to change (i.e. "where" we can intervene) and to therapies or techniques that are most appropriate to manage them (i.e. "what" we can do). Specifically, the theory indicates the nature of the techniques (what they are), which should correspond with the nature of the malleable aspects of the problem. It also explains the mechanism of action through which the techniques induce the desired changes, that is, why a causal link is expected between the application of the techniques and the changes leading to the prevention, management, or resolution of the problem (Davidoff et al., 2015; Dohnke et al., 2018; Kok et al., 2016; Mesters et al., 2018). In other words, the theory clarifies why and how the techniques work.

#### 4.2.1.2 Methods

The application of the theoretical approach begins with identifying middle range theories that explain the health problem and gaining an understanding of the theories' propositions. To this end, an extensive search of the theoretical or conceptual literature is conducted. Publications (articles or textbooks) or other sources (e.g. unpublished documents) are selected that describe the propositions of the theories regarding techniques or therapies for addressing the problem. Information on the therapies or techniques is extracted and organized to highlight: the name or label of the technique (what they are called); the aspect(s) of the health problem they are posited to address (what do they target); the essential elements that characterize the techniques and that are hypothesized as responsible for their anticipated effects (what they consist of); and the pathway linking their application to the anticipated improvement in the problem experience. Information obtained from different publication or sources is analyzed qualitatively, using constant comparison, and synthesized to clarify what the techniques consist of and why/how they are expected to work.

Social cognitive theory is an example of middle range theory that identifies techniques to promote engagement in health behaviors. The theory proposes two main determinants of behaviors: beliefs or attitudes and self-efficacy. It also delineates techniques for each determinant. Provision of knowledge about the behavior and its consequences is a technique recommended to enhance beliefs and attitudes.

Persuasion (e.g. use of messages to promote clients' awareness of the capabilities they have), mastery experiences (e.g. give opportunities for clients' performance of the skills or behavior), and modeling (e.g. have clients watch a video showing that others have succeeded in changing the behavior) are techniques expected to strengthen self-efficacy (e.g. Dalager et al., 2019; Direito et al., 2018).

Bartholomew et al. (2016) have compiled a taxonomy of theory-based methods that can be used to delineate the active ingredients of interventions aimed to change behaviors. The methods are listed for a range of behavior determinants derived from different middle range theories of health behaviors.

### 4.2.1.3   Strengths

The advantages of the theoretical approach relate to the delineation of the intervention's active ingredients that are specific and consistent with the nature of the problem and its malleable aspects. The theory points to the aspects of the health problem that can be modified and to techniques to produce the desired changes. This maintains conceptual consistency or match between aspects of the problem and techniques, which enhances the specificity of the theory-based interventions to the health problem and our understanding of what the active ingredients consists of and why or how they work. Understanding of the active ingredients is critical for their accurate operationalization into specific and nonspecific components of the intervention, which is required for the correct delivery of the intervention. Clarification of the intervention's mechanisms of action has the potential to enhance its effectiveness. Effectiveness is improved because the factors contributing most significantly to the health problem are appropriately addressed and not inadvertently missed (Michie et al., 2008). Evidence indicates that theory-based interventions are more effective than those whose design is not explicitly informed by theory, in producing beneficial outcomes (Glanz & Bishop, 2010; Murray, 2012; Painter et al., 2008; Prestwich et al., 2014).

### 4.2.1.4   Limitations

The limitations of the theoretical approach for delineating the intervention's active ingredients are related to the following points: (1) many middle range theories are descriptive and explanatory in that they provide conceptualizations of the health problem, but they fall short of suggesting how to modify the problem; in other words, the theories do not explicitly propose specific techniques to address the problem; (2) each middle range theory offers a unique conceptualization of the problem that specifies a particular set of determinants; reliance on one theory informs the design of interventions that target the respective determinants only and that may be of limited effectiveness because they do not address the most salient factors contributing to the problem as experienced by clients in the context of interest; and (3) some middle range theories may not have adequate and sufficient empirical support, raising concerns about their utility in informing the design of interventions (Lippke & Ziegelman, 2008).

### 4.2.2   Empirical Approach

#### 4.2.2.1   Overview

The empirical approach is the most frequently advocated and used in designing health interventions, consistent with the emphasis on evidence-based practice. The approach is appropriate where evidence is available on the usefulness of interventions in addressing the health problem. The empirical approach relies on evidence to identify and select interventions. The evidence, derived or synthesized from intervention evaluation research, points to therapies or techniques that have been found effective in addressing specific aspects of the problem or the overall problem. Traditionally, empirical evidence is generated in studies that evaluated an intervention as a whole package. Reports of these studies highlight the results pertaining to the direct effects of the intervention on the health problem. The reports fall short of describing: (1) the intervention itself (e.g. DiRuffano et al., 2017; Hoffmann et al., 2014) making it difficult to identify its active ingredients; (2) the delivery of the intervention limiting the understanding of its specific and nonspecific components; and (3) the mechanism through which the intervention (including its specific and nonspecific components) affects the health problem constraining the ability to discern what aspects of the problem are addressed and how the desired changes are achieved (Abraham et al., 2014). Accordingly, the empirical approach assists in identifying interventions, more so than delineating their active ingredients. However, new methods have been used to compile evidence on the mechanisms underlying the intervention's effects (e.g. realist review of the literature) and the active components comprising the intervention (e.g. component analysis). Traditional and new methods for reviewing empirical evidence are discussed next.

### 4.2.2.2   Methods

*General Review Process*

The traditional and new methods for reviewing empirical evidence involve a search of the literature, critical analysis of the studies' reports, and synthesis of the studies' findings. The two types of methods share similar steps to: search the literature; select reports for review; and extract information. They differ in the analysis and synthesis of the extracted data and studies' findings.

*Literature Search*

The search is done in various bibliographic databases (general and specific health-related disciplines) for comprehensiveness. The search uses keywords that capture the health problem, its indicators, and each of its determinants judged as potentially modifiable. The keywords are combined with those reflecting possible interventions or techniques, including: (1) the name/label of generic intervention techniques (e.g. behavioral intervention) or specific therapies or methods (e.g. persuasion), which may have been suggested and/or actually used to address the modifiable aspects of the problem, or (2) words that are synonymous with the term "intervention" such as therapy, technique, method, care, treatment, service, and program. The search may be limited to a recent time period (e.g. past 10 years) to enhance the relevance of interventions to the current context.

*Selection of Reports*

The selection of reports is based on pre-specified criteria. The criteria are related to: (1) the health problem or its aspects addressed by the intervention under evaluation; (2) the characteristics of the client population (e.g. age or gender) and context (e.g. rural areas) of interest; (3) the setting in which the intervention is delivered (e.g. client's home); and (4) the study design (e.g. randomized clinical trials). It may be useful to specify broad criteria (in particular those related to study design) to enhance comprehensiveness of the evidence. In addition to reports of individual studies, those presenting findings of literature reviews (e.g. scoping, narrative, systematic) and/or describing a study protocol are selected because they provide information on the effectiveness and on the nature of the intervention and its components, respectively.

### Data Extraction and Analysis

The information to extract from the selected reports of studies is presented in Table 4.1. It covers methodological and substantive characteristics of the study. Of importance in informing the delineation of the intervention's active ingredients are details on the intervention related to its components, mode and dose of delivery, mechanism of action, and effectiveness in inducing the desired changes in aspects of the problem and in improving the experience of the problem. The analysis and synthesis of the extracted data vary by review methods.

### Traditional Methods

The traditional review methods include scoping reviews, systematic reviews, and meta-analyses. *Scoping reviews* involve a comprehensive search of the literature to identify the types of interventions that have been proposed, used, and/or found

**TABLE 4.1**  Information to extract from selected reports of empirical studies.

| Category | Examples |
|---|---|
| Methodological characteristics | Type of design<br>Number and type of study groups<br>Time points for outcome assessment<br>Sample size<br>Quality of study |
| Intervention characteristics | Goal of intervention<br>Active ingredients, or specific and nonspecific components<br>Content covered or activities in which clients or participants engage<br>Mode of delivery<br>Dose<br>Type and training of personnel or staff involved in intervention delivery |
| Hypothesized outcomes | Type of outcomes<br>Measures used |
| Results | Findings quantifying the intervention's effects on the hypothesized outcomes<br>Additional findings related to:<br>1. Fidelity with which the intervention is delivered<br>2. Participants' exposure (number of sessions attended), adherence (application of treatment recommendations), and satisfaction with the intervention<br>3. Factors that influenced the delivery and/or outcomes of the intervention<br>4. Mechanism underlying the intervention's effects (either tested empirically or perceived by participants and/or staff)<br>5. Unexpected outcomes |

useful to address the health problem or its malleable aspects. For example, Guruge et al. (2017) conducted a scoping review to map out interventions addressing stigma of mental health. *Systematic reviews and meta-analyses* focus on determining the extent to which interventions are effective in improving the health problem. In all types of reviews, content analysis of the selected reports is applied to identify qualitatively similar interventions. Codes are assigned to different categories of intervention (e.g. medication, education, behavioral).

In systematic reviews, vote counting is used to synthesize the evidence on the interventions' effects. This consists of reviewing the findings of each study to determine if the interventions produce: no significant effects; significant effects in the hypothesized direction (i.e. clients or participants exposed to the intervention report improvement in the problem); or significant effects in the non-hypothesized direction (i.e. participants exposed to the intervention reported worsening in the problem). Interventions are considered effective if they produce significant effects in the hypothesized direction in most (more than 50%) studies included in the review (Hong et al., 2017).

In meta-analyses, statistical methods are applied to estimate the effect size, which quantifies the magnitude of the intervention effect on each outcome examined in each study included in the review. The extent of variability in the effect sizes is examined across studies. Low variability suggests that the intervention's effects on the outcomes are consistent; in this case, the effect sizes are aggregated across studies, taking sample size into account, and yielding an average point estimate (with confidence interval) of the intervention's effects. High variability prompts the investigation of possible causes of the heterogeneity in the estimated effect sizes. Possible causes are characteristics of the client population (e.g. gender, age), the intervention (e.g. components, mode or dose of delivery), the context in which the intervention is delivered (e.g. personnel providing it, setting), or the study (e.g. design, outcome measure). Advanced statistical tests (e.g. meta-regression) are used to relate the effect sizes to possible causes (Hong et al., 2017; Paré et al., 2015). The findings may point to variability in the effectiveness of different interventions in different client population and contexts. Such empirical evidence is most informative in selecting interventions as it indicates the intervention or the components that are most successful in the same or similar client population and context of interest.

### New Methods

New methods for reviewing empirical evidence include mixed methods reviews or syntheses that aim to delineate the interventions' active ingredients and mechanism of action. To address the first aim, intervention component analysis is proposed and illustrated in the Distillation and Matching Model (Chorpita et al., 2005). The intervention component analysis consists of several steps: (1) review relevant theory-based interventions to identify their active ingredients and their operationalization into components and techniques; (2) develop a guideline for coding them, where the guideline specifies the name of the components or techniques and describes what they entail; (3) search and select empirical studies that evaluated the interventions, components, or techniques; (4) extract descriptions of the interventions and results of their evaluation; (5) review the extracted descriptions of interventions and code for the presence of components or techniques; (6) generate matrices that summarize the coded component or techniques and the results of evaluation studies; and (7) analyze the data, using appropriate algorithms or statistical tests to explore patterns in the matrices that indicate which combination of theoretically derived components or techniques is associated with beneficial outcomes. A variant of this method was applied by Fox et al. (2013) to identify the most effective components of the acute care for elder (ACE) model.

To address the second aim, mixed methods review and synthesis are recommended. The review focuses on delineating the interventions' mechanism of action. It involves selection and review of studies that evaluated the process of implementing and of the outcomes of interventions. Process evaluation (see Chapter 13) involves the investigation of the fidelity with which the intervention is delivered, of contextual factors affecting the delivery and effectiveness of the intervention, and of clients' perception of the intervention and its impact. Outcome evaluation (see Chapters 14 and 15) is concerned with examining the effectiveness of the intervention in inducing the desired changes in aspects of the health problem (referred to as immediate and intermediate outcomes) and improving the experience of the health problem and preventing its consequences (posited as ultimate outcomes).

The quantitative and qualitative findings pertaining to process and outcome are analyzed separately or concurrently, and integrated to delineate the pathway linking the intervention or its components and techniques to the immediate and intermediate (i.e. desired changes) and the improvement in the ultimate outcomes (i.e. health problem experience) (Edwards & Kaimal, 2016; Gough, 2013; Snilstveit et al., 2012; White, 2018). Examples of mixed methods review are framework synthesis (Carroll et al., 2013) and realist reviews (Pawson et al., 2005). Both involve (1) engagement in an initial exercise to clarify the problem and to model the intervention's mechanism of action and contextual factors that may affect the delivery, mechanism of action, and/or outcomes of the intervention; this initial model is represented in a configuration that links context, mechanism, and outcome of the intervention; (2) review of the theoretical literature and empirical (quantitative and qualitative) evidence and extraction of data reflective of contextual factors, intervention components or techniques, desired changes and effectiveness in addressing the health problem; (3) coding of the extracted data relative to configuration of context, mechanism, and outcome; and (4) analysis and integration of the theoretical and empirical evidence to determine the adequacy or the need to revise the initial model. The application of the realist review is illustrated in the work of Robert et al. (2017).

### 4.2.2.3    Strengths

The empirical approach has the advantage of identifying interventions that have been implemented and evaluated. The evidence suggests that the interventions are feasible and effective in preventing, managing, or resolving the health problem, in different client populations and contexts.

### 4.2.2.4    Limitations

Extant empirical evidence has limitations: (1) the interventions are often poorly or briefly described, which creates difficulty in appropriately coding them, and the potential of lumping variant interventions in the same category; variability within categories may yield underestimated effects for the categorized interventions; (2) there is a rather small number of studies that evaluated the effects of different active ingredients or components comprising an intervention, the fidelity of intervention delivery, and the context and mechanism underlying the intervention's effects; yet this evidence is useful to delineate the intervention's active ingredients and to select the components that are most effective in addressing the potentially modifiable aspects of the health problem; (3) there is growing acknowledgement of publication bias, which threatens the validity of the synthesized empirical evidence; that is, there is a tendency to selectively report positive outcomes (Chan et al., 2014) and publish reports of studies with "statistically significant" effects; when averaged, these effects yield overestimated intervention's effects (van Assen et al., 2015).

The application of the theoretical and empirical approaches requires the availability of relevant theory and theory-based therapies or techniques, and evidence respectively. In situations where theory and evidence are not accessible, the experiential approach is advocated, whereas in situations where theory has not been tested and evidence has not been generated from studies involving the client population and the context of interest, the combined approach is recommended.

### 4.2.3   Experiential approach

#### 4.2.3.1   Overview

In the absence of theoretical and/or empirical guidance for delineating the active ingredients of an intervention, the experiential approach is a plausible alternative. The experiential approach is characterized by consultation with experts. Expertise refers to advanced knowledge related to the health problem experience and skills in its management. The consultation is done with different experts: researchers who have theoretical knowledge; health professionals who have clinical knowledge; and community leaders and clients who have experiential knowledge of the problem (e.g. Berry et al., 2012; Kildea et al., 2019).

Group, rather than individual, meetings are used to promote exchange, questioning, and elaboration on innovative yet plausible and realistic ideas, and to generate collective knowledge of possible interventions, therapies, or techniques addressing the potentially modifiable aspects of the health problem. The consultation may be unstructured or semi-structured involving brainstorming exercises to generate new or innovative solutions to the problem (e.g. Ammendolia et al., 2016). Alternatively, the consultation is structured involving exercises geared toward confirming the appropriateness of evidence-based intervention or co-development of interventions (e.g. Meng et al., 2019; van Mol et al., 2017).

#### 4.2.3.2   Methods

The group meetings should be well planned and facilitated to meaningfully and actively engage the experts in the delineation of the active ingredients, the specification or selection of techniques that operationalize the ingredients. The following are points to consider.

- The meetings can be held separately for different categories of experts (e.g. health professionals, clients, community leaders). This promotes participants' comfort in expressing their ideas, thereby creating an environment in which thinking is creative, bold, and unrestricted (Newby et al., 2019). Having separate meetings helps in capturing the views of each category of experts, untainted by those of others. Scheduling meetings that include different categories of experts may be useful at a later stage in the process. In such meetings, the facilitator clarifies that all participants are equal partners in the intervention design process, and encourages participants to discuss differences in views and reach an agreement on the most appropriate and feasible techniques.

- The experts are selected to represent various subgroups of the respective categories. For health professionals, the subgroups are defined by their professional affiliation and the types of services they provide. For the target client population, the subgroups are defined by their experience of the problem and its determinants, as well as sociodemographic, cultural, and health or clinical characteristics (Leask et al., 2019). For community leaders, the subgroups reflect a range of positions, such as representatives of specific client associations, media or religious figures, and local or national government officials with a track record of advocacy to mobilize resources to address the health problem as experienced by the target client population.
- The number of experts to include in each meeting ranges from 6 to 12. This number is manageable and enables meaningful participation and high-quality discussion by all group members (Leask et al., 2019).
- The meetings are held in locations that are easily accessible to the experts, and in rooms, with seating that is comfortable (particularly if the experts include clients with physical challenges) and promotes group communication and interaction.
- The meetings may extend over a few hours (e.g. Johnson et al., 2017) or one day (e.g. Meng et al., 2019), necessitating the accommodation for breaks and refreshments.
- It is advisable to have facilitators with a particular set of qualifications. The facilitators have to be familiar with group processes; capable of engaging all participants in the discussion and of managing conflict that may arise; respectful of creative ideas (Clark, 2015); experienced in the application of the planned group exercises; and knowledgeable of the health problem as experienced by the client population.
- The meeting proceeds following the steps described in Table 4.2.

Content analysis of the transcribed group discussion is geared toward the development of a map that identifies the collectively agreed upon techniques for addressing potentially modifiable aspects of the problem and achieving the desired changes. The map generated in different group meetings, held either for the same or different categories of experts, are compared and contrasted to identify communalities or convergence in the proposed techniques; common techniques form a solid ground for delineating the intervention's active ingredients. Discrepancies can be discussed and reconciled in meetings with groups of experts who expressed different views.

The group meetings have been applied in different situations. These include the last step of the concept mapping process as illustrated in Kelly et al. (2007); a modified version of intervention mapping as done by Meng et al. (2019); and intervention co-design workshop described by Newby et al. (2019).

### 4.2.3.3   Strengths

The advantages of the experiential approach relate to the involvement of different experts, most notably clients, in the delineation of intervention active ingredients or techniques to address malleable aspects of the problem perceived as most relevant and salient to the client population and context of interest. As such, the intervention ingredients or techniques are consistent with the beliefs and values of the target client population and feasible within the clients' context (Hawkins et al., 2017).

**TABLE 4.2**   Experiential approach: steps for conducting group meeting with experts.

| Step | Activities |
| --- | --- |
| Step 1 | Clarify the tasks at hand, which are to learn about experts or participants' views of the health problem and ideas of ways to address it |
| Step 2 | Describe the health problem of interest, using simple terms that are easy to grasp by experts with different levels of literacy. The description involves depiction of what the problem is |
| Step 3 | Engage experts in group discussion of:<br>1. How the problem is experienced—to identify the range of possible indicators<br>2. What factors, occurring at what (e.g. individual and/or contextual) levels, contribute to the problem as experienced by the target client population—to identify most relevant ones<br>3. How the factors contribute to the problem—to clarify experts' understanding of the interrelationships among determinants and the pathway linking determinants to the problem |
| Step 4 | Involve experts in the identification of aspects of the problem they view as potentially modifiable, and of those, the aspects they consider most important requiring remediation |
| Step 5 | Facilitate a group brainstorming exercise during which experts are encouraged to:<br>1. Specify desired changes<br>2. Share ideas about ways or techniques to address each aspect of the problem and to achieve the respective changes<br>Examples of questions to facilitate this exercise are:<br>For this particular determinant, what changes should take place?<br>What can done to make these changes?<br>What solutions or techniques are you aware of or have you used to address this determinant?<br>Additional questions are used to probe for clarification of proposed solutions/techniques and their perceived appropriateness and utility in inducing the desired changes |
| Step 6 | Have the experts review the list of proposed solutions/techniquess, determine the ones that are relevant to various subgroups of the target client population and feasible within the context of interest, and reach an agreement on the ones to be selected for integration in the intervention |

This consistency among problem and techniques is likely to enhance the acceptability of the intervention (Leask et al., 2019). Accordingly, the experiential approach is highly valuable in designing interventions that are relevant to clients of different ethnic or cultural backgrounds. The resulting interventions are perceived as desirable or acceptable. Acceptability enhances the uptake, engagement, adherence, and satisfaction with treatment and, hence, achievement of beneficial outcomes as discussed in Chapter 11 (Araújo-Soares et al., 2018; Kildea et al., 2019; Smith et al., 2017).

### 4.2.3.4   Limitations

The application of the experiential approach has some drawbacks. It may be time consuming to find participants who represent all subgroups of expertise and who are motivated and able to attend long meetings (Wamsler, 2017). Those who participate may represent select subgroups (e.g. clients who are articulate or experience the problem at a low level of severity), which can potentially limit the acceptability and applicability of the intervention.

### 4.2.4   Combined Approach

#### 4.2.4.1   Overview

The combined approach has the potential to mitigate the limitations of the theoretical, empirical, and experiential approaches for delineating the intervention's active ingredients. It integrates elements of these three approaches to develop interventions that are well grounded in relevant theory and empirical evidence, yet acceptable to the client population in the context of interest. As commonly described in the literature on intervention mapping (e.g. Koutoukidis et al., 2018; van Mol et al., 2017) and intervention co-design/co-production (e.g. Hawkins et al., 2017; Smith et al., 2017), the combined approach consists of sequential application of the theoretical, empirical, and experiential approaches.

#### 4.2.4.2   Methods

The application of the combined approach involves:

1. The generation of a map representing aspects of the problem amenable to change, intervention's active ingredients operationalized in the respective components and strategies, and the proposed desired changes. The content of the map is derived from relevant theory, empirical evidence or a mix of both, as described in steps 1–5 of the intervention design process (Section 4.1).
2. The conduct of group meetings with experts, most notably clients (as described in Section 4.2.3) to elicit their views on the map. The method for conducting the meeting is semi-structured, involving: an overview of the map; detailed description of the techniques that address each aspect of the problem; rating the proposed techniques for their appropriateness, feasibility and utility in achieving the desired changes; and engaging in a discussion of the techniques with the aim to reach an agreement on the most relevant ones. The steps for conducting the group meetings are presented in Table 4.3.

Analysis of the participants' ratings and transcribed discussion, within and across group meetings, helps to identify those strategies commonly viewed as appropriate, useful, and feasible (indicated by high mean ratings and positive comments), and to clarify what and how they can be modified. Differences in perspectives are discussed and reconciled in additional group meetings (as explained in Section 4.2.3).

#### 4.2.4.3   Strengths

The strengths of the combined approach include the incorporation of experts' input to reformulate, complement, and supplement theory- and evidence-based techniques. The resulting techniques are integrated in health interventions. Interventions designed using the combined approach are expected to be effective in resolving the health problem, yet acceptable to the client population and feasible in the context of interest.

**TABLE 4.3**  Combined approach: steps for conducting group meetings.

| Step | Activities |
| --- | --- |
| Step 1 | Clarify the task at hand, which is to learn about participants' views of the strategies proposed to address the health problem |
| Step 2 | Describe the health problem in detail, informed by the theory or logic model of the problem, using simple easy to understand terms. The description clarifies the definition of the problem (what it is), depicts its indicators (how it is experienced), identifies its determinants (what contributes to the problem) and their relationships with the problem (how the factors leads to the problem), and highlights the consequences of the problem (how it impacts health/life) |
| Step 3 | Identify aspects of the problems that are amenable to change and, therefore, can be modified in order to address the health problem and mitigate its consequences |
| Step 4 | Introduce the map as a blueprint for ways to address the problem |
| Step 5 | Review the information in the map pertinent to each potentially modifiable aspect of the problem<br>Clarify the aspect, describe the proposed techniques, and explain the desired changes expected of the use of these techniques |
| Step 6 | Engage participants in a group discussion to elicit their views on the appropriateness, utility, and feasibility of the techniques proposed for each aspect of the problem<br>Participants may be asked to rate each proposed technique for its appropriateness in addressing the respective aspect of the problem, its potential utility or effectiveness in producing the desired changes, and its ease of use in the context of daily life (for clients) and practice (for health professionals), using validated items.<br>Participants are encouraged to express their opinion on the proposed techniques by answering open-ended questions such as:<br>• What makes this technique appropriate/inappropriate? Potentially useful/not useful? Feasible/not feasible?<br>• How can the technique be modified to improve its delivery? |
| Step 7 | Generate a list of techniques rated highly or viewed favorably for each modifiable aspect of the problem |
| Step 8 | Have participants review the list and agree on the techniques to be selected for inclusion in the intervention |

### 4.2.4.4  Limitations

The application of the combined approach is time consuming and labor intensive. It is often difficult to recruit groups of participants representing various subgroups of the respective categories of experts (Ball et al., 2017; Brendryen et al., 2013).

## 4.3  THEORY OF IMPLEMENTATION

### 4.3.1  Overview

The process for designing health interventions, using any or a combination of approaches, yields information on aspects of the health problem amenable to change, the active ingredients to address the aspects of the problem, and the desired changes expected of the active ingredients and that contribute to the prevention, management, or resolution of the problem. It is possible to have the same techniques for addressing different aspects of the problem. For example, education can be used to convey information about determinants of insomnia and about techniques recommended to address each determinant. The techniques can be integrated into a component. A component is a set of inter-related techniques or activities that have a common goal (e.g. relay information) and/or address a particular aspect of the problem (e.g. behavioral techniques to change sleep habits).

The theory of implementation identifies the active ingredients of an intervention, specifies the components that operationalize the ingredients, and describes each component. As such, the theory of implementation is the blueprint that informs what the intervention is about and how it is delivered. Each component is described in detail to show its correspondence with the respective active ingredients and to point to its most appropriate delivery. In the theory of implementation, the description of a component specifies: the desired changes (objective/goal) it is set to achieve; the information (content/topics) to be relayed including the techniques, behaviors or treatment recommendations that clients are recommended to perform in everyday life in order to achieve the desired changes; the activities in which clients are engaged during the delivery of the intervention; and the mode(s) for providing the component. The components are organized in a meaningful way, indicating the sequence for their delivery through the respective mode.

### 4.3.2    Illustrative Example

In the example of insomnia, education is an active ingredient designed to inform clients about: (1) sleep: what is sleep, why we sleep, and what produces sleep (e.g. circadian rhythm); (2) insomnia: what is insomnia and how it can be experienced; and (3) personal factors and behaviors (e.g. pattern of food and fluid intake, worrying in bed) and environmental factors (e.g. exposure to daylight, sleep environment such as bed room temperature, light and noise) that interfere with sleep and keep insomnia going. This information can be integrated into a component, sleep education, and presented in the specified sequence (i.e. sleep, insomnia, factors), within the first intervention session. This timing is essential as this information helps clients understand their sleep problem, appreciate the contribution of their (non) actions or behaviors to the problem, and the rationale for treatment recommendations. Clients who understand the "why" of the treatment are likely to "buy-in" the treatment, judge it as credible, and therefore engage and adhere to it (Davidoff et al., 2015), which has been shown to improve outcomes (e.g. Constantino et al., 2018). Multiple modes are useful to provide the sleep education component in a way that is attractive and effective for clients with different literacy levels and learning styles. The modes of delivery include: (1) oral presentation by the interventionist to relay and clarify the information in simple terms; (2) written booklet that clients can use to follow through the presentation and take notes for future reference; (3) self-reflection exercise inviting clients to reflect on the personal and environmental factors that are salient in their individual context. This exercise assists clients in recognizing and prioritizing the factors that they should address to promote a good night's sleep. The sleep education component is useful to enhance clients' awareness of factors that interfere with sleep and knowledge of how they perpetuate insomnia. However, as described, this component does not help them learn and apply techniques to change these factors.

Support is another active ingredient of the intervention to manage insomnia. Support is operationalized in the component sleep hygiene that consists of: (1) relaying information on the techniques recommended to modify the factors contributing to insomnia; the information is presented for each factor, describing what is to be done by the clients, how and why; (2) having clients develop an individual plan of action for engaging in the techniques recommended for the factors they identify as salient in their life context. Clients' participation in the development of the action plan generates a sense of ownership. In addition, tailoring the plan to the individual's life circumstances or context promotes its acceptability and feasibility, which enhance clients' engagement, motivation, and proper execution of the plan; (3) encouraging clients to apply the action plan in everyday life (also called "homework assignment"); and (4) discussing clients' experience in applying the action plan to identify barriers, enablers, and impact of the applied techniques on sleep. The discussion can also be geared toward generating or exchanging ideas to overcome the barriers and reinforce the enablers. The first three activities of the sleep hygiene component are performed in the specified sequence within the first session of the intervention (e.g. following the sleep education component). The mode of providing these activities includes using oral presentation and written booklet to relay the information to all clients attending the session, and individual or small group activity to develop the action plan. The last activity (i.e. discussion) is done in a subsequent session to give clients the opportunity to execute the action plan and report on their experience, in a group format to support each other in finding ways to overcome the barriers (Paul-Ebhahimhen & Arenell, 2009), persuade each other of their ability to apply the recommended techniques, and exchange ideas or tips on how best to apply them. Further, in a group format, clients who are successful in carrying out the plan and experienced improvement in sleep, serve as role models for others. The content and activities comprising the sleep hygiene component are expected to increase clients' knowledge, self-efficacy, skills, and consistent application of the recommended techniques.

### 4.3.3   Elements of the Theory of Implementation

The information presented in the previous sections illustrates the theory of implementation. The theory of implementation helps in understanding health interventions, as designed, and provides directions for their delivery to the client population in the context of interest (Blamey et al., 2012; Renger et al., 2013). To be useful, the theory of implementation explains the what, how, and why of the intervention. It offers practical guidance on what to do and how to do it when delivering the intervention, which is important for the accurate delivery of the intervention. The theory also provides corresponding conceptual explanations of the techniques to be performed, which are important for appreciating the rationale of the selected intervention components, content, activities, and mode of delivery. In general, understanding the what, how, and why promotes the quality or adequacy of the intervention delivery. Accordingly, the theory of implementation:

1.  Delineates the active ingredients of the intervention in relation to the potentially modifiable aspects of the problem and the desired changes.
2.  Defines the active ingredients at the conceptual level and explains how they are operationalized into components.
3.  Describes the components in detail. The description depicts: (1) the goal or desired change the component is set to achieve; (2) the content to be covered;

(3) the treatment recommendations that clients should carry out in daily life; (4) the activities to be performed by the interventionist and the clients when delivering the component; and (5) the modes for delivering the components. The sequence for providing the content and/or performing the activities is specified for each component. The sequence for giving the components and the dose for the intervention (comprised of all components) are clarified.

4. Explains the rationale for the selected components, activities, and modes of delivery, as well as their linkages to the desired changes.

5. Identifies the dose at which the intervention (including all components) is provided.

The theory of implementation provides the blueprint for detailing the "nuts and bolts" of the intervention (Blamey et al., 2012) in the intervention manual (see Chapter 7).

## 4.4  THEORY OF CHANGE

### 4.4.1  Overview

In the process of designing interventions, desired changes are identified for each aspect of the health problem judged as potentially modifiable. The active ingredients, operationalized in the respective components, are delineated with the expectation that they will produce these desired changes. The desired changes may occur sequentially leading to the alteration of the corresponding aspect of the problem, which in turn, contributes to the prevention, management, or resolution of the problem. The sequence of changes, occurring with or following the delivery of the intervention, forms the mechanism responsible for the intervention's effectiveness in addressing the problem. The theory of change describes the mechanism of action in terms of the sequence of changes in condition and behaviors that take place with exposure to the intervention, and provides conceptual explanations of why and how the intervention induces the changes that result in improvement in the health problem and prevention of its consequences.

### 4.4.2  Illustrative Example

To elaborate on the example of insomnia, clients exposed to the sleep education and the sleep hygiene components of the intervention are expected to:

1. Understand all information relayed to them: This is necessary to recognize what interferes with sleep and perpetuate insomnia, to learn what the recommended techniques are and how they work in promoting a good night sleep.

2. React positively to the information, that is, view the information as relevant to their individual condition and life circumstances: Clients are likely to attend and act upon what they consider as applicable and useful to them.

3. Build intellectual and practical capacity for change: Clients gain the knowledge required to carry out the recommended techniques, including: what are the techniques; how exactly should the techniques be applied, when, and where; how they work; how the techniques may be adapted to their individual context; what are possible barriers and enablers they may encounter; and what can done about the barriers and enablers. This knowledge prepares clients, and enhances their confidence in their ability, to carry out the techniques properly.

4. Apply and adhere to the recommended techniques in the context of everyday life, which are expected to mitigate or weaken the influence of perpetuating factors on insomnia.

5. Experience improvement in the quantity and quality of sleep.

6. Experience reduced severity of insomnia and enhanced daytime functioning.

The series of desired changes, expected of the delivery of the sleep education and the sleep hygiene components, is the mechanism underlying their effects on insomnia.

### 4.4.3  Elements of the Theory of Change

It is through the theory of change that the mechanism through which interventions produce their effects on the health problem. It is important to note that the terms: mechanism, mechanism of action, mechanism of change, causal processes, causal chain, and impact pathway, have been used in the literature to refer to the series of changes linking the delivery of the intervention (comprised of all respective components) to the prevention, management, or resolution of the health problem. For simplicity, the term "mechanism" is used in this book.

In general, the mechanism represents the processes or pathways that account for how and why an intervention works to produce changes in the hypothesized outcomes (Cambon et al., 2019; Carey et al., 2018; Kazdin, 2007; Mayne, 2017; Sridharan et al., 2016; White, 2018; Wilt, 2012). Different terms have been used to describe the processes. As mentioned previously, the processes entail the series of desired changes specified during the intervention mapping exercise. In the program planning and evaluation literature, the processes are described in terms of reactions to treatment, immediate and intermediate outcomes, which are posited to mediate the impact of the intervention on the hypothesized ultimate outcomes; the latter outcomes include improvement in the health problem and prevention of its consequences. In health-related literature, the variables operationalizing the processes are referred to as intervening variables or mediators (e.g. Chen et al., 2018; Vittengl et al., 2014; Wilt, 2012).

Clients' reactions to treatment refer to their understanding and perception of the intervention as-a-whole and/or its components (e.g. Blamey et al., 2012; Dalkin et al., 2015; Mayne, 2017) as illustrated in the first and second changes expected of sleep education and hygiene component (presented in step 3, Section 4.1). *Understanding* reflects clients' awareness of the intervention's goal and comprehension of the specific activities comprising the intervention and of the treatment recommendations they are expected to carry out in everyday life (Borelli et al., 2005). *Perception* entails clients' views of the intervention as-a-whole and/or its components, activities, mode of delivery, and dose, as well as the treatment recommendations. The views relate to the acceptability, credibility (i.e. endorsement of the intervention logic), expectancy (i.e. anticipated helpfulness of the intervention in resolving the health problem), and satisfaction with the intervention (Sidani & Fox, 2020). Clients' reactions are the instigators for the changes in the immediate outcomes. Interventions that are well understood and perceived favorably are enacted properly and adhered to in everyday life (Beatty & Binnion, 2016; Haanstra et al., 2015).

Immediate outcomes are desired changes occurring with the delivery of the intervention or its components. They are exemplified by building capacity as listed for sleep education and sleep hygiene in step 3, Section 4.1. Changes in the immediate outcomes are expected to lead to changes in the intermediate outcomes. These include continued enactment of the treatment recommendations, resulting in the desired changes in the respective aspects of the health problem addressed by the intervention components. Immediate outcomes are illustrated with the fourth and fifth changes (step 3, Section 4.1), that is, application and adherence of the recommended techniques and improvement in sleep. Several immediate and intermediate outcomes may be specified, as anticipated for each component, and relative to the corresponding aspects of the problem.

Changes in the intermediate outcomes lead to changes in the ultimate outcome. Ultimate outcomes operationalize the overall goals of the intervention, which pertain to the prevention, management, or resolution of the health problem; prevention or mitigation of the consequences of the problem; and improvement in general functioning, health and well-being, as illustrated with the sixth change (step 3, Section 4.1), that is, reduced severity of insomnia and enhanced daytime functioning.

In summary, the theory of change clarifies the mechanism explaining the intervention's effects on the ultimate outcomes by:

1. Identifying the series of mediators (reactions, immediate and intermediate outcomes) and defining them at the conceptual level.
2. Explaining why and how the mediators interrelate to produce the ultimate outcomes.
3. Operationalizing the desired changes in the mediators, by specifying the pattern (i.e. magnitude and direction) and the time surrounding the delivery of the intervention at which the changes are expected to occur.

Some authors suggest that the theory of change has also to propose contextual factors that may influence the initiation of the intervention's mechanism of action. Contextual factors include characteristics of the clients receiving the intervention, the interventionist delivering the intervention, the setting or environment in which the intervention is given and the treatment recommendations are applied; as well as concurrent exposure to other treatments. The factors may have a direct impact on specific variables operationalizing the mechanism.

## 4.5    DESIGNING TAILORED INTERVENTIONS

### 4.5.1    Overview

Most of the literature on designing interventions focused on generating interventions to be delivered in a standardized or "one-size-fits-all" approach. Standardized interventions comprise the same set of components (including content, activities, and treatment recommendations) that are delivered in their entirety, in a consistent manner, using the same mode of delivery and at the same dose, to all clients regardless of their personal characteristics, context or life circumstances, and unique experience of the health problem. The delivery of standardized interventions maintains their comparability and repeatability, which is believed to enhance their quality, safety, and subsequently, effectiveness (Mannion & Exworthy, 2017). However, cumulative evidence on the modest effectiveness of standardized interventions and the high valuing of client-centered care have renewed the interest in tailored interventions. Results of studies that evaluated a range of standardized health interventions consistently indicate that these interventions produce statistically significant improvement in the health problem; but the improvement is rarely clinically meaningful (Hekler et al., 2018). For instance, cognitive behavioral therapy is recognized as first-line treatment for insomnia (Riemann et al., 2017); however, evidence shows that the percentages of responders (i.e. clients reporting clinically significant improvement in sleep outcomes) and remitters (i.e. clients demonstrating post-test scores on sleep outcomes corresponding to "good" sleepers) are often low, being less than 50% (e.g. Epstein et al., 2012; Harvey et al., 2014). Individual differences in personal characteristics, life circumstances, experience of the health problem and the perception, reaction and adherence to the interventions are proposed as factors contributing to variability in clients' responses to the intervention and achievement of the desired clinically relevant changes in the problem (e.g. Raue & Sirey, 2011; Reach, 2016).

There is increasing valuing, demand, and support to implement client or person centered care. Clients view this type of care as very important in attending to their individual experience and life circumstances and in resolving their health problem (e.g. de Boer et al., 2013). Health professionals are increasingly engaging in client-centered practice (e.g. Sidani et al., 2017) and embracing personalized medicine (e.g. Recht et al., 2016; Wittink et al., 2013). Research funding agencies such as the Patient-Centered Outcomes Research Institute in the United States of American and the SPOR initiative supported by the Canadian Institutes of Health Research in Canada, and health policy makers such as the Ontario Ministry of Health and Long Term Care in Canada, are supporting initiatives to design, implement, and evaluate client-centered care. Providing tailored interventions that are responsive to clients' characteristics, life context and values or preferences, is an essential element of client-centered care (Sidani & Fox, 2014).

## 4.5.2   Types of Tailored Interventions

The terms targeted, tailored, individually or person centered, individualized, customized, personalized, and adaptive have been used to characterize health interventions that are delivered using the tailored (i.e. individualized structure—see Chapter 2) approach. This approach involves the provision of different treatment options, or different components of an intervention, through modes of delivery and at dose levels that are responsive (i.e. appropriate and consistent) to individual clients' characteristics. The distinction among the types of interventions is based on the number and the timing at which client characteristics are taken into consideration in the tailoring process.

*Targeted interventions* are designed and delivered to be responsive to a single characteristic (such as gender or culture) that differentiates a subgroup of the client population (Beck et al., 2010). In the example of insomnia, the sleep education and the sleep hygiene components could be offered in face-to-face sessions or web-based modules, on the basis of clients' computer literacy level.

*Tailored, individualized, customized, or personalized* interventions address the clients' individuality. The interventions are provided to be responsive to the clients' unique characteristics, including personal profile (e.g. genetic, physiological, psychological) and life context (e.g. sociocultural, resources, environmental) (Beck et al., 2010; Mannion & Exworthy, 2017; Radhakrishan, 2012). For instance, the sleep hygiene component can be tailored in that only the techniques relevant to the particular personal factors experienced by individual clients (e.g. smokers) are discussed and recommended.

*Adaptive interventions* involve the adaptation and readaptation of the intervention's components, mode of delivery and/or dose to the clients' personal characteristics, evolving experience of the health problem, and/or adherence to treatment. The experience of the problem and adherence to treatment vary over the intervention period (Hekler et al., 2018; Lagoa et al., 2014). The sleep restriction therapy for insomnia illustrates adaptive interventions. The therapy is a behavioral intervention that addresses the determinant of irregular sleep schedules. The interventionist and the client review the client's sleep schedules as reported in a daily sleep diary to determine the individual sleep needs (quantified in total sleep time); together, they work out the sleep–wake schedule for the first week of treatment, based on the client's sleep needs and life style. In subsequent weeks, the sleep schedule, in particular bed time, is adjusted on the basis of available guidelines that account for changes in client's sleep quantity and quality (Manber et al., 2012).

The design of tailored and adaptive interventions requires the identification of salient client characteristics for tailoring and of relevant intervention options, components, and mode and dose of delivery. It also demands the development of an algorithm to guide the tailoring process. Important points to consider in the development of these interventions are presented next.

### 4.5.3   Methods

The design of tailored and adaptive interventions rests on a lucid understanding of the health problem (as delineated in the theory of the problem) and of the features of the interventions (as delineated in the theory of implementation and the theory of change) developed to address the problem. Knowledge of the health problem is necessary for identifying the variables on which to tailor the intervention, and knowledge of the intervention provides directions for specifying its features that can be tailored, how and when. This information is then combined to generate the algorithm that guides the tailoring process.

#### 4.5.3.1   Identification of Variables for Tailoring

Logic, empirical evidence, clinical experience, and the theory of the problem are sources for the identification of variables serving as the foundation for tailoring the intervention design and delivery. The theory of the problem is most informative. It describes variations in the experience of the health problem by specifying the possible range of the problem's indicators, level of severity, duration, and determinants. Variations in the experience of the problem within a particular context and time, suggests the need for tailoring. The theory proposes variables that account for the variation in the experience of the problem. These include clients' personal characteristics and life circumstances or contextual factors, and are considered for tailoring (Lei et al., 2012). For example, clients with insomnia may exhibit some but not all health behaviors associated with insomnia and may have different sleep habits that perpetuate insomnia. Accordingly, these behaviors are considered for tailoring of the sleep hygiene component and behavioral intervention for insomnia as suggested by Manber et al. (2012). The theory of the problem proposes that clients' personal characteristics and life circumstances influence their engagement in the intervention and enactment of treatment recommendations, and subsequently achievement of the desired changes; these are also considered for tailoring. Examples include: level of health literacy, computer skills, comorbid conditions and concurrent treatments, beliefs or explanatory model of the health problem, expectations regarding the potential benefit of and level of motivation for the intervention (e.g. Beck et al., 2010; Cohen et al., 2015), work place requirements and availability of resources required for applying the treatment recommendations.

The theory of the problem, in combination with expert consultation, points to the salient variables that form the foundation for tailoring. These have been referred to as the tailoring variables. The tailoring variables should be clearly defined at the conceptual and operational levels. These definitions inform the selection of reliable and valid instruments to measure them. Assessment of the variables is the first step in the tailoring process. Furthermore, awareness of how the variables influence the experience of the health problem and/or the application of the treatment recommendations gives directions for specifying what features of the intervention to tailor, how and when.

### 4.5.3.2  Identification of Intervention Features for Tailoring

Tailoring may involve (1) the selection and provision of different interventions or components of an intervention, to be consistent with the clients' experience of the health problem and the tailoring variables; (2) modification of an intervention's components, mode or dose of delivery, at one or more points in time during the treatment period to account for clients' response to treatment; and (3) provision of additional nonspecific components to support clients in the application of the treatment recommendations. The goal of tailoring is to enhance the responsiveness of the intervention to the client's experiences.

*Selection of Different Interventions or Components*

The first form of tailoring demands the availability of different interventions (e.g. medication, herbal therapies, cognitive behavioral therapy for insomnia) or different components of an intervention (e.g. education and cognitive restructuring as components of cognitive therapy; stimulus control therapy, sleep restriction therapy and relaxation therapy as components of behavioral therapy for insomnia). The list of interventions and components is generated from relevant theories, or empirical and experiential evidence. Specific interventions or components are selected and delivered in a manner that is consistent or responsive to the salient tailoring variables, assessed at one point in time; the time point is usually baseline or prior to intervention delivery for tailored interventions, or at predetermined time points or intervals (e.g. weekly) during the treatment period for adaptive interventions. For example, clients may vary in their beliefs or explanatory model of depression and are offered interventions that correspond with their beliefs. Clients who believe in biological causes of depression are offered medications (e.g. antidepressants) and those who view depression as resulting from life stress are offered psychotherapy. Clients with insomnia may experience different perpetuating factors; they are given different components of cognitive behavioral therapy. As suggested by Espie et al. (1989), clients experiencing physiological arousal are provided relaxation therapy; those presenting with cognitive arousal are provided paradoxical intention to reduce performance anxiety; and those having poor sleep habits are provided stimulus control therapy.

Alternatively, tailoring may be achieved in what has been called stepped care. This is represented with a sequential delivery of the health intervention's components. The sequential delivery begins with the component that is relevant to the most salient client's experience of the health problem, with subsequent components selected based on client's response (i.e. reported improvement in the problem) following completion of the first component, as is done in adaptive interventions. For example, clients with insomnia are exposed to sleep education and sleep hygiene in the first week of treatment to address misconceptions about sleep and health behaviors known to perpetuate insomnia; those showing no improvement in their sleep quantity and quality are then exposed to relaxation or a behavioral therapy to manage arousal and poor sleep habits.

## Modification of Intervention

The second form of tailoring requires the capacity to modify the intervention components and/or the mode and dose of intervention delivery to fit the clients' experiences. The modification is carefully done to minimize major deviation from the specific components that characterize the intervention's active ingredients; the specific components are responsible for initiating the mechanism of action and the intervention's effectiveness in improving the health problem. The combination of theoretical, empirical, and experiential approaches is useful in specifying what modifications can be done, how and when. The following illustrates modifications to the sleep education and sleep hygiene components that can be made to match the characteristics of clients without jeopardizing their integrity and potential effectiveness: (1) clients with full-time employment involving long working hours and sedentary activities are encouraged to explore work-related activities that can be performed at the level to be counted toward daily recommendations for physical activity, and to find "a buddy system" comprising coworkers to promote engagement in physical activity within the work setting (e.g. taking a walk at lunch break); (2) clients with high general and computer literacy, busy schedule, and transportation or travel difficulty are offered the two components in the form of web-based modules to review at their convenience; (3) clients showing a good understanding and ability to apply the recommended sleep hygiene techniques, and reporting improvement in their sleep quantity and quality may be offered the option to not attend later intervention sessions (i.e. reduced dose) that involve face-to-face group discussion of barriers to implementation of the recommended techniques and of strategies to mitigate the barriers.

## Additional Components

The third form of tailoring involves the procurement of additional nonspecific components to support clients facing challenges during the intervention period, such as those with low motivation to engage or adhere to treatment recommendations and/or those with less-than-optimal improvement in the health problem. For instance, clients with low motivation to initiate and continue treatment may require additional counseling or support from the therapist; motivational techniques can be used in this instance.

The identification of the intervention's features that can be tailored and the specification of how the features can be modified inform the development of the algorithm to guide the delivery of tailored interventions.

### 4.5.3.3   Development of Algorithm

The algorithm is the essence of tailored and adaptive interventions. It consists of a set of decision rules that link or match the tailoring variables with the intervention features to enable the customization of the intervention. The decision rules reflect the logic that underpins the customization, that is, the selection of interventions, specific and nonspecific components, mode of delivery, and dose that are appropriate, consistent or responsive, correspond or match clients' experiences of or levels on the tailoring variables. The rules are operationalized in "if-then" statements (Golsteijn et al., 2017), which take the form of: "If the client presents with a particular variable at a specified level, then this intervention, component (i.e., content, activity, treatment recommendation), mode, or dose is recommended."

The way in which decision rules are stated is comparable for tailored and adaptive interventions; however, the type of tailoring variables and the timing for decision-making vary. For tailored interventions, tailoring variables (e.g. experience of the health problem) are assessed at baseline, prior to the intervention delivery. The results of the assessment inform the decision of what intervention to select or what feature of the intervention is to be modified and how. The selected intervention option or the modified intervention feature is provided to the client throughout the treatment period. For adaptive interventions, the same process is followed to select the appropriate intervention or the modified intervention feature to which clients are exposed for a predetermined time period (e.g. one week). Concurrently, clients report on the experience of the problem and adherence to treatment. Toward the end of this predetermined time period, clients' reports are analyzed to determine their response to the intervention (i.e. level of improvement in the experience of the health problem) and adherence to treatment. Clients' responses and adherence become the client characteristics for further customization, whereby other interventions, components, additional support, or higher dose are provided (Hekler et al., 2018; Lei et al., 2012; Lagoa et al., 2014).

The decision rules can be (1) simple, where the customization is done for one feature of the intervention on the basis of one tailoring variable, or (2) complex, where the tailoring is done for two or more features of the intervention, on the basis of two or more tailoring variables and at two or more time points. In the latter case, principles of control system engineering have been used to develop adaptive interventions (for detail, refer to Deshpande et al., 2014; Lagoa et al., 2014; Rivera et al., 2007).

To ensure their replicability and utility in informing interventionists or health professionals in delivering tailored or adaptive interventions, the decision rules should make explicit:

1. The tailoring variables: The variables should be clearly labeled and defined at the conceptual and operational levels.
2. The instruments measuring the variables: The instruments or measures should be described in terms of the attributes of the tailoring variable captured, the scoring procedure (i.e. how the total score is calculated to quantify the clients' level on the variable), and the interpretation of the score (e.g. cutoff score indicating presence or absence, or range of scores indicating different levels, of the variable).
3. The time at which assessment of the tailoring variables is conducted.
4. The set of possible interventions or components that could be offered through a range of modes and at different dose level: These should be clearly identified and described. The way in which the intervention features are modified and how should be clearly delineated.
5. The decision rules: The rules that link the tailoring variable and the level at which each variable is experienced (as represented by the cutoff or range of scores) with the corresponding intervention, component, or modified intervention features should be lucidly presented (Lei et al., 2012).

The algorithm must be reviewed by a panel of experts (researchers, health professionals, and clients) for precision, utility, and clarity. The experts review (1) the tailoring variables for relevance as the basis for customization; (2) the instrument for measuring the variables for content validity and accuracy of score interpretation;

(3) the appropriateness of the time points for assessing the variables; (4) the set of interventions, components, and modified features for relevance, feasibility, and effectiveness in addressing the unique experience of the health problem; and (5) the decision rules for clarity and accuracy. The experts engage in a discussion of what part to change and how in order to clarify or refine the algorithm.

### 4.5.4   Strengths

The advantages of tailored and adaptive interventions are well recognized. Interventions that match or fit with the clients' experiences of the health problem, are adapted to their initial characteristics and life context and/or readapted to their evolving experience or context, are likely perceived as relevant, acceptable, and potentially useful (Netto et al., 2010). Such favorable perceptions entice clients to initiate, engage, and adhere to treatment recommendations and, consequently, experience improvement in the health problem, functioning, and well-being. Further, tailored and adaptive interventions reduce treatment burden, negative effects, and waste associated with interventions, components, and doses that are inappropriate for individual clients (Deshpande et al., 2014; Heron & Smyth, 2010). Evidence indicates that clients value individualized care and prefer it over standardized care (Beck et al., 2010). Tailored interventions were found marginally successful in enhancing self-management in clients with chronic conditions, which may be due to low fidelity in implementing these interventions (Radhakrishan, 2012), but demonstrated clinically significant effects in changing health behaviors including smoking cessation, physical activity, healthy eating, and regular mammography screening (Krebs et al., 2010) and in improving a range of health outcomes (Richards et al., 2007).

### 4.5.5   Limitations

The design of tailored and adaptive interventions is labor intensive, time consuming, and potentially restricted by limited theoretical and empirical evidence required for developing accurate and useful decision rules. That is, there is limited information on what variables can be used for tailoring and on how intervention features can be customized without jeopardizing the intervention's integrity and effectiveness.

## REFERENCES

Abbey, M., Bartholomew, L.K., Chinbuah, M.A., et al. (2017) Development of a theory and evidence-based program to promote community treatment of fevers in children under five in a rural district in Southern Ghana: An intervention mapping approach. *BMC Public Health*, 17, 120–130. doi: 10.1186/s12889-016-3957-1

Abraham, C., Johnson, B.T., de Brui, M., & Luczcynska, A. (2014) Enhancing reporting of behavior change intervention evaluations. *Journal of Acquired Immune Deficiency Syndrome*, 66, S293–S299. doi:10.1097/QAI.0000000000000231

Ammendolia, C., Côté, P., Cancelliere, C., et al. (2016) Healthy and productive workers: Using intervention mapping to design a workplace health promotion and wellness program to improve presenteeism. *BMC Public Health*, 16, 1190–1207. doi: 10.1186/s12889-016-3843-x

Araújo-Soares, V., Hankonen, N., Presseau, J., et al. (2018) Developing behavior change interventions for self-management in chronic illness. *European Psychologist*, 24(1), 7–25.

Ball, L., Ball, D., Leveritt, M., et al. (2017) Using logic models to enhance the methodological quality of primary health-care interventions: Guidance from an intervention to promote nutrition care by general practitioners and practice nurses. *Australian Journal of Primary Health*, 23, 53–60. doi:10.1071/PY16038

Bartholomew, L.K., Kok, G., & Markham, C.M. (2016) *Planning Health Promotion Programs: An Intervention Mapping Approach*, 4th edn. John Wiley and Sons Inc., Hoboken, NJ.

Beall, R.F., Baskerville, N., Golfam, M., et al. (2014) Modes of delivery in prevention intervention studies: A rapid review. *European Journal of Clinical Investigation*, 44(7), 688–696. doi:10.1111/eci.12279

Beatty, L. & Binnion, C. (2016) A systematic review of predictors of, and reasons for, adherence to online psychological interventions. *International Journal of Behavior Medicine*, 23, 776–794. doi:10.1007/s12529-016-9556-9

Beck, D., Been-Dahmen, J., Peeters, M., et al. (2019) A nurse-led self-management support intervention (ZENN) for kidney transplant recipients using intervention mapping: Protocol for a mixed-methods feasibility study. *JMIR Research Protocols*, 8(3), e11856. https://www.researchprotocols.org/2019/3/e11856

Beck, C., McSweeney, J.C., Richards, K.C., et al. (2010) Challenges in tailored intervention research. *Nursing Outlook*, 58(2), 104–110. doi:10.1016/j.outlook.2009.10.004

Belansky, E.S., Cutforth, N., Chavez, R., et al. (2013) Adapted intervention mapping: A strategic planning process for increasing physical activity and healthy eating opportunities in schools via environment and policy change. *Journal of School Health*, 83, 194–205.

Bello, T.K. & Pillay, J. (2019) An evidence-based nutrition education programme for orphans and vulnerable children: Protocol on the development of nutrition education intervention for orphans in Soweto, South Africa using mixed methods research. *BMC Public Health*, 19, 306–315. doi:10.1186/s12889-019-6596-5

Berry, T.R., Chan, C.B., Bell, R.C., & Walker, J. (2012) Collective knowledge: Using a consensus conference approach to develop recommendations for physical activity and nutrition programs for persons with type 2 diabetes. *Frontiers in Endocrinology*, 3, article 161. doi:10.3389/Fendo.2012.00161

Besharati, F., Karimi-Shahanjarini, A., Hazavehei, S.M.M., et al. (2017) Development of a colorectal cancer screening intervention for Iranian adults: Appling intervention mapping. *Asian Pacific Journal of Cancer Prevention*, 18(8), 2193–2199. doi:10.22034/APJCP.2017.18.8.2193

Blamey, A.A.M., MacMillan, F., Fitzsimons, C.F., et al. (2012) Using program theory to strengthen research protocol and intervention design within an RCT of a walking intervention. *Evaluation*, 19(1), 5–23. doi:10.1177/1356389012470681

Bleijenberg, N., de Man-van Ginkel, J.M., Trappenburg, J.C.A., et al. (2018) Increasing value and reducing waste by optimizing the development of complex interventions: Enriching the development phase of the Medical Research Council (MRC) Framework. *International Journal of Nursing Studies*, 79, 86–93. doi:10.1016/j.ijnurstu.2017.12.001

Borelli, B., Sepinwall, D., Ernst, D., et al. (2005) A new tool to assess treatment fidelity and evaluation of treatment fidelity across 10 years of health behavior research. *Journal of Consulting and Clinical Psychology*, 73, 852–860.

Brendryen, H., Johansen, A., Nesvåg, S., et al. (2013) Constructing a theory- and evidence-based treatment rationale for complex eHealth interventions: Development of an online alcohol intervention using an intervention mapping approach. *JMIR Research Protocols*, 2(1), e6. doi:10.2196/resprot.2371

Burrell, B., Jordan, J., Crowe, M., et al. (2019) Using intervention mapping to design a self-management programme for older people with chronic conditions. *Nursing Inquiry*, 26, e12265. doi:`10.1111/nin.12265`

Byrd, T.L., Wilson, K.M., Smith, J.L., et al. (2012) Using intervention mapping as a participatory strategy: Development of a cervical cancer screening intervention for Hispanic women. *Health Education & Behavior*, 39(5) 603–611. doi: `10.1177/1090198111426452`

Cambon, L., Terral, P., & Alla, F. (2019) From intervention to interventional system: Towards greater theorization in population health intervention research. *BMC Public Health*, 19, 389–345. doi:`10.1186/s12889-019-6663-y`

Caminiti, C., Schulz, P., Marcomini, B., et al. (2017) Development of an education campaign to reduce delays in pre-hospital response to stroke. *BMC Emergency Medicine*, 17, 20–38. doi:`10.1186/s12873-017-0130-9`

Carroll, C., Booth, A., Leaviss, J., & Rick, J. (2013) "Best fit" framework synthesis: Refining the method. *BMC Medical Research Methodology*, 13, 37–51.

Carey, R.N., Connell, L.E., Johnston, M., et al. (2018) Behavior change techniques and their mechanisms of action: A synthesis of links described in published intervention literature. *Annals of Behavioral Medicine*, 53(8), 693–707. doi:`10.1093/abm/kay 078`

Chambers, A., MacFarlane, S., Zvonar, R., et al. (2019) A recipe for antimicrobial stewardship success: Using intervention mapping to develop a program to reduce antibiotic overuse in long-term care. *Infection Control & Hospital Epidemiology*, 40, 24–31. doi:`10.1017/ice.2018.281`

Chan, A.-W., Song, F., Vickers, A., et al. (2014) Increasing value and reducing waste: Addressing inaccessible research. *Lancet*, 383(9913), 257–266. doi: `10.1016/S0140-6736(13)62296-5`

Chen, H.-T., Pan, H.-L.W., Morosanu, L., & Turner, N. (2018) Using logic models and the action model/change model schema in planning the learning community program: A comparative case study. *Canadian Journal of Program Evaluation*, 33(1), 49–68. doi:`10.3138/cjpe.42116`

Chennaoui, M., Arnal, P.J., Sauvet, F., & Léger, D. (2015) Sleep and exercise: A reciprocal issue? *Sleep Medicine Review*, 20, 59–72. doi:`10.1016/j.smrv.2014.06.008`

Chorpita, B.F., Daleiden, E.L., & Weisz J.R. (2005) Identifying and selecting the common elements of evidence based interventions: A distillation and matching model. *Mental Health Services Research*, 7(1), 5–20. doi:`10.1007/s11020-005-1692-6`

Clark, M. (2015) Co-production in mental health care. *Mental Health Review Journal*, 20(4), e64331. `http://eprints.lse.ac.uk/64331`

Cohen, J.N., Potter, C.M., Drabick, D.A.G., et al. (2015) Clinical presentation and pharmacotherapy response in social anxiety disorder: The effect of etiological beliefs. *Psychiatry Research*, 228(1), 65–71. doi:`10.1016/j.psyhcres.2015.04.014`

Constantino, M.J., Coyne, A.E., Boswell, J.F., et al. (2018) A meta-analysis of the association between patients' early perception of treatment credibility and their posttreatment outcomes. *Psychotherapy*, 55(4), 486–495. doi:`10.1037/pst0000168`

Czajkowski, S.M., Powell, L.H., Adler, N., et al. (2015) From ideas to efficacy: The ORBIT model for developing behavioral treatments for chronic diseases. *Health Psychology*, 34(10), 971–982. doi:`10.1037/hea0000161`

Dalager, T., Højmark, A., Jensen, P.T., et al. (2019) Using an intervention mapping approach to develop prevention and rehabilitation strategies for musculoskeletal pain among surgeons. *BMC Public Health*, 19, 320–332. doi:`10.1186/s12889-019-6625-4`

Dalkin, S.M., Greenhalgh, J., Jones, D., et al. (2015) What's in a mechanism? Development of a key concept in realist evaluation. *Implementation Science*, 10, 49–55. doi:`10.1186/S13012-015-0237-X`

Davidoff, F., Dixon-Woods, M., Leviton, L., & Michie, S. (2015) Demystifying theory and its use in improvement. *BMJ Quality Safety*, 24(3), 228–238. doi: `10.1136/bmjqs-2014-003627`

de Boer, D., Delnoij, D., & Rademakers, J. (2013) The importance of patient-centered care for various groups. *Patient Education and Counseling*, 90, 405–410. doi: `10.1016/j.pec.2011.10.002`

Deshpande, S., Rivera, D.E., Younger, J.W., & Nandola, N.N. (2014) A control systems engineering approach for adaptive behavioral interventions: Illustration with a fibromyalgia intervention. *TBM*, 4, 275–289. doi: `10.1007/s13142-014-0282-z`

Direito, A., Walsh, D., Hinbarji, M., et al. (2018) Using the intervention mapping and behavioral intervention technology frameworks: Development of an mHealth intervention for physical activity and sedentary behavior change. *Health Education & Behavior*, 45(3), 331–348. doi: `10.1177/1090198117742438`

diRuffano, L.F., Dinnes, J., Taylor-Phillips, S., et al. (2017) Research waste in diagnostic trials: A methods review evaluating the reporting of test-treatment interventions. *BMC Medical Research Methodology*, 17, 32–44. doi:`10.1186/s12874-016-0286-0`

Dohnke, B., Dewitt, T., & Steinhilber, A. (2018) A prototype-targeting intervention for the promotion of healthy eating in adolescents Development and evaluation using intervention mapping. *Health Education*, 118(6), 450–469. doi: `10.1108/HE-11-2017-0065`

Durks, D., Fernandez-Llimos, F., Hossain, L.N., et al. (2017) Use of intervention mapping to enhance health care professional practice: A systematic review. *Health Education & Behavior*, 44(4), 524–535. doi: `10.1177/1090198117709885`

Edwards, J. & Kaimal, G. (2016) Using meta-synthesis to support application of qualitative methods findings in practice: A discussion of meta-ethnography, narrative synthesis, and critical interpretative synthesis. *The Arts in Psychotherapy*, 51, 30–35. doi: `10.1016/j.aip.2016.07.003`

Eidelman, P., Talbot, L., Ivers, H., et al. (2016) Change in dysfunctional beliefs about sleep in behavior therapy, cognitive therapy, and cognitive-behavioral therapy for insomnia. *Behavior therapy*, 47(1), 102–115.

Epstein, D.R., Sidani, S. Bootzin, R.R., & Belyea, M.J. (2012) Dismantling multi-component behavioral treatment for insomnia in older adults: A randomized controlled trial. *Sleep*, 35(6), 797–805.

Espie, C.A., Brooks, D.N., & Lindsay, W.R. (1989) An evaluation of tailored psychological treatment for insomnia. *Journal of Behavioral Therapy & Experimental Psychiatry*, 20(2), 143–153.

Fassier, J.B., Sarnin, P., Rouat, S., et al. (2019) Interventions developed with the intervention mapping protocol in work disability prevention: A systematic review of the literature. *Journal of Occupational Rehabilitation*, 29, 11–24. doi:`10.1007/s10926-018-9776-8`

Fox, M.T., Sidani, S., Persaud, M., et al. (2013) Acute care for elders components of acute geriatric unit care: Systematic descriptive review. *Journal of the American Geriatrics Society*, 61(6), 939–946.

Free, C., Phillips, G., Galli, L., et al. (2013) The effectiveness of mobile-health technology-based health behavior change or disease management interventions for health care consumers: A systematic review. *PLoS Medicine*, 10(1), e1001362. doi:`10.1371/journal.pmed.1001362`

Garba, R.M. & Gadanya, M.A. (2017) The role of intervention mapping in designing disease prevention interventions: A systematic review of the literature. *PLoS One*, 12, e0174438.

Glanz, K. & Bishop, D.B. (2010) The role of behavioral science theory in development and implementation of public health interventions. *Annual Review of Public Health*, 31, 399–418. doi:`10.1146/annurev.pubhealth. 012809.103604`

Golsteijn, R.H.J., Bolman, C., Volders, E., et al. (2017) Development of a computer-tailored physical activity intervention for prostate and colorectal cancer patients and survivors: OncoActive. *BMC Cancer*, 17, 446–464. doi: `10.1186/s12885-017-3397-z`

Gough, D. (2013) Meta-narrative and realist reviews: Guidance, rules, publication standards and quality appraisal. *BMC Medicine*, 11, 22–25.

Guruge, S., Wang, Z.Y., Jayasuriya-Illesinghe, V., & Sidani, S. (2017) Knowing so much, yet knowing so little: A scoping review of interventions that address the stigma of mental health in the Canadian context. *Psychology, Health & Medicine*, 22(5), 507–523. doi: `10.1080/13548506.2016.1191655`

Haanstra, T.M., Kamper, S.J., & Williams, C.M. (2015) Does adherence to treatment mediate the relationship between patients' treatment outcome expectancies and the outcomes of pain intensity and recovery from acute low back pain? *Pain*, 156(8), 1530–1536. doi:`10.1097/j.pain.0000000000000198`.

Harvey, A.G., Bélanger, L., Talbot, L., et al. (2014) Comparative efficacy of behavior therapy, cognitive therapy, and cognitive behavior therapy for chronic insomnia: A randomized controlled trial. *Journal of Consulting & Clinical Psychology*, 82(4), 670–683. doi:`10.1037/a0036606`

Hawkins, J., Madden, K., Fletcher, A., et al. (2017) Development of a framework for the co-production and prototyping of public health interventions. *BMC Public Health,* 17, 689–699. doi:`10.1186/s12889-017-4695-8`

Hekler, E.B., Rivera, D.E., Martin, C.A., et al. (2018) Optimizing adaptive interventions: Tutorial on when and how to use control systems engineering to optimize adaptive mHealth intervention. *Journal of Medical Internet Reseach*, 20(6), e214. doi: `10.2196/jmir.8622`

Heron, K.E. & Smyth, J.M. (2010) Ecological momentary interventions: Incorporating mobile technology into psychosocial and health behaviour treatments. *British Journal of Health Psychology*, 15, 1–39. doi:`10.1348/135910709x466063`

Hoffmann, T., Glasziou, P.P., Boutron, I., et al. (2014) Better reporting of interventions: Template for intervention description and replication (TIDieR) checklist and guide. *BMJ*, 348, 1678–1698. doi:`10.1136/bmj.g1687`

Hong, Q.N., Pluye, P., Bujold, M., & Wassef, M. (2017) Convergent and sequential synthesis designs: Implications for conducting and reporting systematic reviews of qualitative and quantitative evidence. *Systematic Reviews*, 6, 61–74. doi: `10.1186/s13643=017-04545-2`

Irish, L.A., Kline, C.E., Gunn, H.E., et al. (2015) The role of sleep hygiene in promoting public health: A review of empirical evidence. *Sleep Medicine Reviews*, 22, 23–36.

Johnson, K., Markham, C., Smith, R., & Tortolero, S.R. (2017) Be legendary—using intervention mapping and participatory strategies to develop a multi-component teen pregnancy prevention intervention for older teen males of color. *Journal of Applied Research on Children: Informing Policy for Children at Risk*, 8(1), Article 4.

Kazdin, A.E. (2007). Mediators and mechanisms of change in psychotherapy research. *The Annual Review of Clinical Psychology*, 3, 1–27. doi: `10.1146/annurev.clinpsy.3.022806.091432`

Kelly, C.M., Baker, E.A., Brownson, R.C., & Schootman, M. (2007) Translating research into practice: Using concept mapping to determine locally relevant intervention strategies to increase physical activity. *Evaluation & Program Planning*, 30, 282–293.

Kildea, J., Battista, J., Cabral, B., et al. (2019) Design and development of a person-centered patient portal using participatory stakeholder co-design. *Journal of Medical Internet Research*, 21(2), e11371. doi: `10.2196/11371`

Kok, G., Gottlieb, N.H., Peters, G.-J.Y., et al. (2016) A taxonomy of behavior change methods: An intervention mapping approach. *Health Psychology Review*, 10, 297–312. doi: `10.1080/17437199.2015.1077155`

Koutoukidis, D.A., Lopes, S., Atkins, L., et al. (2018) Use of intervention mapping to adapt a health behavior change intervention for endometrial cancer survivors: The shape-up following cancer treatment program. *BMC Public Health*, 18, 415–424. doi:`10.1186/s12889-018-5329-5`

Krebs, P., Prochaska, J.O., & Rossi, J. (2010) A meta-analysis of computer-tailored interventions for behavior change. *Preventive Medicine*, 51(3–4), 214–221.

Krops, L.A., Dekker, R., Geertzen, J.H.B., & Dijkstra1, P.U. (2018) Development of an intervention to stimulate physical activity in hard-to-reach physically disabled people and design of a pilot implementation: An intervention mapping approach. *BMJ Open*, 8, e020934. doi:`10.1136/bmjopen-2017-020934`

Lagoa, C., Bekiroglu, K., Lanza, S.T., & Murphy, S.A. (2014) Designing adaptive intensive interventions using methods from engineering. *Journal of Consulting and Clinical Psychology*, 82(5), 868–878. doi:`10.1037/a0037736`

Lamort-Bouché, M., Sarnin, P., Kok, G., et al. (2018) Interventions developed with the Intervention Mapping protocol in the field of cancer: A systematic review. *Psycho-Oncology*, 27, 1138–1149. doi:`10.1002/pon.4611`

Leask, C.F., Sandlund, M., & Skelton, D.A., (2019) Framework, principles and recommendations for utilising participatory methodologies in the co-creation and evaluation of public health interventions. *Research Involvement and Engagement*, 5, 2–17. doi:`10.1186/S40900-018-0136-9`.

Lei, H., Nahmu-Shani, I., Lynch, K., et al. (2012) A "SMART" Design for building individual treatment requences. *Annual Review of Clinical Psychology*, 8, 21–48. doi: `10.1146/annurev-clinpsy-032511-143152`

Lippke, S. & Ziegelman, J.P. (2008) Theory-based health behavior change: Developing, testing, and applying theories for evidence-based interventions. *Applied Psychology: An International Review*, 57, 698–716.

Manber, R., Carney, C., Edinger, J., et al. (2012) Dissemination of CBTI to the non-sleep specialist: Protocol development and training issues. *Journal of Clinical Sleep Medicine,* 8(2), 209–218. doi:`10.5664/jcsm.1786`

Mannion, R. & Exworthy, M. (2017).. (Re) Making the proscrustean bed? Standardization and customization as competing logics in healthcare. *International Journal of Health Policy Management*, 6(6), 301–304. doi:`10.15171/ijhpm.2017.35`

Mayne, J. (2017) Theory of change analysis: Building robust theories of change. *Canadian Journal of Program Evaluation*, 32(2), 155–173. doi:`10.3138/cjpe.31122`

Meng, A., Borg, V., & Clausen, T. (2019) Enhancing the social capital in industrial workplaces: Developing workplace interventions using intervention mapping. *Evaluation and Program Planning*, 72, 227–236. doi:`10.1016/j.evalprogplan.2018.11.007`

Mesters, I., Gijsbers, B., & Bartholomew, L.K. (2018) Promoting sustained breastfeeding of infants at risk for asthma: Explaining the "Active Ingredients" of an effective program using intervention mapping. *Frontiers in Public Health*, 6, 87. doi: `10.3389/fpubh.2018.00087`

Michie, S., Johnston, M., Francis, J., et al. (2008) From theory to intervention: Mapping theoretically derived behavioral determinants to behavior change techniques. *Applied Psychology: An International Review*, 57(4), 660–680.

Moore, G.F., Evans, R., Hawkins, J., et al. (2019) From complex social interventions to interventions in complex social systems: Future directions and unresolved questions for intervention development and evaluation. *Evaluation*, 25(1), 23–45.

Morin, C. M., Vallières, A., & Ivers, H. (2007) Dysfunctional beliefs and attitudes about sleep (DBAS): Validation of a brief version (DBAS-16). *Sleep*, 30(11), 1547–1554.

Murray, E. (2012) Web-based interventions for behavior change and self-management: Potential, pitfalls and progress. *Medicine*, 1(2), e3. doi: `10.2196/med20.1741`

Netto, G., Bohpal, R., Leberle, N., et al. (2010) How can health promotion interventions be adapted for minority ethnic communities? Five principles for guiding the development of behavioural interventions. *Health Promotion International*, 25(2), 248–257. doi: `10.1093/heapro/daq012`

Newby, K., Crutzen, R., Brown, K., et al. (2019) An intervention to increase condom use among users of chlamydia self-sampling websites (wrapped): Intervention mapping and think-aloud study. *JMIR Formative Research*, 3(2), e11242. doi: `10.2196/11242`

Painter, J.E., Borba, C.P.C., Hynes, M., et al. (2008) The use of theory in health behavior research from 2000-2005: A systematic review. *Annals of Behavioral Medicine*, 35, 358–362.

Paré, G., Trudel, M.-C., Jaana, M., & Kitsiou, S. (2015) Synthesizing information systems knowledge: A typology of literature reviews. *Information & Management*, 52, 183–199. doi: `10.1016/j.im.204.08.008`

Paul-Ebhohimhen, V. & Avenell, A. (2009) A systematic review of the effectiveness of group versus individual treatments for adult obesity. *Obesity Facts*, 2, 17–24. doi: `10.1159/000186144`

Pawson, R., Greenhalgh, T., Harvey, G., & Walshe, K. (2005) Realist review – A new method of systematic review design for complex policy interventions. *Journal of Health Services Research & Policy*, 10(Suppl 1), S21–S34.

Perry, C.K., McCalmont, J.C., Ward, J.P., et al. (2017) Mujeres Fuertes y Corazones Saludables: adaptation of the StrongWomen – healthy hearts program for rural Latinas using an intervention mapping approach. *BMC Public Health*, 17, 982–989. doi: `10.1186/s12889-017-4842-2`

Prestwich, A., Sniehotta, F.F., Whittington, C., et al. (2014) Does theory influence the effectiveness of health behavior interventions? Meta-analysis. *Health Psychology*, 33(5), 465–474. doi: `10.1037/a0032853`

Radhakrishan, K. (2012) The efficacy of tailored interventions for self-management outcomes of type 2 diabetes, hypertension or heart disease: A systematic review. *Journal of Advanced Nursing*, 68(3), 496–510. doi: `10.1111/j.1365-2648.2011.05860.x`

Raue, P.J. & Sirey, J.A. (2011) Designing personalized treatment engagement interventions for depressed older adults. *Psychiatry Clinics of North America*, 34(2), 489–500. doi: `10.1016/j.psc.2011.02.011`

Reach, G. (2016) Simplistic and complex thought in medicine: The rationale for a person-centered care model as a medical revolution. *Patient Preference & Adherence*, 10, 449–457.

Recht, M., Konkle, B.A., Jackson, S., et al. (2016) Recognizing the need for personalization of haemophilia patient-reported outcomes in the prophylaxis era. *Haemophilia*, 22, 825–832. doi: `10.1111/hae.13066`

Renger, R., Bartel, G., & Foltysova, J. (2013) The reciprocal relationship between implementation theory and program theory in assisting program design and decision-making. *Canadian Journal of Program Evaluation*, 28(1), 27–41.

Riemann, D., Baglioni, C., Bassetti, C., et al. (2017) European guideline for the diagnosis and treatment of insomnia. *Journal of Sleep Research*, 26(6), 675–700. doi:`10.1111/jsr.12594`

Richards, K.C., Enderlin, C.A., Beck, C., et al. (2007) Tailored biobehavioral interventions: A literature review and synthesis. *Research and Theory for Nursing Practice: An international Journal*, 21(4), 271–282.

Rivera, D.E., Pew, M.D., & Collins, L. (2007) Using engineering control principles to inform the design of adaptive interventions: A conceptual introduction. *Drug and Alcohol Dependence*, 88S, S31–S40. doi: `10.1016/j.drugalcdep.2006.10.020`

Robert, E., Samb, O.M., Marchal, B., & Ridde, V. (2017) Building a middle-range theory of free public healthcare seeking in sub-Saharan Africa: A realist review. *Health Policy & Planning*, 32, 1002–1014. doi: `10.1093/heapol/czx035`

Sidani, S. (2015). *Health Intervention Research: Advances in Research Design and Methods.* Sage, London, UK.

Sidani, S. & Fox, M. (2014) Patient-centered care: A clarification of its active ingredients. *Journal of Interprofessional Care,* 28(2), 134–141. doi: `10.3109/13561820.2013.86519`.

Sidani, S. & Fox, M. (2020) The role of treatment perceptions in intervention evaluation: A review. *Science of Nursing and Health Practices*.

Sidani, S., Reeves, S., Hurlock-Chorostecki, C., et al. (2017). Exploring differences in patient-centered practices among healthcare professionals in acute care settings. *Health Communication*, 12, 1–8.

Smith, F., Wallengren, C., & Öhlén, J. (2017) Participatory design in education materials in a health care context. *Action Research*, 15(3), 310–336.

Snilstveit, B., Oliver, S., & Vojtkova, M. (2012) Narrative approaches to systematic review and synthesis of evidence for international development policy and practice. *Journal of Development Effectiveness*, 4(3), 409–429. doi:`10.1080/19439342.2012.710641`

Sridharan, S., Jones, B., Caudill, B., & Nakaima, A. (2016) Steps towards incorporating heterogeneities into program theory: A case study of a data-driven approach. *Evaluation and Program Planning*, 58, 88–97. doi:`10.1016/j.evalprogplan.2016.05.002`

Van Assen, M.A.L.M., van Aert, R.C.M., & Wicherts, J.M. (2015) Meta-analysis using effect size distributions of only statistically significant studies. *Psychological Methods*, 20(3), 293–309.

Van Meijel, B., Gamel, C., van Swieten-Duijfjes, B., et al. (2004) The development of evidence based nursing interventions: Methodological considerations. *Journal of Advanced Nursing*, 48(1), 84–92.

van Mol, M., Nijkamp, M., Markham, C., & Ista, E. (2017) Using an intervention mapping approach to develop a discharge protocol for intensive care patients. *BMC Health Services Research*, 17, 837–849. doi: `10.1186/s12913-017-2782-2`

van Straten, A., van der Zweerde, T., Kleiboer, A., et al. (2018) Cognitive and behavioral therapies in the treatment of insomnia: A meta-analysis. *Sleep Medicine Reviews,* 38, 3–16.

Vittengl, J.R., Clark, L.A., Thase, M.E., & Jarrett, R.B. (2014) Are improvements in cognitive content and depressive symptoms correlates or mediators during acute-phase cognitive therapy for recurrent major depressive disorder? *International Journal of Cognitive Therapy*, 7(3), 255–271. doi:`10.1521/ijct.2014.7.3.251`

Wamsler, C. (2017) Stakeholder involvement in strategic adaptation planning: Transdisciplinarity and co-production at stake? *Environmental Science & Policy*, 75, 148–157. doi:`10.1016/j.envsci.2017.03.016`

White, H. (2018) Theory-based systematic reviews. *Journal of Development Effectiveness*, 10(1), 17–38. doi:`10.1080/19439342.2018.1439078`

Wight, D., Wimbush, E., Jepson, R., & Doi, L. (2016) Six steps in quality intervention development (6SQuID). *Journal of Epidemiology and Community Health*, 70, 520–525. doi:`10.1136/jech-2015-205952`

Wilt, J. (2012). Mediators and mechanisms of psychotherapy: Evaluating criteria for causality. *Graduate Student Journal of Psychology*, 14, 53–60.

Wittink, M.N., Morales, K.H., Cary, M., et al. (2013) Towards personalizing treatment for depression. Developing treatment values markers. *Patient*, 6, 35–43.

# CHAPTER 5

# Intervention Theory

The importance of developing the theory of the problem, the theory of implementation, and the theory of change is well recognized and emphasized in recent guidance for the design, delivery, and evaluation of health interventions (Bartholomew et al., 2016; Medical Research Guidance, 2019). The theory of the problem makes explicit the aspects of the health problem amenable to change and addressed by the intervention. The theory of implementation describes and justifies the active ingredients, operationalized into specific components that characterize the intervention. The theory of change delineates the mechanism through which the intervention produces beneficial outcomes related to the prevention, management, or resolution of the health problem and the mitigation of its consequences. Whereas each of these theories is important and useful for designing an intervention, their integration into the intervention theory is critical for a comprehensive understanding of the intervention, the context of its delivery, and its mechanism of action. This understanding forms the foundation for the development of materials and the mobilization of resources needed to deliver the intervention; the actual delivery of the intervention with fidelity, which is necessary to initiate its mechanism of action; and the design and conduct of a study to evaluate the intervention. In this chapter, the elements of the intervention theory are described. The importance of the theory in guiding the actual delivery of the intervention, and the design and conduct of an evaluation study is discussed.

## 5.1  INTERVENTION THEORY

The intervention theory integrates elements of the theory of the problem, the theory of implementation, and the theory of change into a unified comprehensive conceptualization of a health intervention. In general, the elements of the theory provide answers to these questions: What specifically does an intervention address, in what target client population and in what context? What comprises the intervention? How is the intervention to be delivered? How does the intervention work in improving what outcomes? What could influence the implementation, mechanism of action, and outcomes of the intervention?

*Nursing and Health Interventions: Design, Evaluation, and Implementation*, Second Edition.
Souraya Sidani and Carrie Jo Braden.

**TABLE 5.1**  Configurations of intervention theory.

| | Configuration 1 | Configuration 2 | Configuration 3 |
|---|---|---|---|
| **Field** | Program evaluation | Healthcare organization | Realist evaluation |
| **Sources** | Chen et al. (2018) US General Accountability office (2012) | Sidani and Sechrest (1999) | Dalkin et al. (2015) De Souza (2013) Greenhalgh et al. (2015) Pawson and Manzano-Santaella (2012) Wong et al. (2012) |
| **Elements and definitions** | *Situation* = problem that intervention attempts to address and context in which intervention is delivered | *Structure* = characteristics of clients receiving intervention, characteristics of health professionals delivering intervention, characteristics of context in which intervention is delivered | *Context* = conditions or circumstances in which intervention is introduced, encompassing resources and contextual factors that may moderate (enable or prevent) mechanisms and outcomes |
| | *Input* = resources required for intervention delivery | *Process* = intervention components | *Mechanism* = processes through which intervention components produce outcomes |
| | *Activities* = actions, therapies, or processes comprising intervention | *Outcomes* = series of changes leading to ultimate outcomes | *Outcome* = intended and unintended changes in clients' condition |
| | *Outcomes* = changes in clients' condition, including intended and unintended immediate, intermediate, and ultimate outcomes | | |

The intervention theory describes the health problem, the intervention, and the outcomes; explains the associations among them; specifies the conditions that may influence the associations; and offers directions for implementing the intervention (Dalkin et al., 2015; Davidoff et al., 2015; Slater & Kothari, 2014).

Three configurations are proposed to organize the elements of the intervention theory. The terms used in these configurations are presented in Table 5.1. Despite differences in terminology, the following specific elements are commonly identified.

## 5.1.1   Experience of the Health Problem

The intervention theory: (1) identifies and defines, at the conceptual and operational levels, the health problem addressed by the intervention; (2) clarifies and defines, at the conceptual and operational levels, the aspects (indicators, determinants) of the problem that are potentially modifiable and targeted by the intervention; and (3) explains the reasons for focusing on the selected aspects of the problem. For tailored and adaptive interventions, the theory describes variability in clients' characteristics and/or experience of the problem (i.e. tailoring variables) that should be attended and accounted for in the process of customizing the intervention.

## 5.1.2   Client Factors

The intervention theory identifies client factors that influence their: experience of the health problem, perception of the intervention, capacity to engage in the planned intervention activities, ability to enact the treatment recommendations, and experience of the immediate and intermediate (i.e. mediators) outcomes, as well as the ultimate outcomes. The theory explains why and how the factors exert their influence.

Influential client factors can be categorized into personal and health or clinical characteristics, and accessibility of resources, as mentioned and illustrated in Chapter 3. *Personal characteristics* encompass sociodemographic profile, and personal or cultural beliefs about health in general and the health problem and its treatment. *Health or clinical characteristics* represent individuals' physical, cognitive, and psychosocial functioning, presence of concurrent comorbid physical or mental conditions, and receipt of pharmacological and non-pharmacological therapies to manage the health problem and the comorbid conditions. Accessibility reflects the availability and clients' ability to access or use resources required to engage in the intervention (e.g. transportation to attend the group sessions in-person) and to enact treatment recommendations (e.g. physical, social, financial resources). For tailored and adaptive interventions, the theory identifies, in addition to these characteristics, client factors that form the basis for tailoring and explains the rationale for selecting them to inform the customization process.

## 5.1.3   Resources

The intervention theory specifies the material and human resources needed to enable the delivery of the intervention (Ball et al., 2017; Chen et al., 2018). Material resources are inferred from the description of the intervention's components (including content and activities) and mode of delivery (see Chapter 4 for examples). Material resources include the equipment (e.g. projector, models for demonstration of a skill like location of pressure points); infrastructure (e.g. room, access to computer or telephone); supplies (e.g. USB keys, folders) and written documents such as intervention manual that guides health professionals in implementing the intervention, and pamphlets, booklets, or modules that clients refer to when carrying out the treatment recommendations.

Human resources refer to all personnel involved in the delivery of the intervention. The specification of human resources should be consistent with local professional regulations; these indicate the qualifications of health professionals who can be entrusted the delivery of the intervention. The personnel involved in the delivery of the intervention may include: (1) support staff responsible for screening clients; (2) IT personnel responsible for developing technology-based interventions, and for supporting clients in the use of the respective technology; and (3) health professionals responsible for providing the intervention (face-to-face or distance) to clients. The characteristics of health professionals in direct contact with clients are of particular importance because they play a role in the implementation, and consequently the effectiveness of the intervention (see Chapter 8). Accordingly, the intervention theory specifies the salient personal attributes (e.g. communication skills) and professional qualifications (e.g. educational background) of health professionals that enable or limit the adequate implementation and subsequently, the mechanism of action, of the intervention (Dalkin et al., 2015; De Souza 2013; Greenhalgh et al., 2015).

### 5.1.4   Contextual Factors

The intervention theory describes the features in the context that are needed for an optimal implementation of the intervention. The features may be related to the physical, psychosocial, and/or political factors inherent in the setting in which health professionals deliver the intervention and the environment or life circumstances in which clients apply the treatment recommendations. The physical features are exemplified in the seating arrangement, lighting, and ambient temperature in the room where health professionals facilitate a face-to-face group therapy, and the safety of the neighborhood where clients are expected to walk. The psychosocial features are illustrated with effective communication and collaboration among all personnel involved in the delivery of the intervention, and with social support that clients need to carry out the treatment recommendations. The political features are related to decision makers' or community leaders' endorsement of the implementation of the intervention, and enforcement of policies and rules that ensure clients' accessibility to resources required for carrying out the treatment recommendations.

The intervention theory also clarifies the pathways (or how) through which contextual factors affect the implementation of the intervention. It may also explain if and how these factors interfere with the initiation of the intervention's mechanism of action and/or the achievement of the ultimate outcomes.

### 5.1.5   Intervention

The intervention theory describes the intervention at the conceptual and operational levels. At the conceptual level, the intervention is characterized in terms of its overall goal (e.g. prevention, management or resolution of the problem and its consequences) and active ingredients (see Chapter 4). The theory provides the rationale for the selection of the active ingredients. At the operational level, the intervention theory indicates how and why the active ingredients are operationalized into the respective specific components. For each component, the theory specifies its goal, content, activities, and mode of delivery. Furthermore, the theory clarifies the time point in the trajectory of the health problem (before or after its experience) at which the intervention is given; the sequence for providing the components; and the optimal dose at which the intervention is given. For tailored and adaptive interventions, the theory presents an overview of the customization or tailoring algorithm. The algorithm consists of decision rules that match the interventions, components, modes of delivery, and/or dose to the respective tailoring variables (e.g. client characteristics).

### 5.1.6   Mechanism

The intervention theory explains how the intervention's active ingredients, operationalized in the respective specific components, are expected to produce the desired changes in the immediate and intermediate outcomes that mediate the effects of the intervention on the ultimate outcomes (see Chapter 5). The theory provides a conceptual definition of each mediator. It also delineates the anticipated sequence with which the mediators occur with, during, and following exposure to the intervention. In addition, the theory indicates the timing surrounding delivery of the intervention at which the desired changes in the mediators can be observed and the pattern or trajectory (i.e. direction and rate) of change anticipated for these variables. For example, some interventions yield small but incremental changes, whereas others induce large changes in the mediators, within a short time period following intervention delivery, and these changes are maintained over time.

### 5.1.7   Outcomes

The intervention theory identifies the ultimate outcomes expected of the intervention. It delineates and explains how the desired changes in the aspects of the problem and/or the mediator contribute to changes in the ultimate outcomes. In addition, the theory defines the ultimate outcomes at the conceptual and operational levels and indicates the timing at which changes in the ultimate outcomes occur and the expected pattern of change over time.

There is increasing recognition that health interventions could result in unintended outcomes. These could be either beneficial (e.g. developing a more structured lifestyle with sleep restriction therapy) or harmful (e.g. increased anxiety) (Bonell et al., 2015). Where possible (based on theoretical predictions or available empirical evidence), the theory highlights potential unintended outcomes.

The intervention theory is presented in text and depicted in a logic model. The text format provides ample opportunity to describe the elements of the theory in detail, to define the main concepts (health problem, determinants, active ingredients of the intervention, outcomes) at the conceptual level, and to delineate and explain the proposed direct and indirect (moderated and mediated) relationships among the elements. The logic model depicts the relationships in a diagram as illustrated in Figure 5.1 or a flowchart as shown in Figure 5.2. The logic model, traditionally used in program evaluation, has resurged as a tool that is useful for conveying information about the intervention; it provides an overview or blueprint of the intervention which facilitates its understanding by various stakeholder groups. A review of the logic model helps (1) clarify the logic underpinning the intervention; (2) understand the strengths and weaknesses of the intervention as designed, in producing the anticipated outcomes; (3) identify the resources needed for its delivery; and (4) inform the implementation and evaluation of the intervention (Anderson et al., 2011; Ball et al., 2017; Baxter et al., 2014; Brousselle & Champagne, 2011).

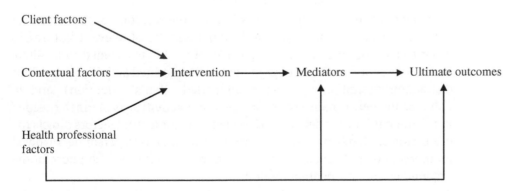

**FIGURE 5.1**   Logic model—diagram of relationships proposed by intervention theory.

Health Problem
[aspects addressed]
Intervention

| Influential factors | Activities | Outcomes | | |
|---|---|---|---|---|
| | | Immediate | Intermediate | Ultimate |
| Resources needed<br>*Human*<br>*Material* | Component 1<br><br>   *a. Goal*<br>   *b. Content / activities*<br>   *c. Model of delivery* | *Name* | *Name* | *Name* |
| Client factors<br>*Personal*<br>*characteristics*<br>*Health status*<br>*Accessibility to*<br>*resources* | Component 2<br><br>   *a. Goal*<br>   *b. Content / activities*<br>   *c. Model of delivery* | ⟹ | ⟹ | ⟹ |
| Contextual factors<br>*Physical*<br>*Psycho-social*<br>*Political* | Component 3<br><br>   *a. Goal*<br>   *b. Content / activities*<br>   *c. Model of delivery* | | | |
| Health professional<br>factors<br>*Personal attributes*<br>*Professional*<br>*qualifications* | Dose | | | |

**FIGURE 5.2**    Logic model—flowchart.

## 5.2    IMPORTANCE OF THE INTERVENTION THEORY

A well-developed and clearly described intervention theory guides the delivery of the intervention, and the design and conduct of its evaluation. The following is a discussion of the utility of the intervention theory:

1. *The preparation for delivering the intervention.*
   - Knowledge of the contextual factors informs the selection of the setting for delivering the intervention and/or the modifications of relevant features, in order to promote the comfort of participating clients (needed to facilitate knowledge acquisition and engagement in the planned activities); to reduce distraction/disruption (to ensure undivided clients' attention); and to enhance the performance of the intervention activities as planned (needed to maintain fidelity of delivery). Knowledge of contextual factors directs the discussion of effective means of communication among personnel involved in intervention delivery and the negotiation of stakeholders' support for the implementation of the intervention.
   - Awareness of environmental factors assists in the discussion, during the intervention delivery, of factors that may influence clients' application of treatment recommendations and of ways or strategies to address them.

- Information on the required material resources is necessary to ensure their availability in appropriate quantity and quality for use in intervention delivery.

- Information on the required human resources is essential to negotiate the personnel or staff complement to hire and to devise staff recruitment strategies. Awareness of the personal and professional profile helps in delineating the focus of the job interview; in selecting the most qualified; and in planning the staff training (see Chapter 8).

- The description of the intervention gives directions for developing the intervention protocol for standardized interventions; delineating the algorithm for tailored and adaptive interventions; and generating the modules for providing technology (web, computer, or mobile)-based interventions. The detailed description of the intervention components, and in particular the treatment recommendations, assists in creating written documents that clients may refer to in carrying out the treatment recommendations properly.

2. *The implementation or actual delivery of the intervention.*

- The specification of the health problem and its aspects addressed by the intervention is critical for identifying the timing within the trajectory of the health problem experience, for providing the intervention. This has implications for recruiting clients and delivering the intervention at the most opportune time, so that clients receive the intervention when it is most needed and benefit from it.

- The description of the intervention's components, mode of delivery and dose, as well as the sequence in which the components are to be given, informs:

  a. The development of the treatment protocol or manual that details the content, activities, and treatment recommendations to be covered in the intervention sessions or modules, and the sequence for providing them within and across sessions or modules (see Chapter 7). Health professionals are expected to follow the manual in delivering the intervention in order to minimize variation and enhance fidelity of delivery. Fidelity is associated with increased effectiveness of the intervention.

  b. The generation of instruments to monitor and assess fidelity with which health professionals deliver the intervention. Results of this assessment are used to provide feedback and support to health professionals.

  c. The creation of measures to assess the extent to which clients apply the treatment recommendations. Results of this assessment determine the need for discussing issues of adherence to treatment during the intervention delivery period.

- Awareness of client and contextual factors that influence implementation of the intervention assists in identifying elements of the intervention that are to be modified, and how. The modifications are necessary for consistency with the characteristics and life circumstances of subgroups of the client population and to fit with the features of the local context in which the intervention is delivered, without jeopardizing fidelity.

3. *The design and conduct of a study to evaluate the intervention's effectiveness.*

- The conceptual definition of the health problem and its aspects addressed by the intervention is important for identifying the target client population, specifying the inclusion criteria, and selecting the instrument for measuring the problem experience.

- Understanding of the client factors that affect the experience of the health problem as well as the intervention's implementation and/or effectiveness guides the specification of: (1) additional exclusion criteria whereby clients with particular characteristics that interfere with their ability to comprehend and apply the treatment recommendations are excluded; and (2) factors that moderate the effectiveness of the intervention; these factors should be assessed and modeled appropriately (e.g. covariate, subgroup analysis) in the data analysis aimed at determining the effects of the intervention.
- Knowledge of the characteristics and life circumstances (e.g. locations or events frequently attended by potentially eligible clients) of the target client population helps in selecting or devising recruitment strategies to reach all subgroups of the client population (see Chapter 15).
- Awareness of contextual factors potentially influencing the delivery and effectiveness of the intervention provides guidance for assessing them (quantitatively or qualitatively) and exploring how they contribute (hinder or enable) to the provision and effects of the intervention.
- Understanding of the intervention's active ingredients is important for selecting and specifying the comparison treatment. The latter treatment should not incorporate components operationalizing the active ingredients of the intervention (see Chapter 15).
- The instruments for assessing the fidelity of intervention delivery by health professionals and treatment adherence by clients are administered at the most appropriate time. The respective data are analyzed to determine the association between level of intervention implementation and improvement in outcomes. This association assists in interpreting the findings related to the effectiveness of the intervention.
- Delineation of the mechanism through which the intervention impacts the ultimate outcomes gives directions for:
  a. Selecting instruments that validly measure the mediators and the ultimate outcomes.
  b. Determining the most appropriate points in time before, during, and following delivery of the intervention, at which the mediators and the ultimate outcomes should be measured. The time points should coincide with those at which changes in the respective variables are expected to take place.
  c. Estimating the anticipated size of the intervention effect on the ultimate outcome; this is helpful in conducting the power analysis for the evaluation study, in particular when the intervention is newly designed.
  d. Planning and performing the data analysis. This involves: (1) specifying the hypothesized pattern of change in the mediators and ultimate outcomes, and testing it empirically; (2) specifying the inter-relationships among the receipt of the intervention or the level of fidelity and adherence, mediators, and ultimate outcomes, as well as the moderating effect of client or contextual factors, and examining these inter-relationships using advanced statistical tests.

4. *The interpretation of the evaluation study's results.*
- The intervention theory proposes the direct and indirect relationships among client and contextual factors, the intervention, the mediators, and the ultimate outcomes to be examined, and provides the frame of reference

for interpreting the results of the evaluation study. It highlights what exactly contribute to the improvement or non-improvement in the ultimate outcomes.

- Results of a theory-informed evaluation study provide answers to the clinically or practice relevant questions (Chapter 1) of: Who would most benefit from the intervention, given in what mode and at what dose, in what context? And how does the intervention work in producing beneficial ultimate outcomes related to improvement in the health problem experience, reduction in its consequences, and enhanced well-being.

## REFERENCES

Anderson, L.M., Petticrew, M., Rehfuess, E., et al. (2011) Using logic models to capture complexity in systematic reviews. *Research Synthesis Methods*, 2(1), 33–42.

Ball, L., Ball, D., Leveritt, M., et al. (2017) Using logic models to enhance the methodological quality of primary health-care interventions: Guidance from an intervention to promote nutrition care by general practitioners and practice nurses. *Australian Journal of Primary Health*, 23, 53-60.

Bartholomew, L.K., Kok, G., & Markham, C.M. (2016) *Planning Health Promotion Programs: An Intervention Mapping Approach* (4th ed). John Wiley and Amp; Sons Inc, New York.

Baxter, S.K., Blank, L., Woods, H.B., et al. (2014) Using logic model methods in systematic review synthesis: Describing complex pathways in referral management interventions. *BMC Medical Research Methodology*, 14, Article Number 62.

Bonell, C., Jamal, F., Melendez-Torres, G. J., & Cummins, S. (2015) "Dark logic": Theorising the harmful consequences of public health interventions. *Journal of Epidemiology and Community Health*, 69, 95-98.

Brousselle, A. & Champagne F. (2011) Program theory evaluation: Logic analysis. *Evaluation and Program Planning*, 34(1), 69–78.

Chen, H.-T., Pan, H.-L.W., Morosanu, L., & Turner, N. (2018) Using logic models and the action model/change model schema in planning the learning community program: A comparative case study. *The Canadian Journal of Program Evaluation*, 33(1), 49–68.

Dalkin, S.M., Greenhalgh, J., Jones, D., et al. (2015) What's in a mechanism? Development of a key concept in realist evaluation. *Implementation Science*, 10, 49–55.

Davidoff, F., Dixon-Woods, M., Leviton, L., & Michie, S. (2015) Demystifying theory and its use in improvement. *BMJ Quality and Safety*, 24(3), 228–238.

De Souza, D.E. (2013) Elaborating the context-mechanism-outcome configuration (CMOc) in realist evaluation: A critical realist perspective. *Evaluation*, 19(2), 141–145.

Greenhalgh, T., Wong, G., Jagosh, J., et al. (2015) Protocol—The RAMESES II study: Developing guidance and reporting standards for realist evaluation. *BMJ Open*, 5, e008567.

Medical Research Council (2019) *Developing and Evaluating Complex Interventions*. Authors

Pawson, R. & Manzano-Santaella, A., (2012) A realist diagnostic workshop. *Evaluation*, 18(2), 176–191.

Sidani, S. & Sechrest, L. (1999) Putting theory into operation. *American Journal of Evaluation*, 20(2), 227–238.

Slater, K.L. & Kothari, A., (2014) Using realist evaluation to open the back box on knowledge translation: A State-of-the-art review. *Implementation Science*, 9,115–128.

US General Accountability Office (2012) *Designing Evaluations*. GAO-12-208G. Washington, DC: The Auhor

Wong, G., Greenhalgh, T., Westhorp, G., & Pawson, R. (2012) Realist methods in medical education research: What are they & what can they contribute? *Medical Education*, 46, 89-96.

# DELIVERING INTERVENTIONS

# CHAPTER 6

# Overview of Intervention Delivery

Carefully designed health interventions, if not delivered as planned, may not induce the desired changes that mediate its effects on the ultimate outcomes. A successful delivery of an intervention rests on applying its components by carrying out the respective activities, in the selected mode, and at the specified dose. For most health interventions, a successful delivery is the responsibility of both (1) the health professionals (also referred to as providers, therapists, interventionists) entrusted the provision of the intervention, and (2) the clients (also referred to as persons and patients in practice, and participants in research) exposed to the intervention and expected to carry out the treatment recommendations.

The intervention theory plays an important role in informing the delivery of the intervention. In particular, elements of the theory of implementation, integrated into the intervention theory and depicted in the logic model (Nelson et al., 2012), guide the specifications of: (1) what is needed in terms of human and material resources, and contextual features, to facilitate the interventionists' and clients' performance of the intervention activities and treatment recommendations, respectively; (2) what are the intervention's specific and nonspecific components, and how they are operationalized into content to be conveyed, activities to be performed by the interventionists and clients during the intervention sessions as well as the treatment recommendations to be carried out by clients in daily life; and (3) how the components are delivered, in what sequence, where, when, and for how long (as explained in Chapters 4 and 5).

To inform the provision of the intervention, the specifications are captured in the intervention protocol or manual. The manual is a document that lists, for each session, the content or topics to be covered, the activities to be performed, and the treatment recommendations for clients to apply in daily life (also called homework) (see Chapter 7). Interventionists are trained (see Chapter 8) and requested to adhere to the manual in order to deliver the intervention with fidelity or integrity. Fidelity means that the intervention is provided as conceptualized (in the intervention theory) and operationalized (in the intervention manual), that is, as intended, designed, or planned. Delivering the intervention with fidelity is essential to initiate its mechanism of action that is responsible for generating the expected improvement in the ultimate outcomes.

*Nursing and Health Interventions: Design, Evaluation, and Implementation*, Second Edition.
Souraya Sidani and Carrie Jo Braden.

Despite extensive efforts at enhancing the delivery of health interventions with fidelity, in research and practice, variations in delivery are highly likely. The variations are introduced by the interventionists and/or the clients, for different reasons. The variations reduce the capacity of the intervention to initiate the mechanism of action and, consequently, its effectiveness in research and practice. In this chapter, possible variations in intervention delivery are described and their impact on the validity of inferences regarding the interventions' effectiveness is discussed. The importance of monitoring fidelity and strategies for promoting fidelity of intervention delivery are introduced. Key points in the fidelity-adaptation debate are highlighted.

## 6.1   VARIATIONS IN INTERVENTION DELIVERY

Variations in the delivery of a health intervention occur at different levels and for several reasons. The variations can take place when the researchers or health professionals engage in the operationalization of the intervention, when the interventionists actually provide the intervention, and when clients or participants apply the intervention. Possible reasons for these variations are presented next.

### 6.1.1   Variations in Operationalization of Interventions by Researchers

Researchers and health professionals, independently or collaboratively, engage in operationalizing the intervention's active ingredients that are identified in the intervention theory. This involves the specification of the components and the development of each component's content, activities, and treatment recommendations (see Chapter 4 and 5). Variations can happen in the operationalization process (Haynes et al., 2016). These variations are reflected in some discrepancy between the intervention's active ingredients as identified in the theory and the components operationalizing them. In other words, the components, specified in terms of content, activities, and treatment recommendations, are not fully in alignment with the active ingredients. This lack of correspondence between the conceptualization and operationalization of the intervention poses a major threat to construct validity of the intervention in that the components, as operationalized, may reflect active ingredients of other (than intended) health interventions. For instance, Keller et al. (2009) reviewed reports of studies that evaluated behavioral interventions to promote physical activity. They found examples of interventions that fell short of incorporating components or activities to promote achievement of the desired changes in key mediators, such as self-efficacy, of improvement in the ultimate outcomes, that is, engagement in physical activity.

Possible reasons for variations in the operationalization of health interventions include:

1. Lack of clarity or comprehensiveness in the conceptualization of the health problem and incomplete analysis of the problem that result in the misspecification of its potentially modifiable aspects. The misspecification contributes to the selection of active ingredients that either address the incorrectly identified aspects of the problem or are incongruent with the intended aspects of the problem (which were inaccurately understood).

2. Limited publication of conceptual knowledge about health interventions, reflected in the theories underpinning them. The limited knowledge presents challenges in delineating the active ingredients that comprise the interventions and in putting them into operation.

3. Scant description of the intervention in published reports, making it difficult to identify the active ingredients of the intervention, and to understand how they are operationalized and delivered (e.g. Abraham et al., 2014; diRuffano et al., 2017).

4. Limited experience in the systematic process for designing interventions and/ or in generating the intervention theory necessary to inform the operationalization of the intervention.

5. Limited time available for theorizing and analyzing the correspondence between the conceptualization and operationalization of the intervention due to social, political, or other types of pressure to find solutions to emerging pressing health problems.

## 6.1.2   Variations in Delivery of Interventions by Interventionists

Although the importance of fidelity is well recognized and its maintenance is emphasized, the chances for variations in the delivery of health interventions, in research and practice, are high. Emerging evidence indicates that interventionists do not fully adhere to the manual when providing interventions in research. A moderate level of adherence has been consistently reported (Hardeman et al., 2008; Toomey et al., 2019), implying that interventionists perform about 50% of the activities comprising the intervention components. Similarly, health professionals do not follow the manual when implementing interventions in practice. It is estimated that less than 50% of health professionals (also called healthcare or service providers, clinicians, practitioners) provide the evidence-based interventions with fidelity, even after training (Wiltsey-Stirman et al., 2015).

Nonadherence to the intervention manual results in variations with which the intervention is delivered to participants in research and clients seen in practice. The variations can take two general forms: adaptations of the intervention's components and/or mode and dose of delivery, and drifts represented in inconsistent delivery of the intervention across participants or clients. Adaptations and drifts are commonly observed in research and practice (DeRosier, 2019; Roscoe et al., 2019). They are often made by interventionists or health professionals delivering the intervention, usually without consultation with the intervention's designers or without reference to the intervention theory and relevant theoretical propositions that guide adaptations (Masterson-Algar et al., 2014; Wiltsey-Stirman et al., 2015).

### 6.1.2.1   Adaptations

Adaptations of the intervention entail modifications to the intervention. The modifications may be extensive so that what clients are exposed to deviates from what is originally designed or planned. The modifications may include:

1. Adding a new specific component; integrating a specific component from other established interventions; or removing a component (Pérez et al., 2016; Wiltsey-Stirman et al., 2015): These modifications result in a combination of components that are not congruent with changes or adaptations of the active

ingredients proposed in the intervention theory. Thus, the intervention as delivered is incongruent with the intervention as designed. This type of adaptation is a threat to construct validity because there is lack of clarity about what exactly is provided to clients and, consequently, what actually produced the intended outcomes.

2. Adding or removing a nonspecific component (e.g. providing feedback) to the intervention: These modifications may not alter the active ingredients but may affect the support that clients need to successfully carry out or enact the treatment recommendations and hence, benefit from the intervention.

3. Use of a different mode for delivering the intervention than the one specified in the intervention theory: This change may impact the size of the intervention effects, as reported in systematic reviews of health interventions. The results indicate that the size of the interventions' effects varies by mode of delivery. For instance, the effect sizes of behavioral therapies for insomnia were smaller with technology-based (self-help modules) delivery than face-to-face group sessions (e.g. van Straten et al., 2018).

Some adaptations of the intervention are made intentionally and formally. This is often done to adapt a generic approach to treatment to a particular health problem or client population including clients of diverse cultural background. For example, cognitive behavioral therapy is a generic approach that has been adapted for the management of insomnia and depression. These adaptations are systematically and carefully done to ensure correspondence of the intervention components with its active ingredients as specified in the intervention theory, while altering specific content, activities, or mode of delivery to accommodate the unique experience of the health problem and/or the characteristics of, the target client population.

Other adaptations of the intervention are not carefully planned, but made for different reasons. These tend to be encountered in several situations:

1. When the intervention is not well defined, its active ingredients are not clearly and explicitly specified: This situation leaves much room for variability in the interpretation of what the intervention comprises and therefore, its operationalization into specific components. In this case, the interventionists or health professionals may use their own frame of reference, expert knowledge or expertise, in articulating the active ingredients of the intervention, specifying its components, and delivering them. This results in deviation of what is provided from what is intended or planned, and variations in what different providers with different frame of references do and convey to clients in different contexts. For example, the intervention "provide psychological support" could be interpreted as any or a combination of the following activities: listen to the client, encourage the client to ventilate his or her feelings, or give positive feedback.

2. When the intervention manual is either not available or its content is not presented in a lucid way: In this situation, there is limited guidance for delivering the intervention. Thus, interventionists or health professionals do not have a clear description of the intervention content to convey and activities to perform, to use as a reference when delivering the intervention. Therefore, they may improvise and drift from what is intended.

3. When the interventionists or health professionals (1) do not have the qualifications required for delivering the intervention, such as expert knowledge of

the health problem and the intervention techniques (Lewis et al., 2019) and (2) do not receive adequate training in the theoretical underpinnings of the intervention and in the process for implementing correctly its components: In this case, interventionists or health professionals do not have the cognitive knowledge and the practical skills to successfully deliver the intervention as planned, leading to less-than-optimal or drifts in performance. Alternatively, providers with the required qualifications and mastery of the intervention protocol may modify components, content, or activities to fit with their expertise (Wiltsey-Stirman et al., 2015). Furthermore, those with unfavorable perceptions of the intervention may make adaptations that are in alignment with their views or beliefs of what would be the most appropriate therapeutic approach or method for the clients.

4. When the resources and the contextual features needed for optimal delivery of the intervention are not readily available: In this situation, interventionists or health professionals are forced to adapt the intervention activities and mode of delivery to be consistent with what is present or can be afforded in local settings. For instance, it may be challenging to provide cognitive behavioral therapy for insomnia in face-to-face sessions in rural remote areas due to the geographical dispersion of providers and clients. In this case, video or teleconferencing is a viable alternative mode of delivery.

The adaptations, if not carefully planned, may alter the intervention in a way that impacts its capacity in initiating the mechanism of action underlying its effects on the ultimate outcomes.

### 6.1.2.2  Drifts

Drifts involve inconsistency in the delivery of the intervention, whereby what the interventionists or health professionals provide varies across clients within or across practice settings. Therefore, clients are exposed to different components, content, activities, and treatment recommendations. Drifts may involve:

1. Customizing some aspects of the intervention to the characteristics, concerns, circumstances, or preferences of individual clients.

2. Loosening the structure of the intervention, whereby more time is permitted to discuss a topic of particular interest to clients, even if the topic is not within the scope of the intervention.

3. Temporarily deviating from the specific components of the intervention (Wiltsey-Stirman et al., 2015).

Drifts are exemplified with flexibility in delivering the cognitive behavioral therapy for insomnia in a group format. For instance, an interventionist may engage clients with cancer in a discussion of their experience of stress. The discussion, although unplanned, is necessary to address the clients' emotional needs. After all, the discussion is beneficial because stress is a determinant of poor sleep.

Drifts are more commonly encountered than adaptations in research and practice. When delivering standardized interventions, drifts are frequently related to the interventionists' or health professionals' perception of the importance of individualizing treatment; this consists of tailoring some intervention's content, activities, and/ or treatment recommendations to the personal profile and life circumstances of clients. Many health professionals are socialized to value person or client-centered care, which involves attending to people's individual needs, collaborating with people to plan care, and providing care that is responsive to people's needs and preferences (Sidani & Fox, 2014). They consider tailoring as an essential element of practice that defines high-quality care (e.g. Aggarwal et al., 2014). Accordingly, health professionals are inclined to drift away from the planned standardized intervention, modifying its content, activities, and treatment recommendations in an attempt to be responsive to clients' needs and life circumstances. They view such modifications as critical to demonstrate understanding and sensitivity to clients, which is the building block for initiating and maintaining a trusting relationship and a working alliance with clients. The relationship is the foundation for clients' satisfaction with, adherence to, and effectiveness of interventions (Waller, 2009).

When delivering tailored interventions in-person, drifts may happen if the customization process is not clearly articulated. In tailored interventions, interventionists or health professionals individualize aspects of the intervention to be responsive to clients' characteristics, based on a well-delineated algorithm, which consists of a set of decision rules. When these rules are not explicit or well described, providers are left with minimal guidance to structure the customization process. They are not clear on: what client characteristics to assess, when, how; how to interpret the results of the assessment; and what intervention component, content, activity, treatment recommendation, or mode of delivery to select. As a result, what is tailored and how it is tailored vary across clients.

When providing standardized or tailored interventions via technology-based modes, drifts may occur if the planned content and activities are not clearly presented and explained, with the potential of misinterpretation.

Drifts affect the reliability of the intervention delivery. This inconsistency is associated with variability in outcome achievement.

### 6.1.3   Variations in Application of Interventions by Clients

Clients are equal partners in the implementation of health interventions. They are expected to (1) attend the planned intervention sessions or review all modules for full exposure to the intervention components; (2) engage in the activities proposed for each session (e.g. discussion of barriers to skill performance) or module (e.g. set goals); and (3) enact or adhere to the treatment recommendations in daily life, correctly and consistently.

Variations in clients' attendance at sessions, engagement in the planned activities, and enactment of treatment recommendations are prevalent in research and practice. These variations are exemplified in situations when clients attend some but not all sessions or review some modules, carry out a select number of treatment recommendations, or inappropriately perform the recommendations. Variations in clients' implementation of the intervention are related to a wide range of reasons, including but not limited to:

1. Challenges in (1) attending the planned intervention in-person sessions—these may be attributed to out-of-control life events (e.g. acute illness, changes in work schedule), transportation or travel issues, forgetfulness, or dissatisfaction with the interventionists' performance or with group dynamics; (2) accessing the modules within the specified time frame due to difficulties with technology. These clients are not exposed to all intervention content and do not engage fully in the planned intervention activities, which may lead to less-than-optimal enactment of the treatment recommendations.

2. Misunderstanding the intervention's content, activities, treatment recommendations and dose, which contributes to inappropriate performance of the skills taught to enact the treatment recommendations in daily life: Misunderstanding may be observed in situations where the intervention is complex requiring many changes in the clients' cognition, behavior, and environment; clients are overwhelmed and may incorrectly apply some treatment recommendations. Misunderstanding can also take place when the content of the intervention is not relayed, orally or written, clearly to clients and in a manner that is meaningful to them (e.g. consistent with their general and health literacy levels).

3. Limited acquisition and sustainability of the skills, whether cognitive or behavioral, required to appropriately carry out the treatment recommendations: This situation may occur when the skills to be learned are complex, demanding, and not well described and explained; when clients are given a limited opportunity to demonstrate the application of the skills; and when clients are provided inadequate feedback on their skill performance, which is necessary to rectify the skills. For example, self-management of a chronic condition such as diabetes requires the acquisition of skills related to monitoring and interpreting changes in signs and symptoms; making decisions on which and how to apply multiple treatments (e.g. adjustment of insulin dose, physical activity, diet); and coping with psychosocial consequences of the condition (e.g. depression). Clients may not be able to grasp what these skills exactly entail and how best to perform them, all at once. Therefore, clients may not gain the skills, not apply them as taught, and lose the ability or will to perform them as recommended over time, which interfere with the achievement of the desired changes in the outcomes.

4. Unfavorable perceptions of the intervention as-a-whole or some of its components (Chapter 11): The perceptions affect clients' attendance, engagement, and enactment of treatment. Clients may perceive the intervention or some of its components (content, activities, treatment recommendations) as inconsistent with their beliefs about the health problem and its treatment, unacceptable (i.e. misaligned with their values), and unsuitable to their lifestyle. For instance, many clients with chronic insomnia view sleep restriction therapy unfavorably. They consider it counterintuitive and at odds with the common belief that people need eight hours of sleep per night (Matthews et al., 2013).

5. Unavailability of material (e.g. availability of vegetable and fruit at affordable price) and human (e.g. support from significant others) resources that clients need to carry out the treatment recommendations in daily life: Obviously, when the resources are not present, clients' engagement and enactment are less than optimal.

Variations in clients' engagement in the intervention are associated with variations in enactment; these, in turn, influence the level of improvement in the outcomes experienced. Overall, variations in providers' and clients' implementation of the intervention impact its effectiveness in the research and practice context.

## 6.2    IMPACT OF VARIATIONS IN INTERVENTION DELIVERY

Unplanned variations in the delivery of the intervention by interventionists and health professionals and in the implementation of the intervention by clients result in differences in what clients, expected to receive the same intervention, are actually exposed to and enact. The differences introduce biases that threaten construct, internal, and external validity of inferences about the effectiveness of the intervention.

### 6.2.1   Impact on Construct Validity

Deviations in the intervention' components that are actually provided from those that are originally designed threaten the construct validity of the intervention. Adding, omitting, or significantly modifying components can alter the active ingredients that characterize the intervention and that are operationalized in its components. These deviations manifest in misalignment or lack of correspondence between the planned content, activities, and treatment recommendations and those to which clients are exposed. Thus, what clients actually receive is dissimilar to what are the intended active ingredients of the intervention, raising the question: What intervention is exactly delivered? Clients are not exposed to and do not enact the intervention as designed; therefore, they may not demonstrate the hypothesized changes in the immediate, intermediate, and ultimate outcomes. The observed nonsignificant improvement in outcomes may lead to type II error, that is, concluding that the intervention as designed is ineffective (when it may have been successful if its components were not drastically modified). The end result is discarding a well-designed and potentially effective intervention (Borrelli, 2011). For example, omitting the sleep hygiene component from a behavioral therapy for insomnia, or not discussing its recommendations such as those related to the intake of caffeine and nicotine, can affect clients' enactment of these sleep-promoting behaviors; these behaviors may interfere with the effectiveness of the behavioral therapy in managing insomnia.

### 6.2.2   Impact on Internal Validity

Deviations in the intervention delivery from its original design, by adding or omitting components, present a threat to internal validity. Drastic changes in the components, particularly those operationalizing the intervention's active ingredients, alter (positively or negatively) the capacity of the intervention to impact the outcomes. In some instances, adding a component, such as activities to promote cohesiveness and support among clients attending a group session, can be beneficial in contributing to positive changes in the outcomes (e.g. Dirksen & Epstein, 2008). However, such deviations, although favorable, confound the intervention's effects and weaken the confidence in attributing the observed improvement in the outcomes solely and uniquely, to the intervention's active ingredients that are reflected in the specific components. In other situations, an intervention may still be found effective even if some of its components are omitted or modified. Although favorable, these findings raise the question: What exactly contributed to the improvement in the outcomes?

Variations in the delivery of the intervention across clients yield differences in the components, mode of delivery, and dose actually received by individuals. Although such variations may be carefully planned and operationalized in tailored and adaptive interventions, this may not be the case in standardized interventions. In instances characterized by variations in the delivery of standardized intervention, clients, unintentionally and informally, are exposed to different sets of components, learn about different contents, engage in different activities, and enact different treatment recommendations in varying ways and at varying dose levels. Thus, not all clients receive the same active ingredients. The inconsistency in the delivery of the intervention by interventionists and health professionals, and the associated inconsistent engagement and enactment of the intervention by clients, result in variations in clients' experience of improvement in the outcomes. Clients exposed to the full intervention (i.e. all its components, as designed) given in the selected mode and at the optimal dose demonstrate the expected pattern of change in the outcomes. Clients who receive some components in the same or different mode and at a less-than-optimal dose show limited improvement in the outcomes. Clients provided a few, if any, components in various modes and at a minimal dose level exhibit no change in the outcomes. Increased variability in the levels of outcome improvement, reported by clients assigned to the intervention group, dilutes the effectiveness of the intervention and reduces the statistical power to detect significant intervention effects (Ibrahim & Sidani, 2015; Stokes & Allor, 2016). The intervention is claimed ineffective. This conclusion is potentially erroneous (type III error) because the observed ineffectiveness is due to inconsistent and/or inappropriate delivery of the intervention (Rixon et al., 2016).

### 6.2.3  Impact on External Validity

Variations in the delivery of the intervention limit external validity. If not made explicit, the variations affect the replicability of the intervention's effects in different research and practice contexts (Campbell et al., 2013; O'Shea et al., 2016; Toomey et al., 2019). With the variations, it would be difficult to (1) determine the active ingredients, reflected in the specific components, that should be provided when the intervention is delivered by different interventionists and health professionals, to different clients, in different settings in order to replicate the intervention's effects on the desired outcomes; (2) identify the intervention's specific and nonspecific components, as well as mode of delivery, that could be modified in order to fit with the characteristics of the client population in different contexts; (3) delineate the most appropriate way to make these modifications without jeopardizing the intervention's integrity and effectiveness; and (4) specify the dose range that is associated with desired changes in the outcomes. This type of information is important to guide the translation and implementation of the intervention in practice.

In summary, variations in the delivery of an intervention by interventionists and health professionals and its implementation by clients can lead to inaccurate conclusions about its effectiveness. Therefore, it is essential to attend to the fidelity with which an intervention is provided.

## 6.3  INTERVENTION FIDELITY

The terms fidelity, integrity, and adherence have been used interchangeably (see Chapter 9) to refer to the extent to which an intervention is delivered as intended, planned, or originally designed (Berkel et al., 2019; Forsberg et al., 2015; French et al., 2015; Haynes et al., 2016; Toomey et al., 2019; Wojewodka et al., 2017). The concern is whether the interventionists and health professionals provide the intervention components; convey the content and the treatment recommendations; and perform the activities in the manner, mode, and dose specified in the intervention theory and described in the intervention manual. Because clients also participate in the implementation of health interventions, the conceptualization of fidelity has been extended to clients' enactment of the treatment recommendations, as intended or planned, in their daily life context (Prowse & Nagel, 2015).

Attendance to fidelity is increasingly emphasized in intervention evaluation (see Chapter 13) and implementation (see Chapter 16) research as a means to address variations in intervention delivery by providers and enactment by clients, which have been reported to contribute to outcome achievement (Roth & Pilling, 2008; Walton et al., 2017; Wang et al., 2015). Therefore, it is important to devise strategies to promote fidelity of intervention delivery; to monitor fidelity regularly throughout the intervention delivery; and to assess and account for the influence of fidelity on the outcomes. Attendance to fidelity has several advantages in research and practice.

1. Promoting fidelity has the potential to reduce variations in intervention delivery by interventionists and health professionals. Providing the intervention as designed and consistently across clients enhances clients' exposure to the content and activities required for their understanding and ability to carry out the treatment recommendations in daily life.

2. Monitoring fidelity with which interventionists and health professionals actually deliver the intervention to clients shed light on:
   - The providers' ability and skills in applying the intervention's components, conveying the content, and performing the activities as planned. Less-than-optimal performance of these skills identifies areas for further training (Lorencatto et al., 2013).
   - The providers' drift away from the intervention as designed at one point in time or over time (Kaye & Osteen, 2011): Monitoring provides an opportunity to observe drifts and to investigate reasons for the drifts. This information assists in early detection of error in delivery and suggests appropriate ways to address drifts, thereby preventing deviations from becoming widespread and long lasting (Borrelli, 2011).
   - Challenges in providers' delivery of the intervention and clients' engagement and enactment of the intervention: Knowledge of these challenges helps to identify aspects of the intervention that require improvement and ways to revise the intervention (Bond et al., 2011; Di Rezze et al., 2013; Lorencatto et al., 2013; Prowse & Nagel, 2015).

3. Assessing fidelity and accounting for its influence on the outcomes generate empirical evidence to support the validity of inferences regarding the effectiveness of the intervention. Specifically:
   a. Assessing the degree to which interventionists and health professionals delivered the intervention with fidelity helps to quantify the components actually given to clients. Comprehensive information on the specific and nonspecific components given and how these components, independently or combined, relate to levels of improvement in outcomes, is useful in determining which components contribute to outcomes. Differences in the association between components and outcomes across subgroups of the target population and/or context indicate the need for adapting the intervention. Similarly, assessment of the extent to which clients apply the treatment recommendations and examination of their contribution to outcomes generates evidence of the most relevant treatment recommendations for different client subgroups and in different contexts. Overall, this knowledge is useful for refining the intervention design, as needed (Wainer & Ingersoll, 2013), and revising the intervention manual; the revised manual identifies what adaptations can be made, how, for whom,

in what context, without jeopardizing fidelity. Detailed descriptions of the adaptations inform the accurate replication of the intervention by different providers, with different clients, in different contexts (Campbell et al., 2013; Di Rezze et al., 2013; O'Shea et al., 2016; Toomey et al., 2019), which enhances external validity.

b. Empirical evidence on fidelity is critical for correct interpretation of the results obtained in intervention evaluation studies.

- When the results indicate that the intervention is effective in producing the hypothesized improvement in the outcomes, evidence on fidelity determines if the observed changes in outcomes are attributable to the intervention's active ingredients represented in the appropriate delivery of the respective specific components.

- When the results indicate that the intervention is ineffective, evidence on fidelity informs the investigation and identification of factors that may account for the findings.

  o If the assessment of fidelity shows that the interventionists and health professionals deliver the intervention as planned, competently and consistently, and that clients engage and enact the intervention as planned, yet the intervention did not produce the anticipated changes in the outcomes, then it can be validly concluded that the intervention as designed is ineffective.

  o If the assessment of fidelity demonstrates variations in the implementation by interventionists and health professionals and clients, as well as in the levels of improvement in the outcomes, then it is clear that inappropriate delivery, rather than the intervention as designed, contributes to its ineffectiveness. Accordingly, evidence on fidelity avoids the commitment of type III error, that is, erroneously inferring that the intervention is not effective when it is poorly implemented (Breitenstein et al., 2010; Rixon et al., 2016).

- The assessment of fidelity could also identify the extent to which contamination or dissemination of the intervention to the comparison treatment group occurred, that is, whether participants in the comparison group were exposed to any component of the intervention. Participants in the comparison group who are exposed to some intervention components experience improvement in the outcomes that may be comparable to the improvement reported by participants in the intervention group. This, in turn, reduces the size of the between-group differences in the outcomes and the power to detect significant intervention effects.

Overall, assessing and accounting for fidelity of intervention delivery in the outcome analysis provide the evidence to determine whether the outcomes are attributable, with confidence, to the intervention's active ingredients, which is an issue of internal validity (e.g. Forsberg et al., 2015; O'Shea et al., 2016; Prowse & Nagel, 2015; Stokes & Allor, 2016). Cumulating evidence supports a positive association between fidelity of delivery and outcomes observed following completion of interventions, implying that optimal implementation generates the hypothesized improvement in the outcomes (e.g. Bond et al., 2011; Dunst et al., 2013; Schwartz et al., 2018; Sundell et al., 2016; Wang et al., 2015).

## 6.4    STRATEGIES TO ENHANCE FIDELITY

The important role of fidelity of intervention delivery in maintaining the validity of inferences about the effectiveness of health interventions imposes the need to integrate, within research and practice contexts, strategies to enhance fidelity and minimize variations in intervention delivery. The following are general strategies, which will be described in more detail in Chapter 9.

### 6.4.1    Strategies to Promote Fidelity

Two general strategies are recommended to promote fidelity and, hence, to minimize variations in the delivery of standardized and tailored interventions (Borrelli, 2011; Campbell et al., 2013; Hardeman et al., 2008).

1. *Development of an intervention manual:*The intervention manual (Chapter 7) covers the theoretical underpinning of the intervention (i.e. intervention theory), its operationalization in components or the tailoring algorithm, the resources required for proper delivery of the intervention, and the overall protocol for delivering the intervention. The manual includes step-by-step guidance for conveying the content and performing the specific activities, as well as for adapting relevant aspects of standardized interventions to meet the need of particular subgroups or individual clients. The manual serves as a reference for training interventionists and health professionals, for generating instruments to assess delivery of the intervention, and for continuous monitoring of intervention delivery.

2. *Careful recruitment, training, and supervision of interventionists:* Recruitment and selection of interventionists (Chapter 8) are informed by personal attributes and professional qualifications identified in the intervention theory as required for or as influencing the delivery of the intervention. Interventionists possessing the required professional qualifications are likely to understand the conceptualization of the intervention and to have the generic skills for the application of its components. Intensive training of providers in the conceptualization and the operationalization of the intervention is critical to deliver the intervention. Continuous supervision of providers' performance and provision of constructive feedback improves their skills and prevent unintended drifts.

### 6.4.2    Strategies to Assess Fidelity

Accurate assessment of fidelity demands the availability of instruments to measure the extent to which interventionists deliver the intervention as planned and described in the manual, and the extent to which clients engage in the intervention and enact the treatment recommendations appropriately. The assessment is done using various methods discussed in Chapter 9.

### 6.4.3    Strategies to Monitor Fidelity

Monitoring fidelity is a form of ongoing surveillance of the interventionists' performance in providing the intervention, the clients' engagement and enactment of treatment, and the factors that may influence implementation of the intervention. Monitoring fidelity is done at regular intervals throughout the intervention delivery, as part of process evaluation. Process evaluation (Chapter 13) aims at understanding how the intervention is given, what influences its implementation, and the capacity of the intervention to initiate its mechanism of action.

## 6.5  FIDELITY—ADAPTATION DEBATE

Despite efforts to promote fidelity (i.e. development of intervention manuals and training of providers), evidence clearly demonstrates variations in intervention delivery in research (e.g. Kyle et al., 2015; Toomey et al., 2019) and in practice (e.g. Brose et al., 2015; Cunningham & Card, 2014). In practice, variations and in particular adaptations of interventions are the rule rather than the exception (Pérez et al., 2016). Asking health professionals to strictly follow the intervention manual has been a challenge, with the potential of poor fidelity. Health professionals express resentment toward strictly adhering to the protocol when delivering interventions, and toward the implementation of standardized interventions. They believe that strict adherence leads to deterioration in the rapport, therapeutic relationship, or working alliance between interventionists and clients (Mignogna et al., 2018; Wallace & von Ranson, 2011). Yet, this relationship is emerging as a significant determinant of clients' engagement and enactment of the intervention, and subsequently experience of improvement in the outcomes (e.g. Webb et al., 2010). Health professionals believe in the importance of adapting or tailoring the intervention to clients' needs, characteristics, and life circumstances, as well as to clients' initial response to the intervention, for achieving successful outcomes. Interventionists' and health professionals' beliefs and attitudes have been found to affect the fidelity with which they deliver health interventions (e.g. Barber et al., 2007; Wang et al., 2015).

The debate between the importance of delivering interventions with fidelity and the perceived necessity of tailoring interventions could account for the reported high prevalence of adaptations in intervention delivery. Adaptations are often done for standardized interventions (DeRosier, 2019). Adaptations can be deliberate/ intentional or accidental/unintentional (Pérez et al., 2016). Their aim is to increase the relevance and applicability of standardized interventions to the characteristics of clients who receive it and/or to the features of the context in which the interventions are given. As such, adaptations are justified and sometimes desirable: They enhance the uptake of the intervention; improve the appropriateness or quality of its delivery by interventionists; and increase the intervention's acceptability, engagement, and enactment by clients, all of which contribute to the intervention's effectiveness (Wainer & Ingersoll, 2013; DeRosier, 2019; Mauricio et al., 2019). However, to achieve their potential benefits, adaptations should be carefully conceptualized within the parameters of the intervention theory and clearly delineated in the intervention protocol and manual that guides intervention delivery (Homel et al., 2019; Lewis et al., 2019).

The adaptation of health interventions should follow a systematic process during which the intervention designers or developers, health professionals, and clients collaborate to identify what needs to be modified, why and how; to specify the principles of adaptation; and to revise the intervention manual accordingly. Basically, the process of adaptation consists of group sessions that involve: (1) presentation of the intervention theory, to contextualize the discussion; (2) description of one intervention component; (3) delineation of how the component reflects the respective intervention's active ingredient and contributes to the desired changes; (4) identification of the resources needed to apply the component; (5) clarification, as needed, of any aspect of the component and its delivery; (6) discussion of the participants' overall perspective on the component as well as on aspects of the component that may not fit the needs or characteristics of the clients or the features of the implementation context—the discussion explores the reasons for the perceived misfit and ways to modify the aspects to improve the intervention's fit, without significantly altering the respective active ingredient; (7) repeating steps 2–6 for each component comprising the intervention; (8) review of the proposed adaptations and generation of clear principles and guidelines for what adaptation can be made, how, when, for what clients, and in what contexts. These principles and guidelines are incorporated in the intervention protocol and manual as suggested by Lewis et al. (2019).

Variants of this systematic process are described for the (1) the cultural adaptation of health interventions (e.g. Sidani et al., 2017), including the behavioral therapies for insomnia (Sidani et al., 2018); and (2) adaptation of interventions to the local target client population and context (e.g. Aarons et al., 2012; Cabassa et al., 2011, 2014; Fox et al., 2019).

## REFERENCES

Aarons, G.A., Green, A.E., Palinkas, L.A., et al. (2012) Dynamic adaptation process to implement an evidence-based child maltreatment intervention. *Implementation Science*, 7, 32.

Abraham, C., Johnson, B.T., de Brui, M., & Luczcynska, A. (2014) Enhancing reporting of behavior change intervention evaluations. *Journal of Acquired Immune Deficiency Syndromes*, 66, S293–S299.

Aggarwal, N.K., Glass, A., Tirado, A., et al. (2014) The development of the DSM-5 cultural formulation interview-Fidelity instrument (CFI-FI): A pilot study. *Journal of Health Care for the Poor and Underserved*, 25(3), 1397–1417.

Barber, J., Sharpless, B., Klostermann, S., & McCarthy, K. (2007) Assessing intervention competence and its relation to therapy outcome: A selected review derived from the outcome literature. *Professional Psychology: Practice*, 38, 493–500.

Berkel, C., Gallo, C.G., Sandler, I.N., et al. (2019) Redesigning implementation measurement for monitoring and quality improvement in community delivery settings. *The Journal of Primary Prevention*, 40, 111–127.

Bond, G.R., Becker, D.R., & Drake, R.E. (2011) Measurement of fidelity of implementation of evidence-based practices: Case example of the IPS Fidelity scale. *Clinical Psychology: Science and Practice*, 18, 126–141.

Borrelli, B. (2011) The assessment, monitoring and enhancement of treatment fidelity in public health clinical trials. *Journal of Public Health Dentistry*, 71, S52-S63.

Breitenstein, S.M., Gross, D., Garvey, C.A., et al. (2010) Implementing fidelity in community-based interventions. *Research in Nursing & Health*, 33, 164–173.

Brose, L.S., McEwen, A, Michie, S, et al. (2015) Treatment manuals, training and successful provision of stop smoking behavioral support. *Behavior Research and Therapy*, 71, 34–39.

Cabassa, L.J., Druss, B., Wang, Y., & Lewis-Fernández, R. (2011) Collaborative planning approach to inform the implementation of a healthcare manager intervention for Hispanics with serious mental illness: A study protocol. *Implementation Science*, 6, 80–89.

Cabassa, L.J., Gomes, A.P., Meyreles, Q., et al. (2014) Using the collaborative intervention planning framework to adapt a health-care manager intervention to a new population and provider group to improve the health of people with serious mental illness. *Implementation Science*, 9, 178.

Campbell, B.K., Buti, A., Fussell, H.E., et al. (2013) Therapist predictors of treatment delivery fidelity in community-based trial of 12-step facilitation. *American Journal of Drug and Alcohol Abuse*, 39, 304–311.

Cunningham, S.D. & Card, J.J. (2014) Realities of replication: Implementation of evidence-based interventions for HIV prevention in real-world settings. *Implementation Science*, 9, 5.

DeRosier, M.E. (2019). Three critical elements for real-time monitoring of implementation and adaptation of prevention programs. *The Journal of Primary Prevention*, 40, 129–135.

Di Rezze, B., Law, M., Eva, K., Pollock, N., & Gortier, J.W. (2013) Development of a generic fidelity measure for rehabilitation intervention research for children with physical disabilities. *Developmental Medicine and Child Neurology*, 55, 737–744.

Dirksen, S.R. & Epstein, D.R. (2008) Efficacy of an insomnia intervention on fatigue, mood and quality of life in breast cancer survivors. Randomized controlled trial. *Journal of Advanced Nursing*, 61(6), 664–675.

diRuffano, L.F., Dinnes, J., Taylor-Phillips, S., et al. (2017) Research waste in diagnostic trials: A methods review evaluating the reporting of test-treatment interventions. *BMC Medical Research Methodology*, 17, 32–44.

Dunst, C.J., Trivette, C.M., & Raab, M. (2013) An implementation science framework for conceptualizing and operationalizing fidelity in early childhood intervention studies. *Journal of Early Intervention*, 35(2), 85–101.

Forsberg, S., Fitzpatrick, K.K., Darcy, A., et al. (2015) Development and evaluation of a treatment fidelity instrument for family-based treatment of adolescent anorexia nervosa. *International Journal of Eating Disorders*, 48, 191–199.

Fox, M.T., Sidani, S., Butler, J.I., Skinner, M.W., & Alzghoul, M.M. (2019) Protocol of a multimethod descriptive study: Adapting hospital-to-home transitional care interventions to the rural healthcare context in Ontario, Canada. *BMJ Open*, 9, e028050.

French, C.T., Diekemper, R.L., & Irwin, R.S., on behalf of the CHEST Expert Cough Panel (2015) Assessment of intervention fidelity and recommendations for researchers conducting studies on the diagnosis and treatment of chronic cough in the adult. Chest guideline and expert panel report. *Chest*, 148(1), 32–54.

Hardeman, W., Michie, S., Fanshawe, T., et al. (2008) Fidelity of delivery of a physical activity intervention: Predictors and consequences. *Psychology and Health*, 23(1), 11–24.

Haynes, A., Brennan, S., Redman, S., et al. & the CIPHER team (2016) Figuring out fidelity: A world example of the methods used to identify, critique and revise the essential elements of a contextualized intervention in health policy agencies. *Implementation Science*, 11, 23–40.

Homel, R., Branch, S., & Freiberg, K. (2019) Implementation through community coalitions: The power of technology and of community-based intermediaries. *The Journal of Primary Prevention*, 40, 143–148.

Ibrahim, S. & Sidani, S. (2015) Fidelity of intervention implementation: A review of instruments. *Health*, 7, 1687–1695.

Kaye, S. & Osteen, P.J. (2011) Developing and validating measures for child welfare agencies to self-monitor fidelity to a child safety intervention. *Children and Youth Services Review*, 33, 2146–2151.

Keller, C., Fleury, J., Sidani, S., & Aisnworth, B. (2009) Fidelity to theory in PA intervention research. *Western Journal of Nursing Research*, 31, 289–311.

Kyle, S.D., Aquino, M.R.J., Miller, C., et al. (2015) Towards standardization and improved understanding of sleep restriction therapy for insomnia disorder: A systematic examination of CBT-I trial content. *Sleep Medicine Reviews*, 23, 83–88.

Lewis, C.C., Lyon, A.R., McBain, S.A., & Landes, S.J. (2019) Testing and exploring the limits of traditional notions of fidelity and adaptation in implementation of preventive interventions. *The Journal of Primary Prevention*, 40, 137–141.

Lorencatto, F., West, R., Christopherson, C., & Michie, S. (2013) Assessing fidelity of delivery of smoking cessation behavioral support in practice. *Implementation Science*, 8(1), 40–49.

Masterson-Algar, P., Burton, C.R., Rycroft-Malone, J., Sackley, C., & Walker, M.F. (2014) Towards a programme theory for fidelity in the evaluation of complex evaluations. *Journal of Evaluation in Clinical Practice*, 20(4), 445–52.

Matthews, E.E., Arnedt, J.T., McCarthy, M.S., Caddihy, L.J., & Aloia, M.S. (2013) Adherence to cognitive behavioral therapy for insomnia: A systematic review. *Sleep Medicine Reviews*, 17, 453–464.

Mauricio, A.M., Rudo-Stern, J., Dishion, T.J., Letham, K., & Lopez, M. (2019) Provider readiness and adaptations of competency drivers during scale-up of the family check-up. *The Journal of Primary Prevention*, 40, 51–68.

Mignogna, J., Martin, L.A., Harik, J., et al. (2018) "I had to somehow still be flexible": Exploring adaptations during implementation of brief cognitive behavioral therapy in primary care. *Implementation Science*, 13, 76–86.

Nelson, M.C., Cordray, D.S., Hulleman, C.S., Darrow, C.L., & Sommer, E.C. (2012) A procedure for assessing intervention fidelity in experiments testing educational and behavioral interventions. *Journal of Behavioral Health Services and Research*, 39, 374–396.

O'Shea, O., McCormick, R., Bradley, J.M., & O'Neill, B. (2016) Fidelity review: A scoping review of the methods used to evaluate treatment fidelity in behavioural change interventions. *Physical Therapy Reviews*, 21, 207–214.

Pérez, D., Van der Stuyft, P., del Carmen Zabala, M., Castro, M., & Lefèvre, P. (2016) A modified theoretical framework to assess implementation fidelity of adaptive public health interventions. *Implementation Science*, 11, 91–103.

Prowse, P.-T. & Nagel, T. (2015) A meta-evaluation: The role of treatment fidelity within psychosocial interventions during the last decade. *Journal of Psychiatry*, 18, 251–257.

Rixon, L., Baron, J., McGale, N., et al. (2016) Methods used to address fidelity of receipt in health intervention research: A citation analysis and systematic review. *BMC Health Services Research*, 16, 263–284.

Roscoe, J.N., Shapiro, V.B., Whitaker, K., & Kim, B.K.E. (2019) Classifying changes to preventive interventions: Applying adaptation taxonomies. *The Journal of Primary Prevention*, 40, 89–109.

Roth, A.D. & Pilling, S. (2008) Using an evidence-based methodology to identify the competences required to deliver effective cognitive and behavioural therapy for depression and anxiety disorders. *Behavioural and Cognitive Psychotherapy*, 36(2), 129–147.

Schwartz, C.L., Seyed-Safi, A., Haque, M.S., et al. (2018) Do patients actually do what we ask? Patient fidelity and persistence to the targets and self-Management for the Control of blood pressure in stroke and at risk groups blood pressure self-management intervention, *Journal of Hypertension*, 36(8), 1753–1761.

Sidani, S. & Fox, M. (2014) Patient-centered care: A clarification of its active ingredients. *Journal of Interprofessional Care*, 28(2), 134–141.

Sidani, S., Ibrahim, S., Lok, J., et al. (2017) An integrated strategy for the cultural adaptation of evidence-based interventions. *Health*, 9, 738–755.

Sidani, S., Ibrahim, S., Lok, J., Fan, L., & Fox, M. (2018) Implementing the integrated strategy for the cultural adaptation of evidence-based interventions: An illustration. *Canadian Journal of Nursing Research*, 50, 1–8.

Stokes, L. & Allor, J.H. (2016) A power analysis for fidelity measurement sample size determination. *Psychological Methods*, 21(1), 35–46.

Sundell, K., Beelmann, A., Hasson, H., & von Thiele Schwarz, U. (2016) Novel programs, international adoptions, or contextual adaptations? Meta-analytical results from German and Swedish intervention research. *Journal of Clinical Child & Adolescent Psychology*, 45(6), 784–796.

Toomey, E., Matvienko-Sikar, K., Heary, C., et al. On behalf of the Choosing Healthy Eating for Infant Health (CHErIsH) study team. (2019) Intervention fidelity within trials of infant feeding behavioral interventions to prevent childhood obesity: A systematic review. *Annals of Behavioral Medicine*, 53, 75–97.

van Straten, A., van der Zweerde, T., Kleiboer, A., et al. (2018) Cognitive and behavioral therapies in the treatment of insomnia: A meta-analysis. *Sleep Medicine Reviews*, 38, 3–16.

Wainer, A. & Ingersoll, B. (2013) Intervention fidelity: An essential component for understanding ASD parent training research and practice. *Clinical Psychology: Science and Practice*, 20, 325–374.

Wallace, L.M. & von Ranson, K.M. (2011) Treatment manuals: Use in the treatment of bulimia nervosa. *Behaviour Research and Therapy*, 49(11), 815–820.

Waller, G. (2009) Evidence-based treatment and therapist drift. *Behaviour Research and Therapy*, 47, 119–127.

Walton, H., Spector, A., Tombor, I., & Michie, S. (2017) Measures of fidelity of delivery of, and engagement with, complex, face-to-face health behaviour change interventions: A systematic review of measure quality. *British Journal of Health Psychology*, 22, 872–903.

Wang, B., Stanton, B., Deveaux, L., et al. (2015) Factors influencing implementation dose and fidelity thereof and related student outcomes of an evidence-based national HIV prevention program. *Implementation Science*, 10, 44–56.

Webb, C.A., DeRubeis, R.J., & Barber, J.P. (2010) Therapist adherence/competence and treatment outcome: A meta-analytic review. *Journal of Consulting and Clinical Psychology*, 78(2), 200–211.

Wiltsey-Stirman, S., Gutner, C.A., Crits-Christoph, P., et al. (2015) Relationships between clinician-level attributes and fidelity-consistent and fidelity-inconsistent modifications to an evidence-based psychotherapy. *Implementation Science*, 10, 115–124.

Wojewodka, G., Hurley, S., Taylor, S.J.C., et al. (2017) Implementation fidelity of a self-management cause of epilepsy: Method and assessment. *BMC Medical Research Methodology*, 17, 100–109.

# CHAPTER 7

# Development of Intervention Manual

Development of an intervention manual is one strategy that is foundational for promoting the fidelity with which a health intervention is delivered in research and practice. Although the terms protocol and manual are often used interchangeably in the literature, they may differ in the level of detail they offer in providing guidance for delivering an intervention. Just like the research design, operationalized in the study protocol, is the blueprint for conducting a study, the intervention protocol is the overall plan for providing the intervention. The protocol gives an overview of the intervention components and lists the topics and activities planned for each intervention session or module. Just like the procedure book or standards available for health professionals in practice, the intervention manual is a structured procedural text that outlines the rationale, goals, and content of an intervention, and details the techniques or actions for administering the intervention (Brose et al., 2015; Lorencatto et al., 2013). The manual is a document that describes the theoretical underpinning of the intervention and specifies what exactly is done, how, where, and when to deliver the intervention. Thus, the manual clarifies the logistics for providing the intervention as designed.

The procedural information presented in a manual differs with the format of health interventions. For standardized health interventions delivered by interventionists in face-to-face or distance format, the manual is available as a book or document that describes the step-by-step procedure for carrying out the activities planned for each session and includes scripts for conveying core content. For technology-based delivery of health interventions, the manual is reflected in the content and other material (e.g. video presentation, exercises) comprising each module. For tailored health interventions, the manual describes the decision rules that interventionists should follow in applying the customization algorithm or that are embedded in the delivery of technology-based adaptive interventions.

In this chapter, the approach for developing a manual is described. The content covered in the manual is specified and illustrated with examples. The potential use of the manual in research and practice is discussed.

*Nursing and Health Interventions: Design, Evaluation, and Implementation*, Second Edition.
Souraya Sidani and Carrie Jo Braden.
© 2021 John Wiley & Sons Ltd. Published 2021 by John Wiley & Sons Ltd.

## 7.1   APPROACH FOR DEVELOPING THE INTERVENTION MANUAL

The intervention theory (Chapter 5) informs the development of the manual. Different elements of the theory provide guidance in detailing what is to be done, why, and how. The theory provides the foundation for describing the theoretical underpinning of the intervention. Including the theoretical underpinning of the intervention assists providers in understanding the health problem and the characteristics of the target client population; in appreciating the importance of the intervention in addressing the problem; and in comprehending how the intervention as-a-whole and its components contribute to the desired changes in the outcomes. This knowledge helps interventionists grasp the significance of the intervention as designed and as operationalized. In fact, when surveyed about parts of intervention manuals most valued, health professionals attached greatest importance to the theoretical overview of the intervention and indicated that this helps them understand the rationale for the intervention (Barry et al., 2008).

The intervention theory identifies the resources required for providing the intervention. Awareness of the human and material resources helps in the specification of and making available/accessible: the particular resources needed for providing each session or module; the features and quality required for the appropriate use of the resources during intervention delivery; the number or quantity with which the resources should be available; and the rationale (i.e. why) and the technique (i.e. how, where, when) for using the resources. For instance, the delivery of web-based health interventions demands the availability of information technology (IT) staff who have expert knowledge and experience in manipulating, monitoring, and regularly checking on the functionality of the technology (which is the medium through which the intervention is given). The staff must have good interpersonal skills and must be accessible, when needed, to assist clients in resolving challenges navigating the system or arising technical difficulties clients may encounter.

The theory describes the contextual factors that affect the delivery of the intervention. The factors are identified and strategies to address them are described in the manual. Physical (e.g. room temperature) and psychosocial (e.g. some participants dominating the group discussion) factors inherent in the setting in which the intervention is delivered are highlighted and strategies to manage them are suggested. This information sensitizes the interventionists of their possible occurrence and the importance of attending to these factors in order to enhance the delivery of the intervention. Similarly, physical and psychosocial factors, inherent in the clients' environment that may affect clients' engagement and enactment of treatment are listed, and ways to handle them are proposed. In detailing the intervention delivery protocol, interventionists are encouraged to discuss the factors with the clients and involve clients in active problem-solving. Alternatively, this information forms the basis for formalizing the adaptation of the intervention's activities and treatment recommendations to fit with the life circumstances of clients who commonly encounter environmental factors. The principles and approaches for adaptations are incorporated in the manual.

Interventionists' personal characteristics (i.e. communication skills, interactional style) represent another set of contextual factors that influence the delivery of an intervention (see Chapter 8). To mitigate their potential influence, the manual describes:

1. The specific content to be covered and the *manner* to convey it: This is often done by preparing scripted text. The scripts advise interventionists on what to say and how, and are a means to standardize the communication of the intervention content.

2. The specific actions or behaviors that are prescribed (i.e. recommended) and proscribed (i.e. unhelpful) in communicating and interacting with clients: This information is reflected in the description of general principles for providing the intervention and the detailed description of how to perform a specific activity.

For example, in the first intervention session, the interventionists are expected to perform the first, conventionally prescribed, activity, which is to introduce themselves to clients. In a research study, the interventionists are advised to state their first name, to clarify their role (i.e. responsible for delivering the intervention), and to share their qualifications that enable them to provide the intervention. The latter may be related to the interventionists' personal experience with the health problem and the intervention. Sharing personal experiences is useful to reinforce the interventionists' qualifications, to provide reassurance to clients, and to develop perceived similarity between the interventionists and the clients. However, interventionists are proscribed from overly disclosing private personal information or experience that is irrelevant, distracting, time consuming, and potentially perceived as shifting the focus away from the clients (Jowers et al., 2019).

The theory delineates the active ingredients and the mechanism of action through which the intervention impacts the ultimate outcomes, which helps interventionists appreciate the contribution of the intervention. The theory identifies the components that operationalize the active ingredients as well as the sequence for providing the components, and the dose for providing the intervention. This information is integrated into a plan that outlines the number of sessions or modules, and the components to be offered within and over sessions or modules.

The theory specifies the goal, content, activities, treatment recommendations, mode of delivery, and the sequence for performing the activities within each component. This knowledge guides the detailing of what is to be done, how, and when. The "what" represents the specific content to be relayed and the specific actions to be carried out. The "how" reflects the selected mode of delivery and the way in which the content is conveyed and the actions are executed. The "when" illustrates the time, within a session or module, at which the specific activity is done. The detailed guide is generated for each session or module, and describes the step-by-step procedure to be followed when offering the sessions or modules.

Although essential for guiding intervention delivery, intervention manuals are not well received or favorably perceived by interventionists in the research context and by health professionals in the practice context. The main concern is that manuals are at odds with the client-centered approach to care that is highly and equally valued by providers and clients. Client-centered care demands flexibility in intervention delivery, which consists of adapting aspects of the intervention and/or its delivery in order to meet the individual characteristics, concerns, and life circumstances of clients. Flexibility is central to the development and maintenance of a good rapport, therapeutic relationship, or working alliance between interventionists and clients. This rapport contributes to clients' engagement, enactment, and satisfaction with the intervention, and consequently experience of improved outcomes (Borrelli, 2011; Brose et al., 2015). To address this tension between delivering intervention a) with fidelity, by strictly adhering to the intervention manual, and b) with flexibility by attending and responding to individual clients' concerns and life circumstances, there are calls to incorporate an additional part in the manual. This part covers principles and methods for adaptations of the intervention's elements that are within the parameters of the intervention theory (Brose et al., 2015; Lewis et al., 2019). The information in this part of the manual specifies what content, activity, treatment recommendation, and mode of delivery can be modified and how, without altering the intervention's active ingredients.

## 7.2   CONTENT OF AN INTERVENTION MANUAL

The intervention manual provides directions for delivering health interventions, in the selected mode, and at the specified dose. It is highly recommended to develop a manual for any intervention, whether comprised of a single or multiple components, and whether using a standardized or tailored approach to delivery. It is advisable to generate a comprehensive manual that gives an overview of the intervention, lists the resources required to deliver the intervention as designed, details the step-by-step procedure for carrying out the activities planned for each intervention session or module, and indicates possible adaptations to address frequently encountered clients' individual needs, concerns, or life circumstances (Barry et al., 2008; Hardeman et al., 2008). Whether available in hard or electronic copy, the intervention manual contains separate sections covering: overview of the intervention, required resources, the procedure for carrying out the intervention activities planned for each session, adaptations, and appendices. The content of these sections is described next and illustrated with examples from the manual for delivering the stimulus control therapy for insomnia.

### 7.2.1   Section 1: Overview of the Intervention

The first section of the manual gives an overview of the intervention theory and of the intervention.

The overview of the intervention theory is described in the text and summarized in a logic model, as mentioned in Chapter 5. The description covers: (1) the definition of the health problem; the aspects of the problem targeted by the intervention; client, interventionist and setting or environmental factors that influence directly or indirectly (moderate) the intervention delivery and outcomes; the immediate and intermediate outcomes that mediate the intervention's effects; and the ultimate outcomes; (2) the specification of the intervention's active ingredients and the respective components, mode and dose of delivery; and (3) the proposed relationships among the contextual factors, intervention, and outcomes. The description is supported by relevant theoretical literature and empirical evidence. Bibliography and additional readings are also cited and referenced (Barry et al., 2008). The overview of the intervention theory serves as a general orientation about what the intervention is about, who receives it, why and how it works. It also identifies the specific components that operationalize the intervention's active ingredients and that should be absolutely provided (under any circumstance) in order to claim the intervention, as designed, is actually given to clients.

The overview of the intervention reiterates the overall goals of the intervention, reviews the components constituting the intervention, and its mode and dose of delivery. The goals and activities characterizing each component are specified. This information is important to clarify the operationalization of the intervention, making explicit the correspondence between the active ingredients and the components. The intervention elements to describe in the overview are illustrated for the stimulus control therapy for insomnia in Table 7.1.

**TABLE 7.1** Overview of stimulus control therapy.

| Element to describe | Specific element | Example |
|---|---|---|
| Name of intervention | | Stimulus control therapy |
| Goals of intervention | Ultimate goals | To reduce the severity of insomnia and promote sleep in clients presenting with chronic insomnia |
| | Desired changes (immediate and intermediate outcomes) mediating intervention's effects on ultimate outcomes | Enhanced understanding of sleep and of factors that influence sleep |
| | | Increased awareness of behaviors that promote sleep and that interfere with sleep |
| | | Reassociation of the bed and the bedroom with sleepiness |
| | | Development of a consistent sleep pattern |
| Components and activities | Component 1: Sleep education | Goal: Inform clients about sleep and about factors that influence sleep. |
| | | Activities: |
| | | Discuss the following topics: |
| | | What is sleep and why do we sleep? |
| | | What is insomnia and what keeps insomnia going? |
| | | What factors influence sleep? |
| | Component 2: Sleep hygiene | Goal: Identify behaviors that promote or interfere with sleep. |
| | | Activities: |
| | | Discuss the general behaviors that affect sleep (i.e. those related to physical activity, fluid and food intake, and use of caffeine and nicotine). |
| | | Explain recommendations to address the behaviors |
| | | Encourage clients to reflect on personal performance of these behaviors and to apply the treatment recommendations that are consistent with their performance. |
| | Component 3: Stimulus control instructions | Goal: Reassociate the bed and bedroom with sleepiness and acquire a consistent sleep–wake pattern. |
| | | Activities: |
| | | Present the instructions related to going to bed only when sleepy, using the bed only for sleep, getting out of bed if cannot sleep and engaging in a quiet activity until sleepy, and waking up at the same time every day; explain reasons for these instructions; and involve clients in finding ways to carry out the instructions. |
| | | Discuss how each instruction works |
| | | Engage clients in generating strategies to promote application of the instructions |
| Mode of delivery | Group format involving four to six persons | Written presentation: |
| | Use combination of written and oral presentation and group discussion | Distribute booklet summarizing content pertaining to sleep education and hygiene and stimulus control instructions, for clients to follow through during verbal presentation and for future reference |
| | | Verbal presentation: Use simple terms to relay information on sleep education and hygiene and stimulus control instructions |
| | | Discussion: Ask questions to get clients to reflect on their beliefs and behaviors, how they relate to insomnia, and what they can do to change general behaviors and sleep habits; assist clients in tailoring instructions to their personal context; explore issues of adherence; involve all clients in responding; and provide feedback to reinforce changes in sleep related behaviors |
| Dose | Two sessions. | |
| | Each session is of 90-minute duration; given once every other week, over a four-week treatment period | |

## 7.2.2  Section 2: Required Resources

The second section of the manual presents a list of the resources required to carry out the activities planned for each session, in the selected mode. The list includes human and material resources.

Human resources relate to persons other than the interventionist who are involved in:

1. Ensuring and/or monitoring the functionality of technology used in delivering the intervention: For instance, IT staff members assist in setting up and ensuring proper operation of equipment to be used when implementing relevant intervention activities such as showing a video or slide presentation.
2. Preparing documents containing client-related information that guides the performance of relevant intervention activities: For example, clients receiving the stimulus control therapy are asked to complete a daily sleep diary. A staff member is expected to compute weekly averages of the treatment recommendations applied and of pertinent sleep or insomnia indicators (e.g. total sleep time). The interventionist reviews this information with clients to reinforce their performance, points to progress made, and addresses challenges in carrying out the treatment recommendations.
3. Providing some aspects of the intervention or assisting in carrying out specific intervention activities: For instance, interventions aimed at improving self-management in clients with chronic diseases consist of multiple components addressing different domains of health and related treatment recommendations such as medications, diet, and physical activities. The components are delivered by different health professionals, based on their expertise, whereby the pharmacist discusses medications, nutritionist discusses diet, and physiotherapist discuses physical activity. Self-management interventions may also include components and activities focusing on enhancing self-efficacy and involve laypersons or other clients who demonstrate high levels of self-efficacy and effective self-management; these clients are requested to share their experience, thereby serving as role models. Role modeling is a behavior change technique for enhancing self-efficacy (Bartholomew et al., 2016).

In this section of the manual, the category of human resources is identified. The role and responsibility of each staff member in providing the intervention are described. Strategies for communication (e.g. contact information) and collaboration between the staff members and the interventionist are presented.

Material resources include all items necessary for carrying out the intervention activities as planned. These resources relate to the environment in which the intervention is given and the objects required for its delivery. Aspects of the environment include:

1. Physical space, such as availability of a room that is of the appropriate size (e.g. medium-sized room to hold group sessions, small room for individual sessions), that minimizes distraction by external noise or events, enhances privacy, and is easily accessible to all clients, including those with physical limitations.
2. Furniture, such as availability of a roundtable to promote group discussion and interaction, comfortable chairs to facilitate relaxation, and fridge to store perishable food items to be used for demonstration.

3. Setting's ambience or features, such as comfortable room temperature and adequate lighting, and capacity to arrange and access items in a way that allows uninterrupted performance of intervention activities.

The objects include:

1. Equipment required for demonstrating access or use of technology-based interventions (e.g. mobile, internet access) or for carrying out specific intervention activities such as laptop, projector, and screen to show a video demonstrating the performance of a skill or behavior; treadmill or cycling machine to perform recommended exercises under the interventionist's supervision.
2. Documents (in hard or electronic copy) to use during an intervention session and to distribute to clients for reference, such as booklets or modules presenting key information that guides clients' application of the treatment recommendations on their own, in daily life.
3. Forms or worksheets to be completed by the interventionists and by the clients during the intervention session, such as instruments measuring the tailoring variables (completed prior to tailoring the intervention), or worksheets to document the individual client's goals and action plans.
4. Forms to be completed by clients to document their implementation of the treatment recommendations and/or their experience of the health problem (e.g. daily sleep diary).
5. Specific supplies needed to carry out the intervention activities, such as pens, food items, or restaurant menu.

The human and material resources required for providing health interventions vary with the type (or nature) of the intervention and its selected mode of delivery. The list of resources mentioned previously is by no means exhaustive; however, it reflects the categories of resources to be mentioned and described in the intervention manual. The list then serves as a reminder for interventionists to (1) contact other staff members and collaborate with them to organize the appropriate and timely delivery of the intervention; (2) ensure the availability of all material items, in the right number (commensurate with the number of clients expected to receive the intervention at the same time). For interventions given in multiple sessions or modules and/or in different modes, it may be useful to specify the resources needed for each session or module, particularly if the specific resources or items differ across sessions or modules. Some items are given only in one session (e.g. hard copy of booklets are distributed to clients attending the first session) and other items are necessary to facilitate the remaining sessions (e.g. forms or documents graphing clients' progress, which are given in subsequent sessions as means to reinforce performance of treatment recommendations or to discuss challenges). An example of material resources needed to deliver the first session of the stimulus control therapy, in a group format, is presented in Table 7.2.

### 7.2.3   Section 3: Procedure

The third section of the intervention manual contains a description of the procedure to be followed when delivering the intervention. The description details the steps for carrying out the activities planned for each intervention session or module, in the selected mode; it also provides scripts for the information (content, treatment recommendations) to be relayed to clients. The detailed description of the procedure

**TABLE 7.2**   Resources needed to deliver the first session of stimulus control therapy.

| Category | Items |
|---|---|
| Staff | Connect with staff to ensure the appropriate room is reserved, the appropriate amount of objects is available |
| Environment | Medium-sized room allowing:<br>• Seating of a group of four to eight clients in a roundtable format to promote group discussion<br>• Good lighting to make it easy to read written information<br>• Comfortable temperature<br>• Good acoustics and minimal external noise to make it easy to hear, particularly for clients with hearing problem, and to reduce distraction. |
| Objects: | Folders to distribute to clients containing:<br>Sleep education and hygiene booklet<br>List of stimulus control instructions<br>List of activities to be completed by clients once they identify quiet activities in which to engage when they cannot sleep<br>Daily sleep diary forms for clients to document the wake-up time agreed upon and to be followed consistently<br>Schedule for the remaining intervention sessions |
| | Form graphing the clients' sleep onset latency, wake after sleep onset, total sleep time, total time in bed, and sleep efficiency reported at baseline; two copies of the form are prepared; the interventionist keeps one and gives one to the client for review during the session |
| | Group session log for interventionist to take clients' attendance at the session |
| | Pens for clients to take notes as needed and to write down information (e.g. list of quiet activities) discussed during the session |

clarifies to interventionists what they are exactly to say or do, how, where, and when. It facilitates the implementation, with fidelity and consistency across clients, of standardized or tailored interventions.

## 7.2.3.1   Standardized Interventions

For standardized interventions, the procedure is described for each session, and the respective steps are presented in a sequence reflecting common logic and the propositions of the intervention theory. Common logic suggests that the sessions are organized into introduction, main part, and conclusion. The intervention theory proposes the sequence for providing the components and activities within the main part of the sessions. The theory indicates if some components and activities are considered foundational or building blocks for providing other components and activities. In the example of stimulus control therapy, it is essential to first give sleep education with an emphasis on factors that control sleep (i.e. sleep drive and biologic rhythms) because some of the stimulus control therapy instructions or treatment recommendations (e.g. avoid napping late in the day and in the evening) are based on these factors (e.g. napping in the evening interferes with sleep drive).

For each session, the step-by-step procedure is described for the introduction, main part, and conclusion. The steps are portrayed in specific actions to be performed by the interventionist and the clients.

## Introduction

The introductory steps of the first intervention session vary from those of remaining sessions. In the first session, the initial steps entail general introductions and provision of an overview of the intervention. General introductions aim to get the interventionist and clients to know each other. The interventionist introduces herself or himself to clients, stating her or his name and role in the delivery of the intervention. Clients are asked to introduce themselves, stating their first name only to maintain confidentiality in group sessions; to share briefly their experience with the health problem; and to express their expectations of treatment. This first step serves as an "ice-breaker" and fosters the development of a rapport between the interventionist and the client in interventions given on an individual basis; in addition, it promotes the development of a supportive relationship and cohesion among clients in interventions given in a group format. The interventionist can point to similarity in clients' experiences as an additional means for promoting group rapport and cohesion.

The second step consists of providing an overview of the intervention. The interventionist follows a script to explain the intervention's goals, components, and dose (i.e. number and duration of sessions), as well as the clients' responsibilities related to engagement in the intervention's activities and enactment of treatment recommendations. The interventionist may emphasize the importance of clients' enactment of treatment recommendations in experiencing beneficial changes in the health problem. The information relayed in this second step helps clients understand the rationale and the general nature of the intervention, as well as what is expected of them. Clarification of expectations at the beginning of the intervention delivery reduces the likelihood of misinterpretation of what the intervention is set to achieve, and consequently a sense of disappointment and dissatisfaction with the intervention, which lead to withdrawal and nonadherence to treatment.

In subsequent sessions, the introductory steps may include: brief introductions if the group membership has changed; an ice-breaking exercise to further enhance rapport or cohesion among group members; self-completion of a brief questionnaire assessing clients' experience of the health problem or perception of progress toward achieving individual goals (the responses to the questionnaire can be discussed later in the session if planned); or general but brief discussion of clients' ability to apply the treatment recommendations, which serves as a leeway for a review of the recommendations and challenges in their implementation and as a strategy for allowing clients to express individual concerns. The fourth section of the manual (adaptations) describes the principles and methods for addressing individual concerns.

## Main Part

The main part of the intervention session consists of the specific actions that represent the application of the intervention components and activities planned for the session. The actions are presented in the sequence proposed in the intervention theory. Each step is specified in a statement that identifies who (interventionist or client) is to do what (action) in what way (how). It may be useful to indicate the time allotted for each component or activity within each session. A time range (e.g. 15–20 minutes) is specified to accommodate for discussion of clients' concerns, while ensuring coverage of all content and performance of all activities planned for the session.

Each step is described in a clear statement of the action to be performed and the qualifiers of the performance of the action, followed by a script clarifying the information to be relayed to clients. The statement may begin with a verb that best reflects the action to be performed. The qualifiers identify the way in which the action is to be performed. It may be useful to mention proscribed behaviors following the description of the action, and to highlight actions that can be modified, if necessary, to meet clients' individual concerns or life circumstances. The modifications are described in the fourth section of the manual.

The script is written in simple, nontechnical language that is easy to understand by clients with different levels of language proficiency or literacy. The scripted sentences are short, presenting one idea or point at a time. The sentences are structured in a way that makes it easy for clients to grasp the content and to follow through; that is, the sentences are prepared in spoken language. For example, the statement of the first introductory step, general introductions, of the stimulus control therapy is described as follows:

*Step 1 – Introduce (action) self as therapist (who)*
- State interventionist's first name.
- Identify role as being responsible for facilitating the sessions (qualifier).
- Review interventionist's professional qualifications and relevant experience.

Note: proscribed behavior: do not disclose private personal information.

*Script*:
- I would like to welcome you to this first session.
- My name is Jane. I am the sleep therapist. I have personally experienced insomnia and understand what you are going through.
- I will facilitate the group sessions and work with you throughout the sessions of this treatment.

## Conclusion

The concluding steps relate to termination of the session. These steps include: (1) recapping the main points discussed during the session; (2) reviewing the treatment recommendations that clients are expected to enact in daily life; (3) explaining assignments or homework or treatment recommendations for clients to do in the time interval between sessions (e.g. setting goals, completing daily sleep diary, applying the stimulus control instructions); and (4) reminding them of the logistics of the next session (i.e. date, time, location). In the last session of health interventions given in multiple sessions or at the end of the session of interventions given in a single session, the concluding steps involve: informing clients of the completion of the intervention, inquiring about questions or concerns clients may have about the intervention, and highlighting the activities or treatment recommendations they are expected to continue carrying out, if necessary, in daily life.

Table 7.3 provides excerpts of the manual for delivering the stimulus control therapy for insomnia, for illustrative purposes. The excerpts were selected to represent the introduction, main part, and conclusion of the first and second sessions of a standardized intervention.

**TABLE 7.3**    Excerpts of manual for delivering sessions 1 and 2 of stimulus control therapy.

**Session 1**

*Introduction* (15–20 minutes)

*Ask* if clients have any questions and address them as needed.

*Main Part*: (60 minutes)

   *Inform* clients of the next topic of presentation: sleep hygiene, using the following script as a guide:

   Now that we have discussed what is insomnia, how it starts, and how it keeps going; we will now discuss what can persons with insomnia do to sleep better.

   In general, persons with insomnia have to get rid of habits that hurt sleep and develop habits that help sleep.

   I will present recommendations that help you be prepared to make the most of your night's sleep.

   *Explain* where clients can find information about these recommendations and what clients are expected to do with these recommendations, using the following script as a guide:

   You will find information on these recommendations in the booklet available in your folder.

   I would like you to read the booklet when you go home. Then see which of these recommendations are appropriate to you, and start applying the appropriate recommendations tonight.

   *Review* each recommendation by explaining what it is about and how it contributes to good sleep, using the following script as a guide:

   Let us review the recommendations. I will explain what each one is about and you can follow through in the booklet.

   The first recommendation is: develop a regular schedule of daytime activity or exercise.

   Activity or exercise may help improve the quality of your sleep.

   Select the type of activity or exercise that you like/enjoy doing, such as walking, gardening, or swimming.

   Do the activity or exercise on a regular basis.

   It is preferable to schedule the activity during the day, late afternoon, or early evening but not immediately before bedtime. This is because activity or exercise stimulates the body and makes falling asleep soon afterward difficult.

   After reviewing all recommendations and responding to clients' questions, *inform* clients of the next topic of presentation: stimulus control instructions, using the following script as a guide:

   Now, we will discuss the stimulus control instructions.

   There are six instructions.

   *Explain* where clients can find information about the instructions, using the following script as a guide:

   You have a list of these six instructions in your folder.

   You may want to pull this list out and follow through while I explain what each instruction is about.

   *Discuss* each instruction, using the following script as a guide:

   I am going to explain each of the six instructions, but I have to emphasize that all are important.

   The first instruction states: go to bed only when you are sleepy.

   It is often the case that persons with insomnia start thinking about bedtime right after dinner. They go to bed too early just to be sure they fall asleep at the desired time. However, since they are not sleepy, they are awake in bed. They start to do things they hope will bring on sleep, like reading, watching TV or just resting. These things seem logical solutions to the sleep problem. But they are counterproductive and contrary to what persons with insomnia need to improve sleep.

   So, persons with insomnia, like you, spend a lot of time in bed awake. This gets you to associate the bed and bedroom with wakefulness or being awake, rather than signals for sleepiness.

   It does not pay to go to bed when you are not sleepy. Therefore, you need to stay up until you are sleepy and then go to bed.

   It is helpful that you start to be aware of when you actually feel like you are getting sleepy. You can start to develop a sense of what sleepiness feels like and use that as a signal to go to bed rather than the clock time.

   There are signals that tell you that you are sleepy, such as yawning, heavy eyelids, and rubbing your eyes.

   You need to pay attention to these signals and if you feel them, then this means you are sleepy. It is only at the time that you feel sleepy that you go to bed with the intent to sleep.

   Have clients *identify* signals or cues for sleepiness; ask each client to think about the signals they feel when sleepy and state them, using the following script as a guide:

   Now, let us see how each one of you know that you are sleepy.

   I would like you to think of the time you feel sleepy; what signals, of the ones I just listed or other ones you may notice, tells you that you are sleepy?

**TABLE 7.3**   (Continued)

Once all clients *identify* their signals for sleepiness, summarize the discussion as follows:
You can see that the signals for sleepiness differ from one person to the other.
So, you need to monitor yourself, starting tonight, to learn more your personal signals for sleepiness.
Remember that when you feel these signals, you know that you are sleepy. You go to bed only when you feel sleepy.

*Conclusion*: (10 minutes)

*Assign* homework as follows:
I am going to ask you, starting tonight to: (1) read the information in the booklet and start following the recommendations that are applicable to you; (2) follow the six stimulus instructions we discussed; and (3) continue to complete the sleep diaries every day. The diary is important to monitor your sleep.

**Session 2**

*Introduction*: (20–30 minutes)
Start *discussion* on implementation of the six stimulus control instructions, using the following script as a guide:
Let us discuss how the last two weeks went.
Overall, were you able to carry out the six stimulus control instructions? How tough was it?
Have clients *comment* about their overall experience implementing the instructions; ask clients to share their experience, one at a time, whether "good" or "bad."
Once all clients give their comments, *remind* them:
I have to remind you that you are learning new habits and you are performing new behaviors.
These behaviors must be practiced consistently over the treatment period to work and to become routine.

*Main part*: (45–50 minutes)
Engage clients in a *discussion* of each stimulus control instruction, with a focus on getting clients to think about their behaviors and to link their performance of the behaviors with the quality and quantity of their sleep, using the following script as a guide:
Now, let us see how you did on each instruction.
How about the first instruction: Go to bed only when you are sleepy?
Use the following questions as *prompts* for discussion: Were you able to follow this instruction? Were you able to know that you are sleepy? That is, did you pay attention to how you feel when you get sleepy?
Tell me how you feel when you get sleepy.
Have clients *state* the signals for sleepiness they noticed.

*Conclusion*: (5–10 minutes)
*Remind* clients that:
This is the last session of the treatment.
They have to (1) follow the six stimulus control instructions, for the treatment to work, (2) monitor their sleep, and (3) continue doing the things or behaviors that helped having a good night sleep and to eliminate those that led to poor night sleep.

## 7.2.3.2   Tailored Interventions

The procedure section in the manual of tailored interventions is comparable to the one described for standardized interventions in terms of organization and detailing the steps. For tailored interventions, there are some procedural variations.

The introductory steps are altered based on the number of clients scheduled to receive the intervention (e.g. brief general introductions of the interventionist and the client is done in individual session) and the mode of delivery (e.g. no introduction is required if clients are expected to access and self-complete web-based intervention modules).

In the main part, an overview of the principles, algorithm and decision rules guiding the tailoring process is provided. This is followed by a description of the key activities in the tailoring process. These delineate the specific actions to be done to assess tailoring variables, to determine the client's level on the variables, and to select the interventions or components that are consistent with the client's level of the tailoring variables as specified in the algorithm.

The last activity entails the actual delivery of the selected intervention options or components. The procedure for implementing each possible intervention or component is detailed as described for standardized interventions. The following is a generic account of the specific actions to be performed in carrying out the first three activities in the tailoring process:

*Activity 1:    Assess tailoring variables*

- Inform clients that they have to complete a questionnaire about some characteristics, which is necessary to guide the delivery of the treatment.
- Remind clients that there are no right or wrong answers to the questions and that the interest is in learning about their condition or perspective.
- Explain that clients take time (i.e. no rush) to complete the questionnaire, and ask for clarification; interventionist can respond, as needed.
- Administer the questionnaire in the selected method.
- Get the completed questionnaire.

*Activity 2:    Determine clients' level on the tailoring variables*

- Review the clients' responses to items assessing each variable.
- Assign appropriate score to each response, following the rules preset for the items.
- Compute the total score for the multi-item scale assessing each variable, following the preset rule.
- Document the total scores for all tailoring variables on the respective forms.
- Interpret the clients' total scores on the tailoring variables, by comparing the scores to normative values or cutoff values preset for the respective scales; this will determine the clients' level on the tailoring variables.

*Activity 3:    Select the interventions or components responsive to clients' levels on the tailoring variables*

- Have the algorithm guiding the tailoring process available.
- Follow the instructions, as specified in the algorithm, to identify the interventions or components to provide to clients.
- Inform clients of the selected interventions.
- Provide the selected interventions as described.

For tailored interventions given via technology, the manual provides the overview of the tailoring algorithm, the scripts of the information to be relayed to clients and the assignment/homework/treatment recommendations that clients are expected to carry out. The application of the tailoring algorithm is embedded in the programming for assessing the tailoring variables, determining clients' levels on the variables, selecting and sending messages informing clients what interventions or components', described in the modules, to access or what activity to engage in and enact.

The scripted information is incorporated in the modules accessed by clients. The suggestions for preparing the information in simple language, short sentences presenting one idea at a time, are highly relevant for this format of intervention delivery. Prompts can be incorporated in interactive programs to highlight the key messages, thereby attracting clients' attention and promoting retention of the information. Exercises can be designed to facilitate the application and retention of the knowledge gained. With advances in technology, videos of healthcare professionals presenting relevant information or laypersons sharing their experiences can be uploaded and reviewed by clients.

## 7.2.4   Section 4: Adaptations

The fourth section of the manual presents information on the principles of adaptations and on possible adaptations that can be made to specific components, content, activities, treatment recommendations, and mode of delivery without altering the active ingredients of the intervention as specified in the intervention theory. The principles reiterate the importance of not modifying the specific components that operationalize the intervention's active ingredients, the reasons for adaptations, and the general guidance for what can be adapted in response to what client concerns or life circumstances. Possible adaptations are described relative to clients' characteristics, concerns, or life circumstances. The description delineates the conditions (e.g. level on a characteristic or a particular life situation) under which the specific content, action, and/or treatment recommendation can be modified and details how it can be modified in a manner that maintains congruence with the intervention's active ingredients.

The following illustrates a concern expressed by clients receiving the stimulus control therapy and a description of strategies that interventionists can use to address the concern without jeopardizing fidelity. The strategies represent modifications for delivering the therapy content and for applying the treatment recommendations. The description of this adaptation, presented in the fourth section of the manual, includes:

*Client concern*: Challenges in implementing the stimulus control instruction (i.e. treatment recommendation) related to: get out of bed if unable to fall asleep within 15–20 minutes.

*Clients' description of concern*: Clients sharing the same bed with their spouse may express concerns with carrying out this instruction; they may indicate that getting out of bed may disturb their spouse's sleep.

*Strategies to address concern*:

- Reiterate the importance of the instruction: Clients are to faithfully and consistently enact this instruction in order to achieve the desired change in reassociating the bed with sleep.
- Encourage clients to engage in problem-solving with their spouse: Clients are advised to discuss the instruction with their spouse and to come up with a mutually agreeable plan for handling the situation (for instance, one of our clients in collaboration with her spouse, made the decision to sleep in a separate room until her sleep problem improves).
- Use cognitive reframing by assisting clients to recognize the long-term benefits of applying this instruction to themselves and to their spouse (e.g. consolidated sleep with minimal interruptions and hence disturbance of the spouse's sleep); and to weigh the short-term disturbance of the spouse's sleep against the long-term benefits of the instruction.

### 7.2.5   Section 5: Appendices

The last section of the manual includes relevant appendices. These represent copy (Barry et al., 2008) of:

- Written materials such as handouts or booklets for use by the interventionist and clients during the intervention sessions, or by clients as a reference to guide the implementation of treatment recommendations.
- Forms to be completed during (e.g. measure of tailoring variables) or in-between (e.g. daily sleep diary) intervention sessions.
- Guidance or references for accessing technology-based materials during or in-between intervention sessions (e.g. video presentation, online modules).

The appended information helps interventionists become familiar with the intervention materials that they or their clients are to use and hence, able to address questions that clients may raise.

## 7.3   USE OF THE INTERVENTION MANUAL

The intervention manual is the means for detailing the operationalization of the intervention's active ingredients. It translates them into specific actions (Lorencatto et al., 2013) and provides a description of what is needed to deliver the intervention; what exactly is to be done, how, where, and when; and ways to modify the intervention to address non-ignorable concerns or life circumstances of clients. It is this detailed description that makes the manual useful in guiding the delivery of the intervention in research or practice.

The manual contributes significantly to the delivery of the intervention with fidelity, across interventionists, clients, and contexts (Borrelli 2011; Brose et al., 2015; Campbell et al., 2013). The manual promotes fidelity through the following (Lorencatto et al., 2013; Wallace & von Ranson, 2011):

- It guides the training of interventionists and/or health professionals responsible for delivering the intervention in research or practice, respectively. The description of specific activities and actions points to the skills that providers have to acquire to properly deliver the intervention. The manual assists in organizing the (1) content of the training, beginning with an overview of the intervention, moving to the resources required for giving it, and ending up with the step-by-step procedure to be followed when implementing it; (2) hands-on demonstration of the skills essential for performing the planned intervention activities; and (3) presentation of case studies representing a range of clients with specific concerns and life circumstances, and of possible adaptations in the intervention activities to address them. In addition, the manual offers the ground for developing theoretical and practical tests to examine the providers' post-training acquisition of the skills needed for intervention delivery. It also serves as a reference for supervisors in supporting interventionists' practical training.
- It forms the basis for developing instruments for monitoring the delivery of the intervention, and for assessing the fidelity with which interventionists and clients implement the intervention (Chapter 9).

- It serves as a guide for interventionists and health professionals in delivering the intervention. Specifically, by reviewing the manual in preparation for delivery, providers are reminded of (1) the resources required for carrying out the intervention in the selected mode, at each planned session; this prompts them to obtain the resources and ensures their proper functioning prior to intervention delivery; and (2) the nature and sequence of the activities to be carried out. Such preparations minimize the potentials for disruption in intervention delivery. Interventionists and health professionals refer to the manual and follow through with the steps as detailed in the manual when actually providing the intervention. This helps them stay focused on the planned content and activities, which maintains the fidelity of intervention delivery.

The development of the intervention manual is demanding. It requires attention to details surrounding delivery of the intervention, clear articulation of the activities to be performed, and description of possible adaptations to address clients' concerns and circumstances. Accordingly, the preparation of the manual is time consuming. It involves careful thinking and efforts to determine the logical sequence for carrying out the intervention components and activities; the appropriateness of the activities in operationalizing the active ingredients; and the feasibility of carrying out the activities in the selected mode of delivery and the selected setting. However, the efforts and time spent in the development of the manual are worthwhile relative to the benefits (i.e. fidelity of intervention delivery) gained in using the manual, whether in research or in practice.

## REFERENCES

Barry, D.T., Fulgieri, M.D., Lavery, M.E., et al. (2008) Research-and-community-based clinicians' attitudes on treatment manuals. *The American Journal on Addictions*, 17(2), 145–148.

Bartholomew, L.K., Kok, G., & Markham, C.M. (2016) *Planning Health Promotion Programs: An Intervention Mapping Approach* (4th ed). John Wiley and Amp; Sons Inc, New York

Borrelli, B. (2011) The assessment, monitoring and enhancement of treatment fidelity in public health clinical trials. *Journal of Public Health Dentistry*, 71, S52–S63.

Brose, L.S., McEwen, A., Michie, S., et al. (2015) Treatment manuals, training and successful provision of stop smoking behavioral support. *Behavior Research and Therapy*, 71, 34–39.

Campbell, B.K., Buti, A., Fussell, H.E., Srikanth, P., & Guydish, J.R. (2013) Therapist predictors of treatment delivery fidelity in community-based trial of 12-step facilitation. *American Journal of Drug and Alcohol Abuse*, 39, 304–311

Hardeman, W., Michie, S., Fanshawe, T., et al. (2008) Fidelity of delivery of a physical activity intervention: Predictors and consequences. *Psychology and Health*, 23, 11–24.

Jowers, C.E., Cain, L.A., Perkey, H., et al. (2019) The relationship between trainee therapist traits with the use of self-disclosure and immediacy in psychotherapy. *Psychotherapy*, 56(2), 157–169.

Lewis, C.C., Lyon, A.R., McBain, S.A., & Landes, S.J. (2019) Testing and exploring the limits of traditional notions of fidelity and adaptation in implementation of preventive interventions. *The Journal of Primary Prevention*, 40, 137–141.

146 Chapter 7 Development of Intervention Manual

Lorencatto, F., West, R., Christopherson, C., & Michie, S. (2013) Assessing fidelity of delivery of smoking cessation behavioral support in practice. *Implementation Science*, 8(1), 40–49.

Wallace, L.M. & von Ranson, K.M. (2011) Treatment manuals: Use in the treatment of bulimia nervosa. *Behaviour Research and Therapy*, 49(11), 815–820.

# CHAPTER 8

# Selecting, Training, and Addressing the Influence of Interventionists

The terms interventionists, therapists, and providers are used interchangeably, referring to the individuals responsible for delivering health interventions. In general, interventionists are health professionals who have the qualifications required by the respective regulatory organizations that enable them to provide an intervention. In some instances, laypersons assume the responsibility of providing health interventions. Lay persons are usually involved in the implementation of interventions in community settings and aimed at enhancing people's self-management of chronic conditions, social connectedness, and/or general health. Nonetheless, the literature focuses on the role and influence of health professionals in delivering interventions, and their influence on the implementation of the intervention.

In this chapter, the role of interventionists is briefly described. Evidence of their influence on the implementation and outcomes of interventions is synthesized. Strategies for selecting and training interventionists are discussed as a means for enhancing their competence for, and promoting fidelity of, intervention delivery. Methodological features for studies aimed at investigating interventionists' effects are highlighted.

## 8.1 ROLE OF INTERVENTIONISTS

In most, if not all, health interventions, the interventionist is the central figure in their delivery, serving as the medium through which the intervention's active ingredients are provided to clients. In educational interventions, the interventionist (e.g. health educator, nurse) relays the information on the health problem and on the treatment recommendations to manage the problem to clients. In cognitive-behavioral interventions, the interventionist (e.g. psychologist) facilitates discussion of the health problem, treatment recommendations to manage it, and ways to address factors that interfere with the implementation of the treatment recommendations in daily life. The interventionist also demonstrates the performance of pertinent cognitive and/or behavioral skills, and assists in monitoring and offers feedback on skill performance. In physical interventions, the interventionist (e.g. physical or occupational therapist) gives instructions on the application of the skills required for applying the treatment recommendations, and provides instrumental support as

*Nursing and Health Interventions: Design, Evaluation, and Implementation*, Second Edition.
Souraya Sidani and Carrie Jo Braden.

needed. Even in the delivery of pharmacological interventions, the interventionist (e.g. pharmacist) is involved not only in dispensing the medication, but also in providing information on its effects, dose, and adverse reactions, and in discussing issues of adherence.

Whether health interventions are offered in an individual or group, face-to-face, in-person or technology-based format, they involve interactions between interventionists and clients. It is through these interactions that interventionists provide, and clients are exposed to the intervention's components. During these interactions, the interventionist conveys, explains, and clarifies the content, that is, the information and instructions on the treatment recommendations that clients are expected to enact. In addition, the interventionist engages clients in the intervention activities (e.g. discussion, performance of a skill) planned for each session, and carries out the nonspecific components (or respective activities) aimed to support clients in implementing the treatment recommendations. Interventionists are requested to provide the specific and nonspecific components as delineated and detailed in the intervention manual in order to minimize deviations or variations in, and to enhance fidelity of, intervention delivery. As mentioned in Chapter 6, fidelity contributes to the achievement of beneficial outcomes.

Interventionists are individuals who vary in their personal and professional qualities, which may affect their capacity and ability to deliver health interventions with fidelity and competence. Such individuality influences interventionists' performance in providing the intervention and, consequently, effectiveness in producing beneficial client outcomes.

## 8.2    INFLUENCE OF INTERVENTIONISTS

Conventionally, interventionists' variability and contribution to the intervention delivery and outcome achievement have often been ignored in intervention research. This is related to the traditional perspective considering the interactions between interventionists and clients as inert, having no influence on the intervention's effectiveness. Cumulating empirical evidence suggests otherwise, that is, interventionists' influence is not ignorable; it is on par with the effects of the intervention's active ingredients (Horvath et al., 2011). This implies that the interventionists' contribution to outcomes is comparable to the contribution of the intervention's active ingredients to outcomes, whether the intervention is delivered in research or practice.

### 8.2.1    Traditional Perspective On Interventionists' Influence

The traditional perspective informing intervention research acknowledges that the interactions between the interventionist and the clients are the means for delivering the active ingredients of the intervention. It views interventionists as the medium through which the active ingredients are provided; therefore, the interventionists' role is simply to facilitate the delivery of the intervention. Accordingly, just like other modes for delivering the intervention, interventionists are not expected to vary or differ in the way they provide the intervention, to affect clients' engagement in the intervention and enactment of the treatment recommendations and to contribute to outcome achievement. In this traditional perspective, only the active ingredients are posited to be responsible for producing the beneficial changes in the outcomes, and all other aspects inherent in the context of intervention delivery including the interventionists are hypothesized to be inert.

The hypothesized inert nature of the interventionist–client interactions forms the basis of the assumption of "interventionist uniformity" that prevailed in intervention research (Kim et al., 2006). The assumption implies that interventionists are equivalent in their ability to deliver the intervention and, hence, to play no (or minimal) role in the achievement of outcomes. Equivalence means that interventionists are comparable in their qualities, capacity, and skills required for providing the intervention, as well as in their actual performance in delivering the intervention. As such, interventionists are considered intersubstitutable; they can be carefully selected and intensively trained in the implementation of the intervention. The training is expected to enhance and equalize their performance in delivering the intervention, which promotes the competence and fidelity with which they provide the intervention. The expectations of equal performance across interventionists and of their limited, if any, contribution to outcomes resulted in little attention given to the examination of interventionists' influence in intervention research.

Recent experience in intervention evaluation research and in implementation initiatives (aimed at disseminating and integrating interventions in practice) indicates that the assumptions of interventionist uniformity, equal performance, and limited contribution to outcomes are untenable. Cumulating evidence supports the interventionists' influence on outcomes which should be accounted for in order to enhance the validity of conclusions or inferences regarding the intervention's effectiveness (Lutz & Barkham, 2015).

## 8.2.2   Evidence of Interventionist Influence

As mentioned previously, interventionists are individuals who have unique characteristics. They differ in their personal qualities, including their sociodemographic profile; cultural beliefs and values; and interpersonal skills. Interventionists also vary in their professional qualifications such as education, knowledge, theoretical orientation, practical skills, and attitudes toward the health problem, the target population, and treatments. Interventionists' personal and professional characteristics, in particular beliefs, attitudes, and skills, inform their perspectives on health problems and treatments, as well as their behaviors and interactions with clients.

Clinical practice is replete with examples illustrating differences among health professionals. Differences are reported in the technical and relational aspects of care. Health professionals vary in their clinical knowledge, experience, and expertise, which affect the quality of their treatment decision-making and performance in providing treatments. Health professionals differ in their communication, interpersonal and interactional skills, which affect their collaboration with members of the healthcare team, and their ability to develop and maintain a rapport, therapeutic relationship, or working alliance with clients. A *therapeutic relationship* is a nurturing one, in which health professionals and clients trust each other and respect each other's beliefs and values; exchange information that guides the planning of care; explore pressing concerns and preferences; and participate as equal partners in making treatment decisions as well as in implementing, evaluating, and revising treatment, as needed (Kitson et al., 2013; Sidani & Fox, 2014). A *working alliance* is a collaborative relationship in which health professionals and clients develop a common understanding and an agreement on the intervention's goals and tasks (Degnan et al., 2016).

Emerging empirical evidence confirms interventionists' variability in the delivery and effectiveness of interventions. The evidence has been generated primarily in studies evaluating psychotherapy, with a recent surge in the number of studies that investigated the influence of interventionists providing other health interventions implemented in research or practice. Studies have examined interventionists' contribution to client outcomes, difference in performance or in the delivery of interventions, and factors predicting their performance and effectiveness.

### 8.2.2.1 Interventionists' Contribution to Outcomes

The interventionists' contribution to outcomes, also referred to as therapist effects, has been investigated in an increasing number of individual studies and systematic reviews/meta-analyses. The studies used a range of experimental and nonexperimental or naturalistic designs. The interventionists were responsible for delivering specific interventions such as behavioral therapy for depression (e.g. Titzler et al., 2018) in research, or selected evidence-based therapies (e.g. Becker-Haimes et al., 2017) in practice. The number of interventionists included in these studies ranged from less than 10 to more than 100; similarly, the client sample size varied across studies, with those involving a naturalistic design having larger samples of interventionists and clients. The client outcomes frequently examined reflected the experience of the health problem targeted by the intervention, and general health or functioning. Despite these differences (i.e. in study design, intervention, sample size, and outcomes), the findings were consistent in showing differences in client outcomes across interventionists; in other words, clients assigned to different interventionists attained different levels of improvement in the outcomes (e.g. Anderson et al., 2009; Dinger et al., 2008; Goldberg et al., 2018). It has been estimated, in individual studies and meta-analyses, that interventionists account for 3–13.5% of the variance in client outcomes observed following treatment (e.g. Baldwin & Imel, 2013; Del Re et al., 2012; Elkin et al., 2006; Lutz et al., 2007; Saxon et al., 2017; Schiefele et al., 2017; Zimmermann et al., 2017). It is important to note that the amount of variance in client outcomes accounted for by interventionists is equal (Horvath et al., 2011) or larger than the amount of variance in the outcomes explained by the intervention that the clients received; the latter variance ranged between 0 and 2% (Kim et al., 2006; Wampold & Brown, 2005).

Recognizing that achievement of desired outcomes rests on clients' completion of treatment (which may be associated with interventionists' performance), researchers have also investigated client attrition rates across interventionists. In two recent naturalistic studies, differences in the rates of clients' withdrawal from treatment were examined for therapists providing different types of psychotherapy. The results were comparable, showing that the treatment attrition or withdrawal rates varied across therapists. The attrition rates ranged between 1.2 and 73.2% (Saxon et al., 2017), whereas the therapist effects accounted for 6% of the variance in the attrition rates after controlling for other client characteristics known to be associated with attrition such as initial or pre-treatment severity of the health problem (Zimmermann et al., 2017).

Variability in interventionists' contribution to clients' attrition and outcomes underscores the importance of attending to the interventionists' influence or effect in intervention evaluation research. Realizing the interventionists' effects may be attributed to the manner in which they provide treatment, studies were designed to explore interventionists' performance in delivering health interventions and factors that predict their performance and effectiveness.

### 8.2.2.2 Interventionists' Performance in Intervention Delivery

Two aspects of interventionists' performance have been examined: (1) fidelity of intervention delivery, which was operationalized in adherence to the intervention manual (comparable to the technical aspect of care), and (2) ability to build a rapport, therapeutic relationship, or working alliance with clients during intervention delivery, which is often considered as reflecting interventionists' competence (also referred to as common factors, and comparable to the relational aspect of care). Variability was observed in the extent to which interventionists adhered to the intervention in research and practice (e.g. Imel et al., 2011).

Evidence showed that health professionals' levels of adherence to different evidence-based psychotherapies were lower than the level considered acceptable, which is ≥80% (Reichow et al., 2008). Levels of adherence ranged between 4.2 and 27.8% in one study (Tschuschke et al., 2015), and from 6.6 to 90% with a mean of 30% in another study (Verschuur et al., 2019). Detailed analyses showed that levels of adherence differed not only across health professionals but also across clients receiving treatment from the same health professional, across types of psychotherapy, and across sessions of the same therapy (Tschuschke et al., 2015). Similarly, the working alliance was found to consistently vary across interventionists, clients presenting with different health problems, and types of interventions (e.g. Imel et al., 2011; Moyers et al., 2005; Wampold & Imel, 2015).

### 8.2.2.3  Factors Predicting Interventionists' Performance

Several personal factors have been investigated in an attempt to understand what contributes to the variability in interventionists' performance in delivering health interventions. Results of individual studies indicated that interventionists who displayed high levels of adherence were likely to have high levels of education (Campbell et al., 2013); to report high self-efficacy in skills for implementing the intervention components (Campbell et al., 2013); and to perceive the intervention favorably, that is, acceptable, advantageous, and consistent with their theoretical orientation and with their clinical experiences (Borrelli, 2011; McDiamid Nelson et al., 2012; Titzler et al., 2018). There were mixed findings related to interventionists' experience. Experience was not associated with adherence in one study (Mauricio et al., 2019), whereas interventionists with low experience (≤ 5 years) exhibited high levels of adherence (Campbell et al., 2013; McDiamid Nelson et al., 2012). This evidence suggests that interventionists with graduate education may have been exposed to different interventions and had ample opportunities to learn and apply the interventions throughout their educational program, which enhances their comfort and confidence in their skills.

One recent study examined the association of selected personal factors with interventionists' working alliance. One such factor included attachment style and the results suggested that interventionists with attachment security had high level of alliance (Degnan et al., 2016).

### 8.2.2.4  Factors Predicting Interventionists' Effectiveness

Researchers attempted to gain an understanding of the observed interventionists' influence on client outcomes by examining the extent to which interventionists' characteristics and performance were related to client outcomes. The interventionists' characteristics entailed their personal attributes (age, gender) and professional qualifications (education, years of experience, theoretical or treatment orientation) and qualities (empathy). In general, the results were mixed. Whereas earlier studies found nonsignificant associations of interventionists' characteristics with client outcomes (e.g. Dinger et al., 2008; Okiishi et al., 2003; Wampold & Brown, 2005), more recent ones reported the following:

1. Young interventionists had better client outcomes (Berghout & Zevalkink, 2011).

2. Female interventionists had better outcomes, after controlling for caseload (Berghout & Zevalkink, 2011).

3. Interventionists' years of experience and theoretical orientation were not associated with clients' outcomes (Berghout & Zevalkink, 2011; Huppert et al., 2001).

Furthermore, Saxon et al. (2017) found that clients who perceived their interventionists as having no or low empathy were likely to withdraw from treatment.

The contribution of interventionists' performance, including adherence to the intervention manual and competence (or working alliance) in providing treatment, has been examined in individual studies, systematic reviews, or meta-analyses. The results pertaining to the association between interventionists' adherence and clients' outcomes were inconsistent. For instance, Tschuschke et al. (2015) reported that adherence alone did not predict outcomes. Other researchers found that increased adherence is associated with better outcomes (DiGennaro Reed & Codding 2014; Pellecchia et al., 2015; Schoenwald et al., 2011). Evidence from Webb et al.'s (2010) meta-analysis suggests that the effect of adherence on outcomes was small (average effect size: 0.02). This small effect was theoretically unexpected and could be attributed to methodological factors such as differences in the methods used to collect data on adherence, the unreliability of the measures, restricted range (i.e. high levels of adherence), or nonlinear nature of the relationship. Indeed, Barber et al. (2006) observed a curvilinear relationship whereby high and low levels of adherence were associated with poor client outcomes. It appears that a moderate level of adherence is optimal for interventionists' effectiveness. This point reflects interventionists' perception of the importance of providing treatment while being responsive to clients' individual concerns and life circumstance (i.e. adapting interventions). Interventionists' responsiveness may be an essential element of their competence.

The findings pertaining to the contribution of interventionists' competence, operationalized in therapeutic relationship, interpersonal skills, or working alliance, to client outcomes are consistent in supporting its direct effects on outcomes. Evidence synthesized across individual studies and systematic reviews or meta-analyses shows that the way in which interventionists deliver health interventions predicts client outcomes. In particular, the working alliance between interventionists and clients (1) enhances clients' appreciation of the value of the intervention, satisfaction with treatment, and motivation to carry out and adhere to the treatment recommendations (Constantino et al., 2007; Fuertes et al., 2007); (2) is associated with reduced rates of withdrawal from treatment (Alcázar Olán et al., 2010); (3) is positively related with achievement of beneficial client outcomes (Del Re et al., 2012; Dinger et al., 2008; Krukowski et al., 2019). The effects of working alliance on client outcomes were of a small-to-moderate (range: 0.02 to 0.27) size, as estimated in meta-analyses (Cameron et al., 2018; Castonguay et al., 2006; Horvath et al., 2011; Webb et al., 2010). On average, the working alliance accounted for 8% of the variability in the outcome (Horvath et al., 2011), which was higher than the percentage of outcome variance attributable to the intervention's effects (Kaplowitz et al., 2011).

The contribution of the interventionists' interpersonal skills to client outcomes has been recently investigated. Facilitative interpersonal skills, which are the cornerstone of the therapeutic relationship or working alliance, include: verbal fluency, warmth, empathy, persuasiveness, hopefulness, ability to create an accepting and supportive relationship, and being problem-focused (Anderson et al., 2009; Lingiardi et al., 2018). Evidence indicates that interventionists exhibiting these facilitative interpersonal skills were effective in increasing clients' engagement in treatment (Moyers et al., 2005; Tschuschke et al., 2015) and in improving clients' outcomes (Anderson et al., 2009; Berghout & Zevalkink, 2011; Goldberg et al., 2018; Greeson et al., 2009; Gaume et al., 2009; Lingiardi et al., 2018).

Mounting clinical and empirical evidence converge in supporting the interventionists' influence on the delivery and outcomes of health interventions. Interventionists' performance including their level of adherence to the intervention manual, and competence represented in their interpersonal skills and working alliance, more so than their personal characteristics, are significant predictors of client outcomes. It appears that interventionists' performance and competence are more influential than the active ingredients of interventions in accounting for the benefits of treatments (Kaplowitz et al., 2011). Accordingly, it would be useful to carefully select and train interventionists, monitor their performance (discussed in Chapter 9), and investigate their contribution to outcomes in intervention evaluation studies.

## 8.3   SELECTION OF INTERVENTIONISTS

The mounting evidence on the interventionists' influence points to the importance of carefully considering the interventionists' characteristics when selecting them into their role in research or practice. The recommendation is to select interventionists who have the personal and professional qualities known to contribute to their performance and effectiveness, without violating local human resources policies. The general intent is to hire the most competent interventionists, capable of delivering the intervention with fidelity while building a good working alliance with clients. No guidelines are available to inform the selection of interventionists. Following are suggestions for qualities to consider and for strategies to ascertain them.

### 8.3.1   Interventionists' Qualities

It may not be possible to list all qualities considered important for delivering specific health interventions. However, the following is a list of general personal and professional characteristics, generated from empirical and experiential evidence, to be taken into account when selecting interventionists, as also suggested by Borrelli (2011).

#### 8.3.1.1   Personal Characteristics

Whereas recent evidence indicates that interventionists' sociodemographic characteristics do not influence their performance and effectiveness as much as their personal attributes, it may be useful to consider both categories in some instances.

1. Sociodemographic characteristics: These include (but are not limited to) age, gender, and ethnicity. Congruence on these characteristics between interventionists and clients may facilitate the delivery of interventions addressing sensitive topics. For instance, women feel comfortable discussing topics related to sexuality or breastfeeding with female interventionists; persons of a particular culture are at ease expressing their beliefs about the health problem and its treatment (which may affect their enactment of the treatment recommendations) with an interventionist of the same culture (who can understand and appreciate their values and beliefs).

2. Personal attributes: These relate to general personality style and relational or interpersonal skills. Examples of personality style are: extroversion, humor, attachment, reflective and introspective capacities (Degnan et al., 2016; Lingiardi et al., 2018). Interpersonal skills are illustrated with interventionists demonstrating: warmth, empathy, helpfulness, hopefulness, verbal fluency, and persuasiveness (Anderson et al., 2009). These personal attributes affect the nature of the interventionists' interactions with clients during the delivery of the intervention, as well as the development of a therapeutic relationship or working alliance. Facilitative interactions and working alliance contribute to clients' motivation, engagement, and enactment of the treatment recommendations, which lead to improvement in outcomes.

### 8.3.1.2   Professional Characteristics

Despite mixed results (presented in Section 8.2.2), some professional characteristics should be carefully considered in selecting interventionists.

1. Professional qualifications: These represent formal education or training, licensing, and experience. Formal education and training and licensing are required by professional regulatory organizations to practice and/or deliver some interventions. For instance, prescription of medications requires advanced education in medicine or nursing (i.e. nurse practitioners) and the delivery of some types of psychotherapy requires at least a master's degree in clinical psychology. Advanced education or training is believed necessary for high-quality and safe practice and delivery of interventions. With advanced education, interventionists are exposed to different theoretical orientations, therapeutic approaches, and practice opportunities. This in turn, helps them develop an understanding of different health problems and interventions, a positive attitude and flexibility to learn new interventions, and enhanced self-efficacy in the technical and interpersonal skills (Campbell et al., 2013). Professional experience is another quality to consider in light of evidence suggesting that less experienced interventionists are likely to deliver interventions with fidelity. In contrast, more experienced interventionists tend to have a solidified working style, which hinders new learning (Campbell et al., 2013). Further, experienced health professionals embrace flexibility in delivering interventions with the aim to attend to clients' individual concerns. Accordingly, experienced health professionals are not supportive of strict adherence to the intervention manual. They view manuals as conceptually at odds with the principles of care or treatment, which should be tailored to individuals' needs, and as potentially detrimental to the achievement of client outcomes (e.g. Addis & Krasnow, 2000; Brose et al., 2015).

2. Knowledge and attitudes toward the intervention: Interventionists' prior theoretical and practical knowledge of the intervention they are responsible to deliver may enhance their training and delivery of the health intervention under evaluation. Interventionists who are aware of the intervention and who have theoretical orientations compatible with the theoretical underpinning of the intervention may easily grasp the intervention theory. This theoretical understanding helps them appreciate the potential contribution and identify the main components of the intervention. Interventionists who have experience, even if limited, in carrying out the intervention or some of its components, are familiar with and may have some confidence in the technical

skills required to deliver the intervention. The training reinforces their self-efficacy in these skills. Interventionists' attitudes toward, specifically their perceived acceptability or endorsement of, the intervention represent other characteristics to consider. Interventionists who do not embrace the theoretical underpinning of the intervention and who view the intervention as unacceptable to them and to their clients are likely to question its utility, to decline its delivery, or to deviate the delivery of its components toward those they endorse (Becker-Haimes et al., 2017; Borrelli, 2011).

## 8.3.2    Strategies to Ascertain Interventionists' Characteristics

Ascertainment of interventionists' characteristics is an ongoing process. It begins with the recruitment and an initial formal interview, and continues with monitoring of interventionists' performance.

### 8.3.2.1    Recruitment

Different venues and strategies can be used to recruit interventionists in research and practice. Advertisement for the position can be disseminated in local newspapers, professional journals, and organizational newsletters or websites. Flyers can be posted in academic institutions or affiliated healthcare organizations. Information about the position can also be spread through word-of-mouth; for instance, academic researchers may refer graduate students and clinicians may refer health professionals.

Regardless of the venue used, the recruitment information should identify the general category (e.g. cognitive behavioral therapy) or the specific type (e.g. stimulus control therapy) of health interventions to be delivered, as well as the main professional qualifications (i.e. education, licensing) that interventionists should have in order to deliver the intervention, as required by professional regulatory organizations. For example, recruitment of interventionists for the study that evaluated the effectiveness of cognitive behavioral therapy for insomnia specified the following requirements: a master's degrees in nursing, psychology, or other health-related disciplines and knowledge or training in the principles of cognitive-behavioral therapy. Those interested are encouraged to apply for the advertised position. The application contains a cover letter (highlighting their qualifications), a resume or curriculum vita (CV), and letters of references (commenting on their technical and interpersonal skills). A careful review of the applications is necessary to determine those who have the required professional qualifications. These individuals are invited to a formal interview.

### 8.3.2.2    Formal Interview

The individual formal interview is scheduled prior to contracting interventionists and aims to assess the remaining personal and professional characteristics that are preset for selecting interventionists. Although the interview can be done through different modes, the in-person mode is preferable as it enables the assessment of nonverbal behaviors that may be reflective of some characteristics such as ability to listen and communicate clearly. A list of open- and close-ended questions is prepared and asked of all applicants. The questions cover indicators of the personal and professional characteristics deemed as prerequisites for the role of interventionists, while providing applicants the opportunity to elaborate on points of interest.

Open-ended questions explore applicants' theoretical orientation, knowledge and attitudes toward the intervention they are to deliver, as well as prior training in providing the intervention or some of its components. Examples of open-ended questions used in interviewing interventionists for the cognitive behavioral therapy for insomnia are: Have you had any training in cognitive-behavioral therapy in general and/or for the management of insomnia in particular? What are the basic principles and features of this therapy? How useful or effective do you think it is?

Close-ended questions may be developed to assess specific personal or professional qualities. Alternatively, available instruments can be administered to measure some qualities such as interpersonal skills or capacity to build a working alliance with clients. For example, applicants may complete the six-item measure of therapeutic alliance developed by Joyce et al. (2003) during the interview.

Applicants' responses to open- and close-ended questions are clearly documented. In addition, the interviewer may attend to and record comments on the applicants' communication, interactional style, and interpersonal skills exhibited during the interview. As well, during in-person interviews, the interviewer may observe and record applicants' demeanor and nonverbal behaviors. Applicants' responses and interviewer's observations and comments form the basis for selecting interventionists.

Audition-style interviews, also called simulation job interviews, are emerging in a number of fields as an approach to assessing potential hires (Friedman, 2014; Schwantes, 2017; Brooks 2010). Given that intervention research often occurs within academic settings through funded studies, students are commonly recruited for interventionist roles. When this is the case it is possible to offer pre-interview and training about the skills required of an interventionist as a component of the research education program. For example, teaching students enrolled in health professional programs about the importance of fidelity in intervention research (Eymard & Altmiller, 2016) as well as incorporating skills training in interviewing for an interventionist role (Huss et al., 2017) can strengthen the candidate pool.

### 8.3.2.3   Interventionist Selection

Applicants' responses to questions and interviewer's observations are then compared to the applicants' CV and letters of references. These comparisons are done to look for convergence of information regarding the extent to which applicants have the characteristics of interest. For example, the CV may confirm educational background, licensure, training, and experience, whereas letters of support may point to the quality of the applicants' interpersonal skills.

Once interviews with all applicants are completed, the information gathered is compared and contrasted across applicants, for the purpose of identifying those who have the pre-specified personal and professional characteristics. A ranking system is designed and followed to choose applicants demonstrating high levels on all characteristics. It may be useful to select a number of applicants that exceeds (e.g. by one or two) the number of interventionists needed to deliver the interventions to all clients participating in a research study or expected to receive care in practice. The selected applicants are trained in the implementation of the intervention (as discussed in Section 8.4).

Securing a large number of carefully selected and trained interventionists is essential to offset possible interventionists' (1) attrition, where some may withdraw for various reasons such as moving out of town to pursue further education; (2) schedule conflict, where some may not be able to facilitate intervention sessions offered in the evening at clients' convenience, and others may need to take time off (e.g. vacation, maternity leave); and (3) inadequate performance, where some may consistently fail to adhere to the intervention protocol or to develop an acceptable level of working alliance with clients.

### 8.3.2.4   Monitoring Performance

Monitoring interventionists' performance during training and delivery of the intervention is another means for assessing their personal and professional characteristics, as well as the fidelity with which they deliver the intervention (see Chapter 9). Interventionists' participation in training provides an opportunity to note their theoretical orientation and knowledge and attitudes toward the intervention, which can be inferred from the questions they ask, comments they make, or their responses to formal tests administered post-training. This test is administered to examine the effectiveness of training in enhancing the interventionists' theoretical and practical knowledge of the intervention.

Interventionists' interactions with each other during the training session offer a window to confirm their interpersonal style. Post-training, initial supervised delivery of the intervention represents an important opportunity to assess interventionists' competence in delivering the intervention and quality of their interpersonal skills or interactions with clients.

The results of the initial (during training) interventionists' performance are essential in further substantiating their personal and professional characteristics (i.e. in addition to the information obtained in the interview). They are useful in giving interventionists feedback on their performance and areas for improvement, and in taking necessary remedial steps. Remedial steps include additional intensive training, reducing the caseload until improvement in performance is achieved, or asking poorly performing interventionists, specifically those with inappropriate interpersonal skills (as reported by other research staff or by clients), to step down.

## 8.4   TRAINING OF INTERVENTIONISTS

Although interventionists are selected on the basis of well-specified personal and professional characteristics, they may not have the theoretical and practical knowledge to inform the delivery of an intervention to the target client population, in a particular context. Therefore, they should receive training to enable them to provide the intervention with fidelity, which is essential to initiate the mechanism mediating the intervention's effects on the ultimate outcomes. Training is offered at different points in time, and covers theoretical and practical content, using different methods. It also is useful to evaluate the effectiveness of training.

### 8.4.1   Time of Training

Initial training is done prior to entrusting newly selected interventionists the delivery of the intervention to clients. Initial training aims to help interventionists understand the theoretical underpinning of the intervention, and to adequately prepare them in the skills or competencies required for a successful implementation of the intervention (Borrelli, 2011). Ongoing training is offered at regular intervals throughout the research study time frame or within the first year of implementing an evidence-based intervention in practice. Ongoing training is important for reinforcing and maintaining the acquired competencies and preventing drifts in performance (Johnson & Remien, 2003). Initial and ongoing training are essential for a proper and accurate implementation of the intervention's components.

## 8.4.2   Content of Training

The content covered in initial and ongoing training differs slightly, even though both focus on supporting the interventionists' cognitive, behavioral, or practical skills required to provide the intervention's components, in the specified mode and dose.

### 8.4.2.1   Initial Training

Initial training is comprehensive and intensive, providing a balance between didactic and experiential learning if it is to adequately prepare interventionists (Webster-Stratton et al., 2014). The didactic part could be offered first followed by the experiential part. Alternatively, the experiential part can be interwoven with the didactic, whereby each intervention component is described at the conceptual level and pertinent skills for providing it are practiced under supervision of the trainer.

*Didactic Part of Initial Training*

The didactic part of initial training revolves around the theoretical underpinning and the operationalization of the intervention. This involves a review of the intervention theory and the intervention manual, respectively. The review of the theory provides the rationale for the intervention, which helps interventionists appreciate the value of the intervention and understand its active ingredients and mechanism of action. The review of the manual informs interventionists of the way in which the active ingredients are put into operation and of the essential content that must be conveyed and the activities that must be performed, and how, in order to produce the beneficial outcomes. The topics to be presented and discussed include:

1. The theory of the health problem that the intervention addresses: A condensed presentation of the problem and its indicators and determinants, and of relevant empirical evidence and experiential accounts of the problem as experienced by the target client population is useful. This information helps interventionists familiarize themselves with the problem; understand why and how the problem is experienced as well as the aspects of the problem addressed by the intervention; and anticipate variability in clients' experience and perception of the problem.

2. The theory of change and the theory of implementation: This involves a detailed description and discussion of the intervention's goals; active ingredients and respective components; the main content, activities, and treatment recommendations; the mode and dose of delivery; and the mechanism of action that mediates the intervention's effects on the ultimate outcomes. This information promotes interventionists' understanding of the intervention's rationale and appreciation of its significance. Interventionists who realize the importance of the intervention may be able to convince clients of its value in addressing the health problem, particularly if they develop a helpful working alliance. Fuertes et al. (2007) reported that clients who understand treatment and agree to it and trust their interventionists are likely to "buy into" treatment, see it as worthy, and follow through it.

3. The operationalization of the intervention: This entails (1) highlighting the components that represent the intervention's active ingredients, and pointing to the importance of carrying them out as planned; and (2) reviewing the intervention manual, clarifying the key principles guiding interactions with clients with the aim of reinforcing interventionists' interpersonal skills, explaining how the activities are to be performed; and delineating when and how adaptations are to be made. These points inform interventionists of what the intervention is about and how it is to be given.

### Experiential Part of Initial Training

The experiential part of initial training focuses on skill performance. It provides interventionists opportunities to observe and practice the cognitive and behavioral skills needed to carry out the planned intervention activities and to review the resources needed for providing the intervention. Various strategies can be used to promote acquisition of these skills. Examples of strategies include:

1. Case studies or vignettes: These consist of presenting information about hypothetical or actual clients, describing the clients' experience of the health problem and individual concerns. Interventionists are requested to analyze the information and delineate the course of treatment or modifications of the intervention delivery as stipulated in the manual. Other case studies can illustrate clients' reactions to the intervention or challenges in implementing the treatment recommendations; interventionists are asked to devise relevant strategies and apply relevant interpersonal skills to handle these situations. Case studies can be completed on an individual, subgroup, or whole group basis. This is followed by inviting interventionists to reflect on their performance and to discuss their answers to clarify the rationale for their answers. The trainer provides feedback, and reviews how best to address the cases within the parameters of the intervention theory and manual.

2. Demonstration: This can be done by the trainer showing the specific steps for relaying the content and performing the intervention activities. Alternatively, audio or video recordings of previously offered intervention sessions are played. If the recordings are unavailable, transcripts of the taped sessions are reviewed to illustrate the implementation of the intervention. This is followed by a group discussion facilitated by the trainer to highlight accurate performance; suggest ways to improve performance; identify deviations in carrying out specific intervention activities, rationale for the deviations, and impact on fidelity of intervention delivery; and review the appropriateness of strategies used to manage emerging issues.

3. Role play or role modeling: This consists of having the interventionists apply the skills or intervention activities that are demonstrated by the trainer or in the recordings. The trainer then provides feedback to reinforce correct performance or to rectify incorrect performance.

4. Supervised delivery of the intervention: If resources are available, trained interventionists attend a practical, hands-on training session. They are asked to deliver a session of the intervention to actors posing as clients, under the supervision of the trainer. The trainer then comments on their technical and interpersonal skills, and works with interventionists on strategies to help them improve their performance.

### 8.4.2.2   Ongoing Training

Ongoing training is recommended to maintain an adequate level of competence for all interventionists involved in the delivery of the intervention. It also provides opportunities to discuss challenges or drifts in implementation and strategies to address them; to give support and feedback on performance; and to reinforce theoretical and practical knowledge.

Ongoing training can take the form of in-service or booster sessions, or coaching and consultations. Booster sessions are organized into two parts. The first part consists of a review of the intervention theory and of the implementation of the intervention. The second part of booster sessions entails discussion of challenges encountered in delivering the intervention, cases of clients who present with specific concerns, and strategies to manage these challenges and concerns. Coaching and consultations involve supervision of interventionists' performance and regular meetings. The trainer or designate (e.g. other health professional with expertise in the intervention delivery) attends randomly selected sessions facilitated by interventionists. If attendance is not possible or agreeable to clients, then the intervention sessions are audio-recorded and the trainer reviews the audio recordings. The trainer provides support, reinforcement, and detailed feedback on the interventionists' performance. At the meetings, held with individual or group of interventionists, the trainer: discusses challenges (e.g. arising individual clients' concerns, unfavorable clients' reactions, unavailability of resources) faced during the delivery of the intervention; factors contributing to the challenges; strategies that interventionists used to manage the challenges; the appropriateness and consistency of the strategies used with those proposed in the manual; the perceived helpfulness of the strategies used; and additional alternative strategies that can be utilized to manage the challenges.

The initial and ongoing training are necessary to promote interventionists' understanding of the theoretical underpinning and practical competence in delivering the intervention. Interventionists who acquire the cognitive and behavioral skills are well positioned to deliver the intervention with fidelity while appropriately attending (with minimal deviations) to individual clients' concerns, characteristics, and life circumstances.

### 8.4.3   Methods for Training

The initial and ongoing, didactic and experiential, training as described in Section 8.4.2 has been usually advocated and extensively used in research. In this context, the training is given in individual or group, face-to-face sessions, followed by close supervision of interventionists' performance.

With the increasing interest in implementing evidence-based interventions in practice, different methods have been devised and evaluated for their effectiveness in improving the skills of health professionals responsible for delivering the interventions. The training methods are described, and relevant evidence synthesized from a review of the literature (Herschell et al., 2010) and individual studies (McDiamid Nelson et al., 2012; Webster-Stratton et al., 2014) is presented next.

*Review and/or discussion of the intervention manual in in-person sessions:* The review and discussion is led by the trainer, similar to the procedure used in the training of interventionists detailed in Section 8.4.2. The trainer proceeds by reading each section of the manual while interventionists follow through with their own copy of the manual. For each section, the trainer: (1) clarifies the information and details the intervention activities to be performed; (2) reiterates the rationale and the way of carrying out the activities; (3) identifies the required resources; (4) explains possible deviations in performing the activities to address challenging situations and individual client concerns while maintaining fidelity in delivering the intervention's active ingredients; (5) discusses strategies to manage the challenges successfully and gives examples to illustrate the points of discussion; and (6) reiterates the main points to reinforce learning. This method for training is necessary and useful for prompt clarification of theoretical or practical content. It was found effective in increasing interventionists' knowledge and capacity to deliver the intervention in the short term, but insufficient for the acquisition and maintenance of the skills or competence in providing the intervention in the long term.

*Self-directed training techniques:* These entail making the intervention manual and other training materials such as video recordings of intervention sessions available electronically. Interventionists access these materials and review them on their own. Evidence suggests that self-directed techniques are viewed favorably by interventionists and have the advantages of cost-effectiveness (i.e. easily accessible by a large number of interventionists). However, the results of Herschell et al.'s (2010) review indicated that less than 50% of interventionists completed the self-directed training and demonstrated only slight improvement in their theoretical knowledge and practical competence in delivering the intervention.

*Workshops:* The workshops are comparable to the initial training and involve didactic and experiential learning (Section 8.4.2). When offered to health professionals responsible for implementing evidence-based interventions in practice, workshops were found to increase health professionals' knowledge; however, they had a short term and small impact on changing their behaviors or skills needed to implement the interventions.

*Post-workshop supervision and feedback:* These were called workshop supplements by Herschell et al. (2010). These methods are comparable to the supervised delivery of the intervention, coaching, and consultations described in Section 8.4.1. These behaviorally oriented methods were reported as influential in improving interventionists' skills.

*Multicomponent training methods:* These consist of different combinations of: review of the intervention manual, workshops, supervision, and feedback. Multicomponent methods demonstrated effectiveness in improving interventionists' (in research) or health professionals' (in practice) knowledge, competence, and adherence to the intervention protocol (i.e. fidelity) in some but not all studies reviewed by Herschell et al. (2010).

Overall, evidence converges in showing that: (1) training methods involving only lecture-style or self-directed, didactic, passive presentation of content related to the conceptualization and operationalization of the intervention are ineffective in enhancing interventionists' knowledge and behavioral skills; (2) training methods involving active learning strategies (e.g. role play, case studies) are effective; and (3) training methods involving a review of the intervention theory, behavior role play, supervision, and feedback are most effective in improving interventionists' or health professionals' knowledge, skills, and ability to deliver the intervention with fidelity (Herschell et al., 2010; McDiamid Nelson et al., 2012; Webster-Stratton et al., 2014).

### 8.4.4  Evaluation of Training

Regardless of the method used, it is wise to evaluate the helpfulness of training in facilitating acquisition of theoretical and practical knowledge of the intervention. The evaluation results determine the interventionists' level of competence and areas of performance that should be improved; and provide guidance for revising the training content and methods to enhance its effectiveness.

There are no specific guidelines and standard instruments for evaluating training. The following points can be considered. The evaluation can be done upon completion of each part of the training, that is, the didactic and the experiential part, or at the end of all training. The evaluation can cover assessment of the interventionists' knowledge of the intervention and practical competence in providing it. Assessment of knowledge is accomplished by administering a test containing close- and open-ended questions, and vignettes followed by relevant questions. The questions are designed to measure interventionists' understanding of the theory underpinning the intervention, the operationalization of its active ingredients into respective components, and the rationale for specific content and activities. Short vignettes and associated items are generated to assess interventionists' skills at implementing various intervention activities accurately and at handling challenges that may arise during delivery. Additional items can be incorporated to assess the interventionists' interpersonal skills. Formal evaluation of interventionists' skills is planned as part of the supervised delivery of the intervention, or in a separate session scheduled prior to entrusting the delivery of the intervention to clients. The latter session is comparable in content and format to the supervised delivery of the intervention: The interventionists deliver a session to actors posing as clients and the evaluator observes and rates their performance.

## 8.5    INVESTIGATING INTERVENTIONIST EFFECTS

Careful selection is useful in having interventionists who possess the personal and professional characteristics required for delivering the intervention. Comprehensive, multi-method training is important in preparing interventionists for appropriate implementation of the intervention. Although selection and training promote the interventionists' capacity to deliver the intervention with fidelity, they do not guarantee adequate and consistent performance. Evidence (presented in Section 8.2) demonstrates variability in interventionists' performance in delivering the intervention to clients and over time. Interventionists vary in their level of adherence to the intervention protocol and in their interpersonal skills or working alliance, both of which contribute to client outcomes. This evidence suggests that ignoring the interventionists' potential influence in planning intervention evaluation studies and in analyzing outcome data can lead to flawed conclusions (Lutz and Barkham 2015). Results showing no differences between the experimental intervention and the comparison treatment groups, in outcomes assessed following intervention delivery (i.e. post-treatment or post-test), could be associated with variability in the performance of interventionists. Variability in performance yields large differences in the level of outcome improvement experienced by clients within each group, which in turn, reduces the power to detect significant differences in the outcomes between groups. In contrast results of intervention evaluation studies supporting the effectiveness of the intervention could reflect the high-quality performance of the interventionists, that contributed, more so than the intervention, to improvement in clients' outcomes. In this case, the interventionists' performance confounds the observed effects of the intervention on the outcomes. Therefore, it is recommended to examine the interventionist effects, in addition to the intervention effects, in research and practice.

Researchers planning to investigate interventionist effects should consider the following methodological features when designing and analyzing data collected in evaluation studies:

1. The number of interventionists has to be large enough (at least 30) in order to obtain meaningful estimates of the interventionist effects. Large number of interventionists can be easily achieved in naturalistic studies evaluating the implementation of evidence-based interventions by health professionals in practice. When accrual of this number is not feasible, which is often the case in experimental studies or clinical trials, it is advisable to have at least two interventionists deliver the experimental intervention and at least two interventionists provide the comparison treatment. In all studies, each interventionist is assigned to deliver the respective treatment (i.e. experimental intervention or comparison treatment) to a reasonable number of clients (at least 30). The number of clients is balanced across interventionists. Assignment of clients to interventionists is done in a way that minimizes potential selection bias, so that the baseline characteristics (such as level of severity of the problem) of clients assigned to different interventionists are comparable. Differences in the number and characteristics of clients across interventionists may confound the interventionist effects (Lutz et al., 2007).

2. A crossed design is most appropriate to dismantle the interventionist from the intervention effects (Kim et al., 2006). In this design, all selected interventionists are trained in the delivery of all treatments under investigation. The treatments may be distinct interventions (e.g. stimulus control therapy and sleep restriction therapy) or an experimental intervention (e.g. cognitive-behavioral therapy) and a comparison treatment (e.g. standard care) for the management of the health problem. Each interventionist is asked to deliver each treatment to the pre-specified number of clients. In this way, all interventionists have the opportunity to deliver all treatments (Staines et al., 2006). The crossed design minimizes the confounding of interventionists with treatments and permits the examination of the interventionist main effect and the interventionist-by-treatment interaction effect. Confounding occurs when the same interventionist provides the same intervention to all clients assigned to that treatment group. In this situation, improvements in clients' outcomes can be attributable, equally, to the interventionist or to the intervention. By having different interventionists deliver different treatments, variability in interventionists and in treatments is generated. Each source of variability induces its unique influence on client outcomes, thereby allowing to detect the interventionist influence independently from the treatment effects. Use of the crossed design requires the selection of interventionists who are willing to learn, acquire competency in, and deliver interventions with which they may not be familiar or that differ from their theoretical orientation.

3. Collection of data on the interventionists' personal and professional qualifications, as well as performance in delivering the intervention: Data on performance relate to adherence to the intervention protocol and interpersonal skills or working alliance, using pertinent measures (discussed in Chapter 9). Interventionists' level of adherence and working alliance were found to impact clients' outcomes (e.g. Lingiardi et al., 2018; Pellecchia et al., 2015).

4. Tracking and documenting which clients receive which treatment from which interventionist: Code numbers are assigned to interventionists and used in pertinent data entry.

5. Application of multilevel models or hierarchical linear models to analyze the client outcome data. These models are statistical techniques that account for the nesting of clients within interventionists and within treatment when estimating the effects of interventionist and of treatment on client outcomes. The outcomes are those assessed following implementation of the intervention or represented in the level of changes in the outcomes over time. It is recommended to consider the interventionists as a random factor and the treatment as a fixed factor in the data analysis. Representing interventionists as a random factor has the advantage of generalizability of the observed effects to other interventionists with characteristics similar to the qualities of interventionists who were involved in the delivery of treatments (Kim et al., 2006; Lutz et al., 2007).

These methodological features are not always practical and feasible. The number of interventionists needed to examine their effects on client outcomes may exceed the financial resources available for a study, or the human resources that are locally accessible. Similarly, the required client sample size is large. Few competent interventionists may agree to the implementation of different treatments, and those who do agree may not be representative of the general population of health professionals. Investigating interventionist effects is best done in large multicenter experimental studies, or in large cohort studies conducted in the natural, real world, practice setting.

## REFERENCES

Addis, M.E. & Krasnow, A.D. (2000) A national survey of practicing psychologists' attitudes toward psychotherapy treatment manuals. *Journal of Consulting and Clinical Psychology*, 68(2), 331–339.

Alcázar Olán, R.J., Deffenbacher, J.L., Hernández Guzmán, L., et al. (2010) The impact of perceived therapist characteristics on patients decision to return or not return for more sessions. *International Journal of Psychology and Psychological Therapy*, 10(3), 415–426.

Anderson, T., Ogles, B.M., Patterson, C.L., Lambert, M.J., & Vermeersch, D.A. (2009) Therapist effects: Facilitative interpersonal skills as a predictor of a therapist success. *Journal of Clinical Psychology*, 65(7), 755–768.

Baldwin, S.A. & Imel, Z.E. (2013) Therapist effects: Findings and methods. In: M.J. Lambert (ed) *Bergin and Garfield's Handbook of Psychotherapy and Behaviour Change* (6th ed.). Wiley, New York, NY.

Barber, J.P., Gallop, R., Crits-Christoph, P., et al. (2006) The role of therapist adherence, therapist competence, and alliance in predicting outcome of individual drug counseling: Results from the National Institute Drug Abuse Collaborative Cocaine Treatment Study. *Psychotherapy Research*, 16(2), 229–240.

Becker-Haimes, E.M., Okamura, K., Wolk, C.B., et al. (2017) Predictors of clinician use of exposure therapy in community mental health settings. *Journal of Anxiety Disorders*, 49, 88–94.

Berghout, C.C. & Zevalkink, J. (2011) Therapist variables and patient outcome after psychoanalysis and psychoanalytic psychotherapy. *Journal of the American Psychoanalytic Association*, 59(3), 577–583.

Borrelli, B. (2011) The assessment, monitoring and enhancement of treatment fidelity in public health clinical trials. *Journal of Public Health Dentistry*, 71, S52–S63.

Brooks, K. (2010). The simulation job interview [Blog post]. Available on: `http://www.psychologytoday.com/blog/career-transitions/201012/the-simulation-job-interview`.

Brose, L.S., McEwen, A, Michie, S, et al. (2015) Treatment manuals, training and successful provision of stop smoking behavioral support. *Behaviour Research and Therapy*, 71, 34–39.

Cameron, S.K., Rodgers, J., & Dagnan, D. (2018) The relationship between the therapeutic alliance and clinical outcomes in cognitive behaviour therapy for adults with depression: A meta-analytic review. *Clinical Psychology & Psychotherapy*, 25, 446–456.

Campbell, B.K., Buti, A., Fussell, H.E., Srikanth, P., & Guydish, J.R. (2013) Therapist predictors of treatment delivery fidelity in community-based trial of 12-step facilitation. *American Journal of Drug and Alcohol Abuse*, 39, 304–311

Castonguay, L.G., Constantino, M.J., & Holtforth, M.G. (2006) The working alliance: Where are we and where should we go? *Psychotherapy: Theory, Research, Practice, Training*, 43(3), 271–279.

Constantino, M.J., Manber, R., Org, J., et al. (2007) Patient expectation and therapeutic alliance as predictors of outcomes in group cognitive-behavioral therapy for insomnia. *Behavioral Sleep Medicine*, 5, 210–228.

Degnan, A., Seymour-Hyde, A., Harris, A., & Berry, K. (2016) The role of therapist attachment in alliance and outcome: A systematic literature review. *Clinical Psychology & Psychotherapy*, 23, 47–65.

Del Re, A.C., Flückiger, C., Horvath, A.O., Symonds, D., & Wampold, B.E. (2012) Therapist effects in the therapeutic alliance–outcome relationship: A restricted-maximum likelihood meta-analysis. *Clinical Psychology Review*, 32(7), 642–649.

DiGennaro Reed, F.D. & Codding, R.S. (2014) Advancements in procedural fidelity assessment and intervention: Introduction to the special issue. *Journal of Behavioral Education*, 23, 1–18.

Dinger, U., Strack, M., Leichsenrig, F., Wilmers, F., & Schauenburg, H. (2008) Therapist effects on outcome alliance in inpatient psychotherapy. *Journal of Clinical Psychology*, 64(3), 344–35.

Elkin, I., Falconnier, L., Martinovich, Z., & Mahoney, C. (2006) Therapist effects in the National Institute of Mental Health treatment of depression collaborative research program. *Psychotherapy Research*, 16, 144–160.

Eymard, A.S. & Altmiller, G. (2016) Teaching nursing students the importance of treatment fidelity in intervention research: Students as interventionists. *Journal of Nursing Education*, 55(5), 288–291.

Friedman, R. (2014) *The Best Place to Work: The Art and Science of Creating an Extraordinary Workplace*. Perigee, Penguin Group, New York, USA.

Fuertes, J.N., Mislowack, A., Bennett, J., et al. (2007) The physician-patient working alliance. *Patient Education and Counseling*, 66, 29–36.

Gaume, J., Gmel, G., Faouzi, M., & Daeppen, J.-B. (2009) Counselor skill influences outcomes of brief motivational interventions. *Journal of Substance Abuse Treatment*, 37, 151–159.

Goldberg, S.B., Hoyt, W.T., Nissen-Lie, H.A., Nielsen, S.L., & Wampold, B.E. (2018) Unpacking the therapist effect: Impact of treatment length differs for high- and low-performing therapists. *Psychotherapy Research*, 28(4), 532–544.

Greeson, J.K.P., Guo, S., Barth, R.P., Hurley, S., & Sisson, J. (2009) Contributions of therapist characteristics and stability to intensive in-home therapy youth outcomes. *Research in Social Work Practice*, 19(2), 239–250.

Herschell, A.D., Kolko, D.J., Baumann, B.L., & Davis, A.C. (2010) The role of therapist training in the implementation of psychosocial treatments: A review and critique with recommendations. *Clinical Psychology Review*, 30(4), 448–466.

Horvath, A.O., Del Re, A.C., Flückiger, C., & Symonds, D. (2011) Alliance in individual psychotherapy. *Psychotherapy: Theory, Research, & Practice*, 48, 9–16.

Huppert, J.D., Bufka, L.F., Barlow, D.H., et al. (2001) Therapists, therapist variables, and cognitive-behavioral therapy outcome in a multicenter trial for panic disorder. *Journal of Consulting and Clinical Psychology*, 69(5), 747–755.

Huss, R., Jhileek, T., & Butler, J. (2017) Mock interviews in the workplace: Giving intern the skills they need for success. *The Journal of Effective Teaching*, 17(3), 23–37.

Imel, Z.E., Baer, J.S., Martino, S., Ball, S.A., & Carroll, K.M. (2011) Mutual influence in therapist competence and adherence to motivational enhancement therapy. *Drug and Alcohol Dependence*, 115, 229–236.

Johnson, M.O. & Remien, R.H. (2003) Adherence to research protocols in a clinical context: Challenges and recommendations from behavioral intervention trials. *American Journal of Psychotherapy*, 57, 348–360.

Joyce, A.S., Ogradniczuk, J.S., Piper, W.E., & McCallum, M. (2003) The alliance as mediator of expectancy effects in short-term individual therapy. *Journal of Clinical and Consulting Psychology*, 71(4), 672–679.

Kaplowitz, M.J., Safran, J.D., & Muran, C.J. (2011) Impact of therapist emotional intelligence on psychotherapy. *Journal of Nervous and Mental Disorders*, 199, 74–74

Kim, D.M., Wampold, B.E., & Bolt, D.M. (2006) Therapist effects in psychotherapy: A random-effects modeling of the National Institute of Mental Health treatment of depression collaborative research program data. *Psychotherapy Research*, 16, 161–172.

Kitson, A., Marshall, A., Bassett, K., & Zeitz, K. (2013) What are the core elements of patient-centered care? A narrative review and synthesis of the literature from health policy, medicine and nursing. *Journal of Advanced Nursing*, 69, 4–15.

Krukowski, R.A., Smith West, D., Priest, J., et al. (2019) The impact of the interventionist–participant relationship on treatment adherence and weight loss. *TBM*, 9, 368–372.

Lingiardi, V., Muzi, L., Tanzilli, A., & Carone, N. (2018) Do therapists' subjective variables impact on psychodynamic psychotherapy outcomes? A systematic literature review. *Clinical Psychology & Psychotherapy*, 25, 85–101.

Lutz, W. & Barkham, M. (2015) Therapist effects. In: R. Cautin & S. Lilienfeld (eds) *Encyclopedia of Clinical Psychology*. Wiley-Blackwell, Hoboken.

Lutz, W., Leon, S.C., Martinovich, Z., et al. (2007) Therapist effects in outpatient psychotherapy: A three-level growth curve approach. *Journal of Counseling Psychology*, 54, 32–39.

Mauricio, A.M., Rudo-Stern, J., Thomas J., et al. (2019) Provider readiness and adaptations of competency drivers during scale-up of the family check-up. *The Journal of Primary Prevention*, 40, 51–68.

McDiamid Nelson, M., Shanley, J.R., Funderbuk, B.W., & Bard, E. (2012) Therapists' attitudes toward evidence-based practices and implementation of parent-child interaction therapy. *Child Maltreatment*, 17, 47–55.

Moyers, T.B., Miller, W.R., & Hendrickson, S.M.L. (2005) How does motivational interviewing work? Therapist interpersonal skill predicts client involvement within motivational interviewing sessions. *Journal of Consulting and Clinical Psychology*, 73(4), 590–598.

Okiishi, J., Lambert, M.J., Nielson, S.L., & Ogles, B.M. (2003) Waiting for supershrink: An empirical analysis of therapist effects. *Clinical Psychology & Psychotherapy*, 10, 361–373.

Pellecchia, M., Connell, J.E., Beidas, R.S. et al. (2015) Dismantling the active ingredients of an intervention for children with autism. *Journal of Autism and Developmental Disorders*, 45, 2917–2927.

Reichow, B., Volkmar, F.R., & Cicchetti, D.V. (2008) Development of the evaluative method for evaluating and determining evidence-based practices in autism. *Journal of Autism and Developmental Disorders*, 38, 1311–1319.

Saxon, D., Barkham, M., Foster, A., & Parry, G. (2017) The contribution of therapist effects to patient dropout and deterioration in the psychological therapies. *Clinical Psychology & Psychotherapy*, 24(3), 575–588.

Schiefele, A.-K., Lutz, W., Barkham, M., et al. (2017) Reliability of therapist effects in practice-based psychotherapy research: A guide for the planning of future studies. *Administration and Policy in Mental Health*, 44(5), 598–613.

Schoenwald, S.K., Garland, A.F., Chapman, J.E., et al. (2011) Toward the effective and efficient measurement of implementation fidelity. *Administration and Policy in Mental Health and Mental Health Services Research*, 38, 32–43.

Schwantes, M. (2017) The job interview will soon be dead. Here's what the top companies are replacing it with. Available on: `https://www.inc.com/marcel-schwantes/science-81-percent-of-people-lie-in-job-interviews-heres-what-top-companies-are-.html`

Sidani, S. & Fox, M. (2014) Patient-centered care: A clarification of its active ingredients. *Journal of Interprofessional Care*, 28(2), 134–141.

Staines, G.L., Cleland, C.M., & Blankertz, L. (2006) Counselor confounds in evaluations of vocational rehabilitation methods in substance dependency treatment. *Evaluation Review*, 30, 139–170.

Titzler, I., Sarwhanjan, K., Berking, M., Riper, H., & Ebert, D.D. (2018) Barriers and facilitators for the implementation of blended psychotherapy for depression: A qualitative pilot study of therapists' perspective. *Internet Interventions*, 12, 150–164.

Tschuschke, V., Crameri, A., Koehler, M., et al. (2015) The role of therapists' treatment adherence, professional experience, therapeutic alliance, and clients' severity of psychological problems: Prediction of treatment outcome in eight different psychotherapy approaches. Preliminary results of a naturalistic study. *Psychotherapy Research*, 25(4), 420–434.

Verschuur, R., Huskens, B., Korzilius, H., et al. (2019) Pivotal response treatment: A study into the relationship between therapist characteristics and fidelity of implementation. *Autism*, 1, 16–27.

Wampold, B.E. & Brown, G.S. (2005) Estimating therapist variability: A naturalistic study of outcomes in managed care. *Journal of Consulting and Clinical Psychology*, 73, 914–923.

Wampold, B.E. & Imel, Z.E. (2015) *The Great Psychotherapy Debate: The Evidence for What Makes Psychotherapy Work*. Routledge, New York, NY.

Webb, C.A., DeRubeis, R.J., & Barber, J.P. (2010) Therapist adherence/competence and treatment outcome: A meta-analytic review. *Journal of Consulting and Clinical Psychology*, 78(2), 200–211.

Webster-Stratton, C.H., Ried, M.J., & Marsenich, L (2014) Improving therapist fidelity during implementation of evidence-based practices: Incredible years program. *Psychiatric Services*, 65, 789–795.

Zimmermann, D., Rubel, J., Page, A. C., & Lutz, W. (2017) Therapist effects on and predictors of non-consensual dropout in psychotherapy. *Clinical Psychology & Psychotherapy*, 24(2), 312–321.

# CHAPTER 9

# Assessment of Fidelity

The development of an intervention manual, the careful selection of competent interventionists, and the intensive training of interventionists are strategies to promote fidelity of intervention delivery; however, they do not guarantee it. The actual delivery of an intervention may deviate from what is designed and described in the manual, and may vary for different clients. Interventionists, especially those experienced, view intervention manuals as being at odds with the principles of treatment, stating that treatment should be provided with flexibility and tailored to clients' individual characteristics, concerns, and life circumstances. Interventionists also report that strictly adhering to the intervention manual interferes with building and maintaining a good rapport, therapeutic relationship, or working alliance, and with the quality of interactions between interventionists and clients; yet, interventionists value these interactions because they contribute to clients' engagement in and enactment of treatment, and subsequently improvement in client outcomes (Brose et al., 2015). Accordingly, interventionists and health professionals have a tendency to not use or follow the intervention manual in delivering standardized and/or individualized interventions (Lorencatto et al., 2014; Wallace & von Ranson, 2011). This, in turn, leads to variability in intervention delivery, which has been reported widely in research (e.g. Webb et al., 2010) and in practice (e.g. Tschuschke et al., 2015; Verschuur et al., 2019). Variability in intervention delivery results in differences in the active ingredients to which clients are exposed, potentially yielding nonsignificant intervention's effects on outcomes.

Monitoring fidelity is critical for identifying deviations or variability in intervention's delivery and rectifying them as necessary. Assessing fidelity is important for examining the impact of such variability on the outcomes expected of an intervention. Monitoring and assessing fidelity rest on a clear conceptualization of fidelity. The focus of this chapter is on the conceptualization and operationalization of fidelity. Definitions and levels of fidelity are reviewed. Strategies and methods for assessing fidelity are discussed.

*Nursing and Health Interventions: Design, Evaluation, and Implementation*, Second Edition.
Souraya Sidani and Carrie Jo Braden.
© 2021 John Wiley & Sons Ltd. Published 2021 by John Wiley & Sons Ltd.

## 9.1    CONCEPTUALIZATION OF FIDELITY

Traditionally, fidelity has received limited attention in intervention evaluation research. This was based on the assumption that well-trained interventionists strictly follow the treatment manual, which ensures standardization and consistency in providing standardized and tailored interventions to clients. The assumption proved to be untenable in light of evidence showing differences in interventionists' use of manual and performance in delivering interventions (as presented in Chapter 8). Fidelity emerged as a concern in intervention research in various fields of study, most notably program evaluation, psychotherapy, and, recently, behavioral medicine. Differences in theoretical and methodological orientations across fields of study may have contributed to differences in terminology and conceptualization of fidelity (McGee et al., 2018).

### 9.1.1    Terminology

Different terms are used to refer to fidelity. These include: (1) integrity, which appears primarily in the field of program evaluation; (2) adherence to treatment protocol, which is mentioned in the field of psychotherapy; and (3) fidelity, which has recently been reported in the fields of psychotherapy, behavioral medicine and implementation science. These terms are often used interchangeably to refer to the extent to which the delivery (in research) or implementation (in practice) of an intervention is consistent with the original intervention design. Recently, the term "flexible fidelity" has appeared in the literature. It reflects the increasing recognition of the need to adapt the delivery of interventions to fit the characteristics and circumstances of the client population and context, while maintaining fidelity in providing the intervention's active ingredients that are operationalized in the specific or core components (e.g. Mignogna et al., 2018; Shelton et al., 2018) and responsible for its beneficial effects. The term fidelity is used throughout this book as it is the most widely employed in current writings.

### 9.1.2    Frameworks of Fidelity

The widening interest in fidelity in different fields of study led to variability in its conceptualization. An increasing number of frameworks has been published; the recently mentioned ones are listed in Table 9.1. The frameworks present different definitions of fidelity that result in its operationalization in varying domains. The domains have been inconsistently defined and operationalized (McGee et al., 2018). These differences add to much confusion as what actually is fidelity and what domains are to be monitored and assessed (Song et al., 2010; Wainer & Ingersoll, 2013). Commonly used definitions of fidelity and its domains, synthesized from extant literature, are presented next.

### 9.1.3    Definition of Fidelity

The definitions of fidelity, advanced by researchers in different fields, are mentioned in Table 9.2. The first definition is by far the most commonly embraced. The second definition does not actually characterize fidelity but confuses fidelity with the use of strategies to promote it (Song et al., 2010). The third definition emphasizes the consistency between the intervention's theoretically identified active ingredients and

**TABLE 9.1**   Recently mentioned frameworks of intervention fidelity.

| Framework | Source | Definition and domains of fidelity |
|---|---|---|
| Consolidated Framework for Implementation Fidelity | Carroll et al. (2007) | Definition:<br>Fidelity is the degree to which interventions are implemented or delivered as intended<br><br>Domain:<br>Fidelity is operationalized in adherence to the intervention protocol or manual<br><br>Moderating factors:<br>Complexity of intervention, quality of delivery, facilitation strategies, client responsiveness |
| Treatment Fidelity Framework | Originally published by Bellg et al. (2004) on behalf of the National Institutes of Health—Behavioral Change Consortium | Definition:<br>Fidelity encompasses methodological strategies used to monitor and enhance the reliability and validity of interventions<br><br>Domains:<br>Design (or fidelity to theory), training, delivery or implementation, receipt, enactment |
| National Implementation Research Network | | Domains:<br>Context, content, competence (covering interventionists' decision making), client responsiveness |
| Comprehensive Intervention Fidelity Guide | Gearing et al. (2011) | Domains:<br>Design, training, monitoring of intervention fidelity, intervention receipt |
| Fidelity of Technology-Based Interventions | DeVito Dabbs et al. (2011) | Domains:<br>Delivery, receipt, technology acceptance |
| Adapted Model of Fidelity | Wainer and Ingersoll (2013) | Domains:<br>Delivery (i.e. adherence, exposure, differentiation)<br><br>Moderating factors:<br>Complexity of intervention, facilitation strategies, competency, comprehension, social validity |
| Treatment Implementation Model | Lichstein et al. (1994) | Domains:<br>Delivery, receipt, enactment |

their operationalization into specific components. This consistency is foundational for ensuring construct validity of interventions. Accordingly, the first and third definitions are relevant for a comprehensive conceptualization of fidelity. The conceptualization posits two levels of fidelity:

1. Theoretical fidelity: As originally proposed by Bellg et al. (2004), theoretical fidelity has to do with the design of the intervention. It refers to the consistency between the intervention's active ingredients as specified in the intervention theory and the intervention's components as described in the logic model, protocol, or manual. In other words, the content, activities and treatment recommendations comprising the intervention components are congruent, in alignment, and accurately reflective of the active ingredients (Haynes et al., 2016; Keller et al., 2009).

**TABLE 9.2**  Conceptual definitions of intervention fidelity.

| Definition | Source |
| --- | --- |
| 1. Degree or extent to which an intervention is actually delivered or implemented as designed or planned or intended | Aggarwal et al. (2014), Berkel et al. (2019), Breitenstein et al. (2010), Brandt et al. (2004), Campbell et al. (2013), Carroll et al. (2007), Carpinteiro da Silva et al. (2014), DeVito Dabbs et al. (2011), DiRezze et al. (2013), Dunst et al. (2013), Forsberg et al. (2015), French et al. (2015), Hasson (2010), Haynes et al. (2016), Ibrahim and Sidani (2016), Judge Santacrocce et al. (2004); Lorencatto et al. (2014), Mowbray et al. (2003), Prowse and Nagel (2015), Oxman et al. (2006), Roy et al. (2018), Schulte et al. (2009), Seys et al. (2019), Southam-Gerow and McLeod (2013), Toomey et al. (2019), Wojewodka et al. (2017) |
| 2. Methodological (quantitative and qualitative) strategies used to monitor and enhance the reliability and validity of interventions; that is, processes that ensure interventions are consistently implemented as outlined in the protocol | Bellg et al. (2004), Borrelli et al. (2005), Hart (2009), Mars et al. (2013), Resnick et al. (2005), Stein et al. (2007), Swindle et al. (2018) |
| 3. Consistency with the components of the intervention theory | Keller et al. (2009), Pearson et al. (2005) |
| 4. Quality of implementation | Forsberg et al. (2015), Saunders et al. (2005) |

2. Operational fidelity: Operational fidelity has to do with the delivery of the intervention. It refers to the extent to which the intervention, represented in its components, is delivered as originally designed or planned. As such, operational fidelity reflects the degree to which the interventionists adhere to the intervention manual (Aggarwal et al., 2014; Berkel et al., 2019; Forsberg et al., 2015).

Most frameworks (Table 9.1) were primarily concerned with operational fidelity and extended it to cover domains representing the implementation of interventions by the interventionists and the clients. The extension is based on the realization that the implementation of health interventions is the responsibility of both. Interventionists are ascribed the functions of relaying content to and engaging clients in the activities as planned; whereas clients exposed to the intervention are expected to engage and enact treatment in daily life. Accordingly, in the frameworks, operational fidelity is represented in the following domains: adherence, competence and differentiation for interventionists, and responsiveness, exposure, receipt or engagement, and enactment for clients. Each of these domains is defined next.

### 9.1.3.1  Domains of Fidelity—Interventionist

*Adherence*

Adherence to the intervention is the core of fidelity. It refers to whether or not the intervention is delivered as designed or intended (Wainer & Ingersoll, 2013). Adherence implies that the interventionist performs the prescribed activities or behaviors for providing the treatment, as described in the intervention manual (Forsberg et al., 2015; Wojewodka et al., 2017) and avoids proscribed activities or behaviors. Prescribed activities are those reflecting the intervention's active ingredients, represented in the specific components. Proscribed activities include those comprising other treatments such as the use of cognitive reframing in a purely behavioral intervention and general activities that detract from the treatment such as allowing the focus of a treatment session to shift to irrelevant topics (Campbell et al., 2013; DiRezze et al., 2013; Stein et al., 2007). Adherence represents the quantity of intervention delivery (Berkel et al., 2019). It is quantified as the number of the intervention's components that are actually provided or the number of prescribed activities actually performed, out of those planned.

Adherence is enhanced by: 1) having an intervention manual that specifies the activities to be performed and how, and the activities to be avoided; 2) training interventionists in the theory and skills for providing the intervention; and 3) requesting interventionists to follow the intervention manual when delivering the intervention.

## Competence

Competence (also called process fidelity by Dumas et al., 2001) focuses on the manner in which the interventionists deliver the intervention. Competence relates to the interventionists' skillfulness at providing the intervention (Leeuw et al., 2009; Stein et al., 2007). A range of skills have been mentioned in the literature as reflecting interventionists' competence. The most common skills pertain to: delivering the intervention while responding appropriately to client characteristics, concerns, and life circumstances (Hartley et al., 2014; Mars et al., 2013; Carpinteiro da Silva et al., 2014); engaging in nonspecific behaviors such as being flexible; adapting the content or activities to clients' concerns and circumstances (Campbell et al., 2013); being client-centered (Aggarwal et al., 2014); showing empathy (Aggarwal et al., 2014); communicating information clearly, at an appropriate pace and in an engaging or interactive way (Wojewodka et al., 2017); demonstrating understanding of clients' life situation; clarifying information; providing constructive feedback; and collaborating with clients (Berkel et al., 2019; Carpinteiro da Silva et al., 2014; Hartley et al., 2014).

The interventionists' competence skills have been characterized slightly differently. Roth and Pilling (2008) identified them as generic skills and defined them as those exhibited in working collaboratively with clients. Dixon and Johnston (2010) characterized the skills as foundation competencies; these skills involve generic communication skills, ability to engage and collaborate with clients, and capacity to adapt treatment in response to clients' concerns and feedback. Alternatively, these skills encompass communication, interactional style, and development and maintenance of a therapeutic relationship or working alliance, as described in Chapter 8.

In general, competence entails generic (also called common factors) therapeutic skills of interventionists and accounts for the interventionist effects on client outcomes. Competence has been characterized as the quality of intervention delivery (Berkel et al., 2019; Southam-Gerow & McLeod, 2013). It is enhanced with careful selection of interventionist and provision of constructive feedback on these generic skills.

## Differentiation

Differentiation is the domain of fidelity concerned with the distinctiveness of the health intervention and other treatments provided to clients in an evaluation study or in practice. It refers to the extent to which the treatments differ from one another in the intended ways (Hasson, 2010; Wainer & Ingersoll, 2013). This means that the interventionists perform the activities prescribed for each treatment and avoid the proscribed ones (Aggarwal et al., 2014; Forsberg et al., 2015), thereby avoiding contamination of the treatments.

### 9.1.3.2   Domains of Fidelity—Client

*Responsiveness*

Client responsiveness has not been lucidly defined at the conceptual level. At the operational level, client responsiveness encompasses domains of fidelity that pertain to clients' implementation of the intervention. It reflects clients' exposure to, engagement in, and enactment of the intervention.

*Exposure*

Exposure represents the amount of the intervention to which clients are exposed. In other words, exposure is the dose of the intervention that clients actually receive (Hasson, 2010; Ibrahim & Sidani, 2016; Wainer & Ingersoll, 2013), reflecting the level of contact with the intervention content. It is usually quantified as attendance at the intervention sessions or self-completion of the intervention modules.

*Receipt or Engagement*

Both terms are often used interchangeably to denote clients' active involvement in the planned intervention activities, comprehension of the content presented in the intervention sessions or modules, and capacity to employ the skills or perform the behaviors required for applying the treatment recommendations (Leeuw et al., 2009; Wainer & Ingersoll, 2013). Clients' involvement in the intervention activities, such as participation in discussion of the treatment recommendations and reading accompanying materials, helps them to gain a good understanding the intervention and to retain the information. The acquired knowledge promotes their confidence to implement the skills, behaviors, or treatment recommendations in daily life (Prowse & Nagel, 2015; Walton et al., 2017). The results of two literature reviews on fidelity indicated that receipt or engagement is operationalized into: understanding or knowledge of the intervention content, self-efficacy, and acceptability or satisfaction with the intervention (O'Shea et al., 2016; Rixon et al., 2016).

*Enactment*

Enactment is defined as the degree to which clients actually apply the treatment recommendations in their daily life during (i.e. in-between intervention sessions) and following the treatment period (Ibrahim & Sidani, 2016; Prowse &, Nagel 2015; Wainer & Ingersoll, 2013). As defined, enactment has traditionally been discussed under the rubric of client adherence to treatment.

### 9.1.4   Simplified Conceptualization of Operational Fidelity

The frameworks and domains of fidelity presented in Section 9.1.2 and 9.1.3 have been critiqued on conceptual grounds. First, the distinction between theoretical and operational fidelity has not been highlighted and the importance of evaluating theoretical fidelity has not been emphasized. Yet, maintaining theoretical fidelity is a prerequisite for enhancing construct validity of the intervention. Theoretical fidelity is maintained through the systematic process of designing health interventions described in Chapter 4 and 5. Briefly, the process begins by specifying the active ingredients of the intervention, followed by operationalizing the ingredients into components and ending with translating the components into specific activities. Evaluating the correspondence or alignment among activities, components, and active ingredients is important to determine the adequacy and accuracy of the operationalization and to delineate what distinguishes the intervention from others.

Second, most domains of fidelity reflect concepts that have been posited and examined as underpinning the interventionist effects on client outcomes (i.e. competence), the mechanism mediating the intervention's effects on outcomes (i.e. all domains under client responsiveness), or methodological issues (i.e. differentiation) (Gearing et al., 2011; Song et al., 2010). Furthermore, these domains are not in alignment with the conceptual definition of fidelity embraced by a large number of researchers (Table 9.2) and characterizing fidelity as the extent to which an intervention is delivered as designed.

Empirical evidence, synthesized in two reviews, indicates that adherence is the most frequently examined and reported domain of fidelity for interventionist and technology-based delivery of health interventions (Ibrahim & Sidani, 2015; O'Shea et al., 2016). This evidence, in combination with the theoretical points presented in the previous paragraph, has contributed to the increasing use of the Consolidated Framework for Implementation Fidelity (Carroll et al., 2007) to inform research on fidelity (McGee et al., 2018; Roy et al., 2018; Seys et al., 2019; Swindle et al., 2018).

The Consolidated Framework for Implementation Fidelity presents a simplified conceptualization of fidelity that is coherent with the definition of fidelity and addresses the critique of available frameworks presented in the previous paragraphs. The simplified framework focuses on operational fidelity as it pertains to interventionists. The domains of operational fidelity pertaining to clients are viewed as embedded in the mechanism responsible for the intervention's effects on the ultimate outcomes, and investigated as part of process evaluation (Chapter 13).

In the simplified conceptualization, fidelity refers to the degree to which the interventionists deliver the health intervention as intended or designed. It is operationalized in terms of adherence to the intervention manual, which is reflected in the interventionists' performance of prescribed activities and avoidance of proscribed activities. Four categories of factors affect (or moderate) interventionists' delivery of the intervention with fidelity. The first category of factors consists of the characteristics of the intervention, with complexity (e.g. number of components) of the intervention being the most prominent. The second category of factors includes the characteristics of the interventionists that define the quality of the intervention delivery; these are represented in the interventionists' perceptions of the intervention, confidence or self-efficacy in providing the intervention, and competence (which encompasses communication skills, interactional style, and working alliance or therapeutic relationship). The third category of factors entails contextual factors such as the availability and use of supportive strategies (e.g. training) to facilitate intervention delivery. The last category involves characteristics of clients (e.g. severity of health problem, motivation) that impact what is provided and how. Interventionists' delivery of the intervention with fidelity influences clients' responsiveness, that is, clients' exposure to, engagement in, and enactment of treatment (Barber et al., 2007; Hasson et al., 2012; Wang et al., 2015). Preliminary evidence supports some of the framework propositions: A positive moderate association was reported between the interventionists' competence and adherence (Peters-Scheffer et al., 2013).

## 9.2    STRATEGIES AND METHODS FOR ASSESSING THEORETICAL FIDELITY

Assessment of theoretical fidelity is important for ensuring the valid operationalization of the intervention's active ingredients into respective components, content, and activities. The results of such an assessment assist in the interpretation of the findings of an intervention evaluation study. The assessment results suggest whether findings indicating the intervention is ineffective are attributable to faulty intervention design and/or misalignment between the intervention's active ingredients and respective components; this implies that the intervention components are inappropriate for initiating the hypothesized mechanism of action. Alternatively, results of theoretical fidelity assessment increase the confidence in attributing the observed improvement in the outcomes to the intervention.

There are no formal published guidelines for assessing theoretical fidelity. Logically, the assessment should involve a thorough examination of the correspondence among the intervention's active ingredients as identified in the intervention theory, and the components and activities as delineated in the intervention logic model, protocol, or manual. Assessment of theoretical fidelity is done prior to the implementation of the intervention. Two strategies can be applied to conduct this assessment: generation of a matrix and content validation.

### 9.2.1    Generation of a Matrix

The matrix is generated to examine the alignment among the intervention's active ingredients and their operationalization in respective components and activities. Pertinent information is gathered from the intervention theory, logic model, and manual; from relevant published or grey literature; and from discussion with intervention designers (Haynes et al., 2016). The intervention's active ingredients are identified by reviewing the intervention theory and relevant literature, and clarified through discussion with the designers. The intervention's components and activities are abstracted from the intervention logic model and manual.

The matrix is generated to list, for each active ingredient of the intervention: (1) the component that operationalizes it; (2) the activities comprising the component, that is, the activities that reflect the specific components operationalizing the active ingredients and those reflecting the nonspecific components that support the implementation of the active ingredients; and (3) the actions to be performed to carry out the respective activities. Information is also gathered on the activities that can be adapted and how, if mentioned in the reviewed documents. Table 9.3 illustrates the matrix for one active ingredient of the stimulus control therapy for insomnia. The matrix is useful in showing or visualizing the linkages among the theoretically specified active ingredients and their operationalization. A thorough analysis of the content provided in the matrix determines the extent of correspondence among the active ingredients, and respective components, activities, and actions, as well as proposed adaptations.

The matrix is used by the intervention designers and/or by experts involved in the assessment of theoretical fidelity. The intervention designers generate the matrix during the process of developing the intervention and preparing the manual. The matrix serves as "internal check" on the alignment of the intervention ingredients with the respective components, activities, and actions. Experts may be consulted on the conceptualization and operationalization of the intervention (Haynes et al., 2016).

**TABLE 9.3**  Matrix for examining theoretical fidelity of one active ingredient of stimulus control therapy.

| Active ingredient | Component | Activities | Actions |
|---|---|---|---|
| Associate bed and bedroom with sleepiness | Stimulus control instructions | | |
| | Instruction 1: Go to bed only when sleepy | *Specific:*<br>Discuss Instruction 1 | *Specific:*<br>State Instruction 1 and point to written material where it is listed<br>Explain rationale for the instruction<br>Assist in identifying cues for sleepiness: Mention commonly reported cues<br>Ask each participant to reflect on their experience and recognize relevant cues<br>Reinforce the instruction by restating it |
| | | *Nonspecific:*<br>Assign homework | *Nonspecific:*<br>Describe homework:<br>Have participants monitor cues for sleepiness<br>Have participants follow Instruction 1 every night |
| | Instruction 2: Use bed only for sleep | *Specific:*<br>Discuss Instruction 2<br><br>Explore challenges in carrying out Instruction 2 | *Specific:*<br>State Instruction 2 and point to written material where it is listed<br>Explain rationale for the instruction<br>Explore current sleep behaviors and strategies to carry out the change in sleep behaviors and follow Instruction 2<br>Engage in problem-solving as needed (e.g. issues with bed partner) |
| | | *Nonspecific:*<br>Facilitate group discussion<br><br>Assign homework | *Nonspecific:*<br>Involve group in providing instrumental support during problem-solving<br>Describe homework:<br>Have participants follow Instruction 2 every night |

The experts are asked to review the matrix, examine correspondence, and provide feedback in case of misalignment. Experts may also be invited to formally validate the content of the intervention, as described next.

## 9.2.2  Content Validation

Content validation is a strategy for the formal assessment of theoretical validity. This strategy draws on the method used to determine content validity of measures (e.g. Armstrong et al., 2005). It involves having experts validate the correspondence between the conceptualization and the operationalization of the intervention.

Experts are selected to represent researchers and clinicians who have been involved in the development, implementation, and/or evaluation of the health intervention of interest, or of similar interventions. Similarity among interventions is inferred from the general approach, active ingredients, or components of interventions. For instance, to determine the theoretical fidelity of a behavioral intervention designed to promote self-efficacy in diabetes self-management, experts are those who have designed and delivered interventions that comprise components teaching and reinforcing self-management skills to improve self-efficacy; the intervention or components may have been provided to clients with a range of chronic conditions. The number of experts to take part in content validation varies with availability, and could range between 3 and 10 (Polit & Beck, 2006).

Experts are given the matrix that lists the intervention's active ingredients, components, activities, actions, and possible adaptations. They are request to:

1. Review the information presented in the matrix.
2. Comment on the comprehensiveness of the components in capturing all active ingredients.
3. Examine the alignment of each active ingredient with the respective component.
4. Assess the accuracy and/or appropriateness of the activities operationalizing each component.
5. Comment on the adequacy and relevance of the actions in carrying out the activities comprising the components, as well as on the proposed adaptations of the activities.
6. Identify any omission of important components, activities, actions, and adaptations.
7. Suggest ways to revise the intervention's active ingredients, components, activities, actions, and adaptations in order to improve the correspondence among them.

The experts' qualitative comments can be supplemented with overall quantitative ratings of the extent to which the active ingredients, components, activities, and actions are aligned, and the adaptations are useful in addressing particular clients' concerns and life circumstances without altering the intervention's active ingredients. Experts' qualitative feedback guides the refinement of the intervention design to enhance theoretical fidelity.

The two strategies (generation of a matrix and content validation) have not been applied to assess theoretical fidelity. However, they parallel methods used to develop and validate the content of instruments measuring concepts of interest. Since an intervention is the independent variable in evaluation research, it is essential to ensure that it is well conceptualized and operationalized. The application of the two strategies is a means to determine the accuracy of the components, activities, and actions in reflecting the intervention's active ingredients and hence, to enhance construct validity of the intervention as delivered. Delivering interventions with validity has the capacity to induce the desired changes that mediate their effects on the ultimate outcomes. To achieve this, it is equally important to monitor and assess the fidelity with which the intervention is actually delivered.

## 9.3    STRATEGIES AND METHODS FOR ASSESSING OPERATIONAL FIDELITY

Monitoring and assessing operational fidelity in research and practice have been emphasized as means to examine the extent to which the intervention is delivered as designed. As well, they assist in identifying deviations and/or variability in intervention delivery and in determining the nature and degree of variability in intervention delivery and its impact on outcomes. Consistent with the simplified conceptualization, assessment of operational fidelity entails examination of the interventionists' adherence to the manual when providing the intervention to clients. Therefore, this section focuses on strategies and methods for assessing adherence; those for assessing competence are briefly reviewed.

Assessment of interventionists' adherence requires the availability of instruments that capture the components and activities reflective of the unique active ingredients of interventions. Accordingly, most measures of operational fidelity are intervention-specific (Ibrahim & Sidani, 2015). However, efforts have been expanded to develop and validate instrument measuring operational fidelity (including adherence and competence) for some categories of standardized interventions that are comprised of the same active ingredients and operationalized in similar components, even if adapted for particular client populations and health problems. Examples of these measures are the Cognitive Therapy Scale (Blackburn et al., 2001), the Tool for Measurement of Assertive Community Treatment (Monroe-DeVita et al., 2011; Teague et al., 2012), and the Method for Assessing Treatment Delivery of behavioral interventions (Leeuw et al., 2009). The Yale Adherence Competence Scale (Carroll et al., 2000) can be used to assess interventionists' competence in delivering behavioral interventions. If accessible, these instruments or relevant subscales should be selected when their content is consistent with the components and activities that comprise the health intervention of interest. Their use to assess operational fidelity of the intervention of interest is highly recommended because these instruments have demonstrated reliability and validity; therefore, they are likely to enhance the accuracy of the data. Where such instruments are not available, new ones are developed and utilized to collect data on adherence from different sources through different methods.

## 9.3.1    Development of Instruments Measuring Adherence

Instruments assessing interventionists' adherence should capture the intervention's specific and nonspecific components. They consist of a list of activities that interventionists are expected to perform (i.e. prescribed) or avoid (i.e. proscribed) when providing the components (Forsberg et al., 2015). The development of these instruments follows the same systematic process for generating measures of various concepts. The process is deductive in that the generation of items assessing adherence is informed by the intervention logic model, manual, or the matrix described in Section 9.2.1. The process involves five steps (Berkel et al., 2019; Carpinteiro da Silva et al., 2014; Leeuw et al., 2009; Nelson et al., 2012).

*Step 1:* The first step includes *reviewing the intervention*'s components and respective activities mentioned in the logic model, protocol, or matrix, and the actions for carrying out the activities described in detail in the intervention manual. The actions include the specific ones reflecting the unique features of the intervention, and the nonspecific ones reflecting strategies to facilitate the performance of the specific actions. The actions also encompass those that are prescribed and those that are proscribed.

*Step 2:* This step involves *producing a list of all activities* and related actions to be performed when delivering the intervention. The activities and related actions are listed for either each component or each session, and in the sequence in which they are to be performed. Listing the activities per session is logical and useful in organizing the content of the instrument for assessing adherence because the assessment is often done per session.

It is worth noting that the list should maintain a balance between coverage and feasibility (Teague et al., 2012). Coverage has to do with what the list should capture: activities or actions. Feasibility has to do with the number of items comprising the instrument. A list of activities may contain a small number of items that broadly state the activity; this broad statement has the potential for variability in the interpretation of what exactly the activity is about and how to perform it. A list of actions may contain a large number of items that clearly indicate what is to be performed and how; however, completing long measures is demanding in terms of cognitive efforts and time. It may result in response fatigue, which is well known to lower the accuracy of the obtained data (Streiner et al., 2015). One strategy to strike a balance is to list the activities and to provide a description of what they entail. The description delineates the respective prescribed and proscribed, specific and nonspecific actions, as presented in the intervention manual.

*Step 3*: In this step, the *items are generated*. The content of the items should reflect the activities that the interventionists are expected to perform. The statement of each item is followed by a description of the respective actions and of how best to carry them out. The description is comparable to the one provided in the intervention manual (see Chapter 7). The statement of items capturing activities that can be adapted should also indicate the possibility of adaptations and the ways in which the activities or respective actions can be adapted, as specified in the manual.

*Step 4*: This step focuses on *selecting the rating scale*. The rating scale can assess the occurrence, frequency, or quantity with which the activities are performed (Mars et al., 2013). A dichotomous scale is most commonly used to document the occurrence or nonoccurrence of prescribed and proscribed specific and nonspecific activities.

*Step 5*: In this final step, the *items and rating scales are integrated* into a form that will be used to assess and document data on adherence. The form consists of a checklist or table that: (1) identifies the activities; (2) provides the description of the activities and actions to be performed and avoided; and (3) has a column for documenting the occurrence of the activities. The items are organized by intervention component (where the set of items assessing a particular component form a subscale) or by sequence of occurrence within a session (as specified in the manual).

It is recommended to prepare an instrument manual to be used for training the staff responsible for assessing adherence. The manual has two sections. The introductory section highlights the importance of assessing adherence and describes the intervention's components, activities, actions, and permissible adaptations. The second section provides detailed instructions on how to conduct the assessment of adherence and document the data; and explains how to compute total scores that quantify levels of adherence (Carpinteiro da Silva et al., 2014; Forsberg et al., 2015). The total scores are usually computed as the percentage of prescribed activities actually performed, out of the total number planned (Cross & West, 2011).

The instrument is subjected to validity and reliability testing prior to using it in the assessment of adherence. Its content validity is evaluated with experts in the design and/or implementation of the intervention, following the process described by Armstrong et al. (2005). Construct validity is examined by exploring the relationship between the observed level of adherence and client engagement and enactment of the intervention. Inter-rater reliability is assessed by having at least two researchers observe and rate the same interventionist delivering the intervention.

## 9.3.2   Methods for Assessing Interventionist Adherence

Once validated, the instrument is used to gather data on the interventionists' adherence to the intervention. Adherence data can be obtained from different sources (including research or clinical personnel, interventionists, and clients) and through different methods (including observation and self-report by interventionists and clients) (Campbell et al., 2013; McGee et al., 2018; Walton et al., 2017). The methods are described and their strengths or advantages and limitations or disadvantages are discussed.

### 9.3.2.1   Observation of Intervention Delivery

The observation is done of the interventionists while providing the intervention sessions. The application of this method involves training the observers and conducting the observation. Observers' level of agreement or inter-rater reliability is evaluated throughout the training and actual observation (Swindle et al., 2018).

*Training of Observers*

Observers include research staff members or other clinical personnel responsible for assessing the interventionists' or health professionals' adherence to the manual when delivering the intervention in research or practice, respectively. The training is intensive involving didactic and hands-on phases; it aims to prepare observers in conducting the observation and using the instrument to record adherence data. The didactic phase is informed by the instrument manual (Section 9.3.1) and covers information on (1) the intervention, with a particular focus on its components and specific activities that should be performed in each planned session; (2) the instrument content and rating scale, with a detailed explanation of how each activity is exhibited; (3) the observation logistics, that is, what to observe, where and when, and how to document it (Forsberg et al., 2015).

The hands-on phase consists of reviewing video or audio recordings of intervention delivery sessions by the trainee and the trainer. Both conduct the assessment and document performance of the activities on the instrument form, independently. The trainer and trainee compare their responses to determine agreement and disagreement. Disagreements are discussed and resolved. The training is extended, as necessary, until an acceptable (usually ≥80%) level of agreement or inter-observer or inter-rater reliability is attained by the trainee.

*Conducting Observation*

Observation of intervention delivery is usually done for (1) each interventionist providing the intervention to clients individually or in group, via in-person, telephone, or other technology-based methods of offering the intervention; (2) all sessions planned to deliver all intervention's components to clients; and (3) the whole or total duration of each session given. This is essential to comprehensively assess interventionists' performance, particularly when the content of the sessions is cumulative, demanding engagement in different sets of specific and nonspecific activities, as well as to enable meaningful computation of adherence scores that quantify the percentage of activities actually performed out of the total planned. Although the ideal is to conduct the observation on all interventionists providing all sessions to all clients, this may not be feasible. Therefore, the observation can be done on each interventionist for 10–25% of her or his clients or of the sessions she or he delivers (Mars et al., 2013; O'Shea et al., 2016; Swindle et al., 2018).

Observation of intervention delivery can be either direct or indirect, and done by trained observers.

### Direct Observation

In direct observation, the observers are physically present during the intervention delivery. They attend the sessions with individual or group of clients; however, they do not participate in any intervention-related activities. Thus, they assume the non-participant observer role. Observers are expected to follow through the interventionist's presentation of the content or information, performance of specific and nonspecific activities, and adaptation of content/activities as needed. The observer should be alert and cognitively able to recognize what the interventionist does, to evaluate the adequacy or consistency of performance with the activities as delineated in the instrument for assessing adherence, and to record accurately the observations.

Direct observation has logistics challenges. Observers' attendance at the sessions requires clients' oral approval or formal written consent (as demanded by the research ethics board or committee). Observers' presence may not be logistically possible such as when the sessions are held with individual clients, in geographically dispersed areas, and at a place and a time convenient to clients (e.g. in client's home, in the evening). Some observers may be overwhelmed with their responsibilities of simultaneously following through, interpreting, and documenting the interventionist's performance. Two observers are needed to overcome this challenge and to reduce potential observer bias. Consequently, direct observation is resource intensive, time consuming, and costly (Toomey et al., 2016).

Direct observation is advantageous. It is considered a valid method for assessing interventionist's adherence (DiRezze et al., 2013). It enables objective assessment of performance that is not tainted by social desirability bias. Specifically, the observer's presence is useful in capturing nuances in interventionists' performance of specific activities, and nonverbal responses that may be associated with some nonspecific activities such as eye contact and smile (Toomey et al., 2016; Walton et al., 2017).

Direct observation has several limitations. Despite intensive training, some observers may not correctly recognize, interpret, and document performance of the intervention activities. Observer fatigue may also lead to inaccurate reporting. Observer expectancies may contribute to biased reporting (Gresham, 2009). The observer's presence at the session may be perceived as intrusive by both the interventionist and clients, producing reactivity (Hardeman et al., 2008). In other words, the observer's presence may not be well received by, and may change the behavior of, those observed (Walton et al., 2017). For instance, interventionists exhibit the best performance and behave in a socially expected and appropriate manner, thereby introducing observation bias indicated by high levels of adherence, which is commonly reported in research and practice (e.g. Mars et al., 2013). Clients may limit their engagement in the planned activities and interventionists may use different or additional strategies to engage clients, which may be interpreted as deviations in performance potentially resulting in less-than-optimal adherence. Logistical challenges may constrain direct observation to a few sessions provided by each interventionist. The reliance on data gathered in these sessions leads to incomplete information on interventionists' adherence across clients and over sessions (Berkel et al., 2019; Cross & West, 2011; Gresham, 2009). The use of these data yields inaccurate scores of the interventionists' actual level of adherence.

*Indirect Observation*

Indirect observation is resorted to when the observer's attendance at the intervention sessions is not logistically possible or when clients' approval of observer's presence is not granted. Indirect observation consists of reviewing video or audio recordings of the intervention sessions. Similar to direct observation, trained observers are expected to recognize what the interventionist does, evaluate the consistency of the actual interventionist's performance with the activities as planned, and record their observations on the instrument form. The review of the recordings is done at the required pace, which allows for comprehensive and detailed examination of interventionist's adherence.

Indirect observation generates some challenges. Clients' written consent must be secured prior to the video or audio recording. Video recording can be done in the presence or absence of a staff member; the presence of a staff member may be required to monitor the appropriate functioning of the recording equipment and to manipulate the video recorder, as necessary, to capture the interventionist's performance (e.g. zooming in to capture the demonstration of a particular skill). The staff member's presence is resource intensive, time consuming, and not always feasible. In the absence of a staff member, the video recorder is set to focus on the interventionist, with the drawback of missing performance of some activities when the interventionist moves away from the recorder range. Audio recording is done with high-quality equipment that can clearly record voices of the interventionist and clients participating in face-to-face, telephone, or other technology-based methods of offering the sessions. Additional challenges reported with the use of video and audio recording include: equipment failure or forgetting to turn on the recording equipment, resulting in the loss of adherence data (Hardeman et al., 2008; Mars et al., 2013).

Similar to direct observation, indirect observation is considered a valid method for objectively assessing interventionists' performance. Compared to audio recording, video recording captures the performance of specific activities such as demonstration of skills and nonverbal behaviors reflecting nonspecific behaviors (Toomey et al., 2016). Indirect observation shares the same limitations (i.e. observer bias, reactivity, incomplete adherence data) as direct observation.

## 9.3.2.2   Interventionist Self-report on Adherence

Interventionist self-report is another method for gathering data on adherence. The method is useful to complement and supplement the adherence data collected through observation. Self-report is utilized to obtain relevant data in situations when observation is not feasible or appropriate such as interventions addressing sensitive topics and requiring maintenance of clients' privacy and confidentiality. With the self-report method, the interventionists are requested to document the intervention activities they perform when providing each session to individual or group of clients (Campbell et al., 2013). This should be done immediately following completion of each session in order to minimize recall bias (Melder et al., 2006).

The documentation or reporting on the activities performed can be unstructured or structured. With unstructured documentation, interventionists list the activities they carried out during the session, in their own words. This may take some time as the interventionists have to recall the activities and to find the appropriate wording to describe the activities. Further, the description of the activities performed may not be quite consistent with the ones delineated in the intervention manual and the instrument measuring adherence, potentially contributing to an underestimation of levels of adherence. Nonetheless, the interventionists' description could be useful in identifying adaptations of the activities.

The structured documentation consists of having interventionists complete a hard or electronic copy (DeRosier, 2019) of the instrument assessing adherence. This may be less time consuming; the content of the items makes it easier for interventionists to recall and report the performance of all specific and nonspecific activities (Cross & West, 2011).

There are advantages to interventionist self-report on adherence. Compared to observation, having interventionists document performance of activities is a practical, easy to implement strategy to obtain comprehensive data on adherence by all interventionists and for all intervention sessions they provide. Further, it requires less resources in terms of personnel and time (Cross & West, 2011; Swindle et al., 2018). In addition, when completing the documentation, interventionists may reflect on their performance, which may serve as a reminder or cue to provide all planned activities, thereby improving adherence (Borrelli, 2011; Swindle et al., 2018). With these advantages, interventionist self-report is increasingly used to collect data on adherence (Toomey et al., 2016; Walton et al., 2017).

Interventionist self-report has some disadvantages. The after-session documentation takes time. There is the potential for missing or omitting report of some activities for some sessions provided to some clients, which results in low or underestimated levels of adherence (Swindle et al., 2018). Social desirability and self-report bias are likely because the interventionists desire to show high performance, which result in high or overestimated levels of adherence (Berkel et al., 2019; DiRezze et al., 2013; Toomey et al., 2019). Evidence indicates a weak but positive correlation between levels of adherence reported through observation and interventionist self-report (e.g. Swindle et al., 2018). The evidence has been considered as supportive of the (superior) validity of observation. However, the correlation should be interpreted with caution: The positive direction indicates consistency in the levels of adherence obtained through the two methods; the small magnitude may be related to differences in what is assessed, that is, activities or actions, and in the number of sessions from which the adherence data were obtained, that is, few and often randomly selected sessions for observations compared to almost all (or all) sessions for self-report. Logically, the latter provides a more comprehensive account of the activities performed.

### 9.3.2.3   Client Report on Adherence

Clients who receive the intervention are in a position to report on the occurrence of activities performed by the interventionist providing the intervention session. Clients can also identify content and activities covered in self-completed intervention modules. Clients are capable of recognizing main content covered such as information on treatment recommendations, and main activities or exercises in which they engage such as discussion of challenges in implementing the treatment recommendations or goal setting. Clients may be requested to indicate whether or not the content was presented and the activities performed. This can take place by:

1. Having clients complete a checklist toward the end of each session or module: The checklist is formatted in a way comparable to that described for the instrument measuring interventionist adherence, with the exception that the key activities are only mentioned. The activities are described in lay, simple, and easy to understand terms. Completing the checklist at the end of the session or module minimizes recall bias and enhances accuracy of reporting (Borrelli, 2011). However, it takes time away from clients' schedule

(e.g. those who have to leave promptly upon session completion due to other commitment) and may increase response fatigue that jeopardizes the quality or accuracy of the data.

2. Holding an "exit interview" (Campbell et al., 2013), scheduled immediately following treatment completion, that is, after attending all planned sessions or completing all modules: The interview can be structured whereby the interviewers administer the checklist or semi-structured whereby the interviewers pose open-ended questions inquiring about clients' exposure to the main content and engagement in the main activities. Although feasible, convenient, and less burdensome (compared to completing the checklist repeatedly) to clients, the timing of the exit interview has the potential to introduce recall bias.

Adherence data gathered through client self-report complement and supplement data obtained through observation and interventionist self-report. Convergence of findings enhances validity as the bias inherent in each method of data collection is counterbalanced by the bias inherent in the others. Nonetheless, clients are inclined to report favorably on the interventionist's performance of all activities, in order to please or show gratitude to the interventionist. This contributes to high (overestimate) adherence levels (Borrelli, 2011). However, clients represent a valuable source of information on the interventionists' competence.

## 9.3.3    Methods for Assessing Interventionists' Competence

Overall, interventionists' competence reflects the quality with which interventionists deliver the intervention (Berkel et al., 2019). Quality of delivery has been conceptualized and operationalized in different ways. These differences make it difficult to devise clear guidance on how best to assess competence (Forsberg et al., 2015). Nonetheless, it is highly recommended to follow a systematic process in selecting the measures of competence.

When competence is operationalized in the skills presented in Section 9.1.2, then a review of relevant literature is conducted to select the most appropriate measures. Communication skills, interactional style, therapeutic relationship, and working alliance are the competence skills most commonly referred in the literature and measured with validated instruments. For example, Carroll et al. (2000) developed the Yale Adherence and Competence Scale; the competence subscale captures relationship and alliance building skills such as validating, tone of voice, collaboration, and ability to correctly teach and tailor the content and activities planned for a session. The scale is generic and can be used to assess competence in delivering a range of health interventions.

When competence is operationalized in nonspecific activities that are unique to an intervention, then the process starts with a delineation of the interventionists' skills that represent high-quality delivery as identified in the intervention manual or matrix mentioned in Section 9.2.1. The skills are then described in detail. The description then informs the generation of new items to capture the skills, following the steps for developing measures of interventionist adherence described in Section 9.3.1. The systematic process is well illustrated in the work of Mars et al. (2013); the researchers developed a measure to assess competence with which a self-management course for chronic pain is delivered. They defined competence as the extent to which health professionals create an environment in which patients feel comfortable sharing their experience and learn new skills. Consequently, they generated items that reflect the extent to which health professionals: introduce the aim and rationale for each program component; generate group discussion and individual disclosure; consolidate and summarize the key information (or patient learning) at the end of each program component; and link the information presented within different components.

Once the instrument measuring competence is selected, then three versions of the measure are generated. The versions are used to collect competence data through observation by trained staff, self-report by interventionists, and rating by clients. Trained observers are asked to document whether or not the interventionists exhibited the competence skills when providing the intervention. However, there are reports that accurate assessment of these nuanced skills is challenging, in particular for not well-trained observers (e.g. Carroll et al., 2000). Interventionists and clients are requested to complete the respective version of the measure following treatment completion. As explained previously, gathering data from different sources using different methods enhances the validity of the competence data.

## REFERENCES

Aggarwal, N.K., Glass, A., Tirado, A., et al. (2014) The development of the DSM-5 cultural formulation interview-Fidelity instrument (CFI-FI): A pilot study. *Journal of Health Care for the Poor and Underserved*, 25(3), 1397–1417.

Armstrong, T.S., Cohen, M.Z., Erikson, L., & Cleeland, C. (2005) Content validation of self-report measurement instruments: An illustration from the development of a brain tumor module of the M.D. Anderson symptom inventory. *Oncology Nursing Forum*, 3, 669–676.

Barber, J., Sharpless, B., Klostermann, S., & McCarthy, K. (2007) Assessing intervention competence and its relation to therapy outcome: A selected review derived from the outcome literature. *Professional Psychology: Practice*, 38, 493–500.

Bellg, A.J., Borrelli, B., Resnick, B., et al. (2004) Enhancing treatment fidelity in health behavior change studies: Best practices and recommendations from the NIH behavior change consortium. *Health Psychology*, 23, 443–451.

Berkel, C., Gallo, C.G., Sandler, I.N., et al. (2019) Redesigning implementation measurement for monitoring and quality improvement in community delivery settings. *The Journal of Primary Prevention*, 40, 111–127.

Blackburn, I.M., James, I.A., Milne, D.L., & Reichelt, F.K. (2001) The revised cognitive therapy scale (CTSR): psychometric properties. *Behavioural and Cognitive Psychotherapy*, 29, 431–447.

Borrelli, B. (2011) The assessment, monitoring and enhancement of treatment fidelity in public health clinical trials. *Journal of Public Health Dentistry*, 71, S52–S63.

Borrelli, B., Sepinwall, D., Ernst, D. et al. (2005) A new tool to assess treatment fidelity and evaluation of treatment fidelity across 10 years of health behavior research. *Journal of Consulting and Clinical Psychology*, 73, 852–860.

Brandt, P.A., Kirsch, S.D., Lewis, F.M., & Casey, S.M. (2004) Assessing the strength and integrity of an intervention. *Oncology Nursing Forum*, 31, 833–837.

Breitenstein, S.M., Gross, D., Garvey, C.A., et al. (2010) Implementing fidelity in community-based interventions. *Research in Nursing & Health*, 33, 164–173.

Brose, L.S., McEwen, A., Michie, S., et al. (2015) Treatment manuals, training and successful provision of stop smoking behavioral support. *Behaviour Research and Therapy*, 71, 34–39.

Campbell, B.K., Buti, A., Fussell, H.E., Srikanth, P., & Guydish, J.R. (2013) Therapist predictors of treatment delivery fidelity in community-based trial of 12-step facilitation. *American Journal of Drug & Alcohol Abuse*, 39, 304–311.

Carpinteiro da Silva, T.F., Lovisi, G.M., & Conover, S. (2014) Developing an instrument for assessing fidelity to the intervention in the critical time intervention—Task shifting (CTI-TS)—Preliminary report. *Archives of Psychiatry and Psychotherapy*, 1, 55–62.

Carroll, K.M., Nich, C., Sifry, R.L., et al. (2000) A general system for evaluating therapist adherence and competence in psychotherapy research in the addictions. *Drug & Alcohol Dependence*, 57(3), 225–238.

Carroll, C., Patterson, M., Wood, S., et al. (2007) A conceptual framework for implementation fidelity. *Implementation Science*, 2, 40.

Cross, W.F. & West, J.C. (2011) Examining implementer fidelity: Conceptualizing and measuring adherence and competence. *Journal of Child Services*, 6(1): 18–33.

DeRosier, M.E. (2019) Three critical elements for real-time monitoring of implementation and adaptation of prevention programs. *The Journal of Primary Prevention*, 40, 129–135.

DeVito Dabbs, A., Song, M-K., Hawkins, R., et al. (2011) An intervention fidelity framework for technology-based behavioral interventions. *Nursing Research*, 60(5), 340–347.

DiRezze, B., Law, M., Eva, K., Pollock, N., & Gortier, J.W. (2013) Development of a generic fidelity measure for rehabilitation intervention research for children with physical disabilities. *Developmental Medicine and Child Neurology*, 55, 737–744.

Dixon, D. & Johnston, M. (2010) Health behaviour change competency framework: Competences to deliver interventions to change lifestyle behaviours that affect health. Public Health Online Resource for Careers, Skills and Training. Available on: www.phorcast.org.uk/document_store/1318587875_wBBR_health_behaviour_change_competency_framework.pdf

Dumas, J.E., Lynch, A.M., Laughlin, J.E., et al. (2001) Promoting intervention fidelity. Conceptual issues, methods and preliminary results from the EARLY ALLIANCE prevention trial. *American Journal of Preventive Medicine*, 20, 38–47.

Dunst, C.J., Trivette, C.M., & Raab, M. (2013) An implementation science framework for conceptualizing and operationalizing fidelity in early childhood intervention studies. *Journal of Early Intervention*, 35(2), 85–101.

Forsberg, S., Fitzpatrick, K.K., Darcy, A., et al. (2015) Development and evaluation of a treatment fidelity instrument for family-based treatment of adolescent anorexia nervosa. *International Journal of Eating Disorders*, 48(1), 91–99.

French, C.T., Diekemper, R.L., & Irwin, R.S., on behalf of the CHEST Expert Cough Panel (2015) Assessment of intervention fidelity and recommendations for researchers conducting studies on the diagnosis and treatment of chronic cough in the adult. CHEST guideline and expert panel report. *Chest*, 148(1), 32–54.

Gearing, R.E., El-Bassel, N., Ghesquiere, A., et al. (2011) Major ingredients of fidelity: A review and scientific guide to improving quality of intervention research implementation. *Clinical Psychology Review*, 31, 79–88.

Gresham, F.M. (2009) Evolution of the treatment integrity concept: Current status and future directions. *School Psychology Review*, 38(4), 533–540

Hardeman, W., Michie, S., Fanshawe, T., et al. (2008) Fidelity of delivery of a physical activity intervention: Predictors and consequences. *Psychology and Health*, 23(1), 11–24.

Hart, E. (2009) Treatment definition in complex rehabilitation interventions. *Neuropsychological Rehabilitation*, 19(6), 824–840.

Hartley, S., Scarratt, P., Bucci, S., et al. (2014) Assessing therapist adherence to recovery-focused cognitive behavioural therapy for psychosis delivered by telephone with support from a self-help guide: Psychometric evaluations of a new fidelity scale. *Behavioural and Cognitive Psychotherapy*, 42, 435–451.

Hasson, H. (2010) Systematic evaluation of implementation fidelity of complex interventions in health and social care. *Implementation Science*, 5, 67–75.

Hasson, H., Blomberg, S., & Dunér, A. (2012) Fidelity and moderating factors in complex interventions: A case study of a continuum of care program for frail elderly people in health and social care. *Implementation Science*, 7, 23.

Haynes, A., Brennan, S., Redman, S., et al., the CIPHER team (2016) Figuring out fidelity: A world example of the methods used to identify, critique and revise the essential elements of a contextualized intervention in health policy agencies. *Implementation Science*, 11, 23–40.

Ibrahim, S. & Sidani, S. (2015) Fidelity of intervention implementation: A review of instruments. *Health*, 7, 1687–1695.

Ibrahim, S. & Sidani, S. (2016) Intervention fidelity in interventions: An integrative literature review. *Research and Theory for Nursing Practice: An International Journal*, 30(3), 258–271.

Judge Santacrocce, S., Maccarelli, L.M., & Grey, M. (2004) Intervention fidelity. *Nursing Research*, 53, 63–66.

Keller, C., Fleury, J., Sidani, S., & Ainsworth, B. (2009) Fidelity to theory in PA intervention research. *Western Journal of Nursing Research*, 31, 289–311.

Leeuw, M.E.J.B., Goossensa, H.C.W., de Vetc, J.W.S. et al. (2009) The fidelity of treatment delivery can be assessed in treatment outcome studies: A successful illustration from behavioral medicine. *Journal of Clinical Epidemiology*, 62, 81–90.

Lichstein, K.L., Riedel, B.W., & Grieve, R. (1994) Fair tests of clinical trials: A treatment implementation model. *Advances in Behaviour Research and Therapy*, 16(1), 1–29.

Lorencatto, F., West, R., Bruguera, C., & Michie, S. (2014) A method for assessing fidelity of delivery of telephone behavioral support for smoking cessation. *Journal of Consulting and Clinical Psychology*, 82(3), 482–491

Mars, T., Ellard, D., Carnes, D., et al. (2013) Fidelity in complex behaviour change interventions: A standardized approach to evaluate intervention integrity. *BMJ Open*, 3, e003555.

McGee, D., Lorencatto, F., Matvienko-Sikar, K., & Toomey, E. (2018) Surveying knowledge, practice and attitudes towards intervention fidelity within trials of complex healthcare interventions, *Trials*, 19, 504–517.

Melder, C., Esbensen, A.-A., & Tusinski, K. (2006) Addressing program fidelity using onsite observations and program provider descriptions of program delivery. *Evaluation Review*, 30, 714–740.

Mignogna, J., Martin, L.A., Harik, J., et al. (2018) "I had to somehow still be flexible": Exploring adaptations during implementation of brief cognitive behavioral therapy in primary care. *Implementation Science*, 13, 76–86.

Monroe-DeVita, M., Teague, G.B., & Moser, L.L. (2011) The TMACT: A new tool for measuring fidelity to assertive community treatment. *Journal of the American Psychiatric Nurses Association*, 17, 17–29.

Mowbray, C.T., Holter, M.C., Teague, G.B., & Bybee, D. (2003) Fidelity criteria: Development, measurement, and validation. *American Journal of Evaluation*, 24, 315–340.

Nelson, M.C., Cordray, D.S., Hulleman, C.S., Darrow, C.L., & Sommer, E.C. (2012) A procedure for assessing intervention fidelity in experiments testing educational and behavioral interventions. *Journal of Behavioral Health Services and Research*, 39, 374–396.

O'Shea, O., McCormick, R., Bradley, J.M., & O'Neill, B. (2016) Fidelity review: A scoping review of the methods used to evaluate treatment fidelity in behavioural change interventions. *Physical Therapy Reviews*, 21, 207–214.

Oxman, T.E., Schulberg, H.C., Greenberg, R.L., et al. (2006) A fidelity measure for integrated management of depression in primary care. *Medical Care*, 44, 1030–1037.

Pearson, M.L., Wu, S., Schaefer, J., et al. (2005) Assessing the implementation of the chronic care model in quality improvement collaboratives. *Health Services Research*, 40, 978–996.

Peters-Scheffer, N., Didden, R., Korzilius, H., & Sturmey, P. (2013) Therapist characteristics predict discrete trial teaching procedural fidelity. *Intellectual and Developmental Disabilities*, 51(4), 263–272.

Polit, D.F. & Beck C.T. (2006) The content validity index: Are you sure you know what's being reported? Critique and recommendations. *Research in Nursing and Health*, 29, 489–497.

Prowse, P.-T. & Nagel, T. (2015) A meta-evaluation: The role of treatment fidelity within psychosocial interventions during the last decade. *Journal of Psychiatry*, 18, 251–257.

Resnick, B., Bellg, A.J., Borrelli, B., et al. (2005) Examples of implementation and evaluation of treatment fidelity in the BCC studies: Where we are and where we need to go. *Behavioral Medicine*, 29(Special suppl), 46–54.

Rixon, L., Baron, J., McGale, N., et al. (2016) Methods used to address fidelity of receipt in health intervention research: A citation analysis and systematic review. *BMC Health Services Research*, 16, 263–284.

Roth, A.D. & Pilling, S. (2008) Using an evidence-based methodology to identify the competences required to deliver effective cognitive and behavioural therapy for depression and anxiety disorders. *Behavioural and Cognitive Psychotherapy*, 36(2), 129–147.

Roy, R., Colquhoun, H., Byrne, M., et al. (2018) Addressing fidelity within complex health behavior change interventions: A protocol for a scoping review of intervention fidelity frameworks and models. *HRB Open Research*, 1, 25.

Saunders, R.P., Evans, M.H., & Joshi, P. (2005) Developing a process-evaluation plan for assessing health promotion program implementation: A how-to guide. *Health Promotion Practice*, 6, 134–147.

Schulte, A.C., Easton, J.E., & Parker, J. (2009) Advances in treatment integrity research: Multidisciplinary perspectives on the conceptualization, measurement, and enhancement of treatment integrity. *School Psychology Review*, 38(4), 460–475.

Seys, D., Panella, M., VanZelm, R., et al. (2019) Care pathways are complex interventions in complex systems: New European pathway association framework. *International Journal of Care Coordination*, 22(1), 5–9.

Shelton, R.C., Cooper, B.R., & Wiltsey Stirman, S. (2018) The sustainability of evidence-based interventions and practices in public health and health care. *Annual Review of Public Health*, 39, 55–76.

Song, M., Happ, M.B., & Sandelowski, M. (2010) Development of a tool to assess fidelity to a psycho-educational intervention. *Journal of Advanced Nursing*, 66(3), 673–82.

Southam-Gerow, M.A. & McLeod, B.D. (2013) Advances in applying treatment integrity research for dissemination and implementation science: Introduction to special issue. *Clinical Psychology: Science and Practice*, 20, 1–13.

Stein, K.F., Sargent, J.T., & Rafaels, N. (2007) Establishing fidelity of the independent variable in nursing critical trials. *Nursing Research*, 56, 54–62.

Streiner, D.L., Norman, G.R., & Cairney, J. (2015) *Health Measurement Scales: A Practical Guide to Their Development and Use* (5th ed.) Oxford University Press, Oxford, UK.

Swindle, T., Selig, J.P., Rutledge, J.M, Whiteside-Mansell, L., & Curran, G. (2018) Fidelity monitoring in complex interventions: A case study of the WISE intervention *Archives of Public Health*, 76, 53–62.

Teague, G.B., Mueser, K.T., & Rapp, C.A. (2012) Advances in fidelity measurement for mental health services research: Four measures. *Psychiatric Services*, 63, 765–771.

Toomey, E., Matthews, J., Guerin, S., & Hurley, D.A. (2016) Development of a feasible implementation fidelity protocol within a complex physical therapy-led self-management intervention. *Physical Therapy*, 96, 1287–1298.

Toomey, E., Matvienko-Sikar, K., Heary, C., et al. On behalf of the Choosing Healthy Eating for Infant Health (CHErIsH) study team (2019) Intervention fidelity within trials of infant feeding behavioral interventions to prevent childhood obesity: A systematic review. *Annals of Behavioral Medicine*, 53, 75–97.

Tschuschke, V., Crameri, A., Koehler, M., et al. (2015) The role of therapists' treatment adherence, professional experience, therapeutic alliance, and clients' severity of psychological problems: Prediction of treatment outcome in eight different psychotherapy approaches. Preliminary results of a naturalistic study. *Psychotherapy Research*, 25(4), 420–434.

Verschuur, R., Huskens, B., Korzilius, H., et al. (2019) Pivotal response treatment: A study into the relationship between therapist characteristics and fidelity of implementation. *Autism*, 1, 16.

Wainer, A. & Ingersoll, B. (2013) Intervention fidelity: An essential component for understanding ASD parent training research and practice. *Clinical Psychology: Science and Practice*, 20, 325–374.

Wallace, L.M. & von Ranson, K.M. (2011) Treatment manuals: Use in the treatment of bulimia nervosa. *Behavior Research and Therapy*, 49(11), 815–820.

Walton, H., Spector, A., Tombor, I., & Michie, S. (2017) Measures of fidelity of delivery of, and engagement with, complex, face-to-face health behaviour change interventions: A systematic review of measure quality. *British Journal of Health Psychology*, 22, 872–903

Wang, B., Stanton, B., Deveaux, L., et al. (2015) Factors influencing implementation dose and fidelity thereof and related student outcomes of an evidence-based national HIV prevention program. *Implementation Science*, 10, 44–56.

Webb, C.A., DeRubeis, R.J., & Barber, J.P. (2010) Therapist adherence/competence and treatment outcome: A meta-analytic review. *Journal of Consulting and Clinical Psychology*, 78(2), 200–211.

Wojewodka, G., Hurley, S., Taylor, S.J.C., et al. (2017) Implementation fidelity of a self-management cause of epilepsy: Method and assessment. *BMC Medical Research Methodology*, 17, 100–109.

# EVALUATION OF INTERVENTIONS

# CHAPTER 10

# Overview of Evaluation of Interventions

Evaluation of newly designed health interventions is a necessary step preceding their implementation in practice. Evaluation consists of a systematic process for determining the merit, worth, or value of health interventions. The value of interventions is indicated by their appropriateness, effectiveness, safety, and efficiency in addressing clients' experience of the health problem and in promoting clients' health (Chapter 1).

Traditionally, evaluation research has been concerned with demonstrating the effectiveness of interventions on the ultimate outcomes. To this end, several studies are conducted, with the expectation that convergence of the studies' findings provides the evidence supporting the effectiveness of an intervention. Cumulating evidence, however, shows limited replicability of the results of studies that evaluate the same health intervention (Woodman, 2014). Limited replicability is indicated by mixed findings, with some supporting and others not supporting the effectiveness of the intervention. The literature is replete with examples of studies revealing mixed results and of systematic reviews and meta-analyses reporting heterogeneity in the primary studies' findings; heterogeneity precludes the synthesis of empirical evidence on the effectiveness of a health intervention. Similarly, the results of implementation studies indicate failure of evidence-based interventions to show benefits in practice (Amrhein et al., 2017; Heneghan et al., 2017). For example, Crawford et al. (2016) reviewed the results of trials that evaluated the efficacy (under controlled research conditions) and effectiveness (under real world practice conditions) of the same simple or complex interventions. They found that, although the interventions were initially (in early efficacy studies) reported to be efficacious, 58% of simple interventions and 71% of complex ones returned negative results in subsequent effectiveness trials, implying that the interventions were no longer effective in later studies.

Several factors have been suggested as contributing to the limited replicability of findings on the intervention's effectiveness. The factors are related to weaknesses in the conceptualization of evaluation studies and in the research methodology used in these studies (Crawford et al., 2016). Conceptually, the evaluation studies were informed by a notion of causality that focuses on the direct impact of the intervention on the ultimate outcomes, and does not attend to other factors with the potential to contribute to the outcomes. The factors are inherent in the context in which the

*Nursing and Health Interventions: Design, Evaluation, and Implementation*, Second Edition.
Souraya Sidani and Carrie Jo Braden.
© 2021 John Wiley & Sons Ltd. Published 2021 by John Wiley & Sons Ltd.

intervention is delivered and are associated with: the characteristics of the setting or environment, the interventionist, and the clients; the fidelity with which the intervention is implemented; the clients' perceptions of the treatments included in the evaluation study; and the capacity of the intervention to initiate the mechanism of action. The focus on the direct causal effects of the intervention on the ultimate outcomes results in an emphasis on internal validity, at the expense of other types of validity, and consequently on valuing the experimental design or randomized controlled trial as the most robust in generating evidence of effectiveness.

With the limited attendance to context, the findings of intervention evaluation studies provide answers to the question: Does the intervention work? They fall short of addressing questions of relevance to practice and of importance in guiding treatment decisions: What clients, presenting with which characteristics, benefit from which intervention, given in what mode, at what dose, and in what context? And how does the intervention produce the beneficial effects.

This state of the science has generated some shifts in perspectives underlying intervention evaluation research, accompanied by the acceptance of various designs and methods as appropriate and useful for determining the effectiveness of health interventions in research and practice. The shifts in perspectives are represented in the adoption of the notion of multi-causality, the emphasis on enhancing all types of validity (discussed in this chapter), and the delineation of what to evaluate and in what sequence. The shifts translated into recommendations for evaluating clients' perceptions of health interventions (Chapter 11); the feasibility of interventions (Chapter 12); the contextual factors and the processes contributing to the implementation and effectiveness of interventions (Chapter 13); and a range of research designs (Chapter 14) and methods (Chapter 15) for examining the effects of interventions on a range of outcomes.

In this chapter, the conventional perspectives on causality, validity, and the sequential phases for evaluating health interventions are briefly reviewed. Advances in the field of intervention evaluation are discussed.

## 10.1  NOTION OF CAUSALITY

Underlying the systematic process for determining the effectiveness of health interventions is the notion of causality. Causality implies that the changes in the outcomes, observed following delivery of an intervention, are attributable to, or represent the impact of, the intervention. The notion of causality is evolving from the traditional perspective of single causality to the more recent view of multiple or multi-causality.

### 10.1.1  Traditional Perspective

Demonstrating the effectiveness of health interventions involves the generation of evidence indicating that the intervention causes the ultimate outcomes. A cause is something that creates an effect or produces a change in a state or condition that would not happen without it (Powell, 2019). Causality refers to a structural relationship that underlies the dependence among phenomena or events (Stanford Encyclopedia of Philosophy, 2008), whereby the occurrence of one phenomenon or event is contingent on the occurrence of another. As applied to intervention evaluation, causality implies an association between the intervention (i.e. cause) and the outcome (i.e. effect). The association is characterized by the dependence of the changes in the outcome on the receipt of the intervention. In other words, the changes in the outcome take place in the presence (or exposure, receipt) of the intervention and do not occur in the absence of the intervention. This association enables the attribution of the outcomes solely and uniquely to the intervention.

This notion of causality focuses on the single, deterministic, and direct association between the intervention and the ultimate outcome. It rests on the counterfactual claim that if an intervention occurs, then the effect would occur or take place and conversely, if an intervention does not occur, then the effect would not occur (Cook et al., 2010). This notion of causality and the way in which it is represented in an evaluation study have been criticized on theoretical and empirical grounds. The traditional perspective on causality is considered simplistic, ignoring the potential direct and indirect influence of a range of factors on the delivery, mechanism of action, and outcomes of health interventions (e.g. Greenhalgh et al., 2015; Wong et al., 2012).

## 10.1.2  Recent Perspective

The recent perspective has extended the notion of causality to encompass chains of structural relationships among phenomena or events. The shift was engendered by the widening recognition that multiple factors, in combination with the intervention, contribute to changes in the outcomes (Chapter 5). The factors are experienced in various domains of health (e.g. physical, psychological, social) and at different levels (e.g. client, community, society). The factors, independently and collectively, predict the health problem or other outcomes; they may also interact with the intervention in shaping clients' perceptions of, responses to, the health intervention, as well as improvement in the immediate and intermediate outcomes that mediate the effects of the intervention on the ultimate outcomes.

The recent notion is that of multi-causality. It acknowledges the interdependence among phenomena or events in that they are posited to influence each other, forming a complex system of causal relationships. The application of the notion of multi-causality to intervention evaluation research translates into three propositions. The first is that a set of contextual factors influence directly the delivery of the intervention by interventionists, the implementation of treatment recommendations by clients, the initiation of the intervention's mechanism of action, and the outcomes. The second suggests that contextual factors moderate the causal effects of the intervention on the outcomes. The third proposition indicates that the effects of the intervention on the ultimate outcomes are indirect, mediated by the immediate and intermediate outcomes that operationalize the hypothesized mechanism of action. The direct and indirect relationships are tested empirically to determine what exactly causes the beneficial effects of health interventions on the ultimate outcomes. The resulting evidence provides answers to the practice or clinically relevant questions of who benefits from the intervention and how does the intervention work, in what context. The intervention theory (see Chapter 5) plays an important role in delineating the complex system of causal relationships.

## 10.1.3  Criteria for Inferring Causality

The criteria for inferring causality commonly mentioned across fields of study (e.g. epidemiology, psychology, program evaluation) are comparable for the traditional and recent perspectives on causality. They include temporality, covariation, contiguity, congruity, and ruling out other plausible alternative causes of the intervention effects (Larzele et al., 2004). The evidence required to support each of these criteria differs slightly for the traditional and the recent perspectives.

*Temporality (or temporal sequence).* This criterion reflects the temporal order of the cause and the effect. It is applicable to both, traditional and recent, perspectives on causality. It is typical and logical to think that the changes in the mediators (representing the mechanism of action) and in the ultimate outcomes should occur with or after the delivery of the intervention. If the changes precede delivery, then they cannot be attributed to the intervention because they occurred irrespective of the intervention. Accordingly, it is necessary to assess the mediators and outcomes before, during, and after the intervention is provided. Finding changes in the mediators and the outcomes during and following treatment is ground for inferring causality, especially when the patterns of change are consistent with the propositions of the intervention theory.

*Covariation.* This criterion operationalizes the structural relationship and counterfactual claim that underpin simple and multi-causality. Ideally, covariation is demonstrated when, the same clients are subjected to two conditions: (1) non-exposure to the health intervention and (2) receipt of the intervention. Evidence supporting covariation shows no changes in the ultimate outcomes under the first condition and improvement in the outcomes under the second condition.

In most situations, meeting this ideal requirement is unrealistic and logistically impossible. For instance, it may not be feasible (or ethically acceptable) to withhold treatment when the health problem is acute and experienced at high levels of severity. Therefore, it is recommended to create two groups of participants who experience the health problem addressed by the intervention under evaluation. One group receives and the other is not exposed to the intervention. Participants in both groups have to be comparable in their experience of the health problem and in their personal, health, or clinical characteristics. Evidence supporting covariation is represented in the following pattern of findings: Participants in the two groups are comparable before delivery of the intervention; participants who receive the intervention show the hypothesized changes in the mediators and the ultimate outcomes during and following the treatment period; participants who do not receive the intervention exhibit no changes in the mediators and the ultimate outcomes; participants in the two groups differ in the levels of mediators and the ultimate outcomes reported during or following the treatment period (Cook et al., 2010).

*Contiguity and congruity.* These two criteria of causality are inter-related. The criterion of contiguity reflects the time lag between delivery of the intervention and the occurrence of changes in the ultimate outcomes. Traditionally, the changes were expected to occur within a rather short time interval following intervention delivery. With longer time frames, other factors may take place and influence the impact of the intervention on the outcomes. Contiguity is supported by observing the hypothesized changes in the outcomes in participants who were provided the intervention, immediately (e.g. within one to two weeks) following treatment completion.

The criterion of congruity has to do with the magnitude, size, or amount of the changes in the ultimate outcomes. Traditionally, the magnitude of these changes was expected to be commensurate with the nature and dose of the intervention. For instance, interventions that are highly specific to the health problem, intense, and of high dose can be logically anticipated to yield large changes in the outcomes.

With the acknowledgement of multi-causality, the contiguity and congruity criteria are reframed to account for the indirect impact of health interventions on the ultimate outcomes, mediated through the hypothesized mechanism of action. As detailed in Chapter 4 and 5, the mechanism of action proposes that a health intervention is expected to induce changes in the immediate and intermediate outcomes that mediate its effects on the ultimate outcomes. Accordingly, the time lag reflecting contiguity and the magnitude of change quantifying congruity differ for the mediators and the ultimate outcomes. For the mediators, small-to-moderate changes are anticipated during and following either immediately or within a relatively short time, such as one to two weeks after, treatment completion. For the ultimate outcomes, changes are expected to increase within a longer time frame after treatment completion, once changes in the mediators are produced. Therefore, the criteria of contiguity and congruity are examined simultaneously.

Generating evidence supporting contiguity and congruity requires the collection of data on the mediators and the ultimate outcomes before, during, and after the intervention delivery. Relevant statistical tests are used to analyze the data. Evidence supporting these two criteria should be consistent with the following pattern of findings (see Chapter 4 and 5 for illustrative examples):

1. Changes in the mediators: Small-to-moderate levels of change in the mediators may take place early in the treatment period. These levels may increase over this period, culminating in moderate-to-large changes immediately following treatment completion; the latter levels of change are maintained or additional changes are reported over time (i.e. at follow-up).

2. Changes in the ultimate outcomes: No or minimal levels of change in the ultimate outcomes are expected over the treatment period. Small-to-moderate levels of change take place immediately following treatment completion. The levels of change increase, gradually or sharply, over time.

3. Magnitude of change: The magnitude of change is usually represented in the association between the intervention and the outcomes. The association is quantified in the difference, on the mediators and the ultimate outcomes, between the group of participants who did receive the health intervention and the group of participants who did not. With the hypothesized mechanism of action, the magnitude of the association between the intervention and the mediators is expected to be larger than the association between the intervention and the ultimate outcomes. This expectation is congruent with the notion of mediation where the effects of the intervention on the ultimate outcomes are indirect, mediated by the immediate and intermediate outcomes (MacKinnon & Fairchild, 2009).

*Ruling out other plausible causes of the intervention effects.* This criterion is applicable to both the traditional and the recent perspectives on causality, and is considered the most important or defensible warrant of causality (Cook et al., 2010). This criterion implies that the intervention effects on the mediators and consequently the outcomes are not confounded by other factors. This implies that the changes in the mediators and outcomes can be solely and uniquely attributed to the intervention. Other factors that could contribute to changes in mediators and outcomes include conceptual or substantive (e.g. characteristics of clients) or methodological (e.g. measurement). These factors introduce bias or present threat to the validity of conclusions or inferences regarding the effectiveness of the intervention (discussed in Section 10.2).

Ruling out these plausible threats is done in two ways. The first entails the application of experimental control over the conditions under which the intervention is delivered. This control consists of eliminating (i.e. holding constant) possible sources of bias, as is done in the randomized controlled or clinical trial (RCT) or experimental design. For instance, the control is exerted through the selection of clients with similar characteristics and random assignment of participants to treatment conditions. Elimination of biases increases the confidence in validly attributing changes in the mediators and outcomes to the intervention. The second way to rule out possible threats involves the a priori identification of potentially confounding factors (based on the propositions of the intervention theory); collection of data on these factors; and examination of their influence on the implementation of the intervention and changes in mediators and outcomes (Nock et al. 2007; Schafer & Kang, 2008). The influence of these factors is examined in the recently proposed pragmatic approach to intervention research, as explained in Chapter 15.

## 10.2    VALIDITY

The primary concern in evaluation studies is to generate evidence that would support the validity of inferences or conclusions on the causal effects of the intervention. Validity refers to the approximate truth of the inferences (Shadish et al., 2002; Tengstedt et al., 2018). In other words, validity has to do with the correctness of the claim that changes in the mediators and outcomes are attributable to or caused by the intervention; that is, the claim accurately corresponds with reality (Salimi & Ferguson-Pell, 2017; Sidani, 2015). Many conceptual and methodological factors introduce biases that threaten validity, which leads to erroneous conclusions.

### 10.2.1    Types of Erroneous Inferences

Three types of erroneous or incorrect inferences are frequently mentioned in the literature.

*Type I error.* This type of error is committed when the intervention is claimed to be effective, when in reality it is not. These positive findings instigate additional research to further evaluate the effectiveness of the intervention within the same or different client populations and contexts. However, the beneficial effects found in the initial study are not reproduced or are refuted in subsequent studies. Lack of replicability is increasingly reported for different health interventions (Amrhein et al., 2017; Crawford et al., 2016; Woodman, 2014). The end result is a waste of research and related resources (Yordanov et al., 2015).

*Type II and III error.* These two types of error are committed when the intervention is claimed to be ineffective, when in reality it is. However, they differ in the types of factor considered as contributing to the findings. A variety of factors operate in contributing to type II error, such as small sample size and unreliable measures of the mediators and the ultimate outcomes. Less-than-optimal delivery of the intervention (i.e. with low fidelity) is the main factor leading to type III error. Both types of error result in the abandonment of a potentially effective intervention.

### 10.2.2    Types of Biases

The term "bias" and "threat to validity" are used interchangeably to refer to any factor or process that tends to systematically (i.e. above and beyond chance) deviate or distort the inferences about the effects of the intervention, away from truth/reality (Chavalarias & Ioannidis, 2010; Kumar & Yale, 2016). Conceptual and methodological factors may introduce bias.

Conceptual factors are related to the characteristics (e.g. literacy level) and behaviors (e.g. withdrawal) of clients who are exposed to the intervention; the characteristics (e.g. therapeutic relationship) of interventionists who provide the intervention; and the characteristics (e.g. accessibility of resources) of the context or environment in which the intervention is applied. The intervention theory identifies possible conceptual factors and outlines their direct or indirect (e.g. moderating) influence on the delivery, mechanism of action (i.e. mediators), and outcomes of the intervention (see Chapter 5 for examples).

Methodological factors are related to the design and conduct of the evaluation study that have the potential to distort the findings, which is manifested in an over- or underestimation of the intervention's effects. A wide range of methodological factors has been identified, such as those associated with attrition, measurement, and sample size.

Indeed, a very large number of biases has been identified in the context of research (e.g. Shadish et al., 2002) and of practice (e.g. Lilienfeld et al., 2014). In research, the biases have been listed for different types of validity, and recently for different stages of an evaluation study. The stages and examples of biases include:

1. Preparation or design (i.e. prior) of the study, where the choice of research question is affected by funding opportunities or hidden agendas.
2. Execution (i.e. during) of the study, where the choice of methods shapes the characteristics and number of accrued participants, the implementation of the intervention and comparison treatment, and the participants' responses to the allocated treatment and to the measures of mediators and ultimate outcomes.
3. Reporting and publication (i.e. after) of the study findings, where the benefits are more likely to be reported than the risks associated with the intervention (Heneghan et al., 2017; Ioannidis, 2008; Kumar & Yale, 2016; McGauran et al., 2010; Wilshire, 2017).

Chavalarias and Ioannidis (2010) reviewed the literature to map out the types of bias. They found that 235 terms are mentioned to represent different types of bias; the most common biases can be categorized as associated with the execution of the study (e.g. confounding) and publication of findings. It is beyond the scope of this book to review all types of bias. However, the most commonly mentioned categories of bias threatening each type of validity during the study execution stage are discussed next.

## 10.2.3   Types of Validity and Related Bias

Four types of validity are delineated to reflect the ways in which conceptual and methodological factors weaken the accuracy of the claim regarding the causal effects of the intervention on the mediators and the ultimate outcomes. These include construct, internal, statistical, and external validity. In addition, the term "social validity" is resurging in the extant literature. The definition of each type of validity is presented. The biases that threaten each type of validity and the pathway through which the biases operate are discussed. It is important to note that different terms (used in different disciplines) are sometimes used to refer to the same bias; these are identified. Strategies to address the bias and thus to enhance validity are briefly mentioned next, and detailed in later chapters in this section of the book.

### 10.2.3.1    Construct Validity

*Definition*

Construct validity has to do with the operationalization of the concepts investigated in an evaluation study, with a primary focus on the intervention, mediators, and ultimate outcomes. The operationalization should be congruent with the conceptualization of the intervention, mediators, and ultimate outcomes as specified in the intervention theory. Nonalignment may introduce contamination or confounding that may result in incorrect inferences about the hypothesized intervention effects (Tengstedt et al., 2018). The biases threatening construct validity are: inaccurate implementation of the intervention, researcher expectancies, inaccurate measurement of the mediators and the ultimate outcomes, and clients' reactivity to treatment and measures.

### Inaccurate Implementation of the Intervention

*Overview*. As discussed in Chapter 5, the intervention theory specifies the active ingredients characterizing the intervention, and the components operationalizing them. Inadequate explication of the active ingredients may result in the delineation of components (including content, activities, and treatment recommendations) that either are not well aligned with the intended active ingredients or reflect components comprising other interventions. Accordingly, the intervention as implemented may be contaminated with components reflecting other interventions (Tengstedt et al., 2018). The deviations in the operationalization of the intervention contribute to incorrect inferences about the intervention's causal effects because the observed changes in the mediators and the ultimate outcomes cannot be accurately attributed to the intervention as intended.

    *Strategies*. This bias can be minimized by systematically developing the intervention theory (Chapter 4 and 5) and conducting a thorough assessment of theoretical fidelity (see Chapter 9). Inaccurate implementation of the intervention also extends to its actual delivery by interventionists to participants. Shifts or variations in providing the interventions represent issues of operational fidelity, leading to type III error of inferences. These issues and strategies to address them have been discussed in detail in Chapter 6 and 9.

### Researcher Expectancies

*Overview*. Different terms have been used to refer to this bias: researcher or experimenter expectancy (Shadish et al., 2002), researcher therapeutic allegiance (Wilshire, 2017), and performance bias (Mansournia et al., 2017). This bias illustrates the researchers' enthusiasm for the intervention under evaluation and their expectation that it will be successful in achieving the hypothesized beneficial effects. The enthusiasm is, intentionally or unintentionally, transferred to research staff.

    Research staff's behaviors may be altered. For example, interventionists deliver the favored (by the researchers) intervention optimally and the comparison treatment poorly. Data collectors over-rate participants' performance on the mediators and the ultimate outcomes, and detect fewer failures or side effects among participants in the intervention group (Hróbjartsson et al., 2012). Data collectors also interact positively with participants, which translates into participants' favorable research experience and desire to please the researchers. Data analysts conduct additional unplanned analyses to identify statistically significant effects of the favored intervention; this is well illustrated in the statement: "if you torture your data long enough, they will confess" (Fleming, 2010).

The researchers' and research staff's enthusiasm is positively transferred to participants. Participants' responses to the intervention are explained in detail in the section on client reactivity.

Overall, researchers' expectancies yield differences in the delivery of the intervention and the comparison treatment. Consequently, these differences in performance, more so than the intervention itself, are responsible for the observed effects quantified in the differences in the mediators and the ultimate outcomes between the intervention and comparison treatment groups. Furthermore, researcher expectancies could contribute to an overinterpretation of the results while overlooking the study limitations (Wilshire, 2017).

*Strategies.* Three strategies are proposed to minimize this bias. First is the provision of adequate training to research staff in the skills required to assume their responsibilities and to interact with clients participating in the study, and frequent monitoring of their performance over the study period. Second is the application of the principle of blinding where possible. At a minimum, blinding involves not divulging to research staff and participants, which treatment is the experimental intervention under evaluation and which is the comparison treatment (Chapter 15). The third strategy is to consider the results of additional analyses as exploratory (rather than definitive indicators of intervention effects), requiring confirmation in future studies.

### Inaccurate Measurement of Mediators and Ultimate Outcomes

Similar to the inaccurate implementation of the intervention, inaccurate measurement of the mediators and the ultimate outcomes is related to the lack of congruence between the theoretical definitions of these concepts advanced in the intervention theory and the instruments selected to measure them. Inaccurate measurement is also reflected in systematic error inherent in the methods and measures used to collect relevant data.

### Lack of Congruence

*Overview.* The theoretical definition delineates the key attributes and respective indicators that characterize each mediator and ultimate outcome. This definition guides the selection of available instruments or the development of new ones. The content of the items comprising the instruments should accurately and comprehensively reflect the specified attributes and indicators. Lack of correspondence yields situations where the instrument either does not measure the attributes defining the respective mediator or ultimate outcome as specified in the intervention theory, or reflects the attributes of other related concepts. For example, measures of depressive symptoms may also capture symptoms of anxiety and insomnia. Consequently, inaccurate instruments cannot capture the mediators and the ultimate outcomes at a particular point in time as well as the hypothesized changes in these concepts over time that quantify the intervention effects.

*Strategies.* A strategy to minimize the potential of this bias is to generate a matrix that identifies the attributes of each concept (mediator and outcome) and indicators advanced in the theory and those captured in available instruments. The information is compared and contrasted prior to selecting the instrument that contains items reflecting the theoretically specified attributes and indicators.

### Systematic Bias

*Overview.* Carefully selected instruments may still be tainted by systematic measurement bias. This bias is associated with:

1. Characteristics of participants that may affect the way in which they complete the instruments: The characteristics frequently mentioned include: level of literacy (potentially leading to misinterpretation of the items' content), cultural background (making the content of some items irrelevant because of differences in beliefs or experiences of the concept), tendency for acquiescence (selecting the same response options for all items), and social desirability (desire to please the researcher or interventionist).

2. Characteristics of the instruments that may influence the accuracy of participants' responses: Common characteristics include: ambiguity or use of negative wording (leading to misunderstanding of the content covered in the items), inclusion of a large number of items (leading to response burden or fatigue), restricted range of response options (leading clients to make forced choices that do not reflect their true responses), and broad categorization of behaviors or activities or events to be observed (making it difficult to discern which one to observe and document).

3. Methods for collecting data, which have inherent error: Methods of data collection are: self-report by participants, observation by research staff, and use of equipment. Self-report is prone to over- or under-reporting, which affects the accuracy of the estimates of the intervention effects (Tengstedt et al., 2018). Observation is associated with observation bias. Observation bias reflects the observers' skills in recognizing and documenting accurately the behaviors of interest, as well as enthusiasm for or expectancy, as discussed in the previous section. Enthusiastic observers have a tendency for over-estimation, also known as ascertainment or detection bias (Hróbjartsson et al., 2012). Some equipment or devices can lead to technical problems, resulting in loss of data.

Overall, systematic bias generates artificially inflated or deflated responses to the instruments measuring the mediators and ultimate outcomes. The responses result in the over- or under-estimation of the intervention's effects.

*Strategies.* Strategies to minimize this bias include:

- Using multiple instruments and methods for collecting data on each mediator and ultimate outcome, if available, while attending to the need to reduce response burden for clients and observation fatigue for raters.
- Selecting self-report instruments whose content is easy to understand and applicable to different subgroups comprising the target client population.
- Intensively training and closely monitoring observers.

### Client Reactivity

Clients participating in an evaluation study react to the treatment (intervention or comparison) to which they are assigned, and to the assessment of the mediators and the ultimate outcomes.

## Reaction to Treatment

*Overview.* Participants' reactions to treatment are related to their perceptions and responses to the intervention and its nonspecific components that facilitate the delivery of the active ingredients. Those who perceive the allocated treatment favorably, that is, as acceptable and credible, develop high expectancy of its effectiveness. Participants who are satisfied with the interventionist's competence in initiating and maintaining a good rapport (nonspecific component) react positively and participate in the collaborative alliance. Participants exhibiting these positive reactions demonstrate improvement in the mediators and the ultimate outcomes. The improvement mimics or masks the improvement anticipated for the intervention; it is traditionally referred to as placebo response, which confounds the intervention effects because it is the placebo responses, more so than the intervention, that are responsible for the beneficial outcomes.

The distribution of participants with favorable perceptions and positive responses in the experimental intervention and the comparison treatment groups affect the estimates of the intervention's effects. If the percentage of this subgroup of participants is higher in the intervention group, then the effects are overestimated. In contrast, if the percentage of this participant subgroup is higher in the comparison treatment group, then the intervention effects are underestimated (Sidani, 2015).

*Strategies.* Strategies to address participants' perceptions and reactions to treatment are discussed in more detail in Chapter 11. The most commonly recommended strategy to address this source of bias is the application of blinding.

## Reaction to Assessment

*Overview.* Participants' reactions to the assessment of mediators and ultimate outcomes reflect their apprehension to evaluation, guessing of the study hypothesis, and learning. There is some evidence supporting the existence, but small influence, of these reactions (McCambridge et al., 2011, 2014).

Evaluation apprehension refers to clients' alterations in their responses to self-report measures or in their behaviors assessed through observation, because of their awareness that they are being evaluated and monitored. Clients change their responses or behaviors in a way that is consistent with their desire to be viewed as competent or that is socially acceptable. These types of reactivity have been traditionally termed Hawthorne effect or social desirability, respectively (Sidani, 2015) and recently, participation effects (McCambridge et al., 2014). Evaluation apprehension contributes to positive responses to measurement that contribute to improvement in the mediators and the ultimate outcomes. This improvement translates into: (1) overestimated intervention effects if the enhanced improvement is reported by a large percentage of participants receiving the intervention; and (2) underestimated intervention effects if the enhanced improvement is reported by all participants (Sidani, 2015).

*Strategies.* Strategies to reduce the potential for this bias include: emphasizing to clients that there are no right or wrong answers; and assessing the tendency for social desirability and accounting for its influence in the data analysis.

## Guessing of Study Hypothesis

*Overview.* Guessing of study hypothesis, also called demand characteristics, illustrates clients' responses or behaviors that conform to their awareness of what is being studied and their anticipation of the findings (McCambridge et al., 2012). Their responses or behaviors underlie the observed changes in mediators and the ultimate outcomes, resulting in overestimation of the intervention effects.

*Strategy*. Blinding is the strategy highly recommended to minimize this bias.

### Learning

*Overview*. Learning is associated with pretesting. Pretesting is the assessment of the mediators and the ultimate outcomes prior to the provision of the intervention. It may induce some learning that affects participants' responses or behaviors measured upon completion of the intervention. The latter responses or behaviors reflect the hypothesized improvement in the mediators and the ultimate outcomes, and can be mistaken for the effects of the intervention.

*Strategies*. Suggested strategies to address this bias include: use of alternate forms of the instrument measuring the same concepts, if available, with one form used at pretest and the alternate form used at post-test; and use of the Solomon four-group design. In this design, subgroups of clients assigned to each of the intervention and the comparison groups complete the measures at both pretest and post-test and other subgroups complete the measures only at post-test. Evidence indicates that this design is rarely used because it is difficult and expensive to carry out, and that the effects of pretesting were inconsistently detected (McCambridge et al., 2011).

### 10.2.3.2 Internal Validity

#### Definition

Internal validity is concerned with the causal effects of the intervention on the mediators and the ultimate outcomes. It refers to the extent to which changes in the mediators and outcomes can be confidently attributed to the intervention, and not to other plausible factors (Salimi & Ferguson-Pell, 2017; Tengstedt et al., 2018). Plausible factors confound the intervention effects: They may be directly associated and are responsible for inducing changes in the mediators and outcomes, or they may moderate (strengthen or weaken) the effects of the intervention (Flannelly et al., 2018). Thus, the factors offer alternative explanations of the findings. Common factors represent characteristics of clients, the context, and the treatments included in the evaluation study. They introduce specific biases.

#### Characteristics of Clients

Clients participating in an intervention evaluation study differ, to varying extent, in their personal profile (demographic, sociocultural), health-related beliefs and behaviors, lifestyle, and clinical condition or experience with the health problem addressed by the intervention. Participant characteristics may lead to selection bias, attrition bias, and spontaneous changes in the mediators and the ultimate outcomes (Sidani, 2015). These biases pose potential threats to internal validity.

#### Selection Bias

*Overview*. Selection bias refers to differences in the characteristics, assessed prior to exposure to treatment, of participants assigned to the intervention and those allocated to the comparison treatment group. These differences influence improvement in the mediators and the ultimate outcomes through two possible pathways.

The first pathway represents the direct impact of client characteristics on the mediators and the ultimate outcomes. The specific characteristics showing differences between the experimental intervention and the comparison treatment groups may be directly associated with mediators and ultimate outcomes, in the absence of the intervention. In other words, the characteristics are known predictors of the mediators and the ultimate outcomes assessed at one point in time (i.e. post-test) or of the level of changes observed in the mediators and the ultimate outcomes from pretest to post-test. For example, gender and age differences have been reported in the experience of insomnia (Sidani et al., 2018, 2019) and may affect how much client subgroups (defined by gender or age) improve following a behavioral therapy for insomnia.

The second pathway illustrates the indirect effects of client characteristics on the mediators and the ultimate outcomes. The characteristics may influence participants' level of exposure, engagement, and enactment of the treatment to which they are assigned. For instance, clients who are physically active are able to and actually engage in the level of physical activity recommended to promote sleep.

In general, differences in participant characteristics confound the intervention effects, that is, the reported changes in the mediators and the ultimate outcomes are attributable to the participant characteristics rather than the intervention (Mansournia et al., 2017; Skelly et al., 2012).

*Strategies*. Selection bias represents a major threat to validity and is minimized by randomly assigning clients to the intervention and the comparison treatment. Where randomization is not used, it is advisable to identify client characteristics (based on the intervention theory) with the potential to confound the intervention effects, measure them, and examine or adjust for their influence in the data analysis (Shadish et al., 2002; Skelly et al., 2012). Randomization and adjustment are explained in detail in Chapter 15.

### Attrition Bias

*Overview*. Attrition or mortality occurs in two situations. In the first, participants withdraw or drop out of the study at any time after providing consent for various reasons. In the second, participants are excluded from the study for reasons related to changes in their health or clinical condition, or violation of the study protocol, after randomization. Attrition threatens statistical conclusion validity. When a large number of participants withdraw, the sample size available for analysis is decreased. The reduced sample size lowers the statistical power to detect significant intervention effects (see Section 10.2.3.3).

Attrition weakens internal validity through two pathways. First, participants who drop out may differ from those who complete the study on some personal and health characteristics. Therefore, clients who complete the study are no longer representative of all subgroups of the target client population. Participants who complete the study may possess characteristics that confound the intervention effects on the mediators and the ultimate outcomes. The second pathway refers to differential attrition. This is a situation where the number and/or characteristics of participants who drop out from the intervention group may differ from those who withdraw from the comparison group. Differential attrition alters the characteristics of participants assigned to both groups, leading to selection bias and, subsequently, confounding of the intervention effects (Mansournia et al., 2017; Nüesch et al., 2009).

*Strategies.* Several strategies (see Chapter 15 for details) are recommended to prevent attrition, including training research staff in communication skills; clarifying expectations related to clients' involvement in the study; maintaining regular contacts with participants throughout the study period; expressing appreciation for clients' involvement; and making involvement in the study convenient and rewarding. Other strategies are proposed to handle attrition, such as maintaining a system to track clients; comparing the characteristics of participants who drop out and who complete the study to delineate the profile of completers and to ascertain the comparability of the study groups on potential confounders; and accounting for these confounders in the data analysis or using intent-to-treat, also called intention-to-treat analysis. The intention-to-treat analysis consists of imputing values on the mediators and the ultimate outcomes for participants who withdraw from the study. It aims to minimize selection bias resulting from differential attrition.

### Spontaneous Changes in Mediators and Outcomes

*Overview.* Participants may experience changes in their condition over the course of treatment. These changes occur for three possible reasons. First, the changes are spontaneous when they are related to natural progression or recovery of the health problem addressed by the intervention. Natural recovery may happen with acute conditions such as reduced severity of postoperative pain within a few days following surgery. The naturally occurring changes confound the effects on the mediators and the ultimate outcomes of health interventions provided within the same time frame. Second, spontaneous changes include normally anticipated changes in the experiences of participants presenting with particular characteristics taking place over the study period; they are also referred to as maturation. Maturation is exemplified by deterioration in the cognitive function of clients with dementia. Third, the changes reflect a phenomenon called regression to the mean. This phenomenon is seen among participants presenting with a particular profile associated with extreme levels on the mediators and the ultimate outcomes measured prior to intervention delivery. Participants with extreme levels at baseline may show spontaneous changes in that they become closer to the average level reported at post-test. The reason for this phenomenon is unclear. Taylor and Asmundson (2008) attributed regression to the mean to the unreliability of measures, at least partially.

*Strategies.* Possible strategies to address the biases associated with spontaneous changes include:

- Incorporating a no-treatment control group which is useful to determine if the intervention had an effect above and beyond the spontaneous changes: This strategy assumes that the spontaneous changes are comparable in direction and magnitude in the comparison treatment group.
- Conducting repeated assessments of the mediators and the ultimate outcomes prior to delivering the intervention, which allows the phenomenon of regression to the mean to take place before exposure to treatment.
- Adjusting statistically for client characteristics associated with extreme levels on the mediators and the ultimate outcomes: The adjustment is done using the characteristics as covariates in the data analysis.

- Conducting subgroup or sensitivity analysis to determine the effects of the intervention for clients with different levels (high, average, low) on the respective characteristics.

### Context

*Overview.* Context (also called history) refers to factors external or unrelated to the protocol of the evaluation study and that influence the mediators and the ultimate outcomes. The factors may occur at different time points: during the delivery of the intervention, during the assessment of the mediators and the ultimate outcomes, or during the period between the delivery of the intervention and the assessment of the mediators and the ultimate outcomes at post-test. A range of external factors may operate in influencing and potentially confounding the intervention effects. As mentioned in Chapter 5, external factors include physical, psychological, and sociopolitical features of the setting in which the interventionists deliver the intervention and the environment in which participants apply the treatment recommendations; these factors are identified in the intervention theory. In addition, unexpected events such as participants' loss of a job, changes in healthcare policy, or natural disasters may happen during the study period. These external factors affect the implementation of the intervention or the way clients' react and respond to the intervention.

The context (time, location) in which the mediators and the ultimate outcomes are assessed at pretest and post-test influences clients' responses to the measures assessing them. These responses may mimic the intervention effects. The influence of context is likely for mediators and outcomes whose levels naturally vary with the time of the day (e.g. diurnal changes in the levels of some hormones) and with the season (e.g. severity of asthma or seasonal affective disorders differs across seasons). Differences in the context of measurement may capture natural variations in the mediators and the ultimate outcomes, rather than the effects of the intervention. For instance, the severity of asthma is higher at pretest if assessed in the spring and lower at post-test if assessed in the summer). Accordingly, context may moderate (i.e. facilitate or hinder) the implementation of and the participants' responses to the instruments measuring the mediators and the ultimate outcomes. In both cases, the influence of context weakens the confidence in attributing changes in the mediators and outcomes directly and solely to the intervention (Sidani, 2015).

*Strategies.* Whether identified in the intervention theory or unexpected, external factors could be monitored, documented, and accounted for in the data analysis. The time of data collection should be carefully planned to avoid diurnal and seasonal variations.

### Study Treatments

*Overview.* In most evaluation studies, two categories of treatment are included. The first category consists of the experimental treatment (traditional term) or the intervention (recent term) of interest. The second category consists of a control condition where any treatment is withheld, thereby meeting the covariation criterion for causality. In light of ethical concerns with withholding treatments, other treatments are used and called "comparators" (Chapter 15). Examples are placebo treatment and treatment-as-usual. The comparison treatment or comparator serves as a reference in the comparison with the intervention on the mediators and the ultimate outcomes, whereby participants assigned to the comparison treatment are not expected to show the hypothesized improvement; this is because the comparison treatment should not comprise the active ingredients distinctive of the intervention. When clients assigned to the control condition or comparison treatment realize that they are assigned to a less-than-optimal or non-beneficial treatment, they express dissatisfaction with the allocated treatment. This situation has been recently called comparator bias (Dawson & Zwerski, 2015; Mann & Djulbegovic, 2013). Dissatisfied clients behave in any of the following manner:

1. They withdraw from the assigned comparison treatment or from the study, thereby introducing attrition bias.
2. They complete the study but exhibit low adherence to the assigned comparison treatment, which yields no change or even worsening in the levels on the post-test mediators and ultimate outcomes. Worsening levels widen the differences on the post-test mediators and ultimate outcomes between the intervention and comparison groups, resulting in overestimates of the intervention effects.
3. They complete the study but inquire about the intervention from clients assigned to the intervention or seek the intervention from other sources (e.g. health professionals, internet). They apply the intervention or some of its components—a situation referred to as contamination, diffusion, imitation, or dissemination of the intervention (Kumar & Yale, 2016; Schellings et al., 2009; Taylor & Asmundson, 2008). Thus, these clients experience improvement in the mediators and the ultimate outcomes. The improvement reduces the differences on the post-test mediators and ultimate outcomes between the intervention and the comparison groups, which results in underestimated intervention effects.
4. They complete the study and actively seek any type of treatment for the health problem from sources outside the study. These clients receive additional treatments (also called co-intervention), which may be effective, yielding improvement in the mediators and the ultimate outcomes. Such effective treatments could also be embedded in usual care. Similar to contamination, co-intervention yields underestimated intervention effects.

Similarly, interventionists or health professionals may consider it unacceptable to withhold treatment or deny clients access to a desirable and potentially useful intervention. Consequently, they attempt to compensate by providing participants allocated to the control condition or the comparison treatment, widely available treatments or components of the intervention, or by enhancing usual care—a situation called compensatory equalization. In this case, clients in the comparison treatment group experience improvement in the mediators and the ultimate outcomes, which underestimates the intervention effects.

In all instances where clients in the comparison group show improvement in the mediators and the ultimate outcomes, the differences between the intervention and comparison groups are reduced at post-test, leading to the inference that the intervention is ineffective (type II error). In situations where participants assigned to the intervention group seek and apply additional treatments (for different reasons), then these treatments may (1) have direct beneficial effects on the mediators and the ultimate outcomes, thereby confounding the effects of the intervention; (2) interact positively with the intervention, thereby contributing to large improvement in the mediators and outcomes, which results in overestimated intervention effects; or (3) interact negatively with the intervention, thereby weakening its impact on the mediators and the ultimate outcomes, which is manifested in underestimated intervention effects (Sidani, 2015).

*Strategies.* The traditional strategies to address biases associated with treatment consist of excluding from the data analysis clients who violated the allocated treatment protocol and of conducting intent-to-treat analysis. Alternative recently proposed strategies include: (1) minimizing opportunities for interactions among participants assigned to the intervention and comparison treatment; (2) explaining and reminding participants in both groups of the importance of not sharing treatment-related information among them; (3) monitoring operational fidelity and participants' adherence to the allocated treatment's recommendations, in both the intervention and comparison treatment groups; and (4) assessing and accounting for participants' use of additional treatments. For example, in the study evaluating the behavioral therapy for insomnia, clients are asked to report on the use of sleep medication and the application of stimulus control therapy in daily sleep diary.

### 10.2.3.3 Statistical Conclusion Validity

*Definition*

Statistical conclusion validity has to do with the covariation between the intervention on one hand, and the mediators and the ultimate outcomes on another hand. It is an issue of the accuracy in the results of statistical analyses. The goals of the analysis are twofold: to examine the occurrence and magnitude of the change in the mediators and the ultimate outcomes within the group of participants exposed to the intervention and to determine the presence and extent of differences in the mediators and the ultimate outcomes between the intervention and the comparison treatment groups, assessed at post-test. Inaccuracy in the results of statistical analysis leads to type I or II error of inference (Tengstedt et al., 2018) as well as over- or underestimation of the intervention effects. Two categories of bias affect the detection of the intervention effects: inadequate statistical power and inappropriate use of statistical tests.

*Inadequate Statistical Power*

*Overview.* Statistical power is related to the sample size, the preset p-level or value, the effect size, and random error (Chapter 15). Sample size is the number of participants assigned to the intervention and the comparison treatment groups. The p-value has been used as a way to quantify how often one would expect to see a result as extreme as the one found in a particular study, due solely to chance (Staggs, 2019). Traditionally, the p-value is preset at 0.05 or 0.01, with p-values less than this criterion indicating that the results of the accompanying statistical tests are not due to chance. The effect size quantifies the magnitude of the intervention effects. Random error represents variation in participants' levels on the mediators and the ultimate outcomes that is not related to the intervention. The variation is often associated with unreliability of measures, random (i.e. due to chance) inconsistency in treatment delivery, random variability in context, and natural heterogeneity of participants. Taken together, sample size, p-value, effect size, and random error affect the power to detect intervention effects.

*Strategies*. Using reliable measures and having a large sample size, an evaluation study would be well powered to detect small intervention effects at p-values $\leq 0.05$ (Lowenstein & Castro, 2009). Conversely, and under the same conditions, a very small sample size reduces the chances to detect the hypothesized effects (Schmidt, 2010), potentially leading to type II error of inference (Tengstedt et al., 2018). Conducting a power analysis is a recommended strategy to minimize this bias.

Recent literature emphasizes the point that scientific inferences should not be based only on p-values. Rather, scientific inferences should also be informed by theory, critical analysis of patterns of findings across studies, and the practical meaningfulness of the intervention effects (Hubbard et al., 2019; Staggs, 2019).

### Inappropriate Use of Statistical Tests

Inappropriate use of statistical tests may happen in two situations: violation of assumptions and repeat testing.

### Violation of Assumptions

*Overview*. Statistical tests are based on a set of assumptions such as independence of observations and equality of variance between groups. Severe violations of these assumptions reduce the chance of detecting the hypothesized intervention effects.

*Strategies*. Alternative statistical techniques can be used to address violations, such as hierarchical linear or multilevel modeling to account for the nesting of clients within treatment and interventionist, that is, the nonindependence of observations. Refer to Norman and Streiner (2014) for more information on statistical tests.

### Repeat Testing

*Overview*. In studies with a large number of mediators and ultimate outcomes, repeat testing is done to examine the effects of the intervention on each. This practice increases the likelihood that between-group differences are observed at different points in time post-treatment. However, these differences may be due to chance, resulting in type I error, that is, inferring that the intervention is effective when it may not be.

*Strategies*. The traditional strategy to minimize this bias is to adjust type I error rate (or p-value) for the number of tests to be performed (e.g. Bonferroni adjustment) or to conduct a multivariate (or multivariable) test followed by planned comparisons. The latter strategy limits the number of tests to be performed to the planned comparisons. Recent advances in multivariate (or multivariable) statistical tests allow for the simultaneous examination of the direct and indirect effects of the intervention on multiple mediators and ultimate outcomes, as hypothesized by the intervention theory.

#### 10.2.3.4   External Validity

### Definition

External validity has to do with the generalization (traditional term) and applicability (recent term) of the intervention's causal effects. Generalizability pertains to whether the effects hold, in general, over variations in persons, contexts, and times

(Shadish, 2010; Tengstedt et al., 2018). Applicability refers to the extent to which the intervention is relevant and its effects are reproducible in particular contexts (Williams et al., 2017). Threats to external validity are discussed in terms of the interactions between the intervention on one hand, and the characteristics of clients and contexts on the other hand (Salimi & Ferguson-Pell, 2017). Recently, evaluation of external validity and internal validity has been informed by the RE-AIM framework, which covers Reach (of the target client population), Efficacy or Effectiveness (of the intervention in improving outcomes), Adoption (of the intervention by health professionals), Implementation (of the intervention with fidelity), and Maintenance (of the intervention effects over time). The framework guided systematic reviews of studies that evaluated various health interventions, such as those promoting physical activity (e.g. Blackman et al., 2013; Craike et al., 2017; McMahon & Fleury, 2012), vegetable intake (e.g. Nour et al., 2016), and management of venous leg ulcerations (e.g. Gethin et al., 2019). Reach, adoption, and implementation are of relevance to external validity.

### Client Characteristics

*Overview.* Participants in an evaluation study should be representative of the target client population in order to generalize the intervention effects to various subgroups comprising the population. The sample representativeness is influenced by recruitment strategies, eligibility criteria and selection procedures, and consent to participate in the study (Steckler & McLeroy, 2008; Rothwell, 2006). These methodological aspects (Chapter 14 and 15), in addition to participants' personal and health characteristics, contribute to the inclusion of particular subgroups of the target client population. Some recruitment strategies may be more effective with specific subgroups of clients than others. Strict eligibility criteria may exclude particular client subgroups. Clients who enroll in the evaluation study may differ from those who decline, resulting in what is termed as self-selection bias (Shadish et al., 2002) or non-consent bias (Kaptchuck, 2001). Non-consent bias, combined with a small sample size, results in a selective sample that responds to the intervention (i.e. level of improvement in the mediators and the ultimate outcomes) in a unique way.

*Strategies.* Strategies to minimize the potential threats to external validity include: using multiple recruitment strategies, exploring reasons for non-enrollment; comparing participants to non-participants where data on nonparticipants are accessible (Gim, 2019; Yang et al., 2017); and reporting the study enrollment or participation rate, as well as detailed information on participants' personal, health, and clinical profiles. Examination of these profiles helps determine the applicability of the findings to clients in other research studies and in practice.

### Context

*Overview.* Context represents both the setting or the environment in which the intervention is implemented and the interventionists or health professionals providing the intervention. As mentioned in Chapter 5, 8, and 9, features of the setting; availability and accessibility of resources; personal qualities and professional qualifications of interventionists affect the delivery of the intervention with fidelity. Fidelity of intervention delivery contributes to the level of improvement in the mediators and the ultimate outcomes observed in a particular study, which may not be generalizable or applicable to other contexts.

*Strategies.* Strategies to address the potential influence of context include the careful selection and training of interventionists (Chapter 8), monitoring fidelity (Chapter 9), and the reporting on the features of the setting and the qualifications of the interventionists (Chapter 13) involved in the evaluation study. This descriptive information helps in determining comparability to other research and practice contexts.

### 10.2.3.5   Social Validity

*Definition*

Social validity reflects clients' perceived acceptance of health interventions (Kazdin, 2006). It is regaining attention for two reasons. The first is the increasing emphasis on client-centeredness and client engagement in the design and implementation of health interventions and healthcare services (Greenhalgh et al., 2016). The second reason is related to cumulating evidence showing the influence of treatment acceptance on clients' and health professionals' use of evidence-based interventions in practice (e.g. Park & Cho Blair, 2019) and on clients' behaviors in intervention evaluation studies (Sidani & Fox, 2020). The pathways through which perceived acceptance of interventions affects clients' behaviors, and subsequently validity of inferences regarding the intervention effects, and strategies to address acceptance, are discussed in Chapter 11.

## 10.3   PHASES FOR INTERVENTION EVALUATION

The evaluation of newly designed health interventions has traditionally been conceived as a systematic process involving four sequential phases. The phases are briefly described in Table 10.1. The results of each phase shed light on a specific aspect of the intervention. The aspects reflect the intervention's acceptance, feasibility, and effects on outcomes. The results of each phase are useful in informing the design and conduct of the research activities planned for the next phase. The cumulative evidence across phases provides support to incorporate effective interventions in practice, with the ultimate goal to benefit the target client population.

Recent perspectives consider this four-phase, stepwise approach to evaluation of interventions as costly and time consuming (Steckler & McLeroy, 2008). The approach is characterized by slow progression (Dawson & Zwerski, 2015) in generating the evidence supporting the benefits of interventions and in making potentially useful interventions accessible to clients who need prompt management of the health problem. Furthermore, the reported limited replicability of findings across evaluation studies and limited reproducibility of the intervention's effects in practice highlight the importance of examining feasibility, perceptions of interventions and process of delivery or implementation in studies evaluating the effects of interventions on the ultimate outcomes.

The remaining chapters in this section of the book focus on the evaluation of different aspects of health interventions: perceptions (Chapter 11), feasibility (Chapter 12), process (Chapter 13), and outcomes. Each aspect of evaluation is defined at the conceptual and the operational levels. Research designs (Chapter 14) and methods (Chapter 15) for examining them are described, and their strengths and limitations are discussed.

**TABLE 10.1**   Phases for intervention evaluation.

| Phase | Focus | Research activities | Accomplishments |
|---|---|---|---|
| Phase 1—Modeling | Development of optimal intervention:<br>Define and understand health problem<br>Identify active ingredients of intervention<br>Operationalize ingredients into components<br>Delineate mechanism of action | Conceptual work:<br>Critical review of theoretical, empirical, and experiential literature<br><br>Empirical work:<br>Quantitative and qualitative studies to determine adequacy of the conceptualization and operationalization of the health problem and intervention (see Chapter 3–5) | Generation of intervention:<br>Theory<br>Protocol/logic model/manual |
| Phase 2—Pilot | Examination of:<br><br>1.Intervention's:<br>Acceptability<br>Feasibility<br>Capacity to initiate or induce the mechanism of action and changes in outcomes<br>2.Research design and methods' feasibility | Pilot studies:<br><br>Small-scale studies:<br><br>1.Mixed-methods designs to explore the intervention's acceptability, feasibility, and capacity to induce change<br><br>OR<br><br>2.Design planned for next phase to examine the feasibility of methods | Validation of the conceptualization and operationalization of the intervention<br>Identification of challenges in the delivery of the intervention<br>Refinement of the intervention protocol or manual to address challenges<br>Determination of the adequacy of the research design and methods (recruitment, screening, randomization, measurement, data collection)<br>Estimation of enrollment and attrition rates<br>Revision of methods as necessary |
| Phase 3—Efficacy | Demonstration of the intervention's causal effects on the ultimate outcomes, under controlled conditions | Randomized controlled trials:<br>Enable testing intervention effects under "ideal conditions" that control for factors (related to client, setting, interventionist) influencing the delivery and the ultimate outcomes of the intervention | Determination of the causal impact of the intervention |
| Phase 4—Effectiveness (also called implementation) | Demonstration of the intervention's effects on ultimate outcomes, under conditions of real-world practice | Practical or pragmatic trials:<br>Enable testing intervention effects under conditions characterized by variability in: client, setting, interventionist, provision of intervention component, mode, and dose of delivery | Examination of who benefits from what intervention or components, given in what mode and at what dose, and under what context |

## REFERENCES

Amrhein, V., Korner-Nievergelt, F., & Roth, T. (2017) The earth is flat (p > .05): Significance thresholds and the crisis of unreplicable research. *Peer Journal*, 5, e3544. doi:10.7717/peerj.3544

Blackman, K.C.A., Zoellner, J., Berrey, L.M., et al. (2013) Assessing the internal and external validity of mobile health physical activity promotion interventions: A systematic literature review using the RE-AIM framework. *Journal of Medical Internet Research*, 15, e224. doi:10.2196/jmir,2745

Chavalarias, D. & Ioannidis, J.P. (2010) Science mapping analysis characterizes 235 biases in biomedical research. *Journal of Clinical Epidemiology*, 63, 1205–1215.

Craike, M., Hill, B., Gaskin, C.J., & Skouteris, H. (2017) Interventions to improve physical activity during pregnancy: A systematic review on issues of internal and external validity using the RE-AIM framework. *BJOG*, 124, 573–583. doi:10.1111/1471-0528.14276

Crawford, M.J., Barnicot, K., Patterson, S., et al. (2016) Negative results in phase III trials of complex interventions: Cause for concern or just good science? *The British Journal of Psychiatry*, 209, 6–8.

Cook, T.D., Scriven, M., Coryn, C.L.S., & Evergreen, S.D.H. (2010. Contemporary thinking about causation in evaluation: A dialogue with Tom Cook and Michael Scriven. *American Journal of Evaluation*, 31, 105–117.

Dawson, L. & Zwerski, S. (2015) Clinical trial design for HIV prevention research: Determining standards of prevention. *Bioethics*, 29(5), 316–323. doi:10.1111/bioe.12113

Flannelly, K.J., Flannelly, L.T., & Jankowski, K.R.B. (2018) Threats to the internal validity of experimental and quasi-experimental research in healthcare. *Journal of Health Care Chaplaincy*, 24, 1–24. doi:10.1080/08854726.2017.14210109

Fleming, K. (2010) Synthesis of quantitative and qualitative research: An example using Critical Interpretative Synthesis. *Journal of Advanced Nursing*, 66(1), 201–217. doi:10.1111/j.1365.2648.2009.05173.x

Gethin, G., Ivory, J.D., Connell, L., McIntosh, C., & Weller, C.D. (2019) External validity of randomized controlled trials of interventions in venous leg ulceration: A systematic review. *Wound Repair and Regeneration*, 27, 702–710.

Gim, T-H.T. (2019) Examining the effects of residential self-selection on internal and external validity: An interaction moderation analysis using structural equation modeling. *Transportation Letters*, 11(5), 275–286. doi: 10.1080/19427867.2017.1338544

Greenhalgh, T., Wong, G., Jagosh, J., et al. (2015) Protocol—the RAMESES II study: Developing guidance and reporting standards for realist evaluation. *BMJ Open*, 5, e008567. doi:10.1136/bmjopen-2015-0085

Greenhalgh, T., Jackson, C., Shaw, S., & Janamian, T. (2016) Achieving research impact through co-creation in community-based health services: Literature review and case study. *Milbank Quarterly*, 94(2), 392–429.

Heneghan, C., Goldacre, B., & Mahtani, K. (2017) Why clinical trial outcomes fail to translate into benefits for patients. *Trials*, 18, 122–128. doi:10.1186/s13063-017-1870-2

Hróbjartsson, A., Thomsen, A.S.S., Emanuelsson, F. et al. (2012) Observer bias in randomised clinical trials with binary outcomes: Systematic review of trials with both blinded and non-blinded outcome assessors. *BMJ*, 344, e1119. doi:10.1136/bmj.e1119

Hubbard, R., Haig, B.D., & Parsa, R.A. (2019) The limited role of formal statistical inference in scientific inference. *The American Statistician*, 73, 91–98.

Ioannidis, J.P. (2008) Perfect study, poor evidence: Interpretation of biases preceding study design. *Seminars in Hematology*, 45, 160–166.

Kaptchuck, T.J. (2001) The double-blind randomized, placebo-controlled trial: Gold standard or golden calf? *Journal of Clinical Epidemiology*, 54, 541–549.

Kazdin, A.E. (2006) Arbitrary metrics: Implications for identifying evidence-based treatments. *American Psychologist*, 61(1), 42–49. doi:10.1037/0003-066X.61.1.42

Kumar, C.S. & Yale, S.S. (2016) Identifying and eliminating bias in intervention research studies—a quality indicator. *International Journal of Contemporary Medical Research*, 3(6), 1644–1648.

Larzele, R.E., Kuhn, B.R., & Johnson, B. (2004) The intervention selection bias: An under recognized confound in intervention research. *Psychological Bulletin*, 130(2), 289–303.

Lilienfeld, S.O., Ritschel, L.A., Lynn, S.J., Cautin, R.L., & Latzman, R.D. (2014) Why ineffective psychotherapies appear to work: A taxonomy of causes of spurious therapeutic effectiveness. *Perspectives on psychological Science*, 9(4), 355–387. doi:10.1177/1745691614535216

Lowenstein, P.R. & Castro, M.G. (2009) Uncertainty in the translation of preclinical experiments to clinical trials: Why do most Phase III clinical trials fail? *Current Gene Therapy*, 9(5), 368–374.

Mann, H. & Djulbegovic, B. (2013) Comparator bias: Why comparisons must address genuine uncertainties. *Journal of the Royal Society of Medicine*, 106, 30–33. doi:10.1177/0141076812474779

Mansournia, M.A., Higgins, J.P.T., Sterne, J.A.C., & Hernán, M.A. (2017) Biases in randomized trials. A Conversation between trialists and epidemiologists. *Epidemiology*, 28, 54–59.

MacKinnon, D.P. & Fairchild, A.J. (2009) Current directions in mediation analysis. *Current Directions in Psychological Science*, 18, 16–20.

McCambridge, J., Butor-Bhavsar, K., Witton, J., & Elbourne, D. (2011) Can research assessments themselves cause bias in behaviour change trials? A systematic review of evidence from Solomon 4-group studies. *PLoS ONE*, 6(10), e25223. doi:10.1371/journal.pone.0025223.

McCambridge, J., de Bruin, M., & Witton, J. (2012) The effects of demand characteristics on research participant behaviours in non-laboratory settings: A systematic review. *PLoS One*, 7(6): e39116.

McCambridge, J., Witton, J., & Elbourne, D.R. (2014) Systematic review of the Hawthorne effect: New concepts are needed to study research participation effects. *Journal of Clinical Epidemiology*, 67, 267–277.

McGauran, N., Wieseler, B., Kreis, J. et al. (2010) Reporting bias in medical research—a narrative review. *Trials*, 11, 37–51.

McMahon, S. & Fleury, J. (2012) External validity of physical activity interventions for community-dwelling older adults with fall risk: A quantitative systematic literature review. *Journal of Advanced Nursing*, 60(10), 2140–2154. doi:10.1111/j.1365-2648.2012.05974.x

Nock, M.K., Ferriter, C., & Holmberg, E. (2007) Parent beliefs about treatment credibility and effectiveness: Assessment and relation to subsequent treatment participation. *Journal of Children and Family Studies*, 16, 27–38. doi:10.1007/s10826-006-9064-7

Norman, G.R. & Streiner, D.L. (2014) *Biostatistics: The Bare Essentials*, 4th edn. People's Medical Publishing House, Connecticut, USA.

Nour, M., Chen, J., & Allman-Farinelli, M. (2016) Efficacy and external validity of electronic and mobile phone-based interventions promoting vegetable intake in young adults: Systematic review and meta-analysis. *Journal of Medical Internet Research*, 18(4), e58.

Nüesch, E., Reichenbach, S., Trelle, S. et al. (2009) The importance of allocation concealment and patient blinding in osteoarthritis trials: A meta-epidemiology study. *Arthritis and Rheumatism (Arthritis Care and Research)*, 61(12), 1633–1641. doi:10.1002/art.24894

Park, E.-Y. & Cho Blair, K.-S. (2019) Social validity assessment in behavior interventions for young children: A systematic review. *Topics in Early Childhood Special Education*, 39(3), 156–169. doi:10.1117/0271121419860195

Powell, S. (2019) Theories of change: Making value-explicit. *Journal of Multi Disciplinary Evaluation*, 15(32), 37–52.

Rothwell, P.M. (2006) Factors that can affect the external validity of randomised controlled trials. *PLoS Clinical Trials*, 1, e9. doi:10.1371/journal.pctr.0010009

Salimi, Z. & Ferguson-Pell, M.W. (2017) Validity in rehabilitation research: Description and classification. In: U. Tan (ed) *Physical Disabilities. Therapeutic Implications*. IntechOpen. *Chapter accessed on*: www.intechopen.com.

Schafer, J.L. & Kang, J. (2008) Average casual effects from nonrandomized studies: A practical guide and simulation example. *Psychological Methods*, 13, 279–313.

Schellings, R., Kessels, A.G., ter Riet, G. et al. (2009) Indications and requirements for the use of prerandomization. *Journal of Clinical Epidemiology*, 62, 393e9.

Schmidt, F. (2010) Detecting and connecting the lies that data tell. *Perspectives on Psychological Science*, 5(3), 233–242.

Shadish, W.R. (2010) Campbell and Rubin: A primer and comparison of their approaches to causal inference in field settings. *Psychological Methods*, 15(1), 3–17.

Shadish, W.R., Cook, T.D., & Campbell, D.T. (2002) *Experimental and Quasi-Experimental Design for Generalized Causal Inference*. Houghton-Mifflin, Boston, MA.

Sidani, S. (2015) *Health Intervention Research: Advances in Research Design and Methods*, Sage, London, UK.

Sidani, S., Guruge, S., Fox, M., & Collins, L. (2019) Gender differences in perpetuating factors, experience and management of chronic insomnia. *Journal of gender studies*, 28(4), 402–413. doi:10.1080/09589236.2018.1491394

Sidani, S., Ibrahim, S., Lok, J. et al. (2018) Comparing the experience of and factors perpetuating chronic insomnia severity among young, middle-aged, and older adults. *Clinical Nursing Research*, 105477381880616. doi:10.1177/1054773818806164

Sidani, S. & Fox, M. (2020) The role of treatment perceptions in intervention evaluation: A review. *Science of Nursing and Health Practices*, 3(2), Article 4.

Skelly, A.C., Dettori, J.R., & Brodt, E.D. (2012) Assessing bias: The importance of considering confounding. *Evidence-based Spine-Care Journal*, 3(1), 9–12.

Staggs, V.S. (2019) Why statisticians are abandoning statistical significance. *Research in Nursing and Health*, 42, 159–160. doi:10.1002/nur.21947

Stanford Encyclopedia of Philosophy (2008). *Counterfactual theories of causation*. Available on: http://plato.stanford.edu/ (accessed in January, 2010).

Steckler, A. & McLeroy, K.R. (2008) The importance of external validity. *American Journal of Public Health*, 98(1), 9–10.

Taylor, S. & Asmundson, G.J.G. (2008) Internal and external validity in clinical research (Chapter 3). In: D. McKay (ed) *Handbook of Research Methods in Abnormal and Clinical Psychology*. Sage Publications, Los Angeles, US.

Tengstedt, M.A., Fagerstrøm, A., & Mobekk, H. (2018) Health interventions and validity on social media: A literature review. *Procedia Computer Science*, 138, 169–176.

Williams, A., Duggleby, W., Ploeg, J. et al. (2017) Overcoming recruitment challenges for securing a survey of caregivers of community-dwelling older adults with multiple chronic conditions. *Journal of Human Health Research*, 1(1), 16–24. doi: 10.14302/issn.2576.9383

Wilshire, C. (2017) The problem of bias in behavioural intervention studies: Lessons from the PACE trial. *Journal of Health Psychology*, 22(9), 1128–1133. doi:10.1177/1359105317700885

Woodman, R.W. (2014) The role of internal validity in evaluation research on organizational change interventions. *The Journal of Applied Behavioral Science*, 50(1), 40–49.

Wong, G., Greenhalgh, T., Westhorp, G., & Pawson, R. (2012) Realist methods in medical education research: What are they & what can they contribute? *Medical Education*, 46, 89–96. doi:10.1111/J.1365-2923.2011.04045.X

Yang, R., Carter, B.L., Gums, T.H. et al. (2017) Selection bias and subject refusal in a cluster-randomized controlled trial. *BMC Medical Research Methodology*, 17, 94–103. doi:10.1186/s12874-017-0368-7

Yordanov, Y., Dechartres, A., Porcher, R. et al. (2015) Avoidable waste of research related to inadequate methods in clinical trials. *BMJ*, 350, h809. doi:10.1136/bmj.h809

# CHAPTER 11

# Examination of Interventions' Acceptance

The interest in examining the social validity of health interventions is resurging (Greenhalgh et al., 2016). Social validity reflects clients' perceived acceptance of interventions (Kazdin, 2006). Two observations are driving the increasing attention to interventions' acceptance. First is the realization that, in practice, acceptance contributes to clients' pursuit and use of interventions. Clients will not seek, initiate, engage, and adhere to evidence-based, effective interventions if they do not perceive the interventions favorably (Alessi & Rasch, 2017; De Las Cuevas et al., 2018). Second is cumulating research evidence indicating that participants' perceptions of the treatments (i.e. experimental intervention and comparison treatment) under evaluation affect their behaviors in an evaluation study. The behaviors are related to participants' enrollment and continued participation in the study, which threaten external validity, as well as their engagement and enactment of the allocated treatment. These behaviors affect their experience of improvement in the outcomes, which threaten internal validity (Kendra et al., 2015).

The significant contribution of acceptance to intervention's uptake, engagement, enactment, and outcomes in research and practice resulted in its consideration as an important client-centered parameter denoting the success of health interventions (Gebhardt et al., 2013; Rejas et al., 2013). Accordingly, acceptance demands special attention in intervention evaluation research. It should be explored when:

1. Designing new interventions: As described in Chapter 4, clients are involved in the design of the intervention. Their perspectives help in identifying aspects (e.g. content, activities, mode of delivery) of the intervention that are viewed favorably and aspects that require modification in order to enhance the acceptance and hence, the use of the intervention (Alessi & Rasch, 2017; Brose & Bradley, 2009).

2. Planning to offer evidence-based interventions in a new context: The context reflects a new target client population or a new setting that was not represented in research that evaluated the intervention. Acceptance of the intervention to clients and health professionals is done to examine aspects of the intervention that are acceptable and those that should be revised to improve the fit of the intervention within the new context (Aarons et al., 2012; Bernal et al., 2009).

*Nursing and Health Interventions: Design, Evaluation, and Implementation*, Second Edition.
Souraya Sidani and Carrie Jo Braden.

3. Evaluating the effects of new or evidence-based intervention in small- or large-scale studies: Data on participants' perceptions of the treatments under evaluation are useful in determining the extent to which these perceptions shape their behaviors in the research study and threaten the validity of inferences (Beasly et al., 2017).

In this chapter, explanations of how perceived acceptance is formulated within an intervention evaluation study are presented. The importance of examining clients' perceived acceptance of interventions to enhance validity of inferences is highlighted. Measures and methods for examining acceptance are discussed.

## 11.1  FORMULATION OF INTERVENTION ACCEPTANCE

Acceptance is an umbrella term entailing favorable perceptions of the experimental intervention and the comparison treatment included in an evaluation study. The perceptions have been reflected in treatment acceptability, preferences, credibility, expectancy, and satisfaction. These perceptions are formulated early in an evaluation study and may change over the course of the study. Clients present with the health problem that is addressed by the treatments under evaluation. Clients differ in their personal profile, health status, beliefs about the health problem, and awareness and values of its treatment, all of which shape their acceptance of the intervention and the comparison treatment.

### Personal and health profiles

Clients of diverse socioeconomic backgrounds differ in their acceptability of treatment for the presenting health problem, as illustrated in the results of several studies. For example, older persons find medications as acceptable for managing sleep problems (Omvik et al., 2010). Women consider counseling or psychotherapy as acceptable for treating depression (Houle et al., 2013). Persons self-identifying as non-white indicate higher acceptance of telephone, compared to internet, delivery of programs for self-management of chronic conditions (Sarkar et al., 2008).

Clients' general health and experience of the health problem are reported to influence their perceptions of treatment. For instance, clients experiencing severe levels of the health problem are likely to find intensive or invasive treatments as acceptable for the remediation of a range of problems (e.g. Dobscha et al., 2007; Gum et al., 2006; Omvik et al., 2010).

### Beliefs about health problem

Clients of diverse sociocultural backgrounds hold personal and normative beliefs about health in general and the health problem in particular. Beliefs about the health problem are also referred to as illness representation and etiological model. Clients' understanding of the problem and of its possible causes vary and shape their perspectives on what they consider as appropriate treatments or remedies to manage the problem and improve general health (Cohen et al., 2015). For example, clients' beliefs about the causes of mental health problems are found to influence their acceptance of pharmacological and non-pharmacological therapies. Those who believe in the organic (biological, chemical, or genetic) causes of depression (Kemp et al., 2014;

Steidtmann et al., 2012; Wright et al., 2012) or insomnia (Bluestein et al., 2011) express acceptance of medications; whereas clients who consider life stress as the primary cause of these mental health problems view non-pharmacological or psychological therapies, aimed at reducing stress, as acceptable (Givens et al., 2007).

### Awareness of treatment

Clients are aware of alternative treatments for addressing the health problem they experience. A range of pharmacological, physical, psychological or behavioral, and complementary/alternative treatments are available. Clients acquire knowledge about treatments from many sources. Treatment-related information is accessible through the internet or World Wide Web; reported in short articles published in newspapers, newsletters or magazines; and presented in documentaries, discussed in health-related sections of daily news or in other general talk shows aired on radio or television. Clients may also learn about treatments through discussion with family members, friends, or colleagues, and through interactions with health professionals (Mills et al., 2011). Furthermore, clients may have personal or vicarious experience with treatments, that is, they may have actually used a treatment or witnessed others' use it. They formulate favorable perceptions of treatments reported to be successful and fitting with their beliefs about the health problem.

### Formulation of acceptance in an evaluation study

Similar to clients in practice, participants entering an intervention evaluation study present with preconceived beliefs about the health problem and acceptance or value of possible treatments (Kowalski & Mrdjenovich, 2013), which influence their perceptions of the treatments under evaluation. During recruitment, participants are briefly told of the treatments under evaluation. For instance, advertisement for a study evaluating the behavioral therapies for insomnia can specify the general type of treatment, stating: "the treatment does not involve mediation." When describing the study prior to obtaining consent, and as required by research ethics, participants are provided information on the treatments, without necessarily revealing which is the experimental and which is the comparison treatment. The information covers the treatments' name (e.g. stimulus control therapy); key or main components (e.g. set of recommendations to do during the day, around bedtime, and during night-time awakenings); mode and dose of delivery (e.g. given in four, face-to-face group sessions, offered once a week); benefits (e.g. found effective in promoting sleep); and risks or discomfort (e.g. experience of daytime fatigue in the first couple of weeks). This information clarifies the treatments to participants and contributes to their perception of the treatments. Participants may compare and contrast their understanding of the treatments under evaluation, with their beliefs about the health problem as well as with their awareness and previous experience with other treatments for addressing the problem. This comparison contributes to the identification of the treatment that is most congruent with their beliefs. Congruent treatments are perceived favorably, whereas incongruent treatments are perceived unfavorably. At this early stage of an evaluation study, participants may express *acceptability* and *preferences* for the treatments. Acceptability and preferences reflect two separate but inter-related perceptions of an intervention's acceptance.

Consenting participants are exposed to the treatment to which they are assigned. The treatments, and in particular health interventions, are provided in individual

**TABLE 11.1**    Treatment information covered in first intervention session or module.

| Treatment information | Illustration—stimulus control therapy |
| --- | --- |
| Goal:<br>What is the treatment set to achieve? | To help manage insomnia<br>To improve the quality of sleep and daytime functioning |
| Rationale:<br>Why and how the treatment works? | Reassociating the bed with sleep |
| Components (content and activities):<br>What does the treatment consist of? | Component 1—sleep hygiene<br>Discussion of recommended activities to do or avoid during the day (e.g. engage in physical activity) or evening (e.g. avoid napping)<br>Component 2—stimulus control<br>Discussion of changes to make in the bedroom (e.g. avoid watching television in bed or reading in bed)<br>Discussion of strategies to do if unable to sleep (e.g. get out of bed and engage in relaxing activities) |
| Side effects:<br>What are risks or discomfort associated with the treatment? | Experience of daytime fatigue in the first two weeks of therapy |
| Effectiveness:<br>What are the benefits of the treatment? | This therapy was found, in research, to improve sleep for persons who follow all recommendations |

or group sessions facilitated by an interventionist, or in modules completed by participants. The first session or module is often designed to cover detailed information about the treatment as summarized and illustrated in Table 11.1. The detailed information may reinforce participants' acceptance or alter their perceptions of the treatments. In particular, information on treatments' rationale and effectiveness contributes to the formation of their perceived *credibility* and *expectancy*, respectively. Participants who view the treatment rationale as credible and expect the treatment to be potentially effective in addressing the health problem and in improving health maintain favorable perceptions (or acceptance) of the allocated treatment; otherwise, participants develop unfavorable perceptions of treatment. Both credibility and expectancy influence participants' engagement and enactment of the treatment.

Participants' exposure, engagement, enactment, and experiences with the treatment may or may not be rewarding. Those who appropriately engage and enact the treatment have great potentials of exhibiting the hypothesized improvement in outcomes; others may not benefit from the treatment. These experiences translate into expressed *(dis)satisfaction* with treatment, which reflect continued acceptance or changes in perceptions of the treatment. Satisfaction with treatment affects participants' continued use of the treatment and achievement of ultimate outcomes.

## 11.2    CONTRIBUTION OF PERCEIVED ACCEPTANCE TO VALIDITY

Mounting evidence supports the contribution of perceived treatment acceptance to the validity of inferences in evaluation studies. Acceptance is represented by perceived treatment's acceptability, preference, credibility, expectancy, and satisfaction. The evidence demonstrates direct and indirect associations between treatment perceptions and immediate, intermediate, and ultimate outcomes. The direct associations are reflected in parameters quantifying the correlation or differences in the outcomes reported for participants with varying levels of treatment acceptance. The indirect relationships are explained by participants' behaviors: Participants expressing different perceptions of the treatments under evaluation may behave differently over the course of an evaluation study. Participants' behaviors are related to their enrollment in and withdrawal (or attrition) from the study, as well as engagement and enactment of the allocated treatment. These behaviors influence the achievement of beneficial outcomes (issue of internal validity) and limit the generalizability of findings (issue of external validity). The way in which treatment perceptions influence participants' behaviors and experience of outcomes is explained next. Supporting evidence is also presented.

### 11.2.1    Treatment Perceptions and Outcomes

The direct association between treatment perceptions and outcomes is well supported empirically; however, the exact mechanism explaining it is not clear. The direct association may represent the placebo response. The placebo response may reflect participants' expectancy of the intervention effectiveness or their perceptions and responses to the interventionist.

Participants perceiving the allocated treatment favorably anticipate that it will be helpful in addressing the health problem. This anticipated helpfulness, or expectancy, translates into reported improvement in outcomes following treatment, regardless of the levels of exposure, engagement, enactment, or adherence to treatment (Frisaldi et al., 2017; Gaudiano et al., 2013; Younger et al., 2012). Participants' perceptions and reactions to the interventionists are related to the interventionists' competence, as discussed in Chapter 8. Participants respond positively to interventionists who are able to initiate and build good therapeutic relationships and working alliance, to communicate clearly, and to interact with respect; these participants report improvement in outcomes, regardless of their engagement and enactment of treatment.

The distribution of participants exhibiting these placebo responses in the experimental intervention and the comparison treatment groups affect the validity of inferences in an evaluation study. When only participants assigned to the experimental intervention group exhibit placebo responses, then the level of improvement in the outcome is augmented, demonstrated in overestimated effects of the intervention. In this case, it would be difficult to tease out the true effects of the intervention from the placebo effects; thus, the placebo responses confound the intervention's effects. When only participants allocated to the comparison treatment group show placebo responses, then differences between the experimental and the comparison treatments in the outcomes are small and nonsignificant, resulting in underestimated effects of the intervention; this situation leads to type II error. A similar situation of increased likelihood for type II error is observed when participants in both treatment groups exhibit placebo responses (Colagiuri, 2010).

There is ample evidence linking acceptance, reflected in different treatment perceptions, to outcomes. The results of several studies evaluating psychological, behavioral, and surgical treatments (e.g. Beard et al., 2011; El-Alaoui et al., 2015; Haanstra et al., 2015; Herdman et al., 2012; Mooney et al., 2014; Narimatsu et al., 2016; Nordgreen et al., 2012) were consistent with those of a meta-analysis (Constantino et al., 2018) in demonstrating a direct positive association between credibility and outcomes. This association implies that participants with high credibility ratings reported large improvement in the outcomes. Similar positive direct relationships between expectancy and outcomes (e.g. Beard et al., 2011; Beasly et al., 2017; Boettcher et al., 2013; El-Alaoui et al., 2015; Haanstra et al., 2015) and between satisfaction and outcomes (e.g. Köhler et al., 2015; Peyrot & Rubin, 2009; Schaal et al., 2017; Schulte et al., 2011) were found.

## 11.2.2   Treatment Perceptions and Enrollment

Clients' perceived acceptability and preferences for treatment influence their enrollment in an evaluation study. Some clients may view both the experimental intervention and the comparison treatment as unacceptable. They decline enrollment and seek treatment for their health problem outside the study (Mills et al., 2011). Two situations ensue when a large number of recruited clients refuse enrollment. The first situation is a reduced sample size, which lowers the statistical power to detect significant intervention effects on the outcomes (Kowalski & Mrdjenovich, 2013). The second situation is the demand for additional resources to expand recruitment efforts in order to acquire the required sample size. Additional resources may not always be accessible, thereby limiting the accrual of the required sample size.

Other clients may perceive one or both treatments under evaluation as acceptable and express preferences for the acceptable treatment. They enroll in the study with the hope to receive the treatment they prefer. Clients perceiving treatments as unacceptable and those viewing treatments as acceptable may differ on some personal and health characteristics, as indicated by evidence presented in Section 11.1. Accordingly, clients with unfavorable perceptions who do not enroll may differ in their personal and health profiles from clients with favorable perceptions who participate in the study. These differences result in a sample that is not representative of all subgroups comprising the target client population (Kowalski & Mrdjenovich, 2013); these differences also introduce biased estimates of the intervention effects that do not replicate in other research studies and in practice (Leykin et al., 2007). The biased estimates are due to the actual participants' characteristics that confound or are correlated with the intervention effects.

## 11.2.3   Treatment Perceptions and Attrition

Clients who enroll in an evaluation study become aware of the method used for assignment to treatment, and then of the treatment to which they are assigned. Participants with varying levels of acceptability and preferences to the study treatments may react differently to the method of assignment and to the allocated treatment, contributing to withdrawal from the study or the treatment (Fernandez et al., 2015; Steidtmann et al., 2012). The method of assignment is based on chance (i.e. randomization) or preference (Chapter 15).

Participants who view both the experimental intervention and the comparison treatment as acceptable and have no strong preferences for either, are indifferent to the method of assignment. They realize that, with chance or preference-based methods, they will be allocated to any treatment they perceive favorably. Their reactions to the method of assignment and to the allocated treatment are positive or neutral, contributing to their continued involvement in the treatment and/or study. Thus, these participants do not withdraw from the treatment or the study.

Participants expressing high levels of acceptability and strong preferences for a particular treatment (either experimental or comparison) react in different ways to chance and preference-based methods of allocation. Many react negatively to randomization. They consider it as unacceptable and unfair because it disregards their right to be actively involved in the process of treatment decision-making and their desire to receive their preferred treatment. This group of participants is likely to decline further participation in the study because of discomfort with being randomized to the non- or the least-preferred treatment. Other participants realize that randomization is potentially useful: After all, they have 50% chance of being allocated to their preferred treatment. They may continue their participation in the study (Bradley-Gilbride & Bradley, 2010). In contrast, participants with high acceptability and strong preference for a particular treatment react positively to preference-based method of assignment. They are enthusiastic about the prospect of receiving their preferred treatment and continue their involvement in the study.

Once known, participants are informed of the treatment to which they are assigned. Participants who are allocated to the treatment that matches their preference are content and continue their involvement in the study. Participants allocated to the treatment that does not match their preference (mismatch) are disappointed. They may withdraw from the study to seek their preferred treatment outside the study. If a large number of participants with mismatched treatment drop out, then the study sample size and power to detect significant treatment effects are reduced. Further, the estimated effects are biased, because the estimates are based on outcome data obtained from a subgroup of participants with matched treatment, high enthusiasm and motivation to enact treatment, and possibly with unique personal and health profiles.

Participants who continue their involvement in the evaluation study are exposed to the assigned treatment. Those allocated to a no-treatment control or treatment-as-usual and receive no information or interaction with the study's interventionist may lose enthusiasm for treatment. Loss of enthusiasm is heightened if the allocated treatment does not match their preference. These participants lose interest in the study, and are likely to withdraw at any time during the treatment or the study period. This situation leads to higher attrition rates in the comparison treatment group than in the experimental intervention group. The number of participants who complete the study is unbalanced between the two groups, potentially resulting in unequal within-group variance, which decreases the chance of detecting significant intervention effects if not addressed properly in the statistical analysis (Sidani, 2015).

Participants allocated to the experimental intervention attend the first session and are exposed to detailed information about the intervention's rationale, components, benefits, and risks. Those who continue to hold favorable perceptions, indicated by high credibility and expectancy, of the allocated treatment maintain their enthusiasm and motivation to complete treatment (Kendra et al., 2015; Mooney et al., 2014). This group of participants show low attrition rates. Participants who develop unfavorable perceptions of the allocated treatment, indicated by low credibility and expectancy, may express discontentment and withdraw from the treatment or the study, resulting in high attrition rates in this treatment group.

The distribution of participants having favorable and unfavorable perceptions of the allocated treatment within the experimental intervention and the comparison treatment groups affects the validity of an evaluation study findings. If the number of participants who withdraw is comparable in the experimental intervention and the comparison treatment groups, then the two groups' size and the power to detect significant between-group differences in the outcomes at post-test are reduced. This, in turn, increases the chance of type I error, that is, inferring that the intervention is not effective when it may be. If the number of participants who drop out is not comparable for the experimental intervention and the comparison treatment groups, then differential attrition is likely. Differential attrition refers to the situation where the number and the personal or health profile of participants who withdraw from one group differ from those of participants who drop out of the other group. Differences in profiles could confound the intervention effects.

The contribution of treatment preferences (rather than acceptability), credibility, and expectancy to attrition has been investigated. The results of individual studies and systematic reviews were consistent in showing lower attrition rates for participants allocated to a treatment that matches their preferences (Sidani et al., 2015; Swift et al., 2011, 2013; Wasmann et al., 2019; Winter & Barber, 2013). In addition, participants having low credibility (Boettcher et al., 2013; Merincavage et al., 2017; Narimatsu et al., 2016) and low expectancy (Zimmermann et al., 2017) ratings of the allocated treatment were likely to withdraw.

## 11.2.4  Treatment Perceptions and Implementation

After exposure to treatment information in the first session or module, participants who continue to view the allocated treatment favorably (i.e. high credibility and expectancy ratings) maintain their enthusiasm for the treatment. They attend the remaining sessions or complete the remaining modules, while actively engaging in the planned activities and enacting the treatment recommendations (Beatty & Binnion, 2016; Haanstra et al., 2015). In contrast, participants who no longer view the allocated treatment favorably (i.e. low credibility and expectancy ratings) may lose their motivation. Some may not attend or complete the remaining sessions or modules, but provide outcome data at post-test. Others may be selective in the sessions or modules they complete, in their level of engagement in the planned activities, and in the treatment recommendations they enact. Therefore, participants assigned to each treatment may vary in their level of adherence to treatment recommendations and, consequently, in their experience of improvement in outcomes. High within-group variance in the outcomes assessed at post-test decreases the power to detect significant between-group differences, potentially leading to type II error. Furthermore, some participants with unfavorable perceptions of the allocated treatment may seek and implement additional therapies to manage their health problem. Receipt of additional therapy, concurrently with the allocated treatment (i.e. co-treatment) weakens the confidence in attributing improvements in outcomes, specifically and solely, to the intervention under evaluation. The improvements may be the independent effects of the concurrent therapy or the interaction effects of the concurrent therapy and the allocated treatment.

Several studies examined the association between treatment perceptions (credibility, expectancy and satisfaction) and adherence to treatment recommendations. Despite variability in the type of intervention evaluated (e.g. physiotherapy, cognitive-behavioral therapy), the results were consistent in demonstrating that participants rating the allocated treatment as credible, had high expectancy for its effectiveness. The results also converged in showing that participants satisfied with the allocated treatment reported high levels of engagement (Hundt et al., 2013; Kwan et al., 2010) and enactment or adherence to its recommendations (Alessi & Rasch, 2017; Beatty & Binnion, 2016; Boettcher et al., 2013; De Las Cuevas et al., 2018; Dong et al., 2018; Eaton et al., 2019; El-Alaoui et al., 2015; Narimatsu et al., 2016; Wong et al., 2015). The association between satisfaction and enactment was also found in a systematic review (Barbosa et al., 2012).

Evidence (presented previously) clearly indicates that perceptions of treatment influence participants' enrollment, withdrawal, and engagement and enactment of treatment, which in turn contribute to their experience of improvement in outcomes. As such, treatment perceptions are potential threats to validity. Therefore, it is critical to assess participants' perceived acceptability, preferences, credibility, expectancy, and satisfaction, and to account for their influence in outcome analysis (Beasly et al., 2017; Sidani & Fox, 2020) in intervention evaluation research.

## 11.3   EXAMINATION OF ACCEPTABILITY

### 11.3.1   Conceptualization of Acceptability

Acceptability of health interventions reflects clients' attitudes toward treatments. The formulation of the attitude is guided by an understanding of the treatments and is based on judgments of the treatments' attributes. Participants need to have a clear, accurate, and adequate understanding of the treatments under consideration before they appraise their acceptability. This understanding encompasses knowledge of the treatments' goals, components, mode of delivery, dose, benefits in addressing the health problem, and associated risks or discomfort (Sidani et al., 2006, 2009). This understanding is foundational for making informed judgments of the treatments' attributes. The attributes commonly reported of relevance to participants appraising health interventions are:

1. Appropriateness: the degree to which an intervention is viewed as reasonable in addressing the health problem and is suitable to one's lifestyle.
2. Effectiveness: the degree to which an intervention is viewed as useful in improving the experience of the health problem in the short term and the long term, and in enhancing general functioning or health.
3. Risks: the degree to which adverse effects or discomfort associated with an intervention are considered to be severe or burdensome.
4. Convenience: the degree to which an intervention is appraised as easy to apply and adhere to in daily life (Lengel & Mullins-Sweat, 2017; Miner et al., 2016; Sidani et al., 2018).

Acceptability, therefore, is operationalized as the desirability of an intervention to potential users or clients or participants. It is inferred from their judgment of the extent to which the intervention's techniques or procedures are appropriate, effective, convenient to use, and associated with no or minimal risks (Kazdin, 2006; Sekhon et al., 2017, 2018). This perspective has implications for the assessment of acceptability. Measures of acceptability should be designed to involve participants in the judgment of the treatments' attributes. Assessment of acceptability can be done at different stages of the intervention design and evaluation, using quantitative and qualitative approaches.

## 11.3.2 Measures of Acceptability

A range of self-report instruments and objective indicators have been used to measure acceptability of health interventions. Commonly used ones are briefly reviewed.

### Self-Report Instruments

Several self-report instruments have been developed, adapted, and validated to measure acceptability of a range of interventions. Carter (2007) reviewed instruments frequently used to assess acceptability of educational and psychological interventions. The Treatment Evaluation Inventory (Kazdin, 1980), the Intervention Rating Profile (Witt & Elliott, 1985), and the Treatment Acceptability Rating form (Reimers et al. in 1992) were the most commonly used or adapted to measure acceptability of specific therapies. Other instruments have been recently generated to assess the acceptability of health and behavioral interventions. Examples include the Treatment Acceptability/Adherence Scale (Milosevic et al., 2015), the Acceptability of Intervention Measure (Weiner et al., 2017), and the Treatment Perception and Preference Scale (Sidani et al., 2018). In addition, single items have been used to measure clients' perception of an intervention's overall acceptability (e.g. Schmidt et al., 2015) or specific attributes such as helpfulness or convenience (e.g. Lengel & Mullins-Sweat, 2017; Miner et al., 2016).

### Objective Indicators

Different objective indicators have been used to assess acceptability in intervention evaluation research. The indicators represent participants' behaviors over the course of the study. The behaviors are mentioned in Section 11.2 as associated with perceptions of treatments. The indicators of acceptability commonly reported include: enrollment rates, reasons for declining enrollment, attrition, reasons for withdrawal, attendance at treatment sessions or self-completion of modules, adherence to treatment recommendations, and reasons for nonadherence (Beard et al., 2011; Saracuta et al., 2018). These objective indicators are inconsistent with the conceptualization of acceptability as an attitude toward or perceived desirability of treatment (Section 11.3.1). They represent participants' behaviors in a study that are influenced by perceived acceptability and that may be associated with other factors; the factors are related to the personal and health characteristics of participants (e.g. lack of transportation, functional limitations) and the characteristics of the research study (e.g. burdensome data collection or invasive procedures) (Sidani, 2015). Accordingly, the behaviors are not directly and solely reflective of perceived acceptability of the treatment; they are inaccurate indicators of acceptability.

### Selection of Measures

The selection of measures should be informed by a clear conceptualization and operationalization of acceptability in order to enhance construct validity (Chapter 10). As presented in Section 11.3.1, acceptability is conceptualized as an attitude toward treatments. Attitudes are best assessed with self-report instruments. Acceptability is operationalized as desirability, formed on the basis of judgment of the treatment attributes. Accordingly, self-report instruments should be designed to involve participants in the appraisal of treatments' attributes.

The self-report instruments mentioned previously vary in their content; some inquire about overall acceptability and others capture different combinations of treatment attributes to appraise. The Treatment Evaluation Inventory (Kazdin, 1980) and the Treatment Perception and Preference Scale (Sidani et al., 2018) involve the appraisal of the four attributes (appropriateness, effectiveness, risks, and convenience) commonly reported of relevance to clients.

To adequately assess acceptability, the self-report instruments should provide a description of the intervention being appraised. The description includes what the intervention is set to achieve (i.e. its goals), what it consists of (i.e. components), how it is delivered (i.e. mode and dose), and what are its benefits and risks (Witteman et al., 2015). The information is essential for participants to gain an understanding of the intervention, prior to judging it relative to the four attributes. The description is generated from relevant theoretical literature defining the intervention's active ingredients, clinical or health sources including the manual operationalizing the active ingredients into components, and empirical evidence supporting the intervention's benefits and identifying possible risks or discomfort. The description is structured and presented in sections covering the intervention's name; purpose; components or activities; schedule (i.e. mode of delivery, number, length and frequency of the sessions or modules); benefits; and risks. This structure makes it easy for clients to recognize the different aspects of the intervention. The information is given in factual statements that report on the aspects of the intervention without any implication of their importance or value. In other words, the information should not reflect professional opinion or any bias in presentation. This is necessary to ensure that participants' appraisal is based on facts, on their understanding of the intervention, and on their own values. In addition, nontechnical, clear and simple to understand (at $4^{th}$ to $6^{th}$ reading level) terms are used to describe the intervention (refer to Sidani et al., 2009 for an example of intervention description).

Advances in technology have enabled the presentation of an intervention's information in alternate modes and formats. The description, covering the same content mentioned previously, can be narrated by a research staff member (e.g. interventionist) and video- or audio-recorded. Participants listen to the audio recording before rating the intervention's acceptability. This mode of presentation is useful for participants who have visual challenges in reading, and those who are geographically dispersed and experiencing problems with transportation that prevent them from attending face-to-face data collection sessions. The written or narrated description of the intervention can be supplemented with pictograms. Pictograms are usually one-page documents that briefly mention the intervention's goal and key activities and include pictures that illustrate the activities. The pictures help clarify the activities to participants with low-to-moderate levels of literacy and cognitive impairment. For example interventions focusing on participants' performance of a particular skill (e.g. correct use of an inhaler, ambulation, leg exercise), video recordings of the skill's performance by the interventionist, actors posing as clients, or actual clients, are prepared. Participants watch the video recordings before appraising the intervention. The video recordings represent an easy and efficient manner for describing skills (as compared to potentially long explanation of the step-by-step procedure for the application of the skills) (Fox et al., 2018). Written as well as audio- and video-recorded information can be made available on a website created for a study, and accessed in face-to-face or remotely held data collection sessions.

After reviewing the intervention's description, participants are instructed to respond to items measuring the appropriateness, effectiveness, risks, and convenience of the intervention. The items usually take the form of statements (e.g. the treatment seems suitable) or questions (e.g. how suitable is this treatment to you?). The response options may include visual analogue scales (e.g. Schmidt et al., 2015), numeric rating scale anchored with "not at all" and "very much" (Sidani et al., 2018), or Likert-type scales reflecting different levels of agreement with the statements.

## 11.3.3   Assessment of Acceptability

Acceptability can be examined at different stages in the design and evaluation of health interventions. Because acceptability is an attitude or perceived desirability, it can be assessed independent of and prior to exposure to the intervention. Specifically, acceptability can be explored during the process of designing new interventions or adapting evidence-based interventions to a new context. It can be investigated in large-scale descriptive studies concerned with determining the acceptability of different interventions addressing a health problem, and in evaluation studies aimed to examine the contribution of acceptability to the success of an intervention.

### Examining Acceptability When Designing or Adapting Interventions

In the process of designing a new health intervention, acceptability is examined as a means to develop the intervention or to confirm the desirability of the newly developed intervention.

#### *Development of Intervention*

Acceptability can be examined following an inductive experiential approach to intervention development (Chapter 4). Clients are consulted to elicit their feedback on the acceptability of strategies, therapies, techniques, or components (content, activities) that could comprise the newly designed intervention. Clients represent various subgroups of the target population. The subgroups are defined in terms of personal characteristics (e.g. computer literacy); health profile (e.g. physical function); and experience of the health problem (e.g. determinants, level of severity). These client characteristics may shape their beliefs and values of the health problem and its treatment, and may influence their ability to engage in the intervention and enact its treatment recommendations.

Selected clients are invited to participate in an individual or group discussion of general strategies, or specific therapies or components they perceive as desirable in addressing the health problem. The discussion is prefaced with a clarification of the health problem (i.e. what it is, how it is experienced, what causes it). It proceeds with posing open-ended questions to elicit clients' input on what constitutes acceptable strategies, therapies, or components to address the problem; examples of questions are: what would you consider as an appropriate way to address the problem? Do you think this specific therapy or component would be acceptable and helpful to manage this particular cause of the problem? Additional questions are asked to probe for clarification on the proposed strategies, therapies, or components; the questions explore: aspects of the proposed therapy or component considered acceptable or unacceptable, and ways to modify the aspects to enhance the overall desirability of the intervention. As well, the questions inquire about the suitability of different ways (e.g. mode, format, timing, setting) to deliver the intervention. In group consultation, the discussion also focuses on reaching agreement on the most desirable intervention's components, activities, mode, and dose. The study by MacDonald et al. (2007) illustrates this method for examining acceptability. The researchers conducted qualitative interviews with adolescents (n = 25) to identify smoking cessation services acceptable to this population. The results elucidated adolescents' perspective on who and what could help them quit smoking. The adolescents reported it desirable to engage with their friends in leisure activities as a diversion from smoking, or to attend with their friends a flexible smoking cessation support program facilitated by a leader who was characterized as "friendly, confidential, supportive, and respected" and offered outside the school system.

### Confirmation of Desirability

An experiential deductive approach to elicit clients' feedback on the acceptability of the intervention is applied in two situations. The first is to determine the acceptability of a newly designed intervention; this takes place once the intervention theory is developed and operationalized into a logic model and manual. The second situation involves examination of the acceptability of evidence-based interventions to a new target population in a new context.

The experiential deductive approach involves individual or group session with clients representing various subgroups of the target population (as defined previously). The session begins by reviewing, briefly, the health problem that is addressed by the intervention, followed by an overview of the intervention to clarify its name, goals, components, mode, dose, and, if known, benefits and risks. The session then proceeds in either of two ways:

1. Presenting a detailed description of each component of the intervention: The description highlights the content to be covered, the activities to be performed by the interventionist and by clients, and the setting and timing, within the trajectory of the health problem, for its delivery. The description is based on the information contained in the logic model, and is supported by relevant audiovisual aids.

2. Providing the intervention to clients in the specified mode: For in-person delivery, the interventionist actually delivers the key components of the intervention in an abridged or condensed manner (e.g. review the six instructions of the stimulus control therapy), within the time frame set for the sessions. For interventions to be self-completed, clients are given the opportunity to read the intervention modules (in hard copy) or to access the intervention materials available electronically during the session, as reported by Chung et al. (2009), Collie et al. (2007), and Gwadry-Sridher et al. (2003).

Acceptability of each component is assessed after describing or delivering each component of the intervention. Then clients are requested to rate the acceptability of the overall intervention (see Table 11.2 for example). They are also invited to comment on the intervention's overall relevance, appraise its acceptability, and suggest modifications as necessary. Open-ended questions are posed to engage clients in the discussion, such as: How reasonable or useful is this aspect of the intervention in addressing the health problem? How suitable or easy to apply is it? How can this aspect be changed to make it acceptable? The session concludes by reiterating the aspects of the intervention viewed as acceptable and the modification to be made, and seeking clients' agreement on these.

**TABLE 11.2**   Excerpt of rating of acceptability of sleep education and hygiene.

| Intervention aspects | Rating of acceptability | | | | |
|---|---|---|---|---|---|
| Activities: | 0 | 1 | 2 | 3 | 4 |
| Discuss the following topics: | | | | | |
|   What is sleep | 0 | 1 | 2 | 3 | 4 |
|   Why do we sleep | 0 | 1 | 2 | 3 | 4 |
|   What regulates sleep | 0 | 1 | 2 | 3 | 4 |
|   What is insomnia | 0 | 1 | 2 | 3 | 4 |
|   How does insomnia develop | 0 | 1 | 2 | 3 | 4 |
|   What keeps insomnia going | 0 | 1 | 2 | 3 | 4 |
|   What can be done to manage insomnia | 0 | 1 | 2 | 3 | 4 |
| Mode of delivery: | | | | | |
|   Discussion done in small group of six to eight persons with insomnia | 0 | 1 | 2 | 3 | 4 |
|   Booklet covering topics of discussion given for future reference | 0 | 1 | 2 | 3 | 4 |
| Dose: | | | | | |
| Discussion takes place in one-hour session | 0 | 1 | 2 | 3 | 4 |

Rating of acceptability: 0, not acceptable at all; 1, somewhat acceptable; 2, acceptable; 3, very acceptable; 4, very much acceptable.

## Examining Acceptability in Descriptive Studies

Acceptability of newly designed or evidence-based interventions can be examined in large-scale descriptive studies. The aim is to determine the desirability of the interventions to various subgroups of the target client population. Whether administered in face-to-face or telephone data collection session, or completed online, the questionnaire should introduce the health problem addressed by the intervention, provide a description of the intervention (as explained in Section 11.3.2), and instruct participants to read the description of the intervention and complete the items assessing their perception of the intervention's appropriateness, effectiveness, risks, and convenience. Space can be provided for participants to comment on the overall acceptability of the intervention and on aspects of the intervention that are most or least desirable, and to offer suggestions for modifying the least desirable aspects in order to enhance the acceptability of the intervention to clients. The questionnaire can be expanded to assess the acceptability of two or more interventions, by including additional sections, each providing the description and the items to rate one intervention. The findings of descriptive studies are informative. They point to interventions that clients desire; these interventions can be included in research studies evaluating their effectiveness or comparative effectiveness, and made available and accessible for use in practice. Offering acceptable interventions reduces waste of efforts in training interventionists, recruiting and retaining clients assigned to non-acceptable interventions. In addition, findings of descriptive studies may reveal variability in perceived acceptability of different interventions by different subgroups of clients. The findings suggest the need for tailoring the intervention.

## Examining Acceptability in Evaluative Studies

Acceptability is examined in randomized, preference, or pragmatic trials evaluating the effectiveness of newly developed or established interventions. It is assessed systematically, with a questionnaire that describes the treatments under evaluation and contains items to rate acceptability (as described in Section 11.3.2). The questionnaire is completed prior to exposure to treatment. It can be administered by research staff, allowing for clarification of aspects of the treatments as necessary, or self-completed by participants. The contribution of acceptability to attrition, engagement, and enactment of treatment, as well as outcomes, can be determined; using appropriate statistical analyses. In preference trials and in practice, acceptability is a key element in the process of eliciting clients' preferences for treatment. Preferences are accounted for in allocating participants to treatments in a preference trial, and are the essence of treatment decision-making and client-centered care in practice (Sidani & Fox, 2014).

## 11.4   EXAMINATION OF PREFERENCES

### 11.4.1   Conceptualization of Preferences

Preferences refer to choice of treatment. They represent the particular treatment, among alternative ones, that clients want to have in order to address the presenting health problem (Goates-Jones & Hill, 2008; Joy et al., 2013). Preferences result from clients' understanding of the treatments under consideration and valuation of these treatments' attributes (Clark et al., 2014; Laba et al., 2012). As explained in Section 11.3.1, understanding is gained from information presented about the treatments' goals, components, mode and dose of delivery, benefits and risks. Valuation is derived from appraisal of the treatments' appropriateness, effectiveness, risks, and convenience (Harrison et al., 2014; Lawton et al., 2013; Witticke et al., 2012).

The conceptualization indicates that assessment of preferences should follow a systematic process in order to ensure that clients are well informed when expressing their preferences (Harrison et al., 2014) and that the expressed preferences validly and accurately reflect their choice. Validity of preferences is important for providing the treatment that matches clients' choice (Dimidjian & Goodman, 2014). The process for assessing preferences involves three steps. In the first step, information is provided on each treatment (e.g. experimental intervention and comparison treatment, or two or more interventions addressing the same health problem) under consideration (Bowling et al., 2008). The second step consists of appraisal of each treatment's attributes. The third step focuses on the expression of preferences. The first two steps of this process are similar to those applied in assessing acceptability (Section 11.3.1) and in shared decision-making (Stacey & Légaré, 2015). Rating the treatments' acceptability helps clients clarify to themselves the attributes they value most. It also assists them in comparing and contrasting alternative treatments relative to the most valued attributes. These comparisons support clients in identifying their preferred treatment, that is, the one they appraised as having all or most of the valued attributes. There is some evidence supporting the association between acceptability and preferences; participants are likely to prefer treatments appraised as acceptable (Bluestein et al., 2011; Sidani et al., 2009).

## 11.4.2  Measures of Preferences

Two general methods have been used to assess preferences in research: direct and indirect. Recent initiatives to promote the implementation of shared treatment decision-making have used decision aids as a means to facilitate assessment of clients' preferences in practice (e.g. Muscat et al., 2015; Stigglebout et al., 2015).

### Direct Method

The direct method consists of informing clients of the treatments under consideration and requesting them to indicate their choice. Information about the treatments is presented in the structure and format explained in Section 11.3.2, or in decision aids. Decision aids usually summarize information about the benefits and risks of each treatment, as well as information comparing the alternative treatments under consideration. Participants may review the information independently or collaboratively with health professionals, before they indicate their choice.

Simple measures are used to indicate which treatment is preferred (Mills et al., 2011). These are often single items that request participants to engage in any of the following cognitive tasks: identify the preferred treatment; choose the treatment they want; rank order the treatments under consideration from the most to least preferred; or express willingness to receive a particular treatment (Sidani et al., 2018). Thus, the direct method focuses on determining the preferred treatment and does not involve participants in a formal appraisal of the treatments' attributes. Accordingly, this method is rather simple and not cognitively taxing (Ali & Ronaldson, 2012). However, the simple method is not quite consistent with the current conceptualization of preferences (Section 11.4.1). Omitting the formal appraisal task (i.e. appraisal of treatments relative to the attributes) may limit participants' ability to determine the attributes they value most and the treatment that has the valued attributes, potentially resulting in the expression of inaccurate preferences (Sidani et al., 2018).

### Indirect Method

The indirect method involves the elicitation of clients' perceptions or acceptability of the treatments under consideration, but without explicitly asking them to indicate the preferred treatment. The indirect method is consistent with the assumption that clients prefer treatments they appraise as desirable (Clark et al., 2014). Two categories of measures have been used.

The first category consists of administering self-report measures of treatment acceptability as described in Section 11.3.2. Participants are provided information on each treatment under consideration and are asked to rate each treatment on different attributes (e.g. appropriateness, suitability). The total score is computed to quantify the overall level of acceptability of each treatment. The treatment with the highest acceptability score is considered as the preferred one. This indirect method is simple and easy to administer to participants with different characteristics, in a range of settings. It provides a structured approach to appraise different treatments relative to the same attributes. However, the available measures vary in the set of treatment attributes they capture, with some of the included attributes overlapping (e.g. acceptability and appropriateness). Participants may have difficulty distinguishing among attributes, which may affect the accuracy of the scores, potentially resulting in situations where the treatments under consideration receive the same total scores. These situations make it hard to identify the preferred treatment. To be consistent with the conceptualization of preferences, it is recommended to add one or two items inquiring about participants' preferences to these measures. For instance, the Treatment Perception and Preference scale (Sidani et al., 2018) provides a description and items to rate the acceptability (capturing the attributes of appropriateness, benefits, risks, and convenience) of each treatment under consideration, followed by two questions designed to elicit participants' preferences. The first question asks participants to indicate if they have a preference for any of the treatments they appraised, and the second question inquires about the treatment they prefer and want to have to address the health problem.

The second category of indirect measures consists of trade-off techniques such as the discrete choice experiment. These techniques involve a series of comparisons among treatments under consideration. Participants are presented with a series of scenarios describing different levels of treatment attributes (e.g. range of odds ratios quantifying the treatment effectiveness in preventing a health problem). Participants are asked to weigh treatments that vary on the different attributes. Complex statistical techniques are applied to compute utility scores, which reflect clients' perceptions or ratings of the treatments and, hence, the preferred one. These techniques have been criticized on several grounds: 1) the description of treatments commonly represents hypothetical treatments that are of no relevance to research or practice (Malhotra et al., 2015); 2) the treatment attributes appraised in the comparisons are of relevance to decision makers (e.g. cost) more so than clients (Finkelstein et al., 2015); and 3) the comparison or weighing exercise is time consuming, cognitively taxing, and burdensome (Hall et al., 2014), resulting in response fatigue and inability to complete the exercise. These disadvantages make the trade-off techniques of limited utility in assessing preferences in research and practice.

### 11.4.3   Methods for Examining Preferences

Preferences are often assessed in descriptive and evaluative studies. In large-scale descriptive studies, participants complete the questionnaire (in hard or electronic copy) that provides a description of the treatments and items for appraising the attributes of each treatment under consideration, as well as measures of preferences, on their own, at their convenience. The results indicate which treatment is most preferred by which subgroup of participants (e.g. Simiola et al., 2015).

In evaluative studies, preferences are assessed with similar measures prior to allocating participants to treatment. In randomized trials, this information is useful to determine whether participants were randomized to treatment that matches or mismatches their preferences, and to examine the extent to which receiving matched or mismatched treatment contributes to attrition, treatment enactment, and outcomes. This analysis is useful in enhancing the validity of inferences regarding the effectiveness of the intervention under evaluation (Chapter 14).

## 11.5   EXAMINATION OF CREDIBILITY

### 11.5.1   Conceptualization of Credibility

Credibility reflects clients' endorsement of a treatment's rationale (Nock et al., 2007; Smith et al., 2013). It is the extent to which they view a treatment as reasonable and logical, that is, the principles underlying the treatment make sense to them and the component and activities comprising a treatment are coherent in terms of how a treatment works in addressing the health problem (Sandell et al., 2011). Accordingly, credibility reflects acceptance of a treatment's rationale (Borkovec & Nau, 1972).

This conceptualization implies that credibility is assessed only after clients are exposed to the treatment's rationale. For many health interventions, the rationale is introduced early in the course of their delivery (Mooney et al., 2014).

### 11.5.2    Measures of Credibility

Credibility is measured with self-report instruments comprised of items inquiring about participants' beliefs about how logical, reasonable, convincing, or "believable" a treatment is (Haanstra et al., 2015). Credibility has been assessed with different validated measures, including:

- One item, visual analogue scales, with scores ranging from 0 to 10 (e.g. Schmidt et al., 2015).
- The Credibility subscale of the Treatment Evaluation Questionnaire developed by Borkovec and Nau (1972), in its original or modified version, and/or the revised version called the Credibility/Expectancy Questionnaire (e.g. El-Alaoui et al., 2015; Beard et al., 2011; Haanstra et al., 2015; Narimatsu et al., 2016; Nock et al., 2007; Sandell et al., 2011; Smith et al., 2013).
- The Opinion about Treatment, which is a three-item measure (Mooney et al., 2014).

### 11.5.3    Methods for Examining Credibility

Credibility has been examined in evaluative studies, after the rationale underlying the intervention is discussed, and its components (content, activities, treatment recommendations) are described in detail. Information on the treatment's rationale and components is relayed to participants in the first session given by the interventionist or in the first module self-completed (in hard or electronic format) by participants. Accordingly, credibility is assessed upon completion of the first session or module. For example, the last five minutes of the first session can be devoted to the completion of the credibility measure. This timing is appropriate as it immediately follows the discussion and clarification by the interventionist, of the treatment rationale and components; it minimizes the potential for bias in participants' recalling the information. Participants' responses allow the generation of total scores quantifying their perceived credibility of the allocated treatment (other than the no-treatment control). The influence of perceived credibility on attrition, treatment enactment, and outcomes can be examined using appropriate statistical tests, such as multiple regression or path analysis.

## 11.6    EXAMINATION OF EXPECTANCY

### 11.6.1    Conceptualization of Expectancy

Expectancy or outcome expectation refers to clients' anticipated effectiveness of a treatment. It is their belief or perception of the extent to which a treatment is potentially useful or helpful in addressing the health problem and in improving health (Colagiuri, 2010; Smith et al., 2013; Younger et al., 2012). In other words, expectancy quantifies the improvement in outcomes that participants expect to achieve with the treatment (Nock et al., 2007). The belief or perception of improvement in outcomes is partly generated from an understanding of the treatment's rationale. This explanation is supported empirically: A moderate-to-high positive association has been reported between perceived credibility and expectancy of interventions (e.g. Constantino et al., 2007; Haanstra et al., 2015; Mooney et al., 2014). Therefore, expectancy is assessed once the treatment rationale and components have been presented to clients (Mooney et al., 2014).

### 11.6.2    Measures of Expectancy

Expectancy is measured with self-report, single- or multiple-item instruments. Participants are asked to indicate the extent to which they view the treatment as potentially helpful in improving the experience of the health problem. Examples of single items for assessing expectancy are reported in Beasly et al. (2017) and Lengel and Mullins-Sweat (2017). Several multi-item instruments or subscales have been used to measure expectancy, including:

- The Expectancy subscale of the original Treatment Evaluation Questionnaire (Borkovec & Nau, 1972) or revised Credibility/Expectancy Questionnaire (e.g. Nock et al., 2007; Haanstra et al., 2015).
- The Stanford Expectations of Treatment Scale developed by Younger et al. (2012).
- The Attitudes and Expectations Questionnaire used by Mooney et al. (2014).
- The Therapy Helpfulness Questionnaire used by Smith et al. (2013).

### 11.6.3    Methods for Examining Expectancy

Using relevant instruments, expectancy is measured toward the end of the first treatment session or module, often concurrently with the assessment of credibility. The methods for examining its contribution within evaluative studies are the same as those described for examining credibility as explained in Section 11.5.3.

## 11.7    EXAMINATION OF SATISFACTION WITH TREATMENT

It is important to note that satisfaction with treatments delivered to participants differs from satisfaction with general healthcare or services provided to clients in practice. Satisfaction with care has been extensively discussed in relevant health services literature.

### 11.7.1    Conceptualization of Satisfaction

Satisfaction with treatment is considered a client-reported parameter of a health intervention's success (Rejas et al., 2013). Satisfaction has been conceptualized as an affective response or attitude toward a treatment, as a cognitive appraisal of a treatment relative to personal expectations of treatment (Alessi & Rasch, 2017), and as an appraisal of a treatment's processes and outcomes (Sidani & Epstein, 2016). The latter conceptualization is widely adapted in intervention evaluation research. The conceptualization underpins the content covered in measures of treatment satisfaction, (e.g. Gamble et al., 2013; Oppenshaw et al., 2012; Umar et al., 2013; Wong et al., 2015), which encompasses processes and outcomes as presented in Section 11.7.2.

In recent conceptualizations, satisfaction with treatment is defined as the subjective evaluation of an intervention. The evaluation involves an appraisal of the intervention's performance relative to its processes and outcomes. The processes reflect what comprises (i.e. component, content, activities) an intervention and how it is delivered. The outcomes represent the impact or effects of an intervention (Brédart et al., 2010; George & Robinson, 2010; Lawlor et al., 2017). Accordingly, satisfaction reflects clients' experience with treatment (Sidani & Epstein, 2016). A comprehensive assessment of satisfaction includes clients' appraisal of its components, mode of delivery, and experienced benefits; it is conducted upon treatment completion (Sekhon et al., 2017; Sidani et al., 2017).

## 11.7.2   Measures of Satisfaction

Several categories of self-report measures of satisfaction with treatment have been used in intervention research. The first category consists of single items measuring global satisfaction with the overall intervention (e.g. Waltz et al., 2014). These items are rather simple and easy to use, providing for participants' general perception of the treatment's acceptance. They may be appropriate to use with simple or single-component interventions such as medications.

The second category includes measures that are composed of multiple items assessing a particular process of interventions. The particular intervention processes measured differ across instruments. Some measures require participants to judge the perceived helpfulness of each intervention component (e.g. Alessi & Rasch, 2017; Jennings et al., 2014; McGregor et al., 2014). A few measures request participants to appraise the climate or dynamics in group therapy sessions (e.g. McClendon & Burlingame, 2010). Other measures ask participants to rate the interventionist's competence (e.g. Oppenshaw et al., 2012) and relationships with clients (e.g. Tierney & Kane, 2011). It is worth noting that interventionists represent the mode for delivering many health interventions and, as discussed in Chapter 8, their competence and working alliance influence how they provide treatment. Accordingly, items measuring interventionists' competence and working alliance have been incorporated into measures of satisfaction with treatment. Instruments assessing specific treatment processes are helpful in shedding light on participants' acceptance of how the intervention is delivered; however, they fall short of examining satisfaction with the full range of processes and omit satisfaction with improved outcomes experienced with the receipt of treatment.

The third category of measures incorporates items eliciting participants' perceived values of different treatment attributes such as benefit, discomfort, and convenience of use (e.g. Frick et al., 2012; Gamble et al., 2013; Rejas et al., 2013; Umar et al., 2013; Wong et al., 2015). The Treatment Satisfaction Questionnaire for Medication (e.g. Kucukarslan et al., 2013) and the Client Satisfaction Questionnaire (Attkisson & Greenfield, 1994) have been frequently used to assess participants' appraisal of attributes of pharmacological and behavioral interventions, respectively. These measures are short ($\leq$ 10 items) and easy to administer; however, they do not cover all processes and outcomes of treatment.

A thorough assessment of satisfaction should cover a range of processes and outcomes. The Multi-Dimensional Treatment Satisfaction Measure (Sidani et al., 2017) provides for a comprehensive assessment of satisfaction with multicomponent health interventions. The measure has several subscales for the appraisal of the following treatment processes:

- Suitability or appropriateness of each intervention component in addressing the health problem.
- Utility or helpfulness of each intervention component in understanding the health problem, in learning ways to manage it, and in increasing confidence in applying the treatment recommendations.
- Overall attitude toward the intervention as-a-whole, and desire to continue using it as needed.
- Competence and interpersonal style of the interventionists delivering the intervention.
- Adequacy of the format (or mode) and dose at which the intervention is delivered in helping clients understand the health problem and apply the treatment recommendations.

The measure also contains three subscales for appraising the outcomes. The first subscale focuses on the treatment's benefits (i.e. improvement in the health problem and functioning), whereas the second focuses on discomfort associated with the treatment. The third subscale inquires about clients' perspective on whether or not improvements in outcomes are attributable to the treatment. Although comprehensive, the measure contains a large number of items, with the potential of inducing response fatigue.

### 11.7.3    Methods for Examining Satisfaction

Because satisfaction reflects clients' appraisal of the treatment's processes and outcomes, it is usually assessed upon its completion (Sekhon et al., 2017; Sidani et al., 2017). The selected measure can be administered toward the end of the last treatment session or within the week following the last session. This timing is appropriate as participants still remember the different treatment components to which they were exposed. Further, this timing is adequate for participants to experience improvements in immediate outcomes and some beneficial changes (though small) in intermediate and ultimate outcomes. Analysis of satisfaction data is usually descriptive, aimed at identifying aspects of the intervention most/least valuable. In addition, the analysis can be geared toward determining the influence of satisfaction on continued use (as necessary) of the intervention, using relevant correlational statistics.

## REFERENCES

Aarons, G.A., Green, A.E., Palinkas, L.A., et al. (2012) Dynamic adaptation process to implement an evidence-based child maltreatment intervention. *Implementation Science*, 7, 32–41.

Alessi, S.M. & Rasch, C.J. (2017) Treatment satisfaction in a randomized clinical trial of mHealth smoking abstinence reinforcement. *Journal of Substance Abuse Treatment*, 72, 103–110.

Ali, S. & Ronaldson, S. (2012) Ordinal preference elicitation methods in health economics and health services research: Using discrete choice experiments and ranking methods. *British Medical Bulletin*, 103, 21–41.

Attkisson, C.C. & Greenfield, T.K. (1994) Client satisfaction questionnaire-8 and service satisfaction scale-30. In: M. E. Maruish ed. *The Use of Psychological Testing for Treatment Planning and Outcome Assessment*. Lawrence Erlbaum Associates, Inc, Mahwah, NJ, pp. 402–420.

Barbosa, C.D., Balp, M-M., Kulich, K., Germain, N., & Rofail, D. (2012) A literature review to explore the link between treatment satisfaction and adherence, compliance and persistence. *Patient Preference and Adherence*, 6, 39–48.

Beard, C., Weisberg, R.B., & Amir, N. (2011) Combined cognitive bias modification treatment for social anxiety disorder: A pilot trial. *Depression & Anxiety*, 28, 981–988. doi:10.1002/da/20873

Beasly, M.J., Ferguson-Jones, E.A., Macfarlane, G.J. on behalf of the MUSICIAN Study team (2017) Treatment expectations but not preference affect outcome in a trial of CBT and exercise for pain. *Canadian Journal of Pain*, 1(1), 161–170. doi:10.1080/2 4740527.2017.1384297

Beatty, L. & Binnion, C. (2016) A systematic review of predictors of, and reasons for, adherence to online psychological interventions. *International Journal of Behavior Medicine*, 23, 776–794. doi:10.1007/s12529-016-9556-9

Bernal, G., Jimenez-Chafey, M., & Domenech Rodriguez, M.M. (2009) Cultural adaptation of treatments: A resource for considering culture in evidence-based practice. *Professional Psychology – Research & Practice*, 40, 361–368. doi:10.1037/a0016401

Bluestein, D., Healy, A.C., & Rutledge, C.M. (2011) Acceptability of behavioral treatments for insomnia. *Journal of American board of Family Medicine*, 24, 272–280.

Boettcher, J., Renneberg, B., & Berger, T. (2013) Patient expectations in internet-based self-help for social anxiety. *Cognitive Behaviour Therapy*, 42(3), 203–214. doi:10.108 0/16506073.2012.759615

Borkovec, T.D. & Nau, S.D. (1972) Credibility of analogue therapy rationales. *Journal of Behavior Therapy and Experimental Psychiatry*, 3, 257–260.

Bowling, A., Reeves, B., & Rowe, G. (2008) Patient preferences for treatment for angina: An overview of findings from three studies. *Journal of Health Services Research & Policy*, 13(Suppl. 3), 104–108.

Bradley-Gilbride, J. & Bradley, C. (2010) Partially randomized preference trial design. In: N.J. Salkind (ed) *Encyclopedia of Research Design*. Sage, Newbury Park, CA, Vol 2, pp. 1009–1015.

Brédart, A., Sultan, S., & Regnault, A. (2010) Patient satisfaction instruments for cancer clinical research or practice. *Expert Review of Pharmacoeconomics & Outcomes Research*, 10(2), 129–141. doi:10.1586/erp.10.7

Brose, L.S. & Bradley, C. (2009) Psychometric development of the Retinopathy Treatment Satisfaction Questionnaire (RetTSQ). *Psychology, Health & Medicine*, 14(6), 740–754. doi:10.1080/13548500903431485

Carter, S.L. (2007) Review of recent treatment acceptability research. *Education and Training in Developmental Disabilities*, 42(3), 301–316.

Chung, L.K., Cimprich, B., Janz, N.K., & Mills-Wismeski, S.M. (2009) Breast cancer survivorship program: Testing cross-cultural relevance. *Cancer Nursing*, 32(3), 236–245.

Clark, M.D., Determann, D., Petrou, S., Moro, D., & de Bekker-Grob, E.W. (2014) Discrete choice experiments in health economics: A review of the literature. *Pharmaco Economics*, 32, 883–902.

Cohen, J.N., Potter, C.M., Drabick, D.A.G., et al. (2015) Clinical presentation and pharmacotherapy response in social anxiety disorder: The effect of etiological beliefs. *Psychiatry Research*, 228(1), 65–71. doi:10.1016/j.psyhcres.2015.04.014

Colagiuri, B. (2010) Participant expectancies in double-blind randomized placebo-controlled trials: Potential limitations to trial validity. *Clinical Trials*, 7, 246–255. doi:10.1177/174077451036

Collie, K., Kreshka, A., Ferrier, S., et al. (2007) Videoconferencing for delivery of breast cancer support groups to women living in rural communities: A pilot study. *Psycho-Oncology*, 16, 778–782.

Constantino, M.J., Coyne, A.E., Boswell, J.F., Iles, B.R., & Vîslă, A. (2018) A meta-analysis of the association between patients' early perception of treatment credibility and their posttreatment outcomes. *Psychotherapy*, 55(4), 486–495. doi:10.1037/pst0000168

Constantino, M.J., Manber, R., Ong, J., et al. (2007) Patient expectations and therapeutic alliance as predictors of outcomes in group cognitive-behavioral therapy for insomnia. *Behavioral Sleep Medicine*, 5, 210–228. doi:10.1080/15402000701263932

De Las Cuevas, C., Motuca, M., Baptista, T., & de Leon, J. (2018) Skepticism and pharmacophobia toward medication may negatively impact adherence to psychiatric medications: A comparison among outpatient samples recruited in Spain, Argentina, and Venezuela. *Patient Preference and Adherence*, 12, 301–310. doi:10.2147/PPA.S158443

Dimidjian, S. & Goodman, S. (2014) Preferences and attitudes toward approaches to depression relapse/recurrence prevention among pregnant women. *Behavioral Research and Therapy*, 54, 7–11.

Dobscha, S.K., Carson, K., & Gerrity, M.S. (2007) Depression treatment preferences of VA Primary Care patients. *Psychosomatics*, 48, 482–488.

Dong, L., Soehner, A.M., Bélanger, L., Morin, C.M., & Harvey, A.G. (2018) Treatment agreement, adherence, and outcome in cognitive behavioral treatments for insomnia. *Journal of Consulting and Clinical Psychology*, 86(3), 294–299. doi:10.1037/ccp0000269

Eaton, C.K., Eakin, M.N., Coburn, S., et al. (2019) Patient health beliefs and characteristics predict longitudinal antihypertensive medication adherence in adolescents with CKD. *Journal of Pediatric Psychology*, 44(1), 40–51. doi:10.1093/jpepsy/jsy073

El-Alaoui, S., Ljótsson, B., Hedman, E., et al. (2015) Symptomatic change and adherence in internet-based cognitive behavior therapy for social anxiety disorder in routine psychiatric care. *PLoS ONE*, 10(4), e0124258. doi:10.1371/journal.pone.0124258

Fernandez, E., Salem, D., Swift, J.K., & Ramtahal, N. (2015) Meta-analysis of dropout from cognitive behavioral therapy: Magnitude, timing, and moderators. *Journal of Consulting & Clinical Psychology*, 86(6), 1108–1122. doi:10.1037/ccp000044

Finkelstein, E.A., Bilger, M., Flynn, T.N., & Malhotra, C. (2015) Preferences for end-of-life care among community-dwelling older adults and patients with advanced cancer: A discrete choice experiment. *Health Policy*, 119, 1482–1489.

Fox, M.T., Sidani, S., Brooks, D., & McCague, H. (2018) Perceived acceptability and preferences for low-intensity early activity interventions of older hospitalized medical patients exposed to bed rest: A cross sectional study. *BMC Geriatrics*, 18, 53–61. doi:10.1186/s12877-018-0722-6

Frick, U., Gutzwiller, F.S., Maggiorini, M., & Christen, S. (2012) A questionnaire on treatment satisfaction and disease specific knowledge among patients with acute coronary syndrome. II: Insights for patient education and quality improvement. *Patient Education and Counseling*, 86, 366–371.

Frisaldi, E., Shaibani, A., & Benedetti, F. (2017) Why we should assess patients' expectations in clinical trials. *Pain Therapy*, 6(1), 1–4.

Gamble, S.A., Talbot, N.L., Cashman-Brown, S.M., et al. (2013. A pilot study of interpersonal psychotherapy for alcohol-dependent women with co-occurring major depression. *Substance Abuse*, 34, 233–241.

Gaudiano, B.A., Hughes, J.A., & Miller, I.W. (2013) Patients' treatment expectancies in clinical trials of antidepressants versus psychotherapy for depression: A study using hypothetical vignettes. *Comprehensive Psychiatry*, 54, 28–33

Gebhardt, S., Wolak, A.M., & Huber, M.T. (2013) Patient satisfaction and clinical parameters in psychiatric inpatients—the prevailing role of symptom severity and pharmacologic disturbances. *Comprehensive Psychiatry*, 54, 53–60.

Givens, J. L, Houston, T.K., van Voorhees, B.W., Ford, D.E., & Cooper, L.A. (2007) Ethnicity and preferences for depression treatment. *General Hospital Psychiatry*, 29, 182–191.

Goates-Jones, M. & Hill, C.E. (2008) Treatment preferences, treatment-preference match, and psychotherapist credibility: Influence on session outcome and preference shift. *Psychotherapy: Theory, Research, Practice, Training*, 45(1), 61–74. doi:10.1037/0033-3204.45.1.61

George S.Z. & Robinson M.E. (2010) Preference, expectation, and satisfaction in a clinical trial of behavioral interventions for acute and sub-acute low back pain. *Journal of Pain*, 11(11), 1074–1082. doi:10.1016/j.jpain.2010.02.016

Greenhalgh T., Jackson C., Shaw S., & Janamian T. (2016) Achieving research impact through co-creation in community-based health services: Literature review and case study. *Milbank Quarterly*, 94(2), 392–429

Gum, A.M., Arean, P.A., Hynkeler, E., et al. (2006) Depression treatment preferences in older primary care patients. *The Gerontologist*, 4, 14–22.

Gwadry-Sridher, F., Guyatt, G.H., Arnold, M.O., et al. (2003) Instruments to measure acceptability of information and acquisition of knowledge in patients with heat failure. *The European Journal of Heart Failure*, 5, 783–791.

Haanstra, T.M., Tilbury, C., Kamper, S.J., et al. (2015) Can optimism, pessimism, hope, treatment credibility and treatment expectancy be distinguished in patients undergoing total hip and total knee arthroplasty? *PLoS ONE*, 10(7), e0133730. doi:10.1371/journal.pone.0133730

Herdman, E., Andersson, E., Ljótsson, B., et al. (2012) Clinical and genetic outcome determinants of internet- and group-based cognitive behavior therapy for social anxiety disorder. *ActaPsychiatryScandinavia*, 126, 126–136. doi:10.1111/j.1600-0447.2012.01834.x

Kazdin, A.E. (2006) Arbitrary metrics: Implications for identifying evidence-based treatments. *American Psychologist*, 61(1), 42–49. doi:10.1037/0003-066X.61.1.42

Kazdin, A.E. (1980) Acceptability of alternative treatments for deviant child behavior. *Journal of Applied Behavior Analysis*, 13, 259–273.

Kendra, M.S., Weingardt, K.R., Cucciare, M.A., & Timko, C. (2015) Satisfaction with substance use treatment use treatment and 12-step groups predict outcomes. *Addictive Behaviors*, 40, 27–32.

Kemp, J.J., Lickel, J.J., & Deacon, B.J. (2014) Effects of a chemical imbalance causal explanation on individuals' perceptions of their depressive symptoms. *Behaviour Research & Therapy*, 56, 47–51. doi:10.1016/j.brat.2014.02.009

Köhler, S., Unger, T., Hoffman, S., Steinacher, B., & Fydrich, T. (2015) Patient satisfaction with in patient psychiatric treatment and its relation to treatment outcome in unipolar depression and schizophrenia. *International Journal of Psychiatry in Clinical Practice*, 19(2), 119–123. doi:10.3109/13651501.2014.988272

Kowalski, C.J. & Mrdjenovich, A.J. (2013) Patient preference clinical trials: Why and when they will sometimes be preferred. *Perspectives in Biology and Medicine*, 56 (1), 18–35. doi:10.1353/pbm.2013.0004

Kucukarslan, S.N., Lee, K.S., Patel, T.D., & Ruparetia, B. (2013) An experiment using hypothetical patient scenarios in healthy subjects to evaluate the treatment satisfaction and medication adherence intention relationship. *Health Expectations*, 18, 1291–1298. doi: 10.1111/hex.12103

Kwan, B.M., Dimidjian, S., & Rizvi, S.L. (2010) Treatment preferences, engagement, and clinical improvement in pharmacotherapy versus psychotherapy for depression. *Behavior Research & Therapy*, 48, 799–804.

Hall, J., Kenny, P., Hossain, I., Street, D.J., & Knox, S.A. (2014) Providing informal care in terminal illness: An analysis of preferences for support using a discrete choice experiment. *Medical Decision Making*, 34, 731–745.

Harrison, M., Rigby, D., Vass, C., et al. (2014) Risk as an attribute in discrete choice experiments: A systematic review of the literature. *Patient*, 7, 151–170.

Houle, J., Villagi, B., Beaulieu, M.-D., et al. (2013) Treatment preferences in patients with first episode depression. *Journal of Affective Disorders*, 147, 94–100.

Hundt, N.E., Armento, M.E.A., Porter, B., et al. (2013) Predictors of treatment satisfaction among older adults with anxiety in a primary care psychology program. *Evaluation Program Planning*, 37, 58–63. doi:10.1016/j.evalprogplan.2013.01.003

Jennings, C.A., Vandelanotte, C., Caperchione, C.M., & Mummery, W.K. (2014) Effectiveness of a web-based physical activity intervention for adults with Type 2 diabetes—a randomised controlled trial. *Preventive Medicine*, 60, 33–40.

Joy, S.M., Little, E., Maruthur, N.M., Purnell, T.S., & Bridges, J.F.P. (2013) Patient preferences for the treatment of type 2 diabetes: A scoping review. *Pharmaco Economics*, 31, 877–892.

Laba, T.-L., Brien, J.-A., & Jan, S. (2012) Understanding rational non-adherence to medications. A discrete choice experiment in a community sample in Australia. *BMC Family Practice*, 13, 61–70.

Lawlor, C., Sharma, B., Khondoker, M., et al (2017) Service user satisfaction with cognitive behavioural therapy for psychosis: Associations with therapy outcomes and perceptions of the therapist. *British Journal of Clinical Psychology*, 56(1), 84–102. doi:10.1111/bjc.12122.

Lawton, T., Rankin, D., & Elliott, J. for the United Kingdom National Institute for Health Research Dose Adjustment for Normal Eating (DAFNE) Study Group (2013) Is consulting patients about their health services preferences a useful exercise? *Qualitative Health Research*, 23, 876–886.

Lengel, G.J. & Mullins-Sweat, S.N. (2017) The importance and acceptability of general and maladaptive personality trait computerized assessment feedback. *Psychological Assessment*, 29(1), 1–12. doi:10.1037/pas0000321.

Leykin, Y., DeRubeis, R.J., Gallop, R., et al. (2007) The relation of patients' treatment preferences to outcome in a randomized clinical trial. *Behavior Therapy*, 38, 209–217.

MacDonald, S., Rothwell, H., & Moore, L. (2007) Getting it right: designing adolescent-centred smoking cessation services. *Addiction*, 102,: 1147–1150. doi:10.1111/j.1360-0443.2007.01851.x

Malhotra, C., Farooqui, M.A., Kanesvaran, R., Bilger, M., & Finkelstein, E. (2015) Comparison of preferences for end-of-life care among patients with advanced cancer and their caregivers: A discrete choice experiment. *Palliative Medicine*, 29, 842–850.

McClendon, D.T. & Burlingame, G.M. (2010) Group cli-mate: Construct in search of clarity. In: R. Conyne (ed) *The Oxford Handbook of Group Counseling*. Oxford University Press, New York. pp. 164–181.

McGregor, M., Coghlan, M., & Dennis, C. (2014) The effect of physician-based cognitive behavioural therapy among pregnant women with depressive symptomatology: A pilot quasi-experimental trial. *Early Intervention in Psychiatry*, 8, 348–357.

Merincavage, M., Wileyto, E.P., Saddleson, M.L., et al. (2017) Attrition during a randomized controlled trial of reduced nicotine content cigarettes as a proxy for understanding acceptability of nicotine products standards. *Addiction*, 112(6), 1095–1103. doi:10.1111/add/13766

Mills, N., Donovan, J.L., Wade, J., et al. (2011) Exploring treatment preferences facilitated recruitment to randomized controlled trials. *Journal of Clinical Epidemiology*, 64, 1127e36.

Milosevic, I., Levy, H.C., Alcolado, G.M., & Radomsky, A.S. (2015) The treatment Acceptability/Adherence Scale: Moving beyond the assessment of treatment effectiveness. *Cognitive Behaviour Therapy*, 44(6), 456–469.

Miner, A., Kuhn, E., Hoffman, J.E., et al. (2016) Feasibility, acceptability, and potential efficacy of the PTSD Coach App: A pilot randomized controlled trial with community trauma survivors. *Psychological Trauma: Theory, Research, Practice & Policy*, 8(3), 384–392. doi:10.1037/tra000092.

Mooney, T.K., Connolly Gibbons, M.B.C., Gallop, R., Mack, R.A., & Crits-Christoph, P. (2014) Psychotherapy credibility ratings: Patient predictors of credibility and the relation of credibility to therapy outcome. *Psychotherapy Research*, 24(5), 565–577. doi:10.1080/10503307.2013.847988

Muscat, D.M., Morony, S., Shepherd, H.L., et al. (2015) Development and field testing of a consumer shared decision-making program for adults with low literacy. *Patient Education & Counseling*, 98, 1180–1188.

Narimatsu, H., Høifødt, R., Alfonsson, S., Olsson, E., & Hursti, T. (2016) Motivation and treatment credibility predicts dropout, treatment adherence, and clinical outcomes in an Internet-based cognitive behavioral relaxation program: A randomized controlled trial. *Journal of Medical Internet Research*, 18 (3), e52. doi:10.2196/jmir.5352

Nock, M.K., Ferriter, C., & Holmberg, E. (2007) Parent beliefs about treatment credibility and effectiveness: Assessment and relation to subsequent treatment participation. *Journal of Children and Family Studies*, 16, 27–38. doi:10.1007/s10826-006-9064-7

Nordgreen, T., Havik, O.E., Ost, L.G., et al. (2012) Outcome predictors in guided and unguided self-help for social anxiety disorder. *Behavior Research & Therapy*, 50, 13–21. doi:10.1016/j.brat.2011.10.009

Omvik, S., Pallesen, S., Bjorvatn, B., et al. (2010) Patient characteristics and predictors of sleep medication use. *International Clinical Psychopharmacology*, 25(2), 91–100.

Oppenshaw, D.K., Morrow, J., Law, D., et al. (2012) Examining the satisfaction of women residing in rural Utah who received therapy for depression through teletherapy. *Journal of Rural Mental Health*, 36(2), 38–45.

Peyrot, M. & Rubin, R.R. (2009) How does treatment satisfaction work? Modeling determinants of treatment satisfaction and preference. *Diabetes Care*, 32(8), 1411–1417.

Reimers, T.M., Wacker, D.P., Cooper, L.J., & De Raad, A. (1992) Acceptability of behavioral treatments for children: Analog and naturalistic evaluations by parents. *School Psychology Review*, 21:4, 628–643. doi:10.1080/02796015.1992.12087371

Rejas, J., Ruiz, M., Pardo, A., & Soto, J. (2013) Detecting changes in patient treatment satisfaction with medicines: The SATMED-Q. *Value in Health*, 16, 88–96.

Sarkar, U., Piette, J.D., Gonzales, R., et al. (2008) Preferences for self-management support: findings from a survey of diabetes patients in safety-net health systems. *Patient Education and Counseling*, 70(1), 102–110. doi:10.1016/j.pec.2007.09.008

Sandell, R., Clinton, D., Frövenholt, J., & Bragesjö, M. (2011) Credibility clusters, preferences, and helpfulness beliefs for specific forms of psychotherapy. *Psychology & Psychotherapy: Theory, Research & Practice*, 84(4), 425–441. doi:10.1111/j.2044-8341.2010.02010.x

Saracuta, M., Edwards, D.J., Davies, H., & Rance, J. (2018) Protocol for a feasibility and acceptability study using a brief ACT-based intervention for people from Sothwest Wales who live with persistent pain. *BMJ Open*, 8, e021866. doi: 10.1136/bmjopen-2018-021866

Schaal, T., Schoenfelder, T., Klewer, J., & Kugler, J. (2017) Effects of care, medical advice and hospital quality on patient satisfaction after primary total knee replacement: A cross-sectional study. *PloS One*, 12(6), e0178591. doi:10.1371/journal.pone.0178591

Schmidt, U., Magill, N., Renwick, B., et al. (2015) The Maudsley Outpatient Study of treatments for anorexia nervosa and related conditions (MOSAIC): Comparison of the Maudsley model of anorexia nervosa treatment for adults (MANTRA) with specialist supportive clinical management (SSCM) in outpatients with broadly defined anorexia nervosa: A randomized controlled trial. *Journal of Consulting and Clinical Psychology*, 83(4), 796–807. doi:10.1037/ccp000019.

Schulte, S.J., Leier, P.S., & Stirling, J. (2011) Dual diagnosis clients' treatment satisfaction—a systematic review. *BMC Psychiatry*, 11, 64–75.

Sekhon, M., Cartwright, M., & Francis, J.J. (2017) Acceptability of healthcare interventions: An overview of reviews and development of a theoretical framework. *BMC Health Services Research*, 17, 88–100. doi:10.1186/s12913-017-2031-8

Sekhon, M., Cartwright, M., & Francis, J.J. (2018) Acceptability of health care interventions: A theoretical framework and proposed research agenda. *British Journal of Health Psychology*, 23, 519–531.

Sidani, S. (2015) *Health Intervention Research: Advances in Research Design and Methods.* Sage, London, UK.

Sidani, S., Bootzin, R.R., Epstein, D.R., Miranda, J., & Cousins, J. (2015) Attrition in randomized and preference trials of behavioral treatments for insomnia. *Canadian Journal of Nursing Research*, 47(1), 17–34.

Sidani, S. & Epstein, D.R. (2016) Toward a conceptualization and operationalization of satisfaction with Non-Pharmacological Interventions. *Research & Theory for Nursing Practice: An International Journal*, 30(3), 242–257.

Sidani, S., Epstein, D.R., & Miranda, J. (2006) Eliciting patient treatment preferences: A strategy to integrate evidence-based and patient-centered care. *Worldviews on Evidence-Based Nursing*, 3(3), 116–123.

Sidani, S., Epstein, D.R., Bootzin, R.R., Moritz, P. & Miranda, J. (2009) Assessment of preferences for treatment: Validation of a measure. *Research in Nursing & Health*, 32, 419–431.

Sidani, S., Epstein, D.R., & Fox, M. (2017) Psychometric evaluation of a multi-dimensional measure of satisfaction with behavioral interventions. *Research in Nursing & Health*, 40(5), 459–469. doi:10.1002/nur.21808

Sidani, S., Epstein, D.R., Miranda, J., & Fox, M. (2018) Psychometric properties of the Treatment Perception and Preferences scale. *Clinical Nursing Research*, 27(6), 743–761. doi:10.1177/1054773816654137

Sidani, S. & Fox, M. (2020) The role of treatment perceptions in intervention evaluation: A review. *Science of Nursing and Health Practices*, 3(2), Article 4.

Sidani, S. & Fox, M. (2014) Patient-centered care: A clarification of its active ingredients. *Journal of Interprofessional Care*, 28(2), 134–141. doi:10.3109/13561820.2013.86519

Simiola, V., Neilson, E.C., Thompson, R., & Cook, J.M. (2015) Preferences for trauma treatment: A systematic of the empirical literature. *Psychological Trauma: Theory, Research, Practice, and Policy*, 7(6), 516–524. doi:10.1037/tra.000038

Smith, A.H., Norton, P.J., & McLean, C.P. (2013) Client perceptions of therapy components helpfulness in group cognitive-behavioral therapy for anxiety disorders. *Journal of Clinical Psychology*, 69, 229–239.

Stacey, D. & Légaré, F. (2015) Engaging patients using an interprofessional approach to shared decision making. *Canadian Oncology Nursing Journal/Revue canadienne de soins infirmiers en oncologie*, 25(4), 455–461.

Steidtmann, D., Manber, R., Arnow, B.A., et al. (2012) Patient treatment preference as a predictor of response and attrition in treatment for chronic depression. *Depression & Anxiety*, 29, 896–905.

Stigglebout, A.M., Pieterse, A.H., & De Haes, J.C.J.M. (2015) Shared decision making: Concepts, evidence, and practice. *Patient Education & Counseling*, 98, 1172–1179.

Swift, J.K., Callahan, J.L., & Vollmer, B.M. (2011) Preferences. *Journal of Clinical Psychology: In Session*, 67(2): 155–165.

Swift, J.K., Callahan, J.L., Ivanovic, M., & Kominiak, N. (2013) Further examination of the psychotherapy preference effect: A meta-regression analysis. *Journal of Psychotherapy Integration*, 23(2), 134–145. doi:10.1037/a0031423

Tierney, K.R. & Kane, C.F. (2011) Promoting wellness and recovery for persons with serious mental illness: A program evaluation. *Archives of Psychiatric Nursing*, 25(2), 77–89.

Umar, N., Schaarchmidt, M., Schmieder, A., et al. (2013) Matching physicians' treatment recommendations to patients' treatment preferences is associated with improvement in treatment satisfaction. *Journal of the European Academy of Dermatology and Venerology*, 27, 763–770. doi: 10.1111/j.1468-3083.2012.04569.x

Waltz, T.J., Campbell, D.G., Kirchner, J.E., et al. (2014) Veterans with depression in primary care: Provider preferences, matching, and care satisfaction. *Families, Systems, & Health*, 32(4), 367–377.

Wasmann, K., Wijsman, P., van Dieren, S., Bemelman, W., & Buskens, C. (2019) Influence of patients' preference in randomised controlled trials. *Journal of Crohn's and Colitis*, 13 (Suppl-1), S517–S518. doi:10.1093/ecco-jcc/jjy222.915

Weiner, B.J., Lewis, C.C., Stanick, C., et al. (2017) Psychometric assessment of three newly developed implementation outcome measures. *Implementation Science*, 12(108), 1–12. doi:10.1186/s13012-017-0635-3

Winter, S.E. & Barber, J.P. (2013) Should treatment for depression be based more on patient preference? *Patient Preference and Adherence*, 7, 1047–1057.

Witt, J.C. & Elliott, S.N. (1985) Acceptability of classroom intervention strategies. In: T.R. Kratochwill (ed). *Advances in School Psychology*. Erlbaum. Witt, J. C., & Robbins, Mahwah, NJ, Vol. 4, pp. 251–288.

Witteman, H.O., Chipenda-Dansokho, S., Colquhoun, H., et al. (2015) User-centered design and the development of patient decision aids: Protocol for a systematic review. *BMC Systematic Reviews*, 4, 1–8.

Witticke, D., Seidling, H.M., Klimm, H.-D., & Haefeli, W.E. (2012) Do we prescribe what patients prefer? Pilot study to assess patient preferences for medication regimen characteristics. *Patient Preference & Adherence*, 6, 679–684.

Wright, A.J., Sutton, S.R., Hankins, M., et al. (2012) Why does genetic causal information alter perceived treatment effectiveness? An analogue study. *British Journal of Health Psychology*, 17(2), 294–313. doi:10.1111/j.2044-8287.2011.02038.x

Wong, W.S., Chow, Y.F., Chen, P.P., Wong, S., & Fielding, R. (2015) A longitudinal analysis on pain treatment satisfaction among Chinese patients with chronic pain: Predictors and association with medical adherence, disability and quality of life. *Qualitative Life Research*, 24, 2087–2097. doi:10.1007/s11136-015-0955-1

Younger, J., Ghandhi, V., Hubbard, E., & Mackey, S. (2012) Development of the Stanford Expectations of Treatment Scale (SETS): A tool for measuring patient outcome expectancy in clinical trials. *Clinical Trials*, 9, 767–776. doi:10.1177/1740774512465064

Zimmermann, D., Rubel, J., Page, A.C., & Lutz, W. (2017) Therapist effects on and predictors of non-consensual dropout in psychotherapy. *Clinical Psychology and Psychotherapy*, 24, 312–321. doi:10.1002/cpp.2022

# CHAPTER 12

# Examination of Feasibility: Intervention and Research Methods

Examination of feasibility is critical for the successful conduct of large-scale studies aimed to evaluate the effects of health interventions. Generally, feasibility has to do with the practicality of an intervention delivery and the application of the evaluation research methods. Testing feasibility prior to a large-scale intervention evaluation study helps in identifying potential challenges and in revising aspects of the intervention and research methods and procedures. The revisions ensure that the study's implementation is logical, practical, convenient; the revisions also are done to lower the probability of biases or threats to validity (Tickle-Degnen, 2013). Challenges in the delivery of the health intervention reduce the interventionists' and clients' enthusiasm for the intervention. The challenges also affect the quality and fidelity of the implementation of the intervention and, consequently, its effectiveness in improving the immediate, intermediate, and ultimate outcomes. Similarly, challenges in carrying out research methods and procedures (e.g. recruitment, randomization, data collection) can be detrimental to the validity of inferences about the intervention's effects. For instance, challenges in recruiting participants result in a small sample size, which limits the power to detect meaningful intervention's effects, leading to type II error.

In this chapter, terms used to refer to feasibility, and the distinction between feasibility of the intervention and feasibility of research methods are introduced. Guidance for examining feasibility is presented. Issues with the interpretation of findings related to outcomes in small-scale preliminary or pilot studies are discussed.

## 12.1 TERMS REFLECTING PRELIMINARY STUDIES

Different terms have been used to refer to preliminary (i.e. prior to large-scale evaluation) studies concerned with testing feasibility. For some, the terms are different and for others, the terms are synonymous (Whitehead et al., 2014).

*Nursing and Health Interventions: Design, Evaluation, and Implementation*, Second Edition.
Souraya Sidani and Carrie Jo Braden.
© 2021 John Wiley & Sons Ltd. Published 2021 by John Wiley & Sons Ltd.

Three main terms are mentioned in the literature to refer to preliminary studies: feasibility, pilot, and proof-of-mechanism or proof-of-concept. The features that are claimed to distinguish them include:

- Feasibility studies are primarily concerned with determining the practicality of one or more aspects of the study planned to evaluate the effectiveness of health interventions. The aspects relate to the application of the intervention, methods, procedures, and measures. Feasibility studies utilize quantitative, qualitative, or mixed methods that are most appropriate to determine the practicality of the study aspect(s) of concern (Abbott, 2014). These studies have also been called non-randomized pilot studies (Eldridge et al., 2016a).

- Pilot studies are described as "miniature" or small versions of the large-scale study planned to evaluate the effects of health interventions. As such, pilot studies replicate the methods and procedures planned for the large-scale or main study (Abbott, 2014). These have also been called randomized pilot studies. They can be conducted independently of or before the start of the main randomized trial (called external pilot study), or in the early stage of the trial with the first group of clients who enroll in the trial (called internal pilot study) (Eldridge et al., 2016a, 2016b). The findings of pilot studies inform the modification, if and as necessary, of the methods and procedures planned for the main randomized trial or evaluation study.

- Proof-of-mechanism (i.e. Phase I trial) and proof-of-concept (i.e. Phase II trial) are terms originating in the guidance for the evaluation of drugs, and have recently appeared in the literature on the evaluation of health interventions. As described, proof-of-mechanism studies are concerned with demonstrating that an intervention is capable of inducing the hypothesized changes in the mechanism of action (i.e. mediators) responsible for mediating the intervention effects on the ultimate outcomes. Proof-of-concept studies focus on the safety and potential effectiveness of interventions (Eldridge et al., 2016b). They apply relevant research designs and methods to determine if the intervention is effective and safe for use in the main study.

For many, the purpose and features of the three types of preliminary studies are not quite distinct. Instead, the features overlap and all types of studies are designed to examine the extent to which aspects of the main study, including the intervention and the research methods and procedures, are practical and feasible, and to make necessary changes in the aspects that would facilitate the conduct of the main study. As such, the terms feasibility studies, pilot studies, and proof-of-mechanism or proof-of-concept studies are used interchangeably (Abbott, 2014; Eldridge et al., 2016b; Lancaster, 2015; Leon et al., 2011; Thabane et al., 2010). The primary focus is on examining the practicality of delivering the intervention and of carrying out the research methods and procedures, as well as the extent to which the intervention, as planned and delivered, is effective in initiating the mechanism of action; thus, the outcomes included in these preliminary studies should reflect the immediate and intermediate outcomes, more so than the ultimate outcomes.

Feasibility can be conceptualized in terms of the practicality of providing a health intervention and of applying the research design, methods, and procedures. Accordingly, strategies for examining feasibility of the intervention and feasibility of the research methods are distinct and discussed next.

## 12.2  FEASIBILITY OF INTERVENTIONS

The importance of examining the feasibility of health interventions has been emphasized (e.g. Arain et al., 2010; Lancaster, 2015; Leon et al., 2011; Thabane et al., 2010; Tickle-Degnen, 2013). However, the feasibility of interventions has not been explicitly defined. As a result, the indicators of feasibility are not clearly operationalized and guidance for testing the feasibility of interventions is not well delineated. Some investigators consider the acceptability of interventions as an indicator of feasibility (e.g. Arain et al., 2010; National Center for Complementary and Integrative Health, 2017), ignoring the distinction in the conceptualization of acceptability, which is defined as the perceived desirability of an intervention (see Chapter 11) and the conceptualization of feasibility, which reflects the practicality of implementation of an intervention as explained next.

### 12.2.1  Definition of Feasibility

Feasibility of health interventions refers to the practicality and adequacy of the logistics required for delivering interventions (Becker, 2008). The logistics entail the resources and procedures for providing the intervention. In a feasibility test, the focus is on determining access to the resources and the capability of carrying out the components and activities of the intervention as planned. Challenges are identified in the provision of any component or the performance of any activity of the intervention. The challenges may be related to: (1) the availability in good quality and quantity of materials resources; (2) the availability, in adequate number, of well-trained interventionists; (3) the comprehensiveness and clarity of the manual in guiding the interventionists' delivery of the intervention with fidelity; and (4) the capacity or ability of clients to engage in the intervention and enact the treatment recommendations.

The occurrence of challenges in the main large-scale evaluation study may reduce the interventionists' enthusiasm for the intervention and the participants' perceptions of the intervention and motivation to complete the treatment and/or the study. Interventionists facing repeated challenges may experience frustration. They may modify, informally and spontaneously, aspects of the intervention to overcome the challenges encountered during delivery. These modifications may result in deviations that jeopardize the fidelity of intervention delivery and subsequently, the achievement of beneficial client outcomes (Chapter 6). Similarly, participants encountering challenges may react unfavorably, generating a sense of disappointment and dissatisfaction with the intervention; this in turn, interferes with their willingness to attend and engage in the intervention sessions, to adhere to treatment recommendations, or to continue their participation in the evaluation study, all of which negatively affect the validity of inferences (Chapters 10 and 11).

Examination of the feasibility of intervention delivery is critical to minimize the potential occurrence of these challenges and their consequences in the main large-scale evaluation study. Identifying difficulties in the delivery of the intervention and understanding their nature (i.e. what the challenges are and what contribute to them) are prerequisites for finding the most appropriate ways to address them. Resolution of the challenges should be done prior to the main evaluation study in order to enhance the delivery, engagement, and enactment of the intervention when testing its effects on outcomes. Several indicators of feasibility of interventions can be examined.

## 12.2.2    Indicators of Feasibility

The definition of feasibility highlights aspects of the intervention delivery that are assessed for practicality and adequacy in their execution. These aspects, and respective indicators, reflect material and human resources, contextual features, and intervention delivery. Feasibility is examined with the actual delivery of the intervention by trained and skilled interventionists to a select group of participants representative of the target client population, in the context specified as having the features required to facilitate intervention delivery. Examination of feasibility involves close monitoring of the activities performed in preparation of and throughout the delivery of the intervention. Relevant quantitative and qualitative methods are used to obtain data on the indicators.

### 12.2.2.1    Material Resources

Feasibility is indicated by the availability of all material resources needed for the proper delivery of the intervention (Arain et al., 2010; Tickle-Degnen, 2013). The types of resources differ with the nature of the intervention and its mode of delivery. As mentioned in Chapter 4, material resources are categorized into: (1) equipment such as laptop and projector for the presentation of educational material during a session, and personal computer for accessing online modules by participants; (2) infrastructure such as rooms with adequate seating; (3) supplies such as items for demonstration of a skill (e.g. inhaler) and for use by participants to apply the treatment recommendations (e.g. pedometer); and (4) written document such as booklet or other self-help information guiding participants in the application of treatment recommendations. Material resources should be available in adequate number for all participants and be functioning properly. Strategies for accessing additional resources (e.g. contacting IT staff to resolve computer problems) as needed and promptly should be put in place.

Information on the availability and accessibility of material resources is gathered formally by having the study personnel complete a checklist. The personnel include the research staff preparing for the delivery of the intervention, the interventionist delivering the intervention, or the observer monitoring the fidelity of intervention delivery. The checklist covers all material resources that should be prepared and made available for delivering the intervention as planned. The study personnel refers to the checklist to facilitate the preparation of the items, indicate the availability of the items; and document any challenges encountered with the accessibility and/or use of the items during the delivery of the intervention. In addition, formal interviews with the research staff, interventionists, and participants, scheduled upon completion of the intervention, are useful in identifying additional challenges in accessing and using material resources throughout the course of the intervention delivery. The information can also be obtained informally during regular meetings with research staff and interventionists. The quantitative data gathered by completion of the checklist are analyzed descriptively to determine the frequency of occurrence of challenges. The qualitative data obtained through formal interviews and discussion at meetings are content analyzed to determine the nature of the challenges and their impact on the delivery of the intervention. The quantitative and qualitative findings are integrated to inform the generation of relevant strategies to ensure preparation, availability, and accessibility of the material resources for providing the intervention. The strategies are embedded in the research protocol and intervention manual for use in the main evaluation study.

### 12.2.2.2   Contextual Features

Contextual features contribute to the feasibility of delivering the intervention. The intervention theory delineates features of the physical and psychosocial environment that facilitate provision of the intervention. The theory guides the selection of the setting (e.g. location, room) for giving the intervention and for promoting participants' engagement. It also identifies aspects of the participants' environment and life circumstances that may affect their enactment of treatment recommendations, and suggests ways to adapt the intervention to address them (see Chapter 5). Nonetheless, it is important to assess the logistics and practicality of delivering the intervention in the selected context. Specifically, the following contextual features are examined:

1. The location of the facility in which the intervention is delivered: The location needs to be convenient to research staff, interventionists, and most importantly participants. It should be easy to identify, within reasonable distance, reachable through public transportation or have affordable parking, and in a geographic area perceived as safe at different times of the day. In addition, the location has to be in close proximity to the setting housing other staff or health professionals involved in the provision of some components of the intervention. Challenges in the location interfere with staff's and interventionists' prompt attendance, and with participants' presence at all planned intervention sessions.

2. The room in which the intervention is offered: The room needs to be easily accessible to various subgroups of the target client population, where necessary amenities are in place for clients requiring assistance (e.g. elevator for frail older clients). The room should have features (e.g. seating arrangement, acoustics, light) known to facilitate intervention delivery. Issues of accessibility to the room may limit participants' attendance at the planned intervention sessions. Less-than-optimal features of the room may affect participants' active engagement in the planned intervention activities.

3. The participants' physical, psychological, and social environment or life circumstances: Availability and accessibility of these contextual features (see Chapter 5 for details) are essential to support participants' enactment of the treatment recommendations in daily life. Identifying the nature and prevalence of contextual challenges is helpful in generating and revising principles and strategies for adapting and tailoring treatment recommendations to fit with participants' life circumstances. These principles and strategies are integrated in the intervention manual to minimize potential deviations in delivering the intervention in the main evaluation study.

4. The timing at which the intervention is offered: Timing for offering the intervention has to do with the day (weekdays or weekend) and part of the day (morning, afternoon, evening) on which the intervention (individual or group) sessions are given in face-to-face or distance (e.g. telephone, videoconferencing) are provided. The timing has to be convenient to interventionists and participants to ensure their presence and active engagement in the planned activities.

The methods for obtaining information on the logistics and practicality of the context in which the intervention is provided are similar to those described for gathering information on material resources. A checklist is developed and used to assess the presence and adequacy level of the contextual features, as specified in the intervention theory. Two versions of the checklist are generated. One version focuses on the research staff, interventionists, and observers' appraisal of the presence and adequacy of the features of the location and room in which the intervention is delivered. They complete the checklist prospectively throughout the intervention period. The other version focuses on participants' judgment of the adequacy of the location, room, and timing of the intervention delivery. It also includes items for participants to report on features in their environment and life circumstances that facilitate or hinder the enactment of the treatment recommendations. Formal interviews with research staff, interventionists, and participants; informal discussion at research staff meetings; and complaints reported informally by participants to interventionists or research staff are all helpful in clarifying the nature of the contextual challenges and in delineating their influence, positive or negative, on the implementation of the intervention. Descriptive, quantitative and qualitative, findings point to contextual features that are inconsistent with those identified in the intervention theory and that interfere with the implementation of the intervention by interventionists and participants. Necessary modifications (e.g. selection of a more convenient location and timing, and revision of principles for adaptation or tailoring) are made prior to the delivery of the intervention in the main evaluation study.

### 12.2.2.3   Human Resources

Feasibility of intervention delivery rests on the interventionists' capacity to provide the intervention, as planned, to the predetermined number of participants (Tickle-Degnen, 2013). Capacity is reflected in the availability of an adequate number of well-prepared interventionists. Examination of this indicator of feasibility is founded on the logistics of delivering the intervention. This information is then used to estimate the number of interventionists needed for the main large-scale evaluation study. In addition, assessment of capacity involves a determination of the extent to which training is adequate in preparing interventionists for intervention delivery.

Estimation of the adequacy of the number of available interventionists is partly based on the nature, mode of delivery, and dose of the intervention as specified in the intervention theory. It is also informed by the logistics for providing the intervention, observed in the preliminary study. The logistics are related to:

1. The timing within the trajectory of the health problem at which the intervention is to be given to maximize its benefits: It is anticipated that providing the intervention within a narrow time interval surrounding the experience of a health problem (e.g. acute pain) necessitates the availability of a large number of interventionists to deliver the intervention, promptly, to a large number of participants.

2. The participants' preferences for the location and time of intervention delivery: A large number of interventionists is required to offer the intervention in different locations at the same time, or in the same location at different times deemed convenient to different subgroups (e.g. retired or employed full-time) of participants.

3. The number of participants (sample size) expected to receive the intervention under evaluation: Large samples demand the availability of a large number of interventionists.

4. The number of interventions under evaluation: The provision of several treatments (experimental intervention and comparison treatment) requires a large number of interventionists.

The estimation should also account for the plan to investigate the influence of interventionists (Chapter 8) and for possible interventionists' resignation or withdrawal, and coverage for vacation and sick time.

In addition to their availability in an adequate number, the interventionists should be well prepared to provide the intervention with fidelity. They are expected to attend the didactic part of the training to gain a comprehensive understanding of the intervention theory and protocol, including principles and strategies for adapting intervention content, activities, or treatment recommendations to fit the characteristics and life circumstance of individuals or subgroups of clients. Interventionists should also actively participate in the hands-on training sessions or supervised delivery of the intervention in order to enhance their skills performance (Chapter 8). It is essential to monitor the training sessions for any issues that may arise during training and to assess the adequacy of the training in terms of content and duration, in preparing interventionists.

Issues that may arise during training may be related to the following:

1. Content of training sessions: The content may lack clarity, depth, and breadth of information on the intervention theory and protocol, in particular the content related to allowable adaptations of the intervention. Alternatively, the presentation of the content may not be clear, logical, and effective in relaying the key messages. Furthermore, the training may involve applications of skills using case studies that are not representative of all possible subgroups of the target client population and may provide limited time allotted for the practice of skills and for giving constructive feedback on performance.

2. Design of the intervention: The training provides an excellent opportunity to review the conceptualization and the operationalization of the intervention when reviewing and discussing the intervention manual. During explanation of the nature and sequence of intervention components (content, activities, treatment recommendations), challenges in providing them to specific subgroups of clients in specific context may be identified by the researchers or clinicians who designed the intervention, by the trainers, or by experienced interventionists undergoing training.

3. Interventionists: Some interventionists may experience challenges in appreciating the value of the intervention or in applying particular skills required for the intervention delivery. These challenges may be noted during the didactic training and close supervision. If sustained despite constructive feedback, it may be appropriate to limit these interventionists' involvement in the intervention delivery.

These issues are identified informally through observation or reviewing audio recordings of the training sessions, or formally through discussion with the trainers or interviews with trainees. The interviews are scheduled upon completion of the didactic and the hands-on practice parts of the training. The discussion and interviews focus on strengths and limitations of the intervention and of the training, and on ways to improve both as needed.

Adequacy of the training reflects its effectiveness in enhancing interventionists' theoretical knowledge, practical competence, and confidence in providing the intervention with fidelity. The effectiveness of training is evaluated by administering questionnaires before, during, and after the didactic and the practice sessions, as described in Chapter 8. This quantitative evaluation can be supplemented with interviews, held individually or in group, with the trainers and the trainees. The interviews are semi-structured, concerned with identifying aspects of the training that are helpful and with exploring ways to improve the training. Results of the descriptive analysis of quantitative data and content analysis of qualitative data indicate aspects of the training that are useful or effective. The results may also identify challenges in carrying out the training and in enhancing interventionists' capacity to deliver the intervention, and strategies to resolve the challenges. The feedback is integrated to refine the training sessions in adequately preparing interventionists or health professionals in future application of the intervention in research (main evaluation study) and practice.

### 12.2.2.4   Intervention Implementation

The implementation of health interventions by interventionists and clients is a key indicator of feasibility (Abbott, 2014; Arain et al., 2010; Leon et al., 2011; National Center for Complementary and Integrative Health, 2017; National Institute for Health Research, 2012; Tickle-Degnen, 2013). Monitoring the fidelity with which interventionists deliver the intervention as well as the level of clients' engagement and enactment is instrumental in identifying the adequacy or challenges in the application of the planned intervention activities. Quantitative and qualitative methods for assessing fidelity, engagement (e.g. attendance at intervention sessions), and enactment (e.g. adherence to treatment recommendations) are detailed in Chapters 9 and 13.

When examining feasibility of the intervention, qualitative methods are appropriate. Feasibility is examined in a trial delivery of the intervention by an interventionist to a number of participants, such as four to six individuals or one group sessions. Close monitoring of the intervention delivery provides an excellent opportunity to address the adequacy of the intervention manual in guiding its delivery and the logistics of performing and engaging clients in the planning activities, and to recognize challenges. The challenges may be related to:

1. Clarity, comprehensiveness, and logical sequence of the content or information given to participants: Issues arise: if technical words (medical jargon) are used; if the information is not well explained; if the treatment recommendations are not discussed in simple terms that are understandable to different subgroups of participants (i.e. varying in general and health literacy); if the rationale of the intervention is not clarified; or if the discussion of treatment recommendations does not follow a meaningful sequence (e.g. discussing complex recommendations that build on simple ones before discussing the latter ones).

2. Ease with which the intervention activities are performed in the specified mode: Examples of questions guiding assessment of feasibility include: Is the number of participants in a group session adequate, allowing meaningful participation by all participants? Is the video or telephone conferencing connection stable and of good quality, offering uninterrupted and clear exchange by all participants including those with vision or hearing

problems? Can the planned physical activity be done in the group format within the allotted space?

3. The time it takes to deliver the intervention components while promoting all participants' engagement in the planned activities: The general question is: Does the delivery of one component take longer than anticipated thereby limiting the time to provide the remaining components?

4. Limited relevance of an intervention's component to participants.

5. Difficulties in carrying out treatment recommendations, as reported by participants during their interactions with the interventionist.

For technology-based interventions, examining the feasibility of delivery entails assessment of:

1. Clarity, comprehensiveness, and logical sequence of the content covered in the modules completed by participants, or of information presented in messages.

2. Participants' understanding and perceived relevance of the intervention activities and treatment recommendations they are to apply.

3. Participants' perceptions of the system's functionality: Functionality is reflected in participants' ability to access and navigate the system and to easily find pertinent information, as well as report of any difficulty in doing so.

4. The time it takes to complete the modules and to access the system.

Qualitative data on feasibility can be obtained through: (1) formal observation of the intervention sessions by the researchers or designates; (2) formal interviews with interventionists and participants; (3) review of formal documents (e.g. diary) completed by participants; (4) informal feedback given by interventionists; and (5) informal communication of challenges encountered by participants to either the interventionist or the research staff. Content analysis of the information gathered formally or informally points to aspects of the intervention that are feasible and those that are challenging and need to be modified and how. The modifications are integrated in the manual in order to enhance the ease and quality of providing the intervention in the main evaluation study.

## 12.2.3   Research Design

The preliminary small-scale study aimed to examine the feasibility of delivering a health intervention usually consists of a one-group, mixed quantitative and qualitative methods, design. Interventionists are trained prior to client enrollment and their perspectives on the feasibility of the intervention and their appraisal of the training examined. Eligible consenting clients are all exposed to the intervention under evaluation. The delivery of the intervention is monitored. Participants' attendance and participation in the activities planned for the sessions are documented. In addition, participants are requested to complete relevant measures of their enactment of the treatment recommendations. For technology-based interventions, participants are invited to a session during which they access the system, review the modules, and complete the planned activities, in the presence of the researchers or designates. Participants are encouraged to communicate their views of the content of the modules and the functionality of the system; to identify challenges; and to suggest ways to improve the delivery of the intervention.

Interviews with interventionists and participants are scheduled within a week after delivery to discuss adequacy of the intervention, to identify challenges, and to generate principles and strategies to address challenges.

## 12.3    FEASIBILITY OF RESEARCH METHODS

Determining the feasibility of research methods planned for the main intervention evaluation study is rightfully emphasized (e.g. National Center for Complementary and Integrative Health [NCCIH], 2017; National Institute for Health Research [NIHR], 2012). Preliminary (feasibility or pilot) studies are designed to answer the overall question: Can the main evaluation study be done, and if so, how? (Abbott, 2014; Eldridge et al., 2016a, 2016b). Accordingly, these studies are concerned with examining the practically of research design, methods, procedures, and measures to be utilized in the main study.

### 12.3.1    Definition

Feasibility refers to the adequacy, effectiveness, and efficiency of the study protocol in gathering data that will contribute meaningfully to addressing the research questions, aims, or objectives, in the main evaluation study. Adequacy reflects the suitability of the planned designs and methods, that is: Are they appropriate, satisfactory and logistically convenient to apply? Effectiveness represents the capacity of the methods in achieving what they are set to do, that is: How successful are they? Efficiency has to do with the cost and time associated with the implementation of the planned methods, that is: How much do they cost and how long do they take?

The goal of examining feasibility of the study protocol is to identify: (1) the research methods, procedures, and measures that are appropriate, can be easily or conveniently performed as planned, and yield good-quality data within a reasonable time frame; and (2) challenges in carrying out the planned methods and procedures. Results of feasibility testing give advance warning about possible pitfalls or deficiencies in the design, methods, and logistics planned for the main evaluation study. Deficiencies have the potential to introduce biases that weaken the validity of the study's inferences. A thorough assessment and lucid knowledge about these possible deficiencies in terms of their nature, extent, and determinants guide the search for appropriate solutions and the revisions of the study protocol prior to the conduct of the main evaluation study. This is essential for enhancing the quality and hence the validity of the main evaluation study.

Although every step of the study protocol, starting with recruitment and ending with data analysis, can be subjected to feasibility testing, it is advisable to focus on those that are novel, innovative, untested, or complex. The specific research methods and procedures to test vary with the overall design of the main evaluation, as discussed next.

### 12.3.2    Indicators

For all types of randomized or non-randomized research design planned for the main evaluation study, it is recommended to examine the feasibility of: recruitment, screening, retention, and data collection. For randomized trials or experimental designs, it is highly advisable to test the feasibility of the randomization procedures. Strategies for assessing feasibility are presented for each of these methods or procedures.

### 12.3.2.1 Recruitment

Examining the feasibility of recruitment consists of determining the size of the sampling pool, the adequacy of the recruitment strategies in reaching various subgroups of the target client population, and the effectiveness and efficiency of the recruitment strategies.

#### Size of the Sampling Pool

It is essential to obtain a good estimate of the size of the available sampling pool, in order to determine the need to expand recruitment efforts to accrue the sample size required for the main evaluation study. Estimating the size of the sampling pool is easier when clients are recruited from participating sites or settings that maintain records of the number and key clinical or health characteristics of the clients served, such as those admitted to an acute care, long-term or rehabilitation facilities, or attending a primary care clinic or community care center. The estimation may be more challenging when targeting the general public using campaign-style recruitment strategies such as announcement in radio or television station or advertisement in newspapers or social media. In collaboration with the sites or settings involved in recruitment, the following information is obtained to estimate the size of the sampling pool: the number of clients at each site that experience the health problem addressed by the intervention and of those, the number of clients that are known to have the general eligibility criteria such as age and proficiency in the local language. Otherwise, estimates of the prevalence of the health problem can be extracted from: relevant empirical literature, databases of local health authorities (e.g. public health department), records of nonprofit organizations that maintain registries for specific conditions (e.g. cancer) or that provide services to specific subgroups of the population (e.g. a particular ethno-cultural group), or registry of technology-based companies that keep track of the number of persons using their services (e.g. subscriptions to cellular/mobile phone).

Documenting the total number of clients who respond to the recruitment for the feasibility or pilot study provides some evidence of the number of potentially eligible clients interested in taking part in the study. A lower than anticipated number suggests possible difficulties in accruing a sample size adequate for the main evaluation study. The difficulties can be addressed by expanding recruitment to multiple sites, selecting additional recruitment strategies, and/or extending the time allotted for recruitment in the main evaluation study and therefore, the study time line.

#### Adequacy and Effectiveness of Recruitment Strategies

It is highly advisable to utilize multiple and different strategies for recruitment, and to test their adequacy and effectiveness in reaching various subgroups of the target client population. Recruitment strategies are often categorized as: (1) passive or reactive, involving indirect contact with clients exemplified by advertisement in newspaper; and (2) active or proactive, consisting of direct contact with clients by the researchers or designates, or by health professionals or other service providers, to inform them of the study (Chapter 14). It is important to use combinations of passive and active strategies to reach various subgroups comprising the target client population and to identify the most effective combination that yields the largest number of recruited clients, within the study budget and time line.

## Adequacy

The adequacy of the planned recruitment strategies is assessed informally during research team meetings and formally by interviewing all personnel involved in recruitment. Personnel include research staff, health professionals, or other staff (e.g. clinic clerk) at the recruitment site responsible for referring clients to the study. Clients representing the target population, in particular those participating on the study advisory committee, can also be interviewed. The discussion focuses on the suitability, that is, appropriateness and convenience of use, of the recruitment strategies to: (1) the participating sites, with questions to pose exemplified by: is it acceptable for research staff to be present at the clinic and directly approach clients; or what is the most appropriate location within the facility to post flyers?; (2) the health professionals or other staff, with questions like: are they willing to assist in identifying and referring potentially eligible clients? (Abbott, 2014; NIHR, 2012); (3) various subgroups of the target client population, with questions to ask: would clients with low computer literacy level be able to access advertisement on social media; to what newspapers/newsletters do clients subscribe and what section do they frequently read?; and (4) the research personnel, with questions including: how comfortable are they in providing a short presentation about the study to clients attending an event? The discussion can also be geared toward exploring ways to enhance the planned recruitment strategies and identifying additional suitable ones.

## Effectiveness

The effectiveness of the planned recruitment strategies is operationalized in terms of the number and characteristics of clients who are aware of the study and contact the research staff to learn more about it. The number of clients who contact the research staff is usually referred to as recruitment rate (Tickle-Degnen, 2013). Effective strategies are those that yield high recruitment rates. It is wise to examine the effectiveness of each planned recruitment strategy, which is done in two ways. First, the recruitment strategies are applied sequentially, that is, one at a time. The number of clients who respond to it within a month is documented. For example, research staff can place an advertisement in a newspaper and record the number of inquiries received over the following month, then proceed with posting flyers at the participating sites. This sequential approach is useful when the recruitment strategies are discrete and time limited; however, it is time consuming. The second way for examining effectiveness involves requesting clients who contact the research staff to inquire about the study, to indicate the sources of information about the study. For example, clients can be asked: "How did you learn about the study?" followed by a list of all recruitment strategies applied. Descriptive analysis of the responses identifies the most frequent source of information, which provides empirical evidence to continue using the strategy and to justify the cost of recruitment requested for the main evaluation study.

Effectiveness of the planned recruitment strategies can be inferred from the analysis of the recruited clients' characteristics. Assessment of the clients' characteristics provides evidence of effectiveness of the planned recruitment strategies in reaching various subgroups of the target client population. Data on sociodemographic, health, or clinical characteristics that define the subgroups (e.g. age, severity of the health problem) can be collected at the time of recruitment, if approved by the research ethics board, and only after obtaining clients' consent. This assessment can be done in conjunction with methods used to ascertain initial eligibility based on general, noninvasive, inclusion and exclusion criteria. After informing clients of the study, research staff explain the rationale (e.g. to see if you are a good candidate for the study) and the method (e.g. answering a few questions about yourself) for obtaining relevant data. The staff obtain clients' oral/verbal consent and administer the questions (e.g. how old are you), and record clients' responses verbatim. If administering the questions is not possible at the time of recruitment, then data on participants' characteristics, collected at baseline from eligible clients who consent to the preliminary feasibility study are analyzed descriptively. The results delineate the profile of participants. The profile can be compared qualitatively to that of the target client population reported in previous research or of the accessible population available at the participating sites. Similarity of the sample of participants to the client population on key characteristics is indicative of the effectiveness of the recruitment strategies in reaching various subgroups of clients. For example, in the study of the behavioral therapy for insomnia, a sample consisting of middle-aged (mean = 55 years) women (66%) with moderate level of insomnia severity (mean score on the Insomnia Severity Index = 17) is considered typical of persons with insomnia. Dissimilarity in the profile of the sample and the population raises questions about the effectiveness of the recruitment strategies and requires investigation of the reasons underlying it. This investigation involves reviewing pertinent literature on the effectiveness of the planned strategies in recruiting different subgroups of the client population. The investigation also consists of discussing with expert researchers, health professionals, and clients representing the target population, of possible reasons for the dissimilarity and appropriate strategies for recruiting non-represented subgroups. For instance, analysis of the characteristics of participants in the study evaluating the behavioral therapy for insomnia showed that persons of a Chinese background were not well represented; they formed less than 10% of the sample whereas they comprise 25% of the accessible population. Discussion with some clients suggested to place advertisement in Chinese newsletters and post flyers in Chinese food stores to reach middle-aged and older persons with insomnia.

Qualitative and quantitative findings are integrated to identify the most effective combination of strategies. The latter strategies are then used to recruit clients in the main evaluation study.

## Efficiency of Recruitment Strategies

Efficiency is usually operationalized in the time it takes to recruit clients in the preliminary feasibility or pilot study (NCCIH, 2017). The focus is on the period of time to accrue the total number of participants required for the preliminary study. It is often represented as the length of time (number of days, weeks or months) from the start of recruitment to the enrollment of the last participant, or as the average number of participants recruited within a unit of time, usually a month (Leon et al., 2011). This information is gathered from the preliminary study's administrative records that document the date on which recruitment strategies are applied and the number of inquiries received. Data on recruitment time are most useful in delineating the time frame needed to complete the main evaluation study.

The expenses associated with the application of the recruitment strategies are estimated. The expenses include the hourly wage of research staff actively recruiting clients; cost of transportation incurred by research staff to the recruitment sites; cost of producing and printing recruitment materials such as pamphlet or flyers; and cost of placing advertisement in the selected media outlet. Additional expenses entail reimbursement to health professionals or to the organization in which they are employed, for recruitment efforts. This cost information is important for determining the cost-effectiveness of the recruitment strategies and for justifying the recruitment budget for the main evaluation study.

### Enrollment

Enrollment is often discussed in conjunction with recruitment and/or screening. In testing feasibility, it is advisable to determine the percentage of clients who meet the eligibility criteria and who consent to enroll in the study, out of those recruited. This is referred to as enrollment or consent rate (Leon et al., 2011; Tickle-Degnen, 2013). The enrollment rate is useful in giving directions regarding the recruitment resources and efforts needed for the accrual of the sample size required for the main evaluation study. For instance, if the recruitment rate is low (e.g. <30% of those recruited actually enroll), then additional strategies should be sought to recruit a large number of clients or the time line for recruitment should be expanded.

It is equally helpful to explore factors contributing to non-enrollment. The factors are generally associated with the clients' personal characteristics, health condition, perceptions of the treatments under evaluation, or views of the research methods (Sidani, 2015). Exploration of these factors can be done formally by research staff responsible for recruitment, and after obtaining consent from clients. At the time of recruitment, research staff explain the study to interested clients, clarify the treatments and aspects of the study as needed, and ask clients about their interest or willingness to take part in the study. Clients expressing lack of interest may be asked if they agree to share the reasons for their refusal. Once oral consent is secured, the research staff may pose general open-ended questions (e.g. what are reasons for your lack of interest?) or semi-structured questions (e.g. is your lack of interest related to the treatment? Please elaborate on or tell me what about the treatment prevents you from taking part in the study) inquiring about their perceptions of the treatments and/or the research methods. Content analysis of clients' responses reveals potential challenges with the design of the treatments and the research methods that can be taken into consideration in revising the treatments and study protocols for the main evaluation study. For instance, persons with chronic insomnia indicated that completing the daily sleep diary for two weeks at pretest and two weeks at post-test is burdensome, preventing them from enrolling. In consultation with expert researchers and health professionals, the time for completing the diary at each time point was reduced to one week, without jeopardizing the quality of the data.

### 12.3.2.2    Screening

Feasibility of screening relates to the practicality of the screening procedures and the suitability of the inclusion and exclusion criteria, as well as the adequacy of the resultant number of clients found eligible. Information on feasibility guides revision, as necessary, of the screening procedures and of the eligibility criteria; the goal is to enhance the accrual of a sample representative of various subgroups comprising the target client population and large enough to detect the intervention effects in the main evaluation study.

### Screening Procedures

Practicality of the screening procedures has to do with:

1. The relevance of the measures used for screening the target client population: Examples of questions posed are: Is the content of the screening measures easy to understand and applicable to participants of different backgrounds?

Do participants perceive the items or the questions as inappropriate or invasive leading them to refuse continued participation in the screening?

2. The utility of the measures in identifying eligible clients: Examples of questions are: Have the measures demonstrated content and construct validity? Do the measures have well-established cutoff scores resulting in good sensitivity and specificity, which are necessary to accurately identify eligible and non-eligible clients?

3. The logistics of applying the screening procedures: Examples of questions are: Do the procedures run smoothly? Do the procedures unduly increase burden on research staff and on participants? How long does the screening take to complete? Is the time at which screening scheduled relative to recruitment appropriate—in other words, is the screening done as soon as possible following recruitment to identify eligible clients and prevent ineligible participants from participating in unnecessary research activities?

4. The ethical conduct of screening: Examples of questions are: Is the screening done after obtaining, at the minimum, oral consent of participants, and within a context that ensures the right for self-determination (right to not answer a question) as well as privacy (when administering the screening measures) and confidentiality?

Data on practicality of the screening procedures are collected informally by:

1. Audio or video recording, or observing the actual conduct of screening with clients: This provides information on the average length of time it takes to complete the screening and on difficulties encountered in administering the screening measures such as misunderstanding of terms, participants' refusal to answer a question they perceive as intrusive, or redundancy in the questions posed. Answering redundant questions is burdensome, which lowers the accuracy of the responses.

2. Eliciting feedback from research staff on challenges faced in applying the screening procedures.

3. Reviewing participants' responses to measures for completeness.

4. Reviewing complaints about the content, the length or the timing of screening voiced by participants: The complaints may be identified in the audio or video recording or through observation; they may be reported to and documented by research staff.

The relevance of the screening measures can also be examined formally, along with testing the relevance of other measures to be used (discussed in Section 12.3.2.4). This involves the application of cognitive interviewing techniques (Miller et al., 2014) to determine participants' understanding of the content and response options of the screening measures. Furthermore, participants' responses to the screening measures and to well-established diagnostic criteria are compared to explore the sensitivity and specificity of the screening measures in the target client population, provided the number of participants in the preliminary study is large enough to conduct the analysis.

### Eligibility Criteria

The suitability of the pre-specified inclusion and exclusion criteria has to do with their appropriateness in selecting a sample of participants that is representative of the target client population. The questions to be addressed in appraising the suitability of the eligibility criteria include: Are the criteria clearly defined and operationalized so that they can be appropriately identified and interpreted in the same way by research staff, health professionals, and other personnel actively involved in recruitment and screening? (Tickle-Degnen, 2013). Are the eligibility criteria too stringent, strict, or restrictive to the point they limit the size of the potential pool of clients and the ability to obtain a sample of adequate size and representative of the population, within a reasonable time (as required for the main evaluation study)? Or, are the criteria less restrictive to the point that potential confounding characteristics are introduced?

Data addressing these questions are obtained from logbooks or databases maintained for the study. Data are recorded to identify the number of clients who inquired about the study, agreed to the screening, and found eligible relative to each of the preset criteria. Descriptive analysis of these data is done to determine:

- The percentage of clients who undergo screening, out of those referred to the study; the percentage of clients who refused screening; and if available, the reported reasons for refusal. Information on reasons for refusal is complementary in delineating potential challenges in the screening procedures.
- The percentage of participants who do not meet each criterion and hence are deemed ineligible: These results indicate the most common (e.g. >50%) reasons for ineligibility. The reasons are carefully reviewed and compared to client characteristics identified in the intervention theory, to determine the centrality of the criterion in defining the target client population and the potential of the criterion to introduce confounding. This kind of comparison guides the decision to confirm or modify the inclusion and exclusion criteria for the main evaluation study. For instance, in a study evaluating the contribution of nursing care to outcomes for clients admitted to cardiac inpatient units, the following selection criteria can be preset: 50 years of age or older, fluency in the spoken and written language, no cognitive impairment, and admission for the management of congestive heart failure. If more than 50% of participants had language barrier or cognitive impairment, then these criteria could be altered or ways to address them are integrated in the main evaluation study. The criterion regarding cognitive impairment may not be changed as clients should provide informed consent and be able to understand and to remember to apply the treatment recommendations. However, language barrier can be addressed by translating the screening measures to, and by having research staff fluent in, the languages spoken by clients.
- The percentage of participants who meet all eligibility criteria and hence, are eligible (Abbott, 2014; Tickle-Degnen, 2013). This percentage has implications for revising the eligibility criteria, for modifying the screening procedures, and for determining the need to expand recruitment efforts for the main evaluation study.

### 12.3.2.3   Retention

A range of strategies are integrated in an intervention evaluation study to minimize attrition and enhance retention. Common examples include maintaining frequent contacts with participants, making clients' involvement in the study convenient, and offering incentives (Chapter 15). Examining the feasibility of these strategies focuses on exploring their adequacy, appropriateness, or relevance to the target client population; determining their effectiveness in promoting retention; and assessing reasons for withdrawal. The proper application of the strategies viewed as appropriate by clients, at the preselected point in time over the course of the study, is essential for their effectiveness in retaining participants assigned to the treatments under evaluation.

### Adequacy

Exploration of the retention strategies' adequacy is done through informal discussion with research staff and participants. Research staff are well positioned to identify difficulties in carrying out the planned retention strategies. The types of difficulties encountered vary with the nature of the strategies used. Examples of difficulties include: participants' refusal to identify and provide contact information of persons who know the whereabouts of hard to reach participants; challenges in being flexible to accommodate participants' concerns and make their involvement convenient; and delays in sending or receiving incentives. Participants' perception of the relevance and appropriateness of the retention strategies can be assessed by: (1) asking key informants representing the target client population or community leaders serving as collaborators on the research team, about their views or opinions of the strategies used; and (2) having research staff document participants' comments related to the acceptability of the strategies. For instance, participants in the study evaluating the behavioral therapy for insomnia expressed dissatisfaction with the monetary incentives, stating that the "compensation is not enough."

Content analysis of the research staff's and the participants' comments indicate which retention strategy is frequently reported as challenging and perceived as unacceptable. Modifications of the planned strategies can be made to improve their adequacy or additional ones are sought for use in the main evaluation study.

### Effectiveness

The effectiveness of retention strategies can be inferred from the results of methodological studies designed to evaluate the usefulness of a strategy or to compare the contribution of different strategies. Although the direct and unique effectiveness of each retention strategy cannot be assessed in preliminary feasibility or pilot studies, the extent to which the strategies, taken together, are useful in enhancing retention can be implied from the preliminary study's retention or attrition rate (Leon et al., 2011; Tickle-Degnen, 2013). Retention rate is the percentage of consenting participants who complete the study, whereas attrition rate is the percentage of consenting participants who withdraw at any point in time (prior to or during treatment, or at follow-up) over the course of the study. The retention and attrition rates found in the preliminary study are compared, qualitatively, to those reported in previous studies that evaluated the same or comparable health intervention, in the same or comparable client population. Similarity in the retention or attrition rates across studies supports the effectiveness of the strategies in improving retention or reducing attrition. For instance, the overall attrition rate (37%) in the study evaluating the behavioral therapy for insomnia was comparable to the 40–55% attrition rate estimated for clinical trials of cognitive-behavioral therapy for insomnia (Ong et al., 2008; Sidani et al., 2015).

The retention or attrition rate can be computed for each treatment included in the preliminary study (Abbott, 2014). This information sheds some light on potential retention challenges that are associated with the nature of the treatment.

*Reasons*

Exploring reasons for participants' withdrawal provides another source of information about the adequacy of the retention strategies. It also assists in identifying potential issues with the treatments under evaluation and with the research methods. The reasons can be explored in a formally planned exit interview with participants who drop out. After obtaining their oral consent, participants are asked open-ended, semi-structured questions related to factors that contributed to their withdrawal. The factors (see Chapter 14 for detail) are categorized as personal circumstances (e.g. occurrence of a life event) and those associated with the treatment (e.g. dislike of group interaction) or research methods (e.g. invasive or burdensome assessment) including the retention strategies.

Synthesis of the quantitative and qualitative results obtained in a preliminary study indicates the retention strategies that can be easily applied; appropriate or relevant to the target client population; and useful in promoting retention. These strategies are utilized in the main evaluation study. Additional strategies reported as acceptable to the target population and found in previous research to be effective are also included in the main evaluation study.

### 12.3.2.4  Data Collection

Preliminary studies offer ample and excellent opportunities to examine the suitability of the planned data collection procedures and measures. Data collection procedures represent the methods (e.g. observation, completion of questionnaire, use of recording instruments such as pedometer) for gathering information from participants. Measures encompass all forms (e.g. logbooks, questionnaires) for documenting the information. Challenges in the application of the procedures and use of the measures interfere with the quality (accuracy and completeness), consistency, and timeliness of the data gathered in the main evaluation study. Low-quality data introduce error of measurement that reduces statistical power and the precision of the estimates of the intervention effects, thereby weakening the validity of inferences regarding the effectiveness of health interventions.

*Data Collection Procedures*

Data collection procedures are examined for their adequacy. Adequacy entails the logistics of implementing the procedures by research staff, and their suitability to participants. Logistics reflects the ease of carrying out the procedures as specified in the study protocol. The overall questions guiding the assessment of logistics are: Can the data collection procedures take place in the selected sequence, in the selected location, at the specified time intervals, and within the specified time frame? What challenges are encountered or what are factors that limit or prevent the implementation of the procedures? The factors may be related to:

1. The study protocol: The steps for carrying out the data collection procedures are not described clearly or are not meaningfully sequenced. Ways to adapt the steps to address or manage participants' unique concerns or life circumstances are not specified, resulting in potential deviations or inconsistencies in applying the procedures across research staff and participants.
2. The research staff training: The didactic and hands-on training is not adequate to promote a good understanding of the importance and the principles

guiding the procedures. The training is less than optimal in enhancing the acquisition of the skills needed to apply the procedures correctly as specified in the study protocol and consistently across participants and time points throughout the study. The ongoing training and supervision of research staff are not sufficient to maintain their competence over the course of the study.

3. The availability and accessibility to the required resources: The location of data collection is not convenient or appropriate for maintaining participants' privacy. The materials, supplies, or equipment are not accessible promptly or are not functioning properly, such as bad telephone connection, limited participants' access to online measures, forgetfulness to charge recording equipment, inadequate space to store specimen before sending to laboratory for analysis.

The types of factors vary with the nature of the data collection procedures. The factors are identified through discussion of the challenges encountered by research staff in carrying out the procedures at regular research meetings, and through close monitoring (direct observation or audio or video recording) of research staff in action.

The suitability of the data collection procedures to participants is another factor that interferes with proper implementation. Some participants may perceive the planned procedures as invasive (e.g. collection of blood specimen), intrusive (e.g. observation of a behavior), inconvenient (e.g. wearing an actigraph for 24 hours), and/or burdensome (e.g. completing a daily diary or responding to items inquiring about the craving for smoking at different points in a day). Participants with unfavorable perceptions react negatively: They refuse to engage in the planned procedures resulting in missing data or they withdraw from the study leading to high attrition rates. These reactions may introduce bias that weakens the validity of inferences in the main evaluation study if unaddressed. It is also possible that participants may not have adequate resources to engage in the planned data collection procedures. For example, some participants with limited income may not afford transportation costs to attend face-to-face data collection sessions, and others may have limited access to the internet to complete online questionnaires.

Data on the suitability of the data collection procedures are obtained by (1) computing the percentage of participants who refused performance of a procedure, (2) eliciting the reason for their refusal, or (3) content analyzing concerns or complaints expressed by participants to research staff.

The quantitative and qualitative results point to challenges in implementing the data collection procedures. The challenges are discussed at research team meetings attended by representatives of the target client population, to further clarify the issues. The discussion is then geared toward finding appropriate solutions. The solutions consist of modifying the procedures or identifying alternative ones to collect data in the main evaluation study; the goals are to prevent the occurrence of challenges and to enhance the quality of the data gathered in the main study.

## Data Collection Measures

Data collection measures are examined for their adequacy. The measures include the forms to be used and completed by research staff (e.g. log book to track participants' progress) and interventionists (e.g. session attendance sheets, assessment of individual characteristics required for tailoring). The forms are evaluated for: clarity of instructions; comprehensiveness of content; ease of completion and calculation of total score (required for on-the-spot tailoring of the intervention); and perceived utility in obtaining the needed information. This evaluation can be done in formal interviews with the research personnel. The interviews are held prior to the actual use of the forms. During the interview, research staff and interventionists carefully review the forms and point to possible deficiencies in content, format, structure, and utility. The evaluation of the forms can also be informal. It takes place during research team meetings scheduled after actual use of the forms. During the meeting, research staff and interventionists report on challenges encountered and discuss possible solutions.

The measures to be completed by participants are examined for suitability (Abbott, 2014; Trickle-Degnen, 2013). The measures include:

- Questions about the participants' personal and health characteristics.
- Newly developed items to assess perception and engagement in the treatments under evaluation, preferences for treatment, and enactment or adherence to treatment recommendations.
- Well-established, adapted or translated, instruments for assessing perceptions, preferences, and enactment of treatments, mediators, and outcomes.
- Open-ended questions included in questionnaires or interviews, such as those inquiring about discomfort or side effects that may be experienced with treatment.

All data collection measures are evaluated for: (1) comprehension, that is, ease of understanding the instructions, items' or open-ended questions' content, and response options; (2) relevance, that is, applicability of the content to the target client population; (3) variability in responses, that is, responses represent the range of options and are not limited to specific (e.g. extreme) response options; (4) completeness of responses, that is, the presence and extent of missing data; and (5) duration or time it takes to complete the measures (Abbott, 2014; Leon et al., 2011; NIHR, 2012; NCCIH, 2017).

Two methods can be used to assess comprehension and relevance of measures. The first involves cognitive interview techniques. These techniques involve semistructured individual or group interviews with participants. Participants are asked to read each item and reiterate the content captured in the item (by answering the question: What does this mean to you?); then, participants read the response options, explain what the options mean, and think aloud when formulating their responses and selecting the most appropriate responses. Participants' reiteration of the content and responses to items identify words, phrases, sentences, or response options that are misunderstood or misinterpreted by most (>60%) or particular subgroups of participants. In addition, participants are interviewed to explore the relevance of the items' content to all or particular subgroups of the target client population (Nápoles-Springer et al., 2015; Miller et al., 2014; Willis, 2015). For example, items inquiring about alcohol intake may be irrelevant to participants who do not drink for personal or religious beliefs. Although advantageous in identifying misunderstanding, cognitive interview techniques are time consuming and burdensome.

The second method for assessing comprehension and relevance of measures is partially based on, but less formal than, cognitive interviewing techniques. It involves having participants complete the measures and comment on any content or response option that is unclear or irrelevant. Items and response options found difficult to understand as intended (or misinterpreted) and inappropriate or irrelevant are identified. They are revised prior to using the measures in the main evaluation study.

Failure to do so lowers the quality of the data in reflecting participants' actual level on the variables measured at one point in time and in quantifying their experience of change in outcomes over time.

Variability and completeness of participants' responses to measures, in particular those assessing the hypothesized outcomes, are important to examine in preliminary, feasibility, or pilot studies. This examination is done by having participants complete the measures, as scheduled, before and after exposure to the intervention, and analyzing their responses descriptively. Variability is reflected in the range and variance in responses reported at each time point, and in changes in the responses to outcome measures from pretest to posttest. Lack of changes in outcomes measures may reflect floor or ceiling effects, which limit the detection of change in the outcomes over time (Chapter 15). Outcome measures demonstrating floor or ceiling effects should be replaced to enhance the capacity to detect changes in the outcomes following exposure to the intervention in the main evaluation study. Results of descriptive analysis indicate items, subscales (i.e. subset of items measuring a domain of the concept), or overall measures that were completed or missed by most (>60%) participants. Missing data lower the accuracy of the scores quantifying participants' level on the respective variables, including outcomes. Missing data on outcomes, if not handled appropriately, introduce bias (under or over) in the estimates of the intervention's effects (McKnight et al., 2007). Factors contributing to missing data are explored by conducting (1) additional statistical tests to determine the profile of participants with missing data; and (2) a brief interview with participants with missing data to discuss what led them to not respond to the items. The findings inform the search for ways to minimize missing data, such as rewording items for clarity, translating the measure to participants' preferred language, or replacing the measure with another instrument that is not prone to ceiling or floor effects.

The duration or length of time it takes to complete the measures at each occasion of measurement (e.g. pretest, posttest, and follow-up), is assessed prospectively by noting the start and end time of the data collection session and calculating the total administration time. Longer time increases the likelihood of response fatigue or burden. Response burden negatively influences the quality and completeness of the data. Response burden can be reduced by (1) carefully reviewing the items and eliminating those covering redundant content, and (2) replacing well-established but lengthy versions by validated short versions of the same measure, if available. For instance, the original Medical Outcomes Trust Study measure of physical, psychological, and social functions had been revised into short versions (MOS-SF) containing 36, 20, and 12 items. These short versions demonstrated good reliability and validity, and take less time to complete by various subgroups of (clinically and ethnically) diverse client populations, than the original (50-item) version.

### 12.3.2.5   Randomization

Where the planned main evaluation study involves random assignment of participants to the experimental intervention or the comparison treatment group, the preliminary feasibility or pilot study should examine the feasibility of the randomization procedure (Leon et al. 2011; Trickle-Degnen, 2013). The focus is on determining the logistics of applying the procedure by research staff and the acceptance of randomization to participants and referring health professionals.

Logistics relate to the capacity to apply the randomization procedure as planned. This is of particular concern when the randomization is entrusted to central services. The logistics for transferring data to the services are delineated; agreement is reached on: what participants' data are needed by the services, what is the best mean of communication to relay participants' data, and how is the information regarding treatment assignment given by the services. The timeliness of the services is evaluated, guided by questions like: how long does it take to reach or contact the services to feed in participants' data and to get a response. For other randomization procedures (e.g. research staff accessing a random number generator program or opening opaque sealed envelopes), logistics relate to the accessibility of the resources required to implement the procedure correctly and promptly. Assessment of logistics is often done informally, through discussion at regularly scheduled research team meetings or by reviewing pertinent complaints made by research staff.

Acceptance of randomization is receiving much attention due to cumulating evidence indicating that an increasing number of participants express unwillingness to be randomized (Sidani et al., 2017). It, therefore, is essential to examine participants' acceptability of randomization in preliminary, feasibility or pilot, studies (Abbott, 2014; Arain et al., 2010; NIHR, 2012). The percentage of participants in the preliminary study who are (un)willing to be randomized to treatments has significant implications for the design of the main evaluation study, as well as effort and resources for recruitment. For instance, if a large number of participants decline randomization, then the design of the main evaluation study is modified to incorporate a preference arm (Chapter 14).

Acceptance of randomization is operationalized as the attitude toward allocation to treatment on the basis of chance, held by participants and by health professionals or other service providers responsible for referring clients to the study. The attitude influences participants' behavior related to involvement in the study. Health professionals or service providers accepting of randomization may actively refer clients to the study, whereas those with unfavorable attitude toward randomization may not refer, or even discourage clients from taking part in the study. Accordingly, it is worth monitoring health professionals' and other providers' referral pattern closely. Monitoring involves the generation of a logbook or database to document, at a minimum, the practice setting or site from which clients are referred, and if possible and ethically allowable, the name of the professionals or providers initiating the referral. The data are analyzed descriptively and periodically (e.g. every month) to identify settings or professionals/providers with low referral rates. Meetings are held with the sites' health professionals or providers to explore the reasons for low referral, with specific probing about their attitude and reaction to randomization. The themes emerging from the discussion indicate possible challenges in referral, including the attitude toward randomization. Approaches for addressing health professionals or providers' attitudes are devised with their collaboration, prior to the main evaluation study. The approaches are exemplified with providing an educational session to clarify the principles and importance of randomization. Failure to change health professionals' or providers' attitude demands more drastic approaches such as (1) excluding the setting from further involvement in referral and replacing the site with others where more favorable attitudes prevail; and (2) revising the main evaluation study's design to one that involves only sites receptive of randomization. In this cluster randomized trial (Chapter 14), participating sites (rather than individual participants within sites) are randomized to the experimental intervention and the comparison treatment groups.

Participants with unfavorable attitude toward randomization may decline enrollment in or withdraw from the study (Chapter 14). Evidence of the influence of participants' attitude is derived from reasons given for declining involvement in the study. Participants may decline initial enrollment, once they learn about the study, particularly when randomization is mentioned at the time of recruitment; participants may decline continued enrollment during or after the process of obtaining consent when chance-based allocation to treatment is explained in detail. A tally of the reasons for refusal to take part in the study indicates the percentage of participants who find randomization unacceptable. Additional sources of evidence on participants' acceptability of randomization include individuals serving as collaborators on the research team; these individuals represent the target client population or community leaders. During research team meetings they may raise concerns about randomization. Published literature is another source. Reports of intervention evaluation studies indicate the number or percentage of participants who refused enrollment or withdrew because of discomfort or unwillingness to be randomized. In situations where a large percentage ($\geq$30%) of participants express unwillingness to be randomized, alterative research designs (Chapter 14) should be considered for the main evaluation study such as preference or comprehensive cohort designs where participants refusing randomization are allocated to the preferred treatment (Beasant et al., 2019). Maintaining randomization as the procedure for assigning participants to treatment in the main study, despite indication that a large number of participants decline it, may be associated with: (1) increased effort, time, and costs to recruit a very large number of participants to offset the percentage of those who are unwilling to be randomized and decline enrollment; (2) self-selection bias, where the sample of participants represent only clients accepting randomization, which limits the applicability of the findings to other subgroups of the target client population (Chapter 14); or (3) high attrition rates, which threaten the validity of inferences (Chapter 15).

### 12.3.3 Research Design

To examine the feasibility of research methods, the design selected for the preliminary, feasibility or pilot, study should mimic, that is, be the same as the design to be used in the main evaluation study, be it experimental (randomized controlled trial) or quasi-experimental (non-randomized cohort trial). It should include the health intervention and the comparison treatment under evaluation, and repeated measurement of outcome data (pretest, post-test, follow-up). In other words, the preliminary study should follow/apply the research protocol planned for the main evaluation study. The design of the preliminary study is expanded to collect qualitative data from participants, referring health professionals, and research staff as discussed in the previous sections. The quantitative and qualitative data are analyzed and integrated in order to identify what works, what does not work, what should be modified and how, or what new methods and procedures should be added to enhance the feasibility of conducting the main evaluation study and to minimize potential biases threatening the validity of its findings.

## 12.4 INTERPRETATION OF OUTCOME FINDINGS

In preliminary studies examining the feasibility of health interventions and/or the feasibility of the research methods, data on mediators and ultimate outcomes (consistent with the focus in proof-of mechanism and proof-of-concept studies), as specified in the intervention theory, are collected before and after delivery of the intervention. Conventionally, the focus has been on what is referred to as "primary outcome," which is often the ultimate outcome of interest to researchers, decision makers or policy makers. Data on the primary or ultimate outcome are collected from participants assigned to the treatment groups included in the preliminary study, at pretest and post-test. The goal of outcome analysis is to estimate the size of the intervention effects. Effect sizes are computed as (1) the standardized difference in the ultimate outcome measured at pretest and post-test within the experimental intervention group if the preliminary study consists of a one-group design, or (2) the standardized difference in the outcome measured at post-test between the experimental intervention and the comparison treatment groups if the preliminary study included these two groups. The computed effect sizes are then used, along with results of statistical tests, to (1) determine the effectiveness of the intervention and, therefore, to make a decision on whether or not to proceed with the main evaluation study, and (2) conduct a power analysis for calculating the sample size to achieve adequate power to detect significant intervention effect in the main evaluation study. This interpretation of outcome-related findings and practice is no longer recommended.

Recent literature emphasizes that preliminary pilot studies should not be used for testing the hypothesized effects of health interventions on the primary or ultimate outcomes, and for generating the effect size needed to calculate the sample size for the main evaluation study. The rationale underlying these recommendations is that the number of participants in preliminary studies is small. Thus, the preliminary studies are usually underpowered to detect accurate intervention effects. The results of statistical tests and the computed effect sizes are inherently imprecise and biased; that is, the effect sizes under- or overestimate the intervention effects, leading to type I or II error. Furthermore, the effect sizes of the intervention on the ultimate outcomes may be nonsignificant or small, if they are fully mediated by the immediate and intermediate outcomes. Therefore, the results may not be reproduced in the main evaluation study (Lancaster, 2015; Leon et al., 2011; Thabane et al., 2010). Instead, it is advisable to focus preliminary studies on examining changes in the mediators as reported by participants exposed to the experimental intervention. These within-group changes represent the extent to which the intervention is successful in inducing the anticipated improvement in the mediators (Abbott, 2014). Interventions that do not produce improvement in the mediators are considered ineffective in initiating the mechanism of action responsible for its impact on the ultimate outcomes. Quantitative data on mediators are supplemented with qualitative data. Qualitative interviews are held with the interventionists and the participants in the preliminary study to explore their views on the capacity of the intervention and/or its components to initiate the mechanism of action; on the extent of changes in mediators and outcomes experienced with or as a result of the intervention; on additional non-hypothesized beneficial or harmful effects; and on factors that may affect the success of the intervention. Such interviews are commonly conducted as part of process evaluation, discussed in Chapter 13.

## REFERENCES

Abbott, J.H. (2014) The distinction between randomized clinical trials (RCTs) and preliminary feasibility and pilot studies: What they are and are not. *Journal of Orthopedic Sports Physical Therapy*, 44(8), 555–558. doi:10.2519/jospt.2014.0110

Arain, M., Campbell, M.J., Cooper, C.L., & Lancaster, G.A. (2010) What is a pilot or feasibility study? A review of current practice and editorial policy. *BMC Medical Research Methodology*, 10, 67–72.

Beasant, L., Brigden, A., Parslow, R.M., et al. (2019) Treatment preference and recruitment to pediatric RCTs: A systematic review. *Contemporary Clinical Trials Communications*, 14, e100335. doi:10.1016/j.conctc.2019.100335

Becker, H.S. (2008) *Tricks of the Trade: How to Think About Your Research While You're Doing It.* University of Chicago Press, Chicago.

Eldridge, S.M., Lancaster, G.A., Campbell, M.J., et al. (2016a) Defining feasibility and pilot studies in preparation for randomized controlled trials: Development of a conceptual framework. *PLOS one*, 11(3), e0150205. doi:10.1371/journal.pone.0150205

Eldridge, S.M., Chan, C.L., Campbell, M. J., et al., on behalf of the PAFS consensus group (2016b) Consort 2010 statement: Extension to randomised pilot and feasibility trials. *BMJ*, 355, i5239. doi:10.1136/bmj.i5239

Lancaster, G.A. (2015) Pilot and feasibility studies come of age! *Pilot and Feasibility Studies*, 1, 1–5. doi:10.1186/2055-5784-1-1

Leon, A.C., Davis, L.L., & Kraemer, H.C. (2011) The role and interpretation of pilot studies in clinical research. *Journal of Psychiatric Research*, 45, 626–629. doi:10.1016/j.jpsychires.2010.10.008

McKnight, P.E., McKnight, K.M., Siḍani, S., & Figueredo, A.J. (2007) *Missing Data: A Gentle Introduction.* Guilford Publications, Inc., New York, NY.

Miller, K., Chepp, V., Willson, S., & Padilla, J.L. (Eds) (2014) *Cognitive Interviewing Methodology.* Wiley, Somerset.

Nápoles-Springer, A.M., Santoyo-Olsson, J., O'Brien, H., & Stewart, A.L. (2015) Using cognitive interviews to develop surveys in diverse populations. *Medical Care*, 44(11), S21–S30.

National Institute for Health Research (2012). NHIR Evaluation, Trials and Studies Coordination Centre: Glossary – Retrieved from: www.netscc.ac.uk/glossary/#glos6/

National Center for Complementary and Integrative Health (2017). Pilot studies – Retrieved from: https://nccih.nih.gov/grants/whatnccihfunds/pilot

Ong, J.C., Kuo, T.F., & Manber, R. (2008) Who is at risk for dropout from group cognitive-behavior therapy for insomnia? *Journal of Psychosomatic Research*, 64(4), 419–425. doi:10.1016/j.jpsychores.2007.10.009

Sidani, S. (2015) *Health Intervention Research: Advances in Research Design and Methods.* Sage, London, UK

Sidani, S., Bootzin, R.R., Epstein, D.R., Miranda, J., & Cousins, J. (2015) Attrition in randomized and preference trials of behavioral treatments for insomnia. *Canadian Journal of Nursing Research*, 47(1), 17–34.

Sidani, S., Fox, M., & Esptein, D.R. (2017) Contribution of treatment acceptability to acceptance of randomization: An exploration. *Journal of Evaluation in Clinical Practice*, 23(1), 14–20. doi:10.1111/jep.12423

Thabane, L., Ma, J., Chu, R., et al. (2010) A tutorial on pilot studies: The what, why and how. *BMC Medical Research Methodology*, 10(1), 1–10.

Tickle-Degnen, L. (2013). Nuts and bolts of conducting feasibility studies. *American Journal of Occupational Therapy*, 67, 171–176. doi:10.5014/ajot.2013.006270

Whitehead, A.L., Sully, B.G., & Campbell, M.J. (2014) Pilot feasibility studies: Is there a difference from each other and from a randomised controlled trial? *Contemporary Clinical Trials*, 38(1), 130–133. doi:10.1016/j.cct.2014.04.001

Willis, G.B. (2015). *Analysis of the Cognitive Interview in Questionnaire Design.* Oxford University Press, New York.

# CHAPTER 13

# Process Evaluation

After ascertaining their feasibility, newly designed health interventions are evaluated for their efficacy or effectiveness in addressing the health problem and in improving functioning and health. These evaluation studies usually focus on the examination of the ultimate outcomes expected of the intervention (detailed in Chapter 14). The focus on the ultimate outcomes presents challenges in the interpretation of the studies' findings, whether the findings do or do not support the effectiveness of the intervention under evaluation. The interpretation becomes more challenging when the results of outcome evaluation studies vary, whereby those of some studies indicate the health intervention is effective and those of other studies of the same intervention show that it is ineffective (Grant et al., 2013). The challenge in the interpretation of the results of an individual study or of several studies is related to the plausibility of multiple possible explanations of the results (Pawson & Manzano-Santaella, 2012). Foremost among possible explanations are the adequacy of the research methods used in an individual outcome evaluation study and the variability in the research methods used in different studies. Adequate methods (e.g. research design, sample size, outcome measures) minimize biases that threaten the validity of inferences. Additional explanations are considered. The explanations are associated with factors that include, but are not limited to: the adequacy of the intervention theory; the appropriateness of the intervention delivery; the participants' perceptions and responsiveness to the intervention; contextual factors influencing the delivery of the intervention by interventionists and application of treatment recommendations by participants; and capacity and/or potency of the intervention in initiating the mechanism of action responsible for its effects on the ultimate outcomes (e.g. Brand et al., 2019; Siddiqui et al., 2018; Van de Glind et al., 2017).

Rather than speculating about possible explanations of the results, it would be logical and informative to gather data pertaining to the associated factors advanced as additional explanations. These data provide evidence that indicates what exactly contributes to the ultimate outcomes observed in an evaluation study. The evidence clarifies why a successful intervention "works" or is effective, and what leads to lack of the intervention's success; specifically, is the lack of success due to failure of the intervention theory or the inappropriate delivery of the intervention (Aust et al., 2010; Bakker et al., 2015; Benson et al., 2018; Craig et al., 2008; Foley et al., 2016; Van de

Glind et al., 2017). Process evaluation is advocated as a means to obtain this evidence when evaluating the effectiveness of health interventions (Medical Research Council, [MRC] UK, 2019).

In this chapter, the importance of process evaluation is highlighted. Its definition and elements are clarified. Quantitative and qualitative methods used in process evaluation are described.

## 13.1   IMPORTANCE OF PROCESS EVALUATION

The importance of conducting a process evaluation in studies examining the effectiveness of health interventions is increasingly recognized as essential in interpreting the results of a particular study (MRC, 2019) and making valid inferences regarding the effectiveness of interventions. In general, the results of an outcome-focused evaluation study indicate that the intervention is, overall, effective or ineffective; they fall short of delineating evidence on what exactly contributed to the observed improvement or no change in the outcomes following delivery of the intervention (Benson et al., 2018).

When the results support the effectiveness of the health intervention, it is important to know: (1) whether the expected improvement in outcomes can be confidently attributed to the intervention and not to other factors such as the interventionist–participant working alliance (an issue of internal validity); (2) what components of the intervention are most helpful (an issue of construct validity) and least helpful in inducing the hypothesized changes in the ultimate outcomes, and how can the intervention as-a-whole or its components be refined to optimize effectiveness; and (3) what contextual factors facilitate the delivery of the intervention and enhance clients' experience of the ultimate outcomes and, therefore, should be accounted for in future implementation of the intervention in research and practice (issue of external validity) (Evans et al., 2015; Furness et al., 2018; Griffin et al., 2014; Masterson-Algar et al., 2016; van Bruinessen et al., 2016; Wilkerson et al., 2019).

When the results of an outcome evaluation study do not support the effectiveness of the health intervention, it is important to explain the discrepancies between the hypothesized and the actually observed ultimate outcomes (Grant et al., 2013; Cheng & Metcalfe, 2018; Mars et al., 2013; Van de Glind et al., 2017). The main question guiding the investigation of these discrepancies is: Do the results (i.e. no change in the ultimate outcomes) reflect (1) unsuccessful intervention or theory failure, meaning that the intervention itself does not work or is inherently flawed, inadequate or deficient; or (2) unsuccessful delivery of the intervention or implementation failure, meaning that the intervention is not delivered appropriately, leading to type III error (Biron et al., 2010, 2016; Evans et al., 2015; van Bruinessen et al., 2016).

It may is wise to explore implementation failure in the context of an outcome evaluation study. If ruled out, then intervention theory failure is investigated.

The specific questions informing exploration of implementation failure include:

1. How well is the intervention delivered by interventionists? How effective is the training in preparing interventionists for providing the intervention? Is the intervention delivered with fidelity and good quality? Is the intervention or any of its components adapted? What is the type of adaptation done? Why, how, for whom, or in what conditions is the adaptation done? (Evans et al., 2015; Nurjono et al., 2018; Sharma et al., 2017; Siddiqui et al., 2018; Tama et al., 2018; van Bruinessen et al., 2016).

2. What contextual factors influence the delivery of the intervention by interventionists? Are all resources available and accessible? What are other barriers (e.g. sociopolitical, economic, historical, cultural) to the appropriate delivery of the intervention and its components? (Foley et al., 2016; Morgan-Trimmer, 2015; Siddiqui et al., 2018; Van de Glind et al., 2017).

3. How do participating clients respond to the intervention? How do they view the intervention and its components? Do participants view the intervention as acceptable, helpful, and are they satisfied with it? Are participants exposed to the full intervention (i.e. all its components and sessions) and if not, why? Is the content covered well understood, received, and useful in enhancing participants' understanding and management of the health problem? Do participants engage in the intervention activities? What contextual factors affect participants' engagement and enactment of the intervention? (Al-HadiHasan et al., 2017; Bakker et al., 2015; Hasson et al., 2012; Morgan-Trimmer, 2015; Siddiqui et al., 2018).

Specific questions informing investigation of intervention theory failure relate to: What is the capacity of the intervention and its components in initiating the mechanism of action mediating its effects on the ultimate outcomes? Were there potential interactions among the intervention components or between the intervention and some contextual factors that weaken the potency of the intervention in producing the hypothesized changes in the ultimate outcomes? Is it possible that the intervention and its components generated an un-hypothesized mechanism of action that lead to unintended outcomes.

As implied in the previous questions, the importance of a process evaluation rests on its focus on the intervention itself. Process evaluation provides information on the nature of the intervention (i.e. its constituent components), the extent and quality of its delivery (i.e. fidelity and influence of contextual factors) and participants' response to the intervention (van Bruinessen et al., 2016). Process data are included in the outcome data analysis to determine what exactly contributed to (lack of) improvement in the ultimate outcomes, in what subgroups of participants, under what context (Pawson & Manzano-Santaella, 2012; Rycroft-Malone et al., 2018; Sorensen & Llamas, 2018). Such knowledge is critical for making valid inferences about the effectiveness of the intervention, and for refining it to optimize its effectiveness in different client subgroups and contexts.

## 13.2    DEFINITION AND ELEMENTS OF PROCESS EVALUATION

Although recognized as important, there is no clear conceptualization of process evaluation. Unclear conceptualization resulted in its inconsistent operationalization, and variability in the specification of its operational elements, within and across fields of study. Five approaches or frameworks have frequently been mentioned in recent literature as informing the conduct of process evaluation; these are summarized in Table 13.1. Different operational elements of fidelity are proposed in the five frameworks. Fidelity of intervention delivery is commonly identified in three frameworks. The Consolidated Framework for Implementation Fidelity developed by Carroll et al. (2007) has guided the examination of the fidelity of intervention delivery in recent studies (Hasson et al., 2012). The Steckler and Linnan's (2002) framework is mentioned as guiding the design and conduct of several process evaluation studies (Table 13.1). However, it has been criticized for incorporating elements

**TABLE 13.1**  Approaches/frameworks for process evaluation.

| Approach or framework | Elements | Sources |
|---|---|---|
| RE-AIM Framework | Reach = rate of participation and representativeness of clients<br>Efficacy or Effectiveness<br>Adoption<br>Implementation<br>Maintenance | Grant et al. (2013), Griffin et al. (2014), Planas (2008) |
| Taxonomy of implementation outcomes (developed by Proctor et al.)—for complex interventions provided in practice | Acceptability<br>Adoption<br>Appropriateness<br>Feasibility<br>Implementation cost<br>Penetration<br>Sustainability | Griffin et al. (2014) |
| Dimensions of process evaluation (developed by Baranowski and Stables) | Context = environmental aspects of the intervention setting<br>Reach = proportion of participants who received the intervention<br>Fidelity = whether the intervention is delivered as planned<br>Dose delivered and received = amount of the intervention delivered and extent to which participants respond to it<br>Implementation = a composite score of reach, dose and fidelity<br>Recruitment = methods used to attract participants | Griffin et al. (2014) |
| Steckler and Linnan Framework | Recruitment = utility of recruitment procedures; number and characteristics of clients refusing enrollment<br>Reach = proportion of target client population that participate in the intervention; characteristics of participants; number of participants completing and withdrawing from treatment/study; reasons for withdrawal<br>Context = characteristics of setting or the practice in which the intervention is given and of interventionists delivering the intervention<br>Fidelity = extent to which the intervention is delivered as planned<br>Dose delivered = extent to which the intervention is given at the specified dose (i.e. number of sessions or contacts)<br>Dose received—exposure = extent of participants' active engagement and receptiveness of the intervention<br>Dose received—satisfaction = extent to which participants view the intervention as acceptable and helpful | Den Bakker et al. (2019), Hasson et al. (2012), Masterson-Algar et al. (2014), Nam et al. (2019), Poston et al. (2013), van Bruinessen et al. (2016), Verwey et al. (2016), Wilkerson et al. (2019). |
| Medical Research Council (UK)—guidance | Fidelity or quantity of intervention implementation<br>Quality of intervention implementation<br>Contextual factors influencing delivery and outcomes of the intervention<br>Causal mechanism or how participants respond to the intervention | MRC (2019) |

indicating the research process (e.g. recruitment, reach) and elements reflecting the intervention process (e.g. fidelity, dose received), leading to confusion in the conceptualization and the operationalization of process evaluation. Siddiqui et al. (2018) and van Bruinessen et al. (2016) advocate the need to distinguish between the research process and the intervention process and to focus process evaluation on the delivery of the intervention. The focus on the intervention process is also supported by the work of other researchers, who operationalized process evaluation into three main elements: delivery of the intervention, context of delivery, and mechanism of action.

1. *Delivery of the intervention*

Health interventions are provided by interventionists in research and health professionals in practice, or through technology. This element of process evaluation involves:

- Monitoring the fidelity with which the intervention components are provided: As explained in Chapter 9, fidelity is operationalized as the extent to which the interventionists adhered to the intervention manual.
- Exploring adaptations of the intervention: The exploration seeks to identify what components (content and activities) are modified, why, how, for whom, and in what conditions; whether the mode and dose of delivery are altered; and whether the adaptations are consistent with the principles explained in the intervention theory for guiding tailoring, and with the allowable changes described in the manual.
- Assessing the quality of intervention delivery: As mentioned in Chapter 9, quality is defined as the competence of the interventionists or health professionals in providing the intervention and in interacting with clients (Dillon et al., 2018; Evans et al., 2015; Hasson et al., 2012; Haynes et al., 2014; Hogue & Dauber, 2013; Mars et al., 2013; Moore et al., 2015; Nielson & Abildgaard, 2013; Nurjono et al., 2018; Ruikes et al., 2012; Sharma et al., 2017; Siddiqui et al., 2018; Tama et al., 2018; van den Branden et al., 2015; Van de Glind et al., 2017). For technology-based interventions, fidelity refers to the extent to which the technology functions as planned (Verwey et al., 2016).

2. *Context of delivery*

Context includes anything external to the intervention that may act as a barrier or facilitator to its implementation by the interventionists and participants, or through technology (Evans et al., 2015; Fridrich et al., 2015; Grant et al., 2013; Haynes et al., 2014; May et al., 2016; Moore et al., 2015; Nielson & Abildgaard, 2013; Nurjono et al., 2018; Ruikes et al., 2012; Tama et al., 2018). Context or contextual factors thought to influence the implementation of the intervention range from the country and community, which have particular economic, historical, social, cultural, and political characteristics; through site, setting or practice in which the intervention is provided, which possesses specific features related to resources, sociocultural norms underlying interactions among health professionals; to the environment in which the participants apply the treatment recommendations, which has unique physical, psycho-social and sociocultural attributes (Benson et al., 2018; Morgan-Trimmer, 2015; Sharma et al., 2017; Van de Glind et al., 2017).

In addition to these contextual factors, some researchers categorize characteristics of the interventionists and the participating clients as contextual factors that play out as barriers or facilitators of intervention implementation (Benson et al., 2018;

May et al., 2016; Verwey et al., 2016). As discussed in Chapter 5, the interventionist and client characteristics are stipulated to influence the implementation of the intervention in the intervention theory.

3. *Mechanism*

This element of process evaluation is conceptualized and operationalized in two ways. The first is the intervention's mechanism of action, also referred to as process (Grant et al., 2013; Nurjono et al., 2018). As explained in Chapter 5, the mechanism of action is responsible for the effects of the health intervention on the ultimate outcomes. It is represented by the series of linkages among changes in the immediate, intermediate (or mediators), and ultimate outcomes, as envisioned by Evans et al. (2015), Moore et al. (2015), Sharma et al. (2017), and van de Glind et al. (2017). It is argued that this conceptualization of mechanism, although important, is within the realm of outcome evaluation (Chapter 14).

The second conceptualization of mechanism reflects how clients who are exposed to the intervention react, perceive, and respond to it (Brand et al., 2019; Dalkin et al., 2015; Dillon et al., 2018; Rycroft-Malone et al., 2018; Van Belle et al., 2016). This conceptualization of mechanism is consistent with the notions of: (1) client responsiveness advanced by Carroll et al. (2007); (2) dose received-exposure and enactment, and satisfaction identified in Steckler and Linnann's framework (see Table 13.1 and Chapter 9); (3) perception or appraisal of the intervention as alluded to in the work of Poston et al. (2013), Nielson et al. (2007), and van den Branden et al. (2015) and discussed in Chapter 11. Of particular interest in process evaluation is participants' responsiveness and satisfaction with the intervention (Carroll et al., 2007; Hasson et al., 2012; Haynes et al., 2014). These two concepts represent participants' views of the intervention's processes (Chapter 11). Accordingly, the second conceptualization of mechanism is relevant to process evaluation.

The previously presented points support the integration of the following elements in a process evaluation. The elements are in alignment with the focus of process evaluation on the intervention itself. The elements are:

- Fidelity and adaptations of the intervention delivery by interventionists.
- Competence of interventionists in intervention delivery.
- Contextual factors, operating at the setting level, influencing delivery of the intervention.
- Client responsiveness, that is, exposure, engagement and enactment of the intervention.
- Contextual factors, operating within participants' environment, and affecting exposure, engagement and enactment of the intervention.
- Perception (or satisfaction) of the intervention by participants.

## 13.3   METHODS USED IN PROCESS EVALUATION

Process evaluation is conducted in different studies, including preliminary small-scale studies aimed to examine feasibility of a health intervention, studies focusing on determining the efficacy of a health intervention under controlled conditions, and studies evaluating the effectiveness of an intervention implemented in practice (Benson et al., 2018; Siddiqui et al., 2018). In all cases, the primary concerns are ascertaining the fidelity and the quality of intervention delivery, and identifying factors that affect the delivery. When process evaluation is integrated in an outcome evaluation study, the additional concern is to "unpack the black box" (Wong et al., 2012) to gain a comprehensive understanding of what contribute to the beneficial outcomes, how and under what conditions (Fletcher et al., 2016; Furness et al,. 2018; Nielson & Abildgaard, 2013).

Process evaluation is guided by the intervention theory, which is operationalized in a logic model (Sorensen & Llamas, 2018; Sharma et al., 2017; Van de Glind et al., 2017). As discussed in Chapter 5, the theory clearly defines the intervention's active ingredients and the respective components, and highlights the components responsible for the interventions effects. Knowledge of the components, including content, activities and treatment recommendations informs the assessment of: the fidelity with which the interventionists deliver the intervention and participating clients' responsiveness (Masterson-Algar et al. 2016, 2018; Wells et al., 2012); and participants' perceptions (satisfaction) of the intervention components. The intervention theory points to key contextual factors, including characteristics of clients, interventionists and setting or environment, that affect the implementation of the intervention. Understanding contextual factors informs their assessment. The intervention theory also specifies the immediate and intermediate outcomes and delineates their associations with specific intervention components, thereby providing guidance for analyzing the contribution of the intervention components to the achievement of outcomes, within and across contexts or settings (Biron et al., 2010, 2016; Sridharan & Nakaima, 2012).

The intervention theory presents conceptual and operational definitions of the intervention components, contextual factors, client responsiveness, and ultimate outcomes. These definitions form the basis for selecting or developing measures of the respective elements of process evaluation. The resulting quantitative data are analyzed descriptively and the proposed relationships are tested using advanced statistical tests. However, to gain a comprehensive and in-depth understanding of the intervention implementation within and across contexts, qualitative methods are used (Cheng & Metcalfe, 2018). Qualitative methods are useful to explore different stakeholder groups' (e.g. interventionist, client) views of the intervention, of influential contextual factors, and of the intervention impact, thereby complementing and supplementing the quantitative results. Accordingly, quantitative and qualitative methods are highly valued, and the integration of their respective data is important in enhancing the validity of process evaluation results (De Vlaming et al., 2010; Van de Glind et al., 2017).

Selected quantitative and qualitative methods may have to be adapted to conduct process evaluation of different health interventions. The adaptation is often necessary to accommodate variability in the nature of the intervention components and mode of delivery; the contextual factors operating at the individual client, interventionist, and setting levels; and the perspective of stakeholder groups (including research ethics board), on the methods to be used. For instance, direct observation of intervention delivery may not be relevant for technology-based health interventions or it may not be acceptable or agreeable to clients (e.g. observation of the provision of intimate care for persons with dementia or of individual sessions addressing personal sexual issues). Furthermore, there are a few established measures of the elements of process evaluation. Those available have to be adapted for consistency with the conceptual and operational definitions of relevant concepts proposed in the intervention theory. Because of this variability, general principles and methods for assessing each element of process evaluation are presented next.

### 13.3.1   Fidelity of Intervention Delivery by Interventionists

The importance, principles, methods, and checklists for monitoring and assessing the fidelity with which interventionists deliver the intervention have been discussed in detail in Chapter 9. Few points are reiterated.

- In principle, assessment of fidelity, including adaptations specified in the intervention manual, should be done for each interventionist delivering each session of a health intervention, during the evaluation study period. This is important for an accurate quantification of the level of fidelity and for reaching valid conclusions about the contribution of the intervention to the ultimate outcomes. For technology-based health interventions, there is no clear guidance on how to determine fidelity; however, Verwey et al. (2016) describe fidelity as the extent to which the technology functions as planned; Mohr et al. (2015) propose to examine its workflow. The workflow determines when specific elements of the intervention are provided through the respective technology, the sequence for delivering them, and the duration.

- Assessment of fidelity is based on a clear specification of the intervention components, content to be covered and activities to be performed in each session, mode and dose of delivery, as well as allowable adaptations. This information guides the development of two measures for assessing fidelity or adherence to the intervention manual. The first measure is a checklist reflecting the activities to be performed, sequentially, in each intervention session. The checklist is completed by observers and interventionists, and guides the collection of quantitative data on performance of the planned intervention activities (Sharma et al., 2017; Siddiqui et al., 2018). The checklist also includes a section to document variations or additional adaptations in intervention delivery and the conditions surrounding them. The second measure is an abridged version of this checklist, which is completed by participants. It contains the main content and activities planned for each session that are recognizable by participants. The content and activities are described in lay, simple, and easy to understand terms. Table 13.2 illustrates an excerpt of such a measure used by participants to report on the fidelity of the sleep education component of the behavioral therapy for insomnia. Participants are requested to indicate whether or not they were exposed to the component, content or topics were covered, and the activities were performed in each session.

- Four methods can be used to collect data on fidelity. The first is observation, which can be direct or indirect. In direct observation, the observer attends the delivery of the intervention while assuming a nonparticipant role (Rycroft-Malone et al., 2018) and documenting the performance of the planned activities on the checklist (Dillon et al., 2018). In indirect observation, the rater reviews video or audio recordings of the intervention delivery sessions and document performance of the activities on the checklist. The second method consists of interventionists' self-report of the performance of the intervention activities on the checklist, also called activity log (Rycroft-Malone et al., 2018), logbook (Griffin et al., 2014), or diary (Poston et al., 2013). The third method involves participants' report on performance of the planned intervention activities, using an abridged version of the activity checklist. The fourth method includes semi-structured interviews. The interviews are held with interventionists to further explore conditions that necessitated

**TABLE 13.2**    Description of Sleep Education component of the Behavioral Therapy for Insomnia.

Did you receive the following treatment as part of your program?

Treatment:
Education about sleep

Description of treatment:
  Education about sleep includes information about sleep and instructions on
    strategies you can do in general to improve your sleep

Questions:
Which of the following information about sleep were you given during the class?
- What is sleep?
- Why do we sleep?
- What is insomnia?
- Why do we have insomnia?
- What are body clocks and how do they affect sleep?
- What is sleep deprivation?

Which of the following general strategies to improve sleep were you given during the class?
- Develop regular daytime activity
- Reduce light, excessive temperature and noise during sleep
- Avoid heavy dinner just before going to sleep
- Avoid alcoholic drinks, coffee or tea, and smoking before going to sleep
- Get some light during the day
- Wind down before going to sleep

adaptations of the intervention. To minimize the potential for recall bias, interventionists and participants are requested to complete the respective measure of fidelity immediately following the session (Hogue & Dauber, 2013). Each method has its strengths and limitations (see Chapter 9); therefore, it is recommended to use more than one method in process evaluation so that the bias inherent in one method is counterbalanced by the bias inherent in another, thereby enhancing validity. However, it is important to take into consideration the feasibility of applying the method(s) within a particular study or practice setting and the acceptability of the method(s) to the target client population.

- Total scores are computed to quantify the level of fidelity or adherence with which a health intervention is provided. Total scores represent the percentage of the intervention activities actually performed, by each interventionist, out of those planned for each session, across all sessions to which participants are exposed. The total scores are used in quantitative data analysis aimed to examine the association of fidelity with outcomes (Griffin et al., 2014; Masterson-Algar et al., 2016). Total scores reflecting the observers', the interventionists', and/or the participants' ratings of fidelity are analyzed separately. Alternatively, their convergence is examined (using advanced statistical analyses such as confirmatory factor analysis) and an index is generated to quantify the collective level of fidelity—refer to Nam et al. (2019) or MRC guidance (2019) for examples.

- Qualitative data on variations or adaptations in the intervention delivery, gathered in the checklist or interviews with interventionists, are content analyzed to describe additional patterns of adaptations; these are then integrated in the intervention manual as necessary.

### 13.3.2   Competence of Interventionist

Methods and measures of interventionists' competence in delivering health interventions are discussed in Chapter 9. Key points to consider include:

- It is essential to generate a clear understanding of competence, including generic and specific skills, expected of interventionists in delivering health interventions. The conceptualization of competence drives the search for and the selection of respective measures. A few measures of generic skills such as communication, interactional style, therapeutic relationship, and working alliance have been established. Measures of specific skills may have to be developed and validated prior to administering them in a process evaluation study.

- Data on competence are obtained through observation, self-report by interventionists, and reported by participants (Chapter 9). Obtaining the data from more than one source is recommended to enhance construct validity. This requires the availability of three versions of the same measure to be completed by the observer, the interventionist, and the participant. The measures are completed by (1) the rater during the observation period, (2) the interventionist during the study period (e.g. once the interventionist has provided the intervention to a group of participants), and (3) the participants immediately upon completion of all intervention sessions, in order to reduce recall bias.

- Total scores are computed to quantify the level of competence, as perceived by each of the observer, the interventionist, and the participants. The formula specified by the developers of the measure is followed to calculate the total score (e.g. sum or mean of the items' scores). The total scores are analyzed descriptively and compared to determine differences in competence as perceived by the observer, interventionist, and participants; however, it is often the participants' perception of the interventionist's competence that is included in the analysis examining the process-outcome linkages; it was found to be most influential (see Chapter 8 for relevant evidence).

### 13.3.3   Contextual Factors Influencing Intervention Delivery

A wide range of contextual factors, embedded in the setting in which the interventionist provides the intervention, can influence the intervention delivery. The intervention theory may identify salient contextual factors but may not capture all those operating in a particular situation, specifically if they are unique and/or reflect random occurrences (e.g. fire alarm going on requiring unexpected early ending of a session; changes in leadership affecting the support for the intervention). Therefore, it is highly recommended to use a mix of quantitative and qualitative methods to assess contextual factors (Griffin et al., 2014).

Quantitative methods include:

1. Development of a checklist that represents factors identified in the intervention theory as affecting delivery: The list can categorize the factors into those pertaining to the omnibus or general setting and to the discrete or specific environment (Fridrich et al., 2015). Examples of general setting factors include changes: in policy, staff complement, practice and/support (instrumental or financial) for the intervention. To assess general setting factors, the checklist

can be completed by the researchers (who become aware of these factors through various means) or the setting's administrative or clinical decision makers (who know/experience the factors) on a regular basis (e.g. monthly or quarterly) throughout the process evaluation study period (e.g. Rycroft-Malone et al., 2018). Examples of specific environmental factors include inappropriate seating arrangement, uncomfortable room temperature, or poorly functioning equipment. To assess specific environmental factors, the checklist is completed by the rater involved in direct or indirect observation of the intervention delivery (e.g. Griffin et al., 2014), and by the interventionist responsible for providing the intervention. The checklist is completed prospectively by the rater and immediately following each session by the interventionist. Descriptive (i.e. frequency distribution) analysis of the data gathered with the checklist identifies commonly occurring contextual factors within and across intervention sessions. This information is useful in interpreting variability in intervention delivery and in outcome achievement; in revising the contextual factors identified in the intervention theory and how they affect delivery; and in guiding the selection or the modification to be made in the setting in order to minimize the occurrence and potential influence of the contextual factors on the intervention's delivery and effectiveness.

2. Administration of established measures that assess specific contextual factors identified in the intervention theory: Established measures are available for assessing specific contextual factors. Examples include indices reflecting features of an in-patient unit such as staff complement (e.g. Verwey et al., 2016), measures capturing the availability of guidelines, organizational culture, organizational and professional endorsement for evidence-based practice, and inter-professional collaboration (e.g. Smith & Hasan, 2020), and the Swedish version of the Scheffield Care Environment Assessment Matrix to assess different features (e.g. privacy, comfort, and safety) of the environment in long-term care settings (Nordin et al., 2015). Relevant databases are searched to identify measures with demonstrated reliability and validity, and the one that operationalizes the factor in a way that is consistent with its conceptual definition advanced in the intervention theory, is selected. The measures are completed by the interventionists and the data are analyzed descriptively to assist in the interpretation of variability in intervention delivery and outcome achievement across settings participating in the evaluation study.

Qualitative methods include unstructured or semi-structured interviews with interventionists (Fridrich et al., 2015; Haynes et al., 2014; Rycroft-Malone et al., 2018). The interviews are usually held following delivery of the intervention and regularly (e.g. quarterly) during the process evaluation study period. The interviews explore challenges that interventionists encountered when delivering the intervention and contextual factors they identify as contributing to these challenges (i.e. barriers). The interviews also inquire about uneventful delivery of the intervention (e.g. adherence to the intervention manual) and contextual factors that promote adherence (i.e. facilitators) (Benson et al., 2018). During the interviews, prompts are used to further explore how the factors operated and influenced the provision of the intervention (Aust et al., 2010; Evans et al., 2015). The responses are analyzed thematically to identify barriers and facilitators, and their inter-relationships in affecting the delivery of the intervention (Masterson-Algar et al., 2016; Van de Glind et al., 2017).

Quantitative and qualitative findings are integrated in a convergence coding matrix (Van de Glind et al., 2017). Convergent findings point to influential contextual factors and delineate how and why they influence intervention delivery. The findings are useful to:

- Refine the intervention theory: This involves revising the type and definition of the contextual factors, as well as the nature of their relationships with intervention delivery.
- Revise the intervention manual: This consists of specifying the contextual factors that should be accounted for in selecting the setting for intervention delivery (i.e. the setting that has most of the facilitators) and should be taken into consideration in future delivery of the intervention in research or practice.
- Understand the context of intervention delivery: The understanding is important in the interpretation of variations in intervention delivery and consequently in outcome achievement that may be reported in process-outcome evaluation studies conducted within and across settings.
- Guide the selection and the quantification of the most influential contextual factors, and therefore the multivariable quantitative analyses aimed to examine the impact of these factors on intervention delivery and outcomes: This kind of analysis is feasible when the process-outcome evaluation study includes a large number of settings, interventionists and participants.

## 13.3.4   Client Responsiveness

Client responsiveness is operationalized in terms of exposure, engagement, and enactment of treatment. Client responsiveness plays an important role in initiating the intervention's mechanism of action, which contributes to improvement in the ultimate outcomes. Assessing participants' exposure, engagement, and enactment is critical for reaching valid conclusions on the effectiveness of health interventions.

### 13.3.4.1   Exposure

Exposure to the intervention is logically and commonly quantified in the number of intervention sessions attended or of modules completed by each participant (Berkel et al., 2019). Exposure represents intervention dose as mentioned Chapters 4 and 5, and as illustrated in Furness et al.'s (2018) study.

Different methods and measures (e.g. logs, computerized systems) are used to obtain data on exposure for health interventions provided in different formats (Haynes et al., 2014; Poston et al., 2013). For interventions facilitated by interventionists and provided in in-person or distance (e.g. video or telephone conferencing), a logbook is used to document participants' attendance at each session and the length of attendance (e.g. whole or part of the session). The interventionist or a research staff member completes the attendance log at the beginning of the session (to report on attendance) and at the end of the session (to report on length of attendance). For interventions offered in modules (in hard copy) that are self-completed by participants, participants are asked to complete a logbook. Participants document: whether or not they completed each module, whether they read all or part of the information covered in the module, and the number of times they reviewed the module. For technology-based interventions, a built-in system is designed to track participants' access to the intervention material (e.g. electronically available module, text message) and to count the number of times each part of the material was accessed.

Total scores are computed to represent each participant's level of exposure to the intervention. The total scores are calculated either as the sum (or number) of sessions attended or modules completed, or as the percentage of the sessions attended or modules completed out of those planned. The total scores are analyzed descriptively (frequency distribution, mean) in a study focusing only on process evaluation. The total scores are included in analyses aimed to examine the extent to which variability in exposure is associated with differences in the level of improvement in the outcomes, in a study concerned with process-outcome evaluation (as is done in some per-protocol analysis). In the process-outcome analysis, exposure is represented in either of two ways: (1) total score quantifying exposure as the only independent variable representing the intervention, or (2) total score quantifying exposure in addition to the variable reflecting the treatment to which participants are assigned. In the latter case, the statistical model includes two independent variables, one representing the treatment group (i.e. experimental intervention and comparison treatment) and one representing exposure as predictors of outcomes. This analysis estimates the unique contribution of treatment group and exposure to the outcomes; it is conceptually relevant as it indicates if exposure independently (i.e. above and beyond treatment group) influences the outcomes. However, the variables representing treatment and exposure may be highly correlated (if participants are likely to attend all sessions of one treatment) limiting the ability to discern their unique influence.

To further understand the contribution of exposure to the outcomes, qualitative data are gathered to explore reasons for participants' attendance/completion or non-attendance/ non-completion of sessions/modules. These data are collected by adding open-ended questions (e.g. what made you attend/not attend the sessions) to the post-test questionnaire or by interviewing participants after completing the intervention (e.g. as part of the interview planned to further assess participants' engagement, enactment, and perceptions, as mentioned in subsequent sections).

### 13.3.4.2  Engagement

Engagement reflects active participation in health interventions. It is operationalized in three concepts: involvement in the planned intervention activities, comprehension of the intervention content, and capacity to employ the behaviors or skills taught in the application of the treatment recommendations. Involvement in intervention activities is exemplified by participation in group discussion or in problem-solving. Comprehension entails an understanding of the topics presented in the intervention session or module, and most importantly, of the treatment recommendations. Capacity is often reflected in self-efficacy or sense of confidence in the ability to perform a behavior or to apply the treatment recommendations. Different methods are suggested to collect data on the concepts reflecting engagement. The selection of methods is dependent on its feasibility and acceptance by research ethics boards and participants, and how engagement data will be used in the process-outcome analysis.

*Observation*

Direct or indirect observation of individual or group sessions by trained raters is one method for gathering data on participants' engagement (Van de Glind et al., 2017). It is done in conjunction with observation of interventionists' performance (see Section 13.3.1) and competence (see Section 13.3.2) in providing the intervention. In principle, the observation is done for all sessions, given by all interventionists, to all participants, in order to accurately estimate levels of participants' engagement. The use of observation is contingent on feasibility and on participants' consent to the presence of the rater. In addition, the raters should be intensively trained to recognize participants' exhibition of verbal and/or nonverbal behaviors indicative of engagement. These behaviors are derived from the intervention manual, in which activities to be performed by participants (e.g. discussion, demonstration of skills) are delineated. Behaviors indicative of engagement should be clearly and precisely identified, defined, and operationalized so that they are comprehensively listed and described in a checklist. Raters are then expected to note the behaviors as they are exhibited by participants throughout the intervention sessions and to document their occurrence on the checklist. Possible challenges with this method are related to: (1) increased burden of observation on the raters who are expected to constantly observe the behaviors of each participant throughout the sessions. Burden leads to fatigue and subsequently missing data. Burden can be mitigated by having raters review video or audio recordings of the sessions, which can be done at their convenience and allow them to replay the recordings as needed to accurately note the behaviors; (2) missing verbal or nonverbal behaviors by some participants (e.g. those sitting outside the recorder range) when reviewing the sessions' recordings, potentially lowering the estimated levels of engagement; and (3) level at which engagement data are documented in group sessions. Engagement data are collected either for individual participants or for the whole group. Individual data are required if the plan is to include levels of engagement in the process-outcome analysis. In this case, total scores (total number or percentage) are calculated to represent participants' engagement in the planned intervention activities across sessions; engagement scores are then examined for their association with improvement in outcomes. Group data are adequate if the plan is to describe the general level of participant engagement in the intervention. These descriptive findings can inform the refinement of the intervention activities, as necessary, to promote engagement.

### Interventionist Report

Report by interventionists facilitating individual or group sessions is another method for gathering data on participants' engagement. Interventionists are requested to keep a log, and/or are interviewed to explore their perspective on participants' engagement in the intervention. The log contains close- or open-ended questions. The log entries reflect the interventionists' general sense of participants' expressed interest in the covered content; motivation or enthusiasm for the intervention as-a-whole or specific components; and learning or understanding of the treatment recommendations (Pawson & Manzano-Santaella, 2012; van Bruinessen et al., 2016; van den Branden et al., 2015; Verwey et al., 2016). Interventionists' responses are analyzed thematically to highlight: general levels of participants' motivation and engagement; content that is understood to varying degree, with content that is not well received pointing to the need for refinement to enhance its comprehension; and intervention activities in which clients enthusiastically participate and those demanding modification to promote engagement.

Compared to observation, this method is relatively feasible, acceptable, and less demanding in terms of burden and cost. However, the interventionists' responses may be tainted by some biases associated with (1) their selective recollection of participants' engagement; for example, they may pay attention and, hence, remember behaviors exhibited by a few participants who dominate the group discussion or ask the most questions during a session; (2) recall bias in that interventionists may miss some information because they focus more on the delivery of the intervention than on observing participants' behaviors; and (3) social desirability or performance bias in that interventionists want to portray themselves as capable of engaging participants.

### Participant Report

Report by participants is a commonly used method for collecting data on engagement. Data on engagement are collected with quantitative and/or qualitative methods, immediately following completion of the intervention. Quantitative methods involve the administration of measures assessing relevant concepts or behaviors indicative of engagement. Qualitative methods consist of interviews with participants, (Den Bakker et al., 2019; Haynes et al., 2014; Poston et al., 2013; Verwey et al., 2016).

Comprehension is assessed with instruments testing participants' understanding of the key content covered in the intervention and of the treatment recommendations they are to apply in daily life. It can also be assessed by reviewing a copy of participants' written goals, action plan, or other assignments, for completeness and appropriateness (Walton et al., 2017). Capacity is usually measured with relevant self-efficacy scales. Because of the specificity of health interventions, measures of comprehension and capacity may have to be developed to reflect a particular intervention's content, activities, and treatment recommendations. Where available, measures that have demonstrated reliability and validity are selected to assess these concepts if their content is consistent with the conceptual definitions advanced in the intervention theory. Available measures may have to be adapted to maintain their fit with the specific content and activities of a health intervention. For example, measures of self-efficacy require modifications to reflect the skills targeted by the intervention under evaluation. Generic, close-ended questions (with respective response scale for rating frequency or agreement) have recently been reported in the literature to assess the concepts reflective of engagement. Examples of questions include:

- Have you participated in the group discussion?
- Have you reviewed the materials (e.g. booklet or online module)?
- Have you learned about strategies or treatment recommendations to help manage the health problem?
- Are you able to apply the strategies or treatment recommendations?
- Are you motivated to apply the strategies or treatment recommendations? (van den Branden et al., 2015; Wilkerson et al., 2019).

Total scores are computed to quantify participants' levels on each engagement concept, or an index representing overall level of engagement (as described for fidelity, Section 13.3.1) is generated. The scores are analyzed descriptively or included in process-outcome analysis, as explained previously.

Interviews with participants are semi-structured inquiring about their engagement in the intervention. Open-ended questions are posed to explore their overall interest, motivation or enthusiasm about the intervention; how they understand the intervention; what they have learned that helps them understand and manage their health problem; their participation in the discussion or use of material available through technology-based modes; and their comprehension and ability to carry out the treatment recommendations (Griffin et al., 2014; Pawson & Manzano-Santaella, 2012;

van den Branden et al., 2015; Van de Glind et al., 2017). Additional questions are posed to probe for clarification and explanation of the reported level of engagement.

Results of thematic analysis of participants' responses shed light on the intervention components, content, activities, and treatment recommendations in which they engage most or least. This information extends, supplements, and helps in the interpretation of the quantitative findings related to engagement, and in understanding how engagement contributes to outcome achievement. It also guides the refinement of the intervention to enhance engagement.

### 13.3.4.3  Enactment

Enactment is frequently operationalized in participant adherence to treatment recommendations in daily life. Different methods are used to collect data on adherence to health interventions. The methods include objective assessment and self-report, with the most commonly used being self-report by participants.

Objective assessment is relevant for some indicators of health interventions. Examples include the use of pedometer to track the number of steps or distance walked in an intervention for promoting physical activity, and the use of actigraph to monitor adherence to the sleep–wake schedule in sleep restriction therapy.

Self-report by participants is most feasible and appropriate for monitoring the performance and adherence to treatment recommendations comprising many health interventions. In these interventions, treatment recommendations are often cognitive or behavioral in nature and are to be applied in participants' daily life. Accordingly, their performance under daily life circumstances may not be observed by others (such as researchers, interventionists, or significant others) nor detected objectively through available technology. Two measures of adherence are available. Participants are asked to keep a diary or complete a checklist (in paper or electronic format) of the treatment recommendations they apply over the treatment period, or to respond to a question about their global adherence to treatment after completion of the intervention (e.g. Furness et al., 2018; Kyle et al., 2011).

The diary or checklist contains the treatment recommendations that participants are expected to perform. Each recommendation is clearly and precisely described in terms of the specific action to perform, how, where, and when (e.g. avoid heavy meals within two to four hours before going to bed). Participants are asked to indicate whether they perform the recommendations and the number of times they do so. They are also invited to write any comment related to performance of the treatment recommendations such as difficulties encountered and reasons for alterations in performance of the treatment recommendations. The diary or checklist is completed throughout the intervention period. This has the advantage of prospective data collection, which minimizes recall bias and improves the accuracy of the reported adherence data. However, completing the diary or checklist is not well received. It is burdensome for many participants because it is time consuming and demanding, leading to response fatigue and ensuing low accuracy of the data. Some participants may stop completing the diary leading to missing data. To reduce burden, the checklist can be completed toward the end of a treatment period. At post-test, participants are instructed to report on the performance of each treatment recommendation and the frequency of performance over the treatment period. Although completing the checklist at this time is less demanding or burdensome than keeping a diary, it has the potential for introducing recall bias.

Participants' self-report may introduce bias, reflected in overestimates of adherence. To address this bias, where feasible, adherence data are gathered from

participants' significant others. However, involving significant others in the evaluation study requires approval of participants to contact their significant others and the
significant others' willingness and ability to observe and document participants'
implementation of the treatment recommendations.

Questions on global adherence are increasingly used to inquire about participants' perception of the extent to which they complied with the treatment recommendations (Bellg et al., 2004). Responses to such questions provide a general sense
of adherence but are possibly influenced by recall bias leading to underestimation, or
by social desirability yielding overestimation of levels of adherence.

Based on the measure used, total scores on adherence reflect: (1) the percentage
of treatment recommendations applied out of those prescribed or are applicable to
individual participants; for example, some sleep hygiene recommendations such as
those related to smoking, may not be relevant to nonsmokers. The percentage is
computed based on data collected through the checklist completed at post-test. The
percentage is also computed for data obtained with a diary, for each day and aggregated over the duration of the treatment period, for each participant; or (2) the
reported global adherence level. Similar to other process elements, data on adherence
are analyzed descriptively or included in process-outcome analysis to determine the
contribution of adherence to improvement in outcomes. In addition, open-ended
questions inquiring about reasons for adherence or nonadherence are posed during
participant interviews planned to assess other process elements, following completion of the intervention (Kyle et al., 2011).

### 13.3.5  Contextual Factors Affecting Participants' Exposure, Engagement and Enactment of Intervention

Similar to contextual factors influencing the delivery of the intervention by interventionists, a wide range of factors inherent in the participants' lifestyle and environment affect their exposure, engagement, and enactment of the intervention. For
factors identified in the intervention theory, available established measures are
selected if they fit the factors' conceptual and operational definitions. For instance,
several self-report instruments assessing social support have been validated. The
measures are completed at different points in time over the treatment period to
capture the occurrence at a particular time point or possible changes in the factors
over the treatment period. Changes in the factors can dynamically influence exposure,
engagement, enactment, and improvement in outcomes (Fridrich et al., 2015;
Krauss, 2018; Morgan-Trimmer, 2015). For example, a reduction in perceived social
support over the course of the intervention (e.g. spouse or bed partner no longer
supportive of the changes in bedroom environment or in sleep–wake schedule)
negatively affects a client's ability to enact the stimulus control instructions.

Total scores are computed to quantify the experience of the factors, following the
instructions provided by the instrument developers. The scores are included in the
data analysis. The analysis aims to (1) describe the prevalence of these factors among
participants or the levels at which the factors are experienced, and (2) examine the
factors' associations with exposure, engagement, and enactment of the intervention,
and subsequently improvement in outcomes. The latter analysis is done using
advanced statistical tests such as path analysis and requires large samples.

Two methods are useful to assess other factors proposed in the intervention
theory but for which there are no available measures. First, participants are requested
to report on the occurrence of each factor on a checklist that is completed separately

or integrated in the diary used to assess enactment. The second method consists of interviewing participants at post-test. The interview engages participants in identifying contextual factors they encountered and how the factors influenced exposure, engagement, and enactment. Interviews have the advantages of identifying additional contextual factors (not covered in the intervention theory) and exploring the pathway through which they influence participants' implementation of the intervention. The findings are useful in modifying the intervention's content, activities, or treatment recommendations, or prescribed adaptations to inform participants of the potential influence of the contextual factors and of strategies to handle them in order to promote participants' exposure, engagement, and enactment of the intervention.

### 13.3.6   Perception of the Intervention by Participants

Of the intervention perceptions discussed in Chapter 11, satisfaction is of primary concern in process evaluation (Ruikes et al., 2012; Verwey et al., 2016; Wilkerson et al., 2019). Satisfaction is conceptualized as participants' appraisal of the intervention's processes and outcomes (Sidani & Epstein, 2016). Satisfaction is reflected in participants' ratings of the helpfulness of the intervention as-a-whole and/or its components in understanding the health problem and the treatment recommendations (Al-Hadi-Hasan et al., 2017; Den Bakker et al., 2019; Poston et al., 2013; van Bruinessen et al., 2016; Verwey et al., 2016; Wilkerson et al., 2019); the competence of the interventionists (Van de Glind et al., 2017); and the effectiveness of the intervention in improving outcomes and its overall impact on participants' lives (Siddiqui et al., 2018; Tama et al., 2018; Verwey et al., 2016). Several measures of satisfaction with health interventions have been validated (Chapter 11). The one developed and validated by Sidani et al. (2017) covers a range of domains related to satisfaction with the processes and outcomes of behavioral interventions; it may be of relevance in measuring satisfaction with treatment processes as advocated for process evaluation.

Satisfaction measures are usually completed by participants after receipt of the intervention. Total scale or subscales (reflecting different domains of satisfaction) are calculated following the instructions given by the instrument developers. Analysis of quantitative data aims to describe the extent of satisfaction with the intervention and its components, and to examine its association with outcomes. In addition, open-ended questions can be included in the questionnaire completed at post-test or posed in interviews scheduled at post-test. The questions elicit participants' perceptions of the intervention and its components in terms of their acceptability and usefulness in improving outcomes (Al-HadiHasan et al., 2017; Den Bakker et al., 2019; Haynes et al., 2014; Poston et al., 2013; Siddiqui et al., 2018); experience with the intervention (Griffin et al., 2014); and views on what aspect (component, content, activities, mode of delivery) they like most/least and why, and on how the intervention can be modified to enhance its delivery and effectiveness. Results of thematic analysis of these qualitative data provide guidance for refining the intervention and its delivery, with the goals of making it attractive and satisfying to clients, and enhancing its potency in improving outcomes.

## 13.4   ANALYSIS OF PROCESS DATA

General strategies for analyzing quantitative and qualitative data representing each element of process evaluation are presented throughout the Section 13.3. Overall, the analysis is descriptive and correlational. The descriptive analysis aims to (1) characterize the extent to which interventionists deliver the health intervention with fidelity, and the levels of participants' exposure, engagement, enactment, and satisfaction with the intervention; and (2) to identify contextual factors influencing the implementation of the intervention by both interventionists and participants. For each element of process evaluation, convergence of data obtained through different quantitative methods (e.g. observation, self-report) and through quantitative and qualitative (e.g. completion of a measure and interview) methods is examined using appropriate analytic strategies. These may include confirmatory factor analysis and convergence coding matrix, respectively.

The purpose of correlational analysis is to determine the contribution of the intervention's processes to improvement in outcomes. This is often done by analyzing quantitative and qualitative data separately, then integrating the results. Different statistical approaches can be used for quantitative correlational analysis, including:

1. Bivariate correlation (e.g. Pearson's correlation coefficient) to estimate the magnitude and direction of the association between each process element and either the outcomes reported following the intervention or the level of change (from pretest to post-test) in the outcomes: This approach is appropriate when the sample size is rather small, which limits the use of advanced statistical tests, and when the focus is on examining the independent contribution of each process element to the outcomes. However, with multiple testing, the chance of type I error is increased.

2. Generating indices that reflect the two main process elements: The first index captures the overall delivery of the intervention by interventionists and is generated by aggregating data quantifying fidelity and competence, as suggested by the Medical Research Council guidance and reported by Nam et al. (2019). The second index quantifies the overall adherence to the intervention by participants. It aggregates scores on exposure, engagement, and enactment. The indices are then used in the correlational analysis. This approach is also appropriate when the sample size is small, and has the advantage of reducing the likelihood of type I error. It is also appropriate when the focus is on general levels of interventionists' and participants' performance.

3. Multivariable or multivariate correlational analysis to examine the direct and indirect relationships among process elements and outcomes, as proposed in the intervention theory: This approach is appropriate when the sample size is large and the focus is on the simultaneous contribution of all process elements, which allows the detection of the most influential ones. Multiple regression analysis can be used to examine the direct relationships between the process elements (fidelity, competence, exposure, engagement, enactment) and either the outcomes assessed at post-test or the changes in outcomes (from pretest to post-test). Path analysis or structural equation modeling are used to test the proposed direct (as specified for multiple regression) and indirect relationships. The indirect relationships delineate the influence of contextual factors on implementation of the intervention represented in the respective process elements or their indices, and the influence of these process elements (individual or indices) on the outcomes (quantified in the post-test scores or the changes in outcomes) (Hansen & Jones, 2017).

The qualitative findings are integrated with the results of the correlational quantitative analysis. The qualitative findings are instrumental in interpreting, explaining, or extending the quantitative results. The integrated findings inform the revision of the intervention theory and the refinement of the design and delivery of health interventions; the purpose is to enhance the intervention's acceptability to the target client population, feasibility, effectiveness, and efficiency.

## REFERENCES

Al-HadiHasan, A., Callaghan, P., & Lynn, J.S. (2017) Qualitative process evaluation of a psycho-educational intervention targeted at people diagnosed with schizophrenia and their primary caregivers in Jordan. *BMC Psychiatry*, 17, 68–83.

Aust, B., Rugulies, R., Finken, A., & Jensen, C. (2010) When workplace interventions lead to negative effects: Learning from failures. *Scandinavian Journal of Public Health*, 38(3), 106–119.

Bakker, F., Persoon, A., Schoon, Y., & Olde Rikkert, M.G.M. (2015) Uniform presentation of process evaluation results facilitated the evaluation of complex interventions: Development of a graph. *Journal of Evaluation in Clinical Practice*, 21, 97–102.

Bellg, A.J., Borrelli, B., Resnick, B., et al. (2004) Enhancing treatment fidelity in health behavior change studies: Best practices and recommendations from the NIH behavior change consortium. *Health Psychology*, 23, 443–451.

Benson, H., Sabater-Hernández, D., Benrimoj, S.I., & Williams, K.A. (2018) Piloting the integration of non-dispensing pharmacists in the Australian general practice setting: A process evaluation. *International Journal of Integrated Care*, 18(2), 1–10.

Berkel, C., Gallo, C.G., Sandler, I.N., et al. (2019) Redesigning implementation measurement for monitoring and quality improvement in community delivery settings. *The Journal of Primary Prevention*, 40, 111–127.

Biron, C., Gatrell, C., & Cooper, C. L. (2010) Autopsy of a failure: Evaluating process and contextual issues in an organizational-level work stress intervention. *International Journal of Stress Management*, 17(2), 135–158.

Biron, C., Ivers, H., & Brun, J.-P. (2016) Capturing the active ingredients of multicomponent participatory organizational stress interventions using an adapted study design. *Stress and Health*, 32, 275–284.

Brand, S.L., Callahan, L., Quinn, C., et al. (2019) Building programme theory is to develop rare adoptable & scalable complex interventions: Realist formative process evaluation prior to full trial. *Evaluation*, 25(2), 149–170.

Carroll, C., Patterson, M., Wood, S., et al. (2007) A conceptual framework for implementation fidelity. *Implementation Science*, 2, 40.

Cheng, K.K.F. & Metcalfe, A. (2018) Qualitative methods and process evaluation in clinical trials context: Where to head to? *International Journal of Qualitative Methods*, 17, 1–4.

Craig, P., Dieppe, P., Macintyre, S., et al. (2008) Developing and evaluating complex interventions: The new Medical Research Council guidance. *BMJ*, 337, a1655–1660.

Dalkin, S.M., Greenhalgh, J., Jones, D., Cunningham, B., & Lhussier, M. (2015) What's in a mechanism? Development of a key concept in realist evaluation. *Implementation Science*, 10, 49–55.

De Vlaming, R., Haveman-Nies, A., Veer, P., & de Groot, L.G.P.G.M (2010) Evaluation design for a complex intervention program targeting loneliness in non-institutionalized elderly Dutch people. *BMC Public Health*, 10, 552–560.

Den Bakker, C.M., Huirne, J.A.F., Schaafsma, F.G., et al. (2019) Electronic health program to empower patients in returning to normal activities after colorectal surgical procedures: Mixed-methods process evaluation alongside a randomized controlled trial. *Journal of Medical Internet Research*, 21(1), e10674.

Dillon, L., Clemson, L., Coxon, K., & Keay, L. (2018) Understanding the implementation and efficacy of a home-based strength and balance fall prevention intervention in people aged 50 years or over with vision impairment: A process evaluation protocol. *BMC Health Services Research*, 18, 512–519.

Evans, R., Scourfield, J., & Murphy, S. (2015) Pragmatic, formative process evaluation of comples interventions and why we need more of them. *Journal of Epidemiology & Community Health*, 69, 925–926.

Fletcher, A., Jamal, F., Moore, G., et al. (2016) Realist complex intervention science: Applying realist principles across all phases of the Medical Research Council framework for developing and evaluating complex intervention. *Evaluation*, 22(3), 286–303.

Foley, L., Mhurchu, C.N., Marsh, S., et al. (2016). Screen time weight-loss intervention targeting children at home (SWITCH): Process evaluation of a randomised controlled trial intervention. *BMC Public Health*, 16, 9–24.

Fridrich, A., Jenny, G.J., & Bauer, G.F. (2015) The context, process and outcome evaluation model for organisational health interventions. *BioMed Research International*, 2015, 414832.

Furness, C., Howard, E., Limb, E., et al. (2018) Relating process evaluation measures to complex intervention outcomes: Findings from the PACE-UP primary care pedometer based walking trial. *Trials*, 19, 58–65.

Grant, A., Treweek, S., Dreischulte, T., Foy, R., & Guthrie, B. (2013) Process evaluation for cluster-randomized trials of complex interventions: A proposed framework for design and reporting. *Trials*, 14, 15–24.

Griffin, T.L., Pallan, M.J., Clarke, J.L., et al., and on behalf of the WAVES study trial investigators (2014) Process evaluation design in a cluster randomised controlled childhood obesity prevention trial: The WAVES study. *International Journal of Behavioral Nutrition and Physical Activity*, 11, 112–123.

Hansen, A.B.G. & Jones, A. (2017) Advancing "real world" trials that take accont of social context and human volition. *Trials*, 18, 531–533.

Hasson, H., Blomberg, S., & Dunér, A. (2012) Fidelity and moderating factors in complex interventions: A case study of a continuum of care program for frail elderly people in health and social care. *Implementation Science*, 7, 23–32.

Haynes, A., Brennan, S., Canter, S., et al, & the CIPHER team (2014) Protocol for the process evaluation of a complex intervention designed to increase the use of research in health policy and program organizations (the SPIRIT study). *Implementation Science*, 9, 113–124.

Hogue, A. & Dauber, S. (2013) Assessing fidelity to evidence-based practices in usual care: The example of family therapy for adolescent behaviour problems. *Evaluation and Program Planning*, 27, 21–30.

Krauss, A. (2018) Why all randomized controlled trials produce biased results. *Annals of Medicine*, 50(4), 312–322.

Kyle, S.D., Morgan, K., Spiegelhalder, K., & Espie, C.A. (2011) No pain, no gain: An exploratory within-subjects mixed-method evaluation of the patient experience of sleep restriction therapy (SRT) for insomnia. *Sleep Medicine*, 12, 735–747.

Mars, T., Ellard, D., Carnes, D., et al. (2013) Fidelity in complex behaviour change interventions: A standardized approach to evaluate intervention integrity. *BMJ Open*, 3, e003555.

Masterson-Algar, P., Burton, C.R., Rycroft-Malone, J., Sackley, C.M., & Walker, M.F. (2014) Towards a programme theory for fidelity in the evaluation of complex interventions. *Journal of Evaluation in Clinical Practice*, 20, 445–452.

Masterson-Algar, P., Burton, C.R., & Rycroft-Malone, J. (2016) A mixed-evidence synthesis review of process evaluations in neurological rehabilitation: Recommendations for future research. *BMJ Open*, 6, e013002.

Masterson-Algar, P., Burton, C.R., & Rycroft-Malone, J. (2018) The generation of consensus guidelines for carrying out process evaluations in rehabilitation research. *BMC Medical Research Methodology*, 18, 180–190.

May, C.R., Johnson, M., & Finch, T. (2016) Implementation, context and complexity. *Implementation Science*, 11, 141–152.

Medical Research Council [MRC] (2019) *Guidance for evaluating complex intervention*. The authors, UK.

Mohr, D.C., Schueller, S.M., Riley, W.T., et al. (2015) Trials of intervention principles: Evaluation methods for evolving behavioral intervention technologies. *Journal of Medical Internet Research*, 17, e166.

Moore, G.F., Audrey, S., Barker, M., et al. (2015) Process evaluation of complex interventions: Medical Research Council guidance. *BMJ*, 350, h1258.

Morgan-Trimmer, S. (2015) Improving process evaluations of health behavior interventions: Learning from the social sciences. *Evaluation & the Health Professions*, 38(3), 295–314.

Nam, C.S., Ross, A., Ruggiero, C., et al. (2019) Process evaluation and lessons learned from engaging local policymakers in the B'More healthy communities for kids trial. *Health Education Behavior*, 46(1), 15–23.

Nielson, K. & Abildgaard, J.S. (2013) Organizational interventions: A research-based framework for the evaluation of both process and effects. *Work and Stress*, 27(3), 278–297.

Nielson, K., Randall, R., & Albertsen, K. (2007) Participants' appraisal of process issues and the effect of stress management interventions. *Journal of Organizational Behavior*, 28, 793–810.

Nordin, S., Elf, M., McKee, K., & Wijk, H. (2015. Assessing the physical environment of older people's residential care facilities: Development of the Swedish version of the Sheffield care environment assessment matrix (S-SCEAM). *BMC Geriatrics*, 15, 3.

Nurjono, M., Shrestha, P., Lee, A., et al. (2018) Realist evaluation of a complex integrated care programme: Protocol for a mixed methods study. *BMJ Open*, 8, e01711.

Pawson, R. & Manzano-Santaella, A., (2012) A realist diagnostic workshop. *Evaluation*, 18(2), 176–191.

Planas, L.G. (2008) Intervention design, implementation and evaluation. *American Journal of Health-System Pharmacy*, 65, 1854–1863.

Poston, L., Briley, A.L., Barr, S., et al. (2013) Developing a complex intervention for diet and activity behavior change in obese pregnant women (the UPBEAT trial); assessment of behavioral change and process evaluation in a pilot randomised controlled trial. *BMC Pregnancy and Childbirth*, 13, 148–165.

Ruikes, F.G.H., Meys, A.R.M., van de Wetering, G., et al. (2012) The care well-primary care program: Design of a cluster controlled trails and process evaluation of a complex intervention targeting community-dwelling frail elderly. *BMC Family Practice*, 13, 115–123.

Rycroft-Malone, J., Seers, K., Eldh, A.C., et al. (2018) A realist process evaluation within the facilitating implementation of research evidence (FIRE) cluster randomised controlled international trial: An exemplar. *Implementation Science*, 13, 138–152.

Sharma, S., Adetora, O.O., Vilder, M., et al. (2017) A process evaluation plan for assessing a complex community-based maternal health intervention in Ogun state, Nigeria. *BMC Health Services Research*, 17, 238–247.

Sidani, S. & Epstein, D.R. (2016) Toward a conceptualization and operationalization of satisfaction with non-pharmacological interventions. *Research & Theory for Nursing Practice: An International Journal*, 30(3), 242–257.

Sidani, S., Epstein, D.R., & Fox, M. (2017) Psychometric evaluation of a multi-dimensional measure of satisfaction with behavioral interventions. *Research in Nursing & Health*, 40(5), 459–469.

Siddiqui, N., Gorard, S., & See, B.H. (2018) The importance of process evaluation for randomised control trials in education. *Educational Research*, 60(3), 357–370.

Smith, J.D. & Hasan, M. (2020) Quantitative approaches for the evaluation of implementation research studies. *Psychiatry Research*, 283, 112521.

Sorensen, J. & Llamas, J.D. (2018) Process evaluation of a community outpatient program treating substance use disorders. *Journal of Community Psychology*, 46(7), 844–855.

Sridharan, S. & Nakaima, A. (2012) Towards an evidence base of theory-driven evaluations: Some questions for proponents of theory-driven evaluation. *Evaluation*, 18(3), 378–395.

Steckler, A. & Linnan, L. (eds) (2002) *Process Evaluation for Public Health Interventions and Research*. Jossey-Bass, San Francisco.

Tama, E., Molyneux, S., Waweru, E., et al. (2018) Examining the implementation of the free maternity services policy in Kenya: A mixed methods process evaluation. *International Journal of Health Policy and Management*, 7(7), 603–613.

Van Belle, S., Wong, G., Westhorp, G., et al. (2016) Can "realist" randomised controlled trials be genuinely realist? *Trials*, 17, 313–318.

van Bruinessen, I.R., van Weel-Baumgarten, E.M., Gouw, H., Zijlstra, J.M., & van Dulmen, S. (2016) An integrated process and outcome evaluation of a web-based communication tool for patients with malignant lymphoma: Randomized controlled trial. *Journal of Medical Internet Research*, 18(7), 14–23.

Van de Glind, I., Bunn, C., Gray, C.M., et al. (2017) The intervention process in the European fans in training (EuroFIT) trial: A mixed method protocol for evaluation. *Trials*, 18, 356–369.

van den Branden, S., Van den Broucke, S., Leroy, R., Declerck, D., & Happenbrouwers, K. (2015) Evaluating the implementation fidelity of a multicomponent intervention for oral health promotion in preschool children. *Preventive Science*, 16, 1–10.

Verwey, R., van der Weegen, S., Spreeuwenberg, M., et al. (2016) Process evaluation of physical activity counseling with and without the use of mobile technology: A mixed methods study. *International Journal of Nursing Studies*, 53, 3–16.

Walton, H., Spector, A., Tombor, I., & Michie, S. (2017) Measures of fidelity of delivery of, and engagement with, complex, face-to-face health behaviour change interventions: A systematic review of measure quality. *British Journal of Health Psychology*, 22, 872–903.

Wells, M., Williams, B., Treweek, S., Coyle, J., & Taylor, J. (2012) Intervention description is not enough: Evidence from an in-depth multiple case study on the untold role an impact of context in randomised controlled trials of seven complex interventions. *Trials*, 13, 95–111.

Wilkerson, A.H., Bridges, C.N., Wu, C., et al. (2019) Process evaluation of the BearStand behavioral intervention: A social cognitive theory-based approach to reduce occupational sedentary behavior. *Journal of Occupational and Environmental Medicine*, 61(11), 927–935.

Wong, G., Greenhalgh, T., Westhorp, G., & Pawson, R., (2012) Realist methods in medical education research: What are they & what can they contribute? *Medical Education*, 46, 89–96.

# CHAPTER 14

# Outcome Evaluation: Designs

Outcome evaluation focuses on determining the causal effects of health interventions on the hypothesized ultimate outcomes. The goal is to demonstrate the benefits of interventions in addressing the health problem and in improving general health and well-being in the target client population. As explained in Chapter 10, causal effects imply that the interventions' active ingredients are solely and uniquely responsible for producing the improvement in the ultimate outcomes observed after implementation of the interventions. Thus, changes in the outcomes are attributable, with confidence, to the intervention and not to any other factor that may be operating in the context of intervention delivery such as the characteristics of clients and of their life environment. Logic, intervention theory, experience, and evidence indicate that a range of factors may influence the effects of health interventions on the ultimate outcomes (Cao et al., 2014); therefore, the factors present plausible alternative explanations of the interventions' effects.

There are two general approaches for handling these factors. The first involves an experimental control. The control consists of eliminating or minimizing the potential influence of the factors; it is accomplished by incorporating some features into the design of the evaluation study, as is advocated for examining the efficacy of an intervention. The experimental or the randomized controlled or clinical trial (RCT) design has been considered the most reliable design for determining the efficacy of health interventions (Anglemyer et al., 2014). The second approach entails an account of the factors and investigation of their influence on the intervention's effects. This is usually done by testing the intervention's effects under real-world conditions that represent variability in the factors and in clients' perceptions and responses to the intervention. Relevant data are collected to determine what factors, in addition to or in combination with the intervention, contribute to the ultimate outcomes, as is advocated for examining the effectiveness of interventions. Although the RCT is still considered appropriate, other experimental and non-experimental designs are suggested (Medical Research Council, 2019), and have been found suitable for examining effectiveness.

In this chapter, the features of the conventional RCT design are described; the pathways through which its features control for factors and improve the validity of inferences regarding the causal effects of an intervention are explained. Yet, these

*Nursing and Health Interventions: Design, Evaluation, and Implementation*, Second Edition.
Souraya Sidani and Carrie Jo Braden.
© 2021 John Wiley & Sons Ltd. Published 2021 by John Wiley & Sons Ltd.

same features and the assumptions underlying them are being questioned in light of cumulating evidence indicating the vulnerability of the RCT design to biases that weaken the validity of inferences regarding the causal effects of interventions. The limitations of the RCT design are delineated, supported by relevant empirical evidence. Alternative experimental and nonexperimental designs are presented for examining the effectiveness of health interventions under real-world conditions. The features, advantages or strengths, and disadvantages or limitations of these designs are discussed relative to how they overcome the limitations of the RCT.

## 14.1   TRADITIONAL RCT DESIGN

The traditional experimental or RCT design is considered the most reliable, even the "gold standard" for determining the causal effects (efficacy and effectiveness) of a health intervention on the ultimate outcomes (Winter & Colditz, 2014). The ascribed "high status" emanates from the features of the RCT that are believed to eliminate or minimize the influence of factors (other than the intervention) on the outcomes. The factors reflect the characteristics of clients, interventionists, and contexts; the delivery of the intervention; and the assessment of outcomes. The experimental control of these factors is posited to reduce their likelihood as plausible alternative explanations of the changes in the ultimate outcomes observed post treatment. Ruling out alternative plausible explanations is the most important criterion for inferring causality (see Chapter 10). Therefore, the control increases the confidence in attributing the changes in outcomes to the intervention. The main features of the RCT are careful selection of clients, random assignment to treatment conditions, blinding and concealment of treatment allocation, manipulation of treatment delivery, and outcome assessment and analysis.

### 14.1.1   Careful Selection of Clients

Clients are carefully selected to ensure enrollment of participants that are representative of the target population; yet, the participants should not have characteristics that are known or hypothesized (in the intervention theory) to affect engagement and enactment of treatment, and to confound the intervention effects (i.e. have unique and direct associations with the outcomes). Careful selection is achieved by prespecifying a set of inclusion and exclusion criteria, assessing the criteria with appropriate measures, and ascertaining that participants meet all eligibility criteria prior to exposure to treatment. The inclusion criteria ensure that participants in the RCT belong to the target client population and experience the health problem in a way that is amenable to treatment by the intervention under evaluation. Therefore, the inclusion criteria are delineated to represent the characteristics of the target client population in terms of:

1. The *experience of the health problem* addressed by the intervention under evaluation, and not only a particular medical or health condition. Many health problems are experienced in a comparable way across medical conditions. Clients are deemed eligible if they report having the indicators, level of severity, and determinants of the health problem that are specified in the intervention theory as amenable to change by the intervention. For instance, clients with different medical conditions (e.g. cancer, cardiac disease) experience insomnia

as difficulty falling or staying asleep and would be eligible if they report one or both difficulties for at least 30 minutes per night, for at least 3 nights per week, over at least 3 months; these are the indicators of insomnia.

2. *Personal characteristics* required to participate in treatment such as proficiency in the language in which treatment is provided and the outcomes are measured, and intact cognitive function. Both characteristics are necessary for understanding the treatment.

3. *Sociodemographic characteristics* that also define the target client population such as age, gender, culture or ethnicity, or residence in a particular geographic area.

The exclusion criteria are used to control for clients' characteristics that are hypothesized in the intervention theory (see Chapter 5) to interfere with participants' engagement and enactment of the intervention, and/or to be directly associated with the ultimate outcomes. The direct associations between the characteristics and the outcomes can be present irrespective of exposure to treatment and are illustrated by the well-established gender differences in the experience of depressive symptoms and the relationship between anxiety and knowledge gain. The client characteristics include personal, clinical, or health conditions (1) that may limit participants' engagement and enactment of treatment, such as limited physical functioning that prevents attendance at treatment sessions or optimal adherence to treatment recommendations; (2) for which the intervention is contraindicated, such as pregnancy during which taking a medication may not be safe; and (3) for which the intervention was found ineffective or potentially harmful; for instance, cognitive therapy alone may not be appropriate for managing insomnia associated with dysfunction in circadian rhythm. Two categories of additional exclusion criteria are preset. The first is related to concurrent treatment; the treatment is prescribed for the same health problem targeted by the intervention or for comorbid conditions. Participants are excluded if they are receiving a treatment or if their healthcare providers are unable or unwilling to stop or keep constant the type and dose of concurrent treatment during the trial period. The concurrent treatment can confound or moderate (i.e. strengthen or weaken) the effects of the experimental intervention on the ultimate outcomes, in particular outcomes reflecting resolution of the health problem. The second category is related to clients' tendency for noncompliance. It is assessed during a run-in-period, prior to exposure to treatment. Participants who do not comply with a task (e.g. completing a diary) are excluded in order to minimize variability in their adherence to treatment and consequently, in their level of improvement in the ultimate outcomes.

The selection of participants on the basis of strict eligibility criteria is believed to "guarantee" the exclusion of participants with potentially confounding characteristics. It results in the inclusion of participants who are homogeneous in terms of their experience of the health problem and their personal and health or clinical profiles. The homogeneity of the sample is expected to contribute to the comparability of participants in the experimental intervention group and the comparison treatment group on all characteristics and outcomes measured at baseline or pretest. Participants assigned to each treatment group are also expected to exhibit comparable responses to the allocated treatment. Participants assigned to the experimental group and having similar baseline profile are all expected to show a similar pattern of improvement in the ultimate outcomes; that is, they report change in the outcome of the same direction and amount or level, following delivery of the intervention.

Participants assigned to the comparison group and having a similar baseline profile are all expected to exhibit no change in the outcomes. The comparability in the baseline profile is a means for controlling the potential influence of clients' characteristics on their responses to treatment; the influence is minimized because these characteristics are constant. Furthermore, the comparability of participants' pattern of change in the ultimate outcomes, within each of the experimental group and the comparison group, reduces the individual variability in the level of outcomes achieved post treatment. When the posttest outcomes are compared between the two groups, the difference in the groups' means is larger (which is the numerator in the formula for the independent sample $t$-test or $F$-test) than the within-group variability (that reflects differences across individuals within groups and is the denominator in the formula for the $t$-test and $F$-test). Thus, the large between-to-within group ratio (i.e. $t$-test or $F$-test) increases the power to detect significant intervention effects. The effects can be confidently attributed to the intervention because the groups are similar in their baseline profile, which controls for the potential confounding influence of client characteristics on the ultimate outcomes.

## 14.1.2    Random Assignment

Random assignment or randomization is the hallmark of the experimental or RCT design. It is the feature believed to "ensure or guarantee" the comparability of the baseline profile of participants allocated to the experimental intervention and the comparison treatment groups. Therefore, randomization controls for selection bias that induces confounding and weakens internal validity, that is, the claim that the observed improvement in the ultimate outcomes is solely attributed to the intervention (Borglin & Richards, 2010; Sidani, 2015).

Randomization involves the application of chance-based procedures (see Chapter 15 for details) for allocating participants to the experimental intervention and the comparison treatment groups. The chance-based procedures eliminate human influence, whether unconscious or deliberate, on assignment to group. Humans (e.g. researchers or health professionals) may interfere with the assignment. For instance, researchers favoring the experimental intervention have a tendency to assign to the experimental intervention, participants who are fit and have great potentials to benefit from the intervention. This pattern of assignment compromises the comparability of the study groups on baseline profiles.

Randomization is believed to enhance the comparability of participants in the experimental and the comparison groups on all measured and unmeasured characteristics, before treatment delivery (Donovan et al., 2018). It leads to a situation in which participants with given characteristics assigned to one group will, on the average, be counterbalanced by participants with similar or the same characteristics assigned to the other group (Cook & Campbell, 1979). This translates into an even or balanced distribution of participants in the experimental intervention and the comparison treatment groups, with similar characteristics that may influence engagement and enactment of treatment or that may be associated with the ultimate outcomes. This comparability at baseline is believed to yield two situations. First, it holds client characteristics constant between groups. Therefore, the characteristics cannot contribute to participants' responses to treatment, which increases the confidence in attributing the observed effects solely to the intervention. Second, the comparability reduces the individual variability in the outcomes assessed post treatment within each group. The low variability in posttest outcomes increases the power to detect significant intervention effects.

### 14.1.3 Blinding and Concealment of Treatment Allocation

Blinding (also called masking) entails concealing or not disclosing the nature (whether experimental or comparison) of the treatments included in the RCT to those involved in the trial. These include research staff (i.e. data collectors and interventionists if possible), participants, and health professionals assisting in referring their clients. Blinding requires that the treatments are comparable; they should have the same structure, mode, and dose of delivery, and should be not labeled as experimental or control (Sil et al., 2019; Wartolowska et al., 2018). Rather, the treatments are referred to by their respective label such as sleep education and stimulus control therapy for insomnia; they are described as different strategies that put emphasis on slightly different ways of addressing the health problem (e.g. McCurry et al., 2014) in all study documents and in particular, the consent information form.

Blinding minimizes biases associated with perceptions and reactions to treatments that have the potential to affect the validity of inferences regarding the causal effects of the intervention. Blinding is believed to reduce the following biases: performance bias which is associated with the attention provided to participants in the intervention group, ascertainment or detection bias which is related to knowledge of the treatment that influences judgment in outcome assessment, co-treatment bias where participants in the comparison treatment group seek additional treatment outside the trial, crossover from one treatment group to another, and attrition from treatment or study (Probst et al., 2019; Renjith, 2017; Wartolowska et al., 2018).

Several pathways explain the impact of nonblinding. Participants may perceive the experimental intervention favorably that is, desirable and helpful. If not assigned to this intervention, they may react negatively resulting in attrition, nonengagement and nonenactment of the allocated treatment, resulting in less-than-optimal improvement in the ultimate outcomes. Health professionals' awareness of the treatments under evaluation could affect their decision to refer their clients to the RCT, potentially influencing the size of the sampling pool. If clients enroll in the trial, health professionals' knowledge of the treatment to which their clients (participating in the RCT) are allocated may hold favorable or unfavorable views of that treatment; they may discuss the trial treatment with participants and nudge them to continue or withdraw from treatment, respectively. In addition, health professionals may alter their assessment of participants' condition (e.g. heightened sensitivity toward side effects) and their interactions with participants (e.g. prompting participants for experiences of side effects). This in turn, influences participants' behaviors in the RCT (e.g. withdrawal, adherence to treatment) and responses to the allocated treatment. Research staff who are aware of which treatment is the experimental may be biased in outcome data collection and analysis. They may be tempted to observe and report improvement in the outcomes in the experimental group more so than the comparison group, and to modify the analysis plan to show that the intervention is effective. All these perceptions and reactions could confound the intervention effects and result in their biased (under or over) estimates (Sidani, 2015). Blinding is believed to mitigate these biases.

Concealment of treatment allocation means nondisclosing or hiding the randomization scheme from research staff involved in participant assignment and health professionals referring clients to the RCT. Concealment is done to eliminate research staff's and professionals' potential influence on the assignment of participants to the experimental intervention and the comparison treatment groups. Research staff and health professionals may engage in what is depicted as "gaming the system" in order to allocate participants to a particular treatment they view as most appropriate in addressing the individual participant's needs. For instance, research staff may delay assignment of a participant in need of an active treatment that she or he cannot afford elsewhere (Streiner & Sidani, 2015). This pattern of assignment could compromise the comparability on baseline characteristics, of participants allocated to the experimental intervention and the comparison treatment groups. Between-group differences in characteristics introduce confounding and biased estimates of the intervention effects. Concealment of treatment allocation is best maintained by entrusting the randomization scheme to a central office.

### 14.1.4    Manipulation of Treatment Delivery

Manipulation of treatment delivery involves controlling the context and the actual provision of the experimental intervention and the comparison treatment.

Controlling the context of delivery is achieved through:

The *selection of the setting* in which the experimental intervention and the comparison treatment are delivered. The setting is selected on the basis of physical, psychosocial, and/or political features, hypothesized in the intervention theory to facilitate the delivery of the intervention. Factors that may interfere with the provision of the intervention are eliminated or maintained constant across participants over the treatment delivery period. For instance, the room temperature is kept at the same level when having participants listen to relaxing music in order to minimize potential physical discomfort that affects the achievement of the intended outcome of decreased anxiety. It is believed that providing the experimental intervention and the comparison treatment in the same setting eliminates or minimizes the influence of setting on the delivery and the effects of the intervention.

The *selection and training of interventionists* for delivering the treatments. Interventionists are selected on the basis of clearly specified personal qualities and professional qualifications and intensively trained in the theoretical underpinning and the practical skills required for delivering the treatments. Interventionists are also instructed to give the treatments in a standard and consistent way across participants in order to enhance fidelity of treatment delivery. They are encouraged to maintain the same style of interpersonal interactions and the same demeanor with all participants in order to standardize the nature and level of therapeutic relationship or working alliance. The standardization of interactions is expected to minimize their influence on outcomes.

The *selection and training of research staff* in the study protocol and the interaction with participants. The purpose of training is to maintain high-quality performance of research activities, in particular data collection. Staff are encouraged to be consistent in the manner in which they behave and communicate with participants. Staff are not informed of the RCT hypotheses, the nature of the experimental and comparison treatments, and participants' assignment to treatment, in order to ensure blinding. This is considered essential so that research staff do not develop expectancies or prejudice about treatments, that may affect their perception, observation, or judgment when collecting outcome data, particularly following treatment delivery.

Controlling the actual delivery of the experimental intervention and the comparison treatment is exerted in three ways.

The *provision of the experimental intervention* to one group and withholding it from another group of participants. This is essential to generate differences in exposure to the experimental intervention and to demonstrate differences in outcome achievement post treatment between the groups. These differences present the evidence required for demonstrating the covariation criterion of causality (Chapter 10).

The *specification and the provision of the comparison treatment*. Ideally, participants assigned to the comparison treatment group should not be exposed to any treatment—called no-treatment control condition. The no-treatment condition is required to demonstrate the covariation criterion of causality. Further, participants who may be taking a prescribed treatment to manage the health problem targeted by the experimental intervention are requested to stop taking it or to keep its dose constant throughout the RCT treatment period. Withholding or keeping constant a prescribed treatment minimizes the potential threat of co-treatment because the prescribed treatment may confound or moderate the effects of the experimental intervention on the outcomes. However, the no-treatment control condition presents an ethical dilemma when a much needed treatment is withheld. Other comparison treatments can be and have been used in RCTs (see Chapter 15) such as the placebo treatment and usual care. It is essential that the selected comparison treatment should not incorporate any of the active ingredients that characterize the experimental intervention, in order to minimize potential overlap between the experimental intervention and the comparison treatment. The overlap affects the magnitude of the between-group differences in the posttest outcomes and, hence, the power to detect significant intervention effects. That is, if participants in the comparison group are exposed to some active ingredients of the intervention, then they may experience, to some degree, improvement in the outcomes assessed at posttest. This improvement reduces the magnitude of the between-group differences and increases the variability within the comparison group resulting in nonsignificant intervention effects.

The *standardized and consistent delivery of the intervention*. The same treatment components, content, and activities comprising the intervention are given, with fidelity, in the same way and at the same dose to all participants assigned to this experimental group. Standardized and consistent delivery is expected to reduce variability in levels of exposure to the intervention, and in enactment of the treatment recommendations and subsequently, in responses to the intervention. Thus, participants are expected to demonstrate similar or same levels of improvement in the outcomes measured at posttest. With the decreased variability in posttest outcomes within the experimental group, the power to detect significant intervention effects is increased. Standardized and consistent delivery is also applicable to the comparison treatment if different from no-treatment conditions. Standardized and consistent delivery minimizes variability in levels of exposure to the comparison treatment and the potential for contamination, both of which could yield nonsignificant intervention effects.

## 14.1.5   Outcome Assessment and Analysis

In an RCT, the timing for outcome assessment is well specified relative to the delivery of the experimental intervention. The timing is the same in both the experimental intervention and the comparison treatment groups, which is critical for meeting the temporal order criterion of causality (Chapter 10). Therefore, all outcomes are measured in both groups, at the same occasions: at least once before and once after treatment is given. The outcomes assessed before treatment (baseline or pretest) serve as a reference point for comparison with the outcomes measured after treatment (posttest). The comparison over time delineates the pattern of change, that is, direction (increase, no change, decrease) and magnitude (how much) of change. The pattern of change is important to determine the extent to which participants in the experimental intervention group experience the hypothesized improvement in the outcomes, and to compare this group's changes in outcomes to the comparison treatment group's anticipated report of no changes in the outcomes. Differences in the pattern of change in the outcomes between groups represent the evidence supporting the efficacy or effectiveness of the intervention.

In an RCT, analysis of the outcome data is based on the intention or intent-to-treat principle. In intent-to-treat analysis, all participants randomized to the experimental intervention and the comparison treatment groups are included, whether or not they completed the allocated treatment or the study. As such, the comparability of the two groups (achieved through randomization) on baseline profile is maintained. The baseline comparability controls for selection bias and the influence of any potential confounding variable. To be able to conduct the analysis, outcome data are imputed for participants who withdraw, using the mean of the participants' respective group at posttest or the last observation carried forward. It is believed that the intent-to-treat analysis is the most appropriate, providing valid estimates of the causal effects of the intervention on the outcomes, because it controls for selection and confounding bias.

Traditionally, the features of the experimental or RCT design were considered the strengths of this research design, making it the most appropriate or the gold standard for outcome (efficacy and effectiveness) evaluation. The features are congruent with the conventional notion of causality that focuses on the direct association between the intervention and the outcomes. The RCT features operationalize the criteria for determining conventional causality and are expected to yield unbiased estimates of the intervention effects. However, the RCT features may not align well with the recently acknowledged notion of multicausality (Chapter 10). They are limiting in examining the effectiveness of health interventions delivered in real-world practice and in providing answers to practice-relevant questions: Who most benefit, from what intervention, given in what mode and at what dose? How does the intervention work to produce beneficial outcomes? Furthermore, cumulating experience (in designing and conducting RCTs) and empirical evidence (mainly generated through systematic reviews of RCT findings) have identified limitations of the experimental or RCT design in evaluating outcomes of health interventions.

## 14.2   LIMITATIONS OF THE TRADITIONAL RCT DESIGN

Despite its advantages in controlling for potential confounding factors and hence, in establishing a causal relationship between an intervention and the ultimate outcomes (Deaton & Cartwright, 2018; Frieden, 2017; Holm et al., 2017), the experimental or RCT design has several limitations. The limitations stem from its features that ignore the complexity of the real world, which is characterized by multicausality, heterogeneity, and flexibility. As discussed in Chapter 10, multicausality recognizes that the intervention is not the only determinant of health outcomes (Chavez-MacGregor & Giordano, 2016); rather, a range of factors, inherent in a particular context in which the intervention is delivered and related to the characteristics of participants, interventionists, setting or environment, the nature and method of delivering the intervention, influence directly the ultimate outcomes or interact with the intervention in producing the outcomes (Amaechi & Counsell, 2013; Daniel et al., 2016; Diez-Roux, 2011; Fernandez et al., 2015; Hansen & Tjørnhøj-Thomsen, 2016; Mazzuca et al., 2018; Robins & Weissman, 2016; Tarquinio et al., 2015; Vander-Weele, 2016; WanderWeele et al., 2016). Furthermore, multicausality recognizes the complexity of the mechanism of action for health interventions, whereby several specific and nonspecific processes mediate the effects of the intervention on the ultimate outcomes (Bonell et al., 2012; Fletcher et al., 2016; Midgley et al., 2014). Yet, understanding these processes is the essence of causal explanation or inference (Blackwood et al., 2010; Johnson & Schoonenboom, 2016; Villeval et al., 2016). By focusing on the direct association between the intervention and the ultimate outcomes, and by experimentally controlling for contextual factors, the traditional RCT may not be well suited to capture the complex processes contributing to the intervention's effects in the real-world context.

Heterogeneity and flexibility are other characteristics of the real world that are ignored in the RCT. The broad assumption underlying the RCT is that participants have comparable sociodemographic and health or clinical characteristics, and experience the health problem in a similar way (e.g. same level of severity). Therefore, they can all benefit from the same intervention, given in a fixed mode and dose (Mohr et al., 2015). Participants are also expected to react in a similar manner to the health intervention and to respond to it in the same or similar way. Accordingly, the focus in the RCT is on the "average" effects (Krauss, 2018). Individual variability in responses to treatment is ignored (Nahum-Shani et al., 2012) and is usually represented as "error" variance in outcome data analysis (i.e. denominator in the $t$-test or the $F$-test). The RCT findings are of limited relevance to real-world practice, where the emphasis is on client centeredness. Client centeredness involves accounting for clients' individuality, tailoring treatment to meet their individual experiences of the health problem, concerns and life circumstances, and adapting treatment on the basis of clients' observed responses to treatment (Fernandez et al., 2015; Ling, 2012; Marchal et al., 2013; Mohr et al., 2015; Reynolds et al., 2014).

Ironically, the features of the traditional RCT design reflect both its strengths and limitations. The limitations are serious enough to weaken internal validity and external validity including the meaningfulness of the RCT findings in informing practice. Conceptual arguments and relevant empirical evidence (where available) pointing to the limitations of the traditional RCT are presented next.

## 14.2.1  Careful Selection of Clients

A set of strict, stringent, or restrictive eligibility criteria is specified in the traditional RCT to control for client characteristics that could potentially influence engagement and enactment of treatment, and/or confound the intervention effects on the ultimate outcomes. The application of such criteria contributes to:

1. Reduced pool of potentially eligible clients available at a particular site or setting (e.g. in-hospital unit, health clinic, community catchment area). This necessitates an expansion of recruitment to additional sites. Differences in the characteristics of clients, health professionals, environment, and availability of human and material resources may exist among sites. If not accounted for in the RCT conduct and in the outcome analysis, the differences could influence the intervention delivery and outcomes, yielding biased overall (i.e. average) estimates of the health intervention effects.

2. Need for additional human and material resources for recruiting clients and screening a large number of clients, over a long period of time, to determine eligibility. Thus, the RCT becomes costly and time consuming (Frieden, 2017; Troxel et al., 2016), taking on average, 5.5 years to complete. The results may no longer be relevant in light of other scientific advances (Riley et al., 2013).

3. A small percentage of clients meet the eligibility criteria (Mitchell-Jones et al., 2017). This situation yields a small sample size and a sample that is not fully representative of the target client population, presenting threats to statistical conclusion and external validity, respectively. These two limitations of the traditional RCT are possible explanations for the widely reported nonreplication of the RCT findings (Bothwell et al., 2016; Rigato et al., 2017; Smeeing et al., 2017; Zeilstra et al., 2018).

Results of individual RCTs (e.g. Cha et al., 2016) and systematic reviews indicate that less than 50% of clients recruited for an RCT meet the preset eligibility criteria (e.g. Grapow et al., 2006) and the accrued sample size is, on average, small (Golfam et al., 2015). Small sample sizes reduce the power to detect significant intervention effects and yield unreliable or unstable estimates of the intervention effects (Greenhalgh et al., 2014; Golfam et al., 2015). Furthermore, the sample (small or large) accrued in an RCT is not representative of all subgroups comprising the target client population, leading to sample selection bias (Berger, 2018; Yang et al., 2017). Differences in the personal and health or clinical characteristics of participants and nonparticipants in an RCT have been reported. In general, compared with nonparticipants, participants are depicted as younger; less deprived that is, have higher education and income, and are of the dominant ethnicity (Cha et al., 2016); having fewer comorbid conditions (Chavez-MacGregor & Giordano, 2016) or being high risk (Frieden, 2017); being more motivated to get treatment for the health problem; and open to new treatment (Tarquinio et al., 2015; Troxel et al., 2016). The unrepresentativeness of the RCT samples of the target client population is additionally supported by estimates consistently indicating that less than 40% of clients seen in real-world practice meet the eligibility criteria (Hershkop et al., 2017; Shean, 2014). Accordingly, the RCT findings, based on a selective subgroup of the target client population, are of limited applicability in real-world practice, as the findings are relevant or applicable to a rather small percentage of the client population (Frieden, 2017; Horwitz et al., 2017; Leviton, 2017; Tomlison et al., 2015; Troxel et al., 2016; Woodman, 2014). Non-applicability of findings may account for the slow uptake of RCT-derived evidence in practice (Donovan et al., 2018). The limited generalizability and applicability of RCT findings is further compounded by nonconsent bias, as discussed in the next section.

### 14.2.2   Random Assignment

Although random assignment has been considered the main strength of the RCT in mitigating selection bias and controlling for potential confounding, it has been recently questioned on scientific and practical grounds. There is also evidence linking randomization to some biases, including nonconsent or nonenrollment bias and unfavorable reactions to the allocated treatment (see Chapter 11 for detail) that threaten the validity of inferences.

Scientifically, randomization does not secure valid inferences about the causal effects of the intervention on the ultimate outcomes (Hernán, 2018). Randomization increases the likelihood of the comparability between participants assigned to the experimental intervention group and the comparison treatment group, thereby minimizing selection bias. **This is all it does, nothing else**! Randomization does not prevent, address, or rule out other, equally important, biases that are introduced following randomization and that weaken the confidence in attributing the improvement in the ultimate outcomes, solely, to the intervention (Cook et al., 2010; Hernán,

2018; Krauss, 2018; West & Thoemmes, 2010). These biases include: differential attrition, contamination or crossover, non-adherence to treatment recommendations, co-treatment, interventionists' interactional style, and participants' perceptions and engagement in treatment.

Contrary to common belief, randomization does not guarantee or ensure baseline comparability on all measured and unmeasured or known and unknown characteristics of participants assigned to the experimental intervention and the comparison treatment groups, within a particular RCT, especially when the sample size is small that is, less than 1000 (Berger, 2018; Frieden, 2017; Henry et al., 2017). Accordingly, some known and many unknown factors may not be equally distributed between groups with randomization (Krauss, 2018). Some argue that any between-group differences in participants' baseline characteristics observed with randomization are due to "chance" (and not human influence or interference). The counterargument is that the characteristics showing these differences may affect participants' engagement and enactment of treatment and be directly correlated with the ultimate outcomes. Thus, even if due to chance, differences in baseline characteristics between groups result in selection bias and confound the effects of the intervention on the ultimate outcomes (Rickles, 2009). In addition, the comparability on baseline profile is anticipated, maintained, and examined at the group level, and not at the individual level. Group level comparability is determined by nonsignificant between-group differences in the personal and health or clinical characteristics measured at baseline. However, interindividual differences, within each group, in these characteristics are not controlled with randomization. The interindividual differences are represented in large within-group variance. They can still operate by affecting participants' engagement and enactment of treatment, and experience of improvement in the ultimate outcomes at posttest. The latter point is supported by evidence from two reviews (Heinsman & Shadish, 1996; Sidani, 2006). The reviews' results showed a significant, low-moderate, positive correlation between the effect sizes for outcomes measured at pretest and the effect sizes for the same outcomes measured at posttest. This correlation suggests that baseline variables continue to exert their influence on the outcomes, despite randomization. This point resurged in the literature; Liu and Maxwell (2020) explained that the amount of change in the outcomes is proportional to the baseline values.

At the practical level, randomization is not acceptable to clients. It does not reflect how treatment is provided in practice: treatment is given to meet individual experiences of the health problem and after careful consideration of alternative treatments. As mentioned in Chapter 11, clients participating in an RCT may have preferences for the treatments they view as acceptable. Clients resent randomization as it deprives them their right to actively engage in treatment decision-making and from getting the treatment they desire. This unfavorable perception of randomization contributes to participants' decision to:

1. Not enroll in an RCT, resulting in nonconsent bias or sample selection bias. Clients who are reluctant or refuse randomization and have strong preferences decline participation in the RCT (Sidani et al., 2017). Along with strict eligibility criteria, participants' acceptance of randomization yield a sample that is un-representative of the target client population, limiting the generalizability and applicability of RCT findings to practice (Mitchell-Jones et al., 2017; Mustafa, 2015; Younge et al., 2015).

2. Withdraw from the RCT, resulting in attrition. Attrition reduces the sample size and the power to detect significant intervention effects. Differential attrition introduces confounding (see Chapter 11 for details).

3. Not engage and enact the allocated treatment, resulting in less-than-optimal adherence to treatment. Low engagement and adherence are associated with low levels of improvement in the outcomes and underestimation of the intervention effects.

4. Crossover from the comparison treatment to the experimental treatment group, or seek treatment outside the RCT, resulting in contamination and co-treatment bias, respectively (Younge et al., 2015).

Evidence from several recent meta-analyses that compared the effect sizes for the same intervention, given to the same target client population, obtained in RCT and nonrandomized (e.g. observational) studies, consistently indicates convergence in findings across research designs. The estimated effects reported in RCTs were not significantly different from those found in nonrandomized studies (Anglemyer et al., 2014; Finch et al., 2016; Golfam et al., 2015; Mallard et al., 2016; Nelms & Castel, 2016; Rigato et al., 2017; Smeeing et al., 2017; Soni et al., 2019; Tang et al., 2016). This evidence suggests that well-designed nonrandomized studies that minimize or appropriately account for biases produce results that approximate those of RCTs. Therefore, the important role traditionally ascribed to randomization in ensuring high internal validity and unbiased estimates of the intervention effects, is questionable (Golfam et al., 2015), which led Krauss (2018) to warn again "blind faith" in RCT as they are fallible.

### 14.2.3   Blinding and Concealment of Allocation

Blinding and concealment of allocation may not be feasible in RCTs evaluating health interventions, especially when the comparison treatment is not comparable to the experimental intervention. The noncomparability is obvious when the comparison treatment is a no-treatment control (Younge et al., 2015). The latter treatment condition may not be structurally equivalent to the experimental intervention (see Chapter 15). Even when blinding is possible, it is difficult to maintain once the allocated treatment (whether pharmacological or nonpharmacological) is delivered (Tarquinio et al., 2015). Participants are active agents, capable of interpreting their experiences, making decisions and taking actions. They are able to monitor their experience of the health problem and to correctly guess the treatment they receive, either independently or in collaboration with their healthcare providers (Berger, 2018; Kowalski & Mrdjenovich, 2013). Participants who receive the experimental intervention experience improvement in the health problem and other health outcomes. They may also experience possible side effects associated with the intervention. Participants exposed to the comparison treatment do not experience changes in the health problem. Three systematic reviews (Baethge et al., 2013; Broadbent et al., 2011; Hróbjartsson et al., 2007) examined trials that reported on the success of blinding by asking participants to guess the treatment received. Overall, the findings showed that blinding was unsuccessful in less than 45% of the trials included in the reviews. Baethge et al. (2013) and Broadbent et al. (2011) reported that up to two-thirds of participants assigned to the experimental intervention or the placebo treatment correctly guessed the treatment they received. Further, the evidence on the effects of blinding and concealment is inconsistent. Whereas the findings of systematic reviews (Hróbjartsson et al., 2014; Probst et al., 2019; Saltaji et al., 2018) show that lack of client and healthcare provider blinding was associated with large estimates of the interventions' effects, the results of a review of meta-epidemiologic studies (i.e. review of systematic reviews and meta-analyses) indicated that blinding (or lack of) affected, to a little extent, the estimates of the interventions' effects (Page et al., 2016). The evidence questions the utility of blinding in evaluating a range of health interventions.

### 14.2.4  Manipulation of Treatment Delivery

The nature of the experimental intervention, the type of comparison treatment, and the control exerted in delivering both treatments in an RCT are different from what is offered and what happens in real-world practice. The differences may be grave, rendering the trial findings of no clinical relevance (Johnson & Schoonenboom, 2016).

The *nature of the experimental intervention*: Health interventions evaluated in a traditional RCT are usually discrete, composed of specific active ingredients. They are provided either in isolation of (i.e. participants are asked to stop other prescribed treatments) or on top of other prescribed treatments, to all participants (i.e. regardless of their individual experience of the health problem, concerns and life circumstances), in a standardized way and in fixed mode and dose. Such interventions are described as "unrealistic" (Hernán et al., 2013) and hence, challenging, if not impossible, to integrate in real-world practice. Real-world context is characterized by flexibility: the norm is the provision, by multiple health professionals, of different yet complementary treatments that are selected and tailored to the individual clients' characteristics, and further adapted (in terms of type, mode, and dose) in light of individual responses to treatment. The traditional RCT is ill-suited to evaluate the outcomes of adaptive interventions (Nahum-Shani et al., 2020).

The *type of comparison treatment*: In an RCT, a comparison treatment is included. The capacity of the intervention in inducing the hypothesized changes in the ultimate outcomes is inferred from comparing the posttest outcomes between the experimental intervention and the comparison treatment groups, a situation that is not afforded in real-world practice. In practice, the effectiveness of treatment is examined through within-person comparison over time. Thus, participants serve as their own control as the responses to treatment are individual and dependent on personal baseline profile (Frieden, 2017; Johnson & Schoonenboom, 2016; Liu & Maxwell, 2020). In addition, the comparison treatment in a traditional RCT is typically a no-treatment or placebo treatment. These two types of comparison treatments may introduce biases associated with participants' reactions to treatment. Those allocated to no-treatment or placebo treatment may be disappointed and dissatisfied, and therefore, may withdraw from the trial and seek treatment outside the RCT. Alternatively, clients allocated to the no-treatment or placebo treatment react negatively, expressed as worsening outcomes at posttest. All reactions contribute to biased (under or over) estimates of the intervention effects (Chemla & Hennessy, 2016; Horwitz et al., 2017).

In addition, results indicating that health interventions are more effective than no-treatment or placebo treatment are of limited relevance to practice, because these comparison treatments are not viable options in practice, except where no-treatment watchful waiting or monitoring is an appropriate option (as in early stage prostate cancer). Health professionals and policy makers want information on the comparative effectiveness of different active treatments, that is, how does the new intervention fare in comparison to available treatments in current use, before integrating it in practice.

The *delivery of intervention*: In a traditional RCT, the intervention is provided by carefully selected and intensively trained interventionists. They strictly adhere to the manual in order to deliver treatment in a standardized manner and with fidelity, in a context that has all required material and human resources. Thus, the intervention is delivered in a rigid way and the focus is on isolating its causal effects on the ultimate outcomes, disregarding the potential influence of the context of delivery (Bradley et al., 2009; Leviton, 2017; Shean, 2014; Tomlison et al., 2015).

This is in contrast with the delivery of interventions in practice. In real-world practice, interventions are delivered by health professionals with varying personal qualities and professional qualifications, who often receive brief, mainly didactic training (due to time constraints). Health professionals differ in their acceptability of the intervention, competency in delivering the intervention, ability to initiate and maintain a good rapport with clients, and interpersonal style. They also vary in their success in clearly relaying treatment-related information to clients and in motivating clients to engage in treatment and enact the treatment recommendations. The influence of interventionists or health professionals on the outcomes is well documented, accounting for 69% of the variance in the outcomes of psychotherapy (Mulder et al., 2018). Ignoring interventionists' influence in an RCT yields biased results and estimates of the intervention effects (see Chapter 8).

In practice, interventions must be tailored to fit the individual clients' characteristics and life circumstances. Further, interventions are provided in a flexible manner that is responsive to the clients' changing condition. Standardized interventions are not compatible with the demands of real-world practice. Thus, the experimental control over intervention delivery restricts the type of health interventions to evaluate in a traditional RCT; the interventions in an RCT are usually standardized (Shean, 2014; Tarquinio et al., 2015).

In practice, interventions have to be adapted to fit the physical, sociocultural and political features, as well as the human and material resources available in a particular setting. Nondisclosure of these features and resources, and not accounting for their direct and indirect impact on the outcomes limit efforts to integrate the intervention in practice, appropriate adaptation of the intervention (without affecting its active ingredients), and understanding how the intervention works. Ignoring the influence of context contributes to nonreplication of the intervention effects across research or practice settings (Van Belle et al., 2016). Lastly, interventions are given in conjunction with other treatments that clients need. The latter treatments may interact with the intervention in that they may strengthen or weaken the intervention's effects. Eliminating or ignoring treatment interactions is not useful in fully informing treatment decision-making in practice.

### 14.2.5   Outcome Assessment and Analysis

In a traditional RCT, the ultimate outcomes are assessed before and after intervention delivery; follow-up assessments are scheduled at regular intervals, usually over a rather short time period (one to two years on average). The short term follow-up precludes the assessment of the durability of the intervention effects (Frieden, 2017) and of the safety of the long term use of the intervention. The outcome analysis focuses on the direct association between the intervention and each of the hypothesized ultimate outcomes; it is concerned with group-level comparison; and it follows the intent-to-treat principle. The results of such analysis may be biased and of limited relevance to practice.

The direct association between the intervention and the ultimate outcomes disregards the mechanism of action. This limits the understanding of how the intervention works and what exactly contributed to the ultimate outcomes. Thus, the results fail to address questions of scientific and clinical importance: How does the intervention work and what causal mechanisms operate, where and when (Byrne, 2013). Answers to these questions are essential to inform the refinement, delivery and evaluation of the intervention in research and practice, and to guide decision-making in practice (Van Belle et al., 2016). Furthermore, the direct effects of the intervention on the ultimate outcomes should be carefully interpreted. Consistent with the intervention theory and the hypothesized indirect relationship, the direct effects of the intervention on the ultimate outcomes are expected to be small or nonsignificant, being mediated by the immediate and intermediate outcomes (Wiedermann & von Eye, 2015). In this case, the interpretation of findings related to the direct impact of the intervention is erroneous. Conclusions that the intervention is not effective in improving the ultimate outcomes may be incorrect as the intervention has the capacity to induce the mechanism of action that mediates its impact on the ultimate outcomes.

The focus on group-level comparison ignores the heterogeneity in individual participants' responses to the intervention. Heterogeneity, represented in individual differences, implies that some participants experience improvement in the outcomes (called responders); others show no change in the outcomes; and still others report worsening in the outcomes. Individual differences are reflected in the error term of statistical tests. When large, individual differences reduce the power to detect differences in the outcome between the experimental intervention and the comparison treatment groups, leading to type I error and the inference that the intervention is not effective. Therefore, a potentially useful intervention is abandoned. To minimize error, it is important to acknowledge that interventions do not work universally. It is equally useful to determine who benefit, to what extent, from the intervention to yield results that inform treatment decision-making in practice (Beutler et al., 2016; Boyer et al., 2016).

The intent-to-treat principle translates into analyzing the ultimate outcomes for participants randomized to the experimental intervention and the comparison treatment groups, regardless of their withdrawal, crossover, and adherence to the allocated treatment. The goal is to maintain the comparability of the groups in baseline characteristics and consequently, to control for potential confounding at the data analysis stage (Ranganathan et al., 2016). The logic of intent-to-treat principle has been questioned. Intent-to-treat analysis is believed to estimate the effects of "treatment assignment" (Hernán & Hernádez-Diaz, 2012; West & Thoemmes, 2010), rather than the causal effects of the intervention: an intervention cannot produce changes in the outcomes if the participants are not exposed to it and do not engage and enact it. In addition, evidence consistently demonstrates that results based on the intent-to-treat analysis are biased, often underestimating the intervention effects on the outcomes. Underestimated effects potentially lead to type II error and the incorrect conclusion that the intervention is ineffective (Candlish et al., 2017; Hernán & Hernádez-Diaz, 2012; TenHave et al., 2008). The analysis should be supplemented with per-protocol analysis.

Advances in research designs and methods have been made to address the limitations of the traditional RCT. These are summarized in Table 14.1. Advances in research designs are presented in the next section, and those pertaining to methods for conducting an intervention evaluation study are described in Chapter 15.

**TABLE 14.1**  Overview of designs and methods addressing the limitations of the traditional RCT.

| RCT limitation | Design | Method |
|---|---|---|
| Reduced pool of potentially eligible participants | Multisite RCT and/or cluster RCT | Multiprong recruitment strategy |
| Small percentage of clients meeting eligibility criteria resulting in small, unrepresentative sample | Pragmatic approach informing experimental (e.g. practical clinical trial) or quasi-experimental (e.g. cohort) trials | Specification of broad, less restrictive eligibility criteria. Power analysis to estimate required sample size |
| Participants' declining randomization and preferences for treatment | Preference trials | Assessment of preferences (Chapter 11) Assignment to treatment of choice |
| High attrition | | Integration of strategies to minimize attrition |
| Crossover and contamination within site | Cluster RCT | Conduct of process evaluation (Chapter 13) and of per protocol analysis |
| Delivery of fixed interventions in a standardized manner | Adaptive interventions and designs | Development of protocol or manual to adapt intervention (Chapters 6, 7, and 9) Conduct of process evaluation (Chapter 13) |
| Limited relevance of comparison (no-treatment, placebo) treatment | Comparative effectiveness trials Within-subject designs | Conduct of process evaluation (Chapter 13) |
| Ignoring influence of interventionists | Pragmatic approach guiding experimental and quasi-experimental studies | Assessment of interventionists' characteristics (Chapter 8) Accounting of nesting of participants within interventionists Examining influence of interventionists in outcome analysis |
| Ignoring influence of context and/or concurrent treatment | Cluster RCT Pragmatic approach guiding experimental and quasi-experimental studies Mixed (quantitative and qualitative) method designs | Assessment of contextual factors and concurrent treatment Accounting for nesting of participants within sites Examining influence of sites and of contextual factors in outcome analysis Conduct of process evaluation Subgroup analysis to examine impact of concurrent treatment |
| Ignoring participants' needs and response to treatment | Adaptive interventions and designs Regression-discontinuity design | Assessment of characteristics at baseline Delivery of treatment as specified in tailoring protocol Assessment of outcome (response to treatment) at regular intervals Subgroup or multilevel outcome analysis |
| Ignoring intervention's mechanism of action | Mixed (quantitative and qualitative) method designs | Assessment of mediators (representing the mechanism of action) Integration of process and outcome evaluation Conduct of meditational analysis |

**TABLE 14.1** (Continued)

| RCT limitation | Design | Method |
|---|---|---|
| Ignoring level of exposure to treatment | All types of designs | Assessment of exposure, engagement and enactment (Chapter 9) Conduct of per-protocol analysis and account for level of exposure in outcome analysis |
| Limited capacity to examine long-term effects of intervention | Quasi-experimental design and within-subject design with long-term follow-up | |

## 14.3  ALTERNATIVE DESIGNS

A pragmatic approach to intervention evaluation underpins the advances in research designs. A pragmatic approach calls for examining the effects of health interventions under the real-world conditions, which enables the generation of evidence that is relevant to practice (Methodological Committee of the Patient-Centered Outcomes Research Institute [PCORI], 2012). A pragmatic approach acknowledges the complexity of the real-world and embraces the notions of multicausality, flexibility, and heterogeneity that are inherent in the real world. Consequently, it advocates against the high experimental control that characterizes the traditional RCT design in order to reflect the natural diversity of clients, interventionists, contexts, health interventions and outcomes, and to examine the intricate relationships among multiple factors, occurring at multiple levels and contributing to the effectiveness of interventions. The goal is to provide answers to questions guiding real-world treatment decisions: Who benefit from which health intervention, given by whom, in what mode, format and dose? How does the intervention work, in what context? What are risks or discomforts associated with the intervention?

Intervention evaluation studies that are informed by a pragmatic approach have any or a combination of these features: (1) selection of participants that represent the diversity (personal and health profiles) of the target client population; (2) selection of sites or settings that represent the diversity (physical, sociopolitical, availability of resources) of practice setting; (3) comparison of the health intervention of interest to other active treatments considered as standards of care; (4) involvement of health professionals in the implementation of the intervention in a standard or tailored format; (5) assessment of a range of outcomes, including patient-oriented or -centered health outcomes, over time; and (6) use of random, nonrandom, or a mix of both methods for treatment allocation. Accordingly, different designs are being developed and are considered appropriate for evaluating health interventions under real-world conditions. It is beyond the scope of this book to review all research designs mentioned in the literature. However, the experimental or randomized, quasi-experimental or nonrandomized, and mixed designs that are commonly and recently used in intervention research are discussed next. Where available, different terms used to refer to the same design are presented.

### 14.3.1  Experimental or Randomized Designs

The experimental or randomized category represents designs that extend the traditional RCT. The extensions consist of some modification in the trial's features aimed to address specific limitations or challenges encountered in the conduct of the traditional RCT (Krauss, 2018).

### 14.3.1.1   Waiting-List Control Group Design

The waiting-list control (WLC) group design is also called delayed start design (D'Agostino, 2009) or deferred-treatment design (Campbell et al., 2005). It has been recommended when withholding treatment and randomization of individual participants to treatment groups are unethical or unacceptable. This may be the case when: (1) there is empirical evidence (synthesized from previous research) indicating that the health intervention under evaluation is more beneficial (i.e. demonstrates larger effects) than standard care; (2) the target client population is in pressing need for treatment that is not affordable outside the trial; or (3) clients, health professionals, and decision-makers involved in the trial find it ethically unacceptable to withhold treatment and to provide treatment on the basis of chance (Sidani, 2015). The WLC group design is a viable alternative because it mimics the pattern of treatment delivery followed in practice, where some clients are given the needed treatment at different points in time (i.e. immediately or delayed) as a result of limited resources in a practice setting.

### Features

The WLC group design has features comparable to those characterizing the traditional RCT, except that participants in the comparison or control group are provided the intervention at a delayed time. Thus, at the end of the trial, all participants are exposed to the experimental intervention. The conduct of the WLC group design involves these steps:

1. Assessing the outcomes on all eligible consenting participants at pretest (Time 1).
2. Randomly assigning participants to the immediate or delayed group. The delivery of the experimental intervention takes place once pretest outcome data are collected in the immediate group but is deferred to a later point in time in the delayed group.
3. Providing the experimental intervention to participants in the immediate group. During this time period, participants in the delayed group are not exposed to the intervention. As such they serve as a control group.
4. Assessing the outcomes in participants in both groups once the experimental intervention is completely delivered in the immediate treatment group (Time 2).
5. Delivering the experimental intervention to participants in the delayed group.
6. Assessing the outcomes in participants in the delayed group, following intervention delivery (Time 3). It also is advisable to assess the outcomes at Time 3 in participants allocated to the immediate group, which offers an opportunity to examine the sustainability of the intervention effects.

The outcome data analysis involves:

1. Examining differences in the outcomes assessed at Time 2 between the immediate and the delayed groups, similar to the analysis done in the traditional RCT. The results of this group comparison determine the effectiveness of the experimental intervention in improving the outcomes. Improvement is indicated by the report of the hypothesized changes in the outcomes in the immediate group and no change in the outcomes in the delayed group, from Time 1 to Time 2.
2. Examining differences in the outcomes assessed at the three time points, within each group, to determine the capacity of the intervention to induce the hypothesized

improvement in the outcomes. In the immediate group, it is expected to see significant beneficial changes in the outcomes at Time 2 that are sustained at Time 3; sustainability is indicated by observing no drastic change in the outcomes between Time 2 and Time 3. In the delayed group, no change in the outcomes are anticipated between Time 1 and Time 2 (i.e. in the absence of the intervention) but significant improvement in the outcomes are expected at Time 3;

3. Examining change in the outcomes assessed immediately before (Time 1 for the immediate group and Time 2 for the delayed group) and immediately after (Time 2 for the immediate group and Time 3 for the delayed group) delivery of the intervention, when the respective outcomes data are pooled from both groups. These findings (similar to those obtained in a single group pretest—posttest design) are based on a large sample size (i.e. combination of both groups) and useful in determining the magnitude of improvement in the outcomes that is induced by the experimental health intervention.

## Advantages/Strengths

The WLC group design has some advantages. It addresses the ethical issues related to: (1) withholding any type of treatment in a no-treatment control group (done in some traditional RCT) and (2) denying a potentially beneficial intervention for participants in need of treatment (Cunningham et al., 2013). In the WLC group design, all participants are aware that they will ultimately receive the experimental health intervention, whether immediately or at a later time, as is typically done in practice. This awareness entices them to participate in the trial, thereby increasing trial enrollment rates (Sidani, 2015) and accrual of the required sample size within the study time line. Similarly, health professionals are aware that all participants will receive the experimental intervention. Therefore, they are not compelled to disseminate the experimental intervention (if they are responsible for delivering it) to the WLC group, thereby minimizing the risk of contamination. Also, they are not compelled to enhance usual treatment provided to participants in the control group, thereby reducing the risk of treatment compensation (Campbell et al., 2005).

The WLC group design enables between- and within-group outcome analyses. The between-group comparison (Time 2) reflects the covariation criterion for causality; thus, it is useful in determining the causal effects of the experimental intervention on the outcomes. In the within-group outcome analysis, in particular within the delayed group, individual participants serve as their own control because they are exposed first to no treatment and second to the experimental intervention, a situation reflective of the counterfactual. The comparison on outcomes within the delayed treatment group is important for determining the causal effects of the intervention, unbiased by the potential confounding influence of participants' baseline characteristics (Berry et al., 2006) (further discussed in Section 14.3.2.4). In addition, the analysis examining changes in the outcomes from pretest to posttest, done in the pooled sample, yields reliable estimates of the magnitude of improvement in the outcomes, immediately following completion of the experimental intervention.

## Disadvantages/Limitations

The limitations of the WLC group design stem from the nature of the health problem and its recovery, participants' expectations, and logistical issues. Participants experiencing acute, time-limited health problems (e.g. common cold, acute fatigue or insomnia, skin abrasion) and assigned to the delayed group may spontaneously and naturally recover, resulting in improvement in the outcomes at Time 2. This improvement reduces the size of the between-group differences at Time 2, leading to an underestimation of the intervention effects.

Participants randomized to the delayed group may have different expectations. Some may have desired immediate attention and treatment to manage what they consider as a pressing, severe health problem; those disappointed may withdraw early in the trial (i.e. before Time 2) to seek treatment outside the trial. High attrition rates, in particular in the delayed group, have been reported (Foster, 2012). High attrition rates contribute to reduced sample size and statistical power, and to post-randomization confounding, and subsequently to biased estimates of the intervention effects. Other participants in the delayed group anticipate that their health problem or its severity will improve over time. This expectancy is reflected in reported (even if small) improvement in the outcomes at Time 2, leading to underestimated intervention effects (Sidani, 2015). Still, other participants in the delayed group expressing readiness to change or taking steps to make the change, may halt their change initiative because they perceive that they have to wait to make the change until they receive the experimental intervention, as reported by Cunningham et al. (2013). The logistical problems associated with repeated measurement of outcomes may be viewed as burdensome by participants, contributing to their withdrawal (Berry et al., 2006).

### 14.3.1.2    Crossover Design

The crossover design is similar to the WLC group design in that participants are crossed over from one treatment to another during the study period. However, the treatments consist of either different components of a complex, multicomponent intervention or different interventions addressing the same health problem. The design can be used in two situations: (1) to compare the effects of the selected components or interventions in a situation where it is ethically unacceptable to withhold treatment, and (2) to determine the most appropriate, effective, safe and efficient sequence for providing the components or the interventions. In the latter situation, the findings inform the implementation of a stepped approach to care, which is desirable to reduce the burden of care for participants (e.g. providing intensive treatments to those who may not need it) and for health professionals in practices with limited resources.

*Features*

The features of the crossover design are comparable to those of the WLC group design, except for incorporating washout periods. The washout period is of higher importance for trials aimed to compare the components or the interventions than trials focusing on determining the appropriate sequence of treatments' delivery.

The washout period is scheduled after providing a component or intervention but before exposure to another. During this washout period, the first component or intervention is withheld to allow its effects to dissipate prior to providing the second component or intervention. This is important to prevent the carryover effects of the first component or intervention and to minimize the cumulative influence or the interaction (strengthening or weakening) effects of the first with the second component or intervention. The length of the washout period is informed by available theoretical or clinical knowledge of the duration of each component's or intervention's effects; otherwise, it is logical to specify the duration of the washout period to be equal to the duration for giving the components or interventions (Sidani, 2015). For instance, if it takes four weeks to provide an intervention, then the washout period is four weeks.

The sequence for providing the components or interventions is planned in advance. This is usually done by randomizing the order for exposure to the components or interventions: participants are randomly assigned to different sequences. For example, some participants receive intervention 1 followed by intervention 2, whereas others are exposed to intervention 2 followed by intervention 1, separated by a washout period. When the concern is the development of a stepped approach to intervention delivery, the delineation of the sequences for providing components or interventions can be informed by the intervention theory or relevant clinical knowledge. For instance, foundational, non-intensive components (e.g. sleep education and hygiene) could be offered first, followed by more intensive ones (e.g. stimulus control therapy). Alternatively, the order for giving the intensive components could be randomized (e.g. stimulus control therapy then relaxation therapy then sleep restriction therapy, versus relaxation therapy then stimulus control therapy then sleep restriction therapy).

Conducting a crossover design involves:

1. Randomly assigning participants to receive different sequences of components or interventions (specified either on the basis of chance or relevant knowledge) such as intervention 1 followed by intervention 2, or intervention 2 followed by intervention 1.
2. Assessing the outcomes on all participants (Time 1) serving as baseline for all participants.
3. Delivering the first component or intervention as delineated by the sequence to which participants are allocated.
4. Assessing the outcomes on all participants (Time 2), representing the posttest for the first component or intervention.
5. Allowing for the washout period during which participants are asked to withhold treatment.
6. Assessing the outcomes on all participants (Time 3), representing the pretest for the second component or intervention.
7. Providing the second component or intervention as delineated by the sequence to which participants are allocated.
8. Assessing the outcomes on all participants (Time 4), representing the posttest for the second component or intervention.

The outcome analysis is complex as it should account for the possible carryover and ordering effects when comparing the effects of the components or interventions, as explained by Wellek and Blettner (2012). The analysis includes comparisons between groups after receiving each component or intervention, shedding light on their relative (to each other) effectiveness. The analysis also includes comparisons within group over time. These comparisons generate evidence on the capacity of each component or intervention to induce the beneficial outcomes while controlling for possible confounding associated with participants' characteristics (since participants serve as their own control).

### Advantages/Strengths

The crossover design enables the concurrent evaluation of two or more components or interventions, or the sequence for providing them, thereby generating evidence of relevance to practice. All participants receive treatment, thereby mitigating the ethical dilemma of withholding treatment to those who need it. Since participants receive all components or interventions under evaluation, they serve as their own control, allowing comparison of the same participants under different components or interventions. This comparison controls for or minimizes the potential influence of client characteristics on treatment engagement, enactment, and outcomes (Berry et al., 2006). It yields two advantages: (1) reduced error variance, which increases the statistical power to detect significant intervention effects; and (2) need for a small sample size, estimated to be about one half of that required for traditional RCTs (Hui et al., 2015).

### Disadvantages/Limitations

Several limitations have been reported for the crossover design. The design yields high attrition rates for two reasons (Berry et al., 2006). First, the design is burdensome and demanding in terms of repeated exposures to components or interventions, multiple outcome assessments, and time; the duration of the trial is long, covering treatment and washout periods. Second, participants exposed to the first allocated component or intervention may experience beneficial outcomes; they may lose interest in receiving additional treatment and withdraw from the trial. Alternatively, they may experience side effects associated with the first component or intervention, and therefore, are unwilling to receive additional treatment.

The repeated assessment of the same outcomes generates learning or testing effects, whereby participants' responses to self-report measures early in the trial influence their responses to the same measures at a later time. The latter responses can bias the treatment effects. Some of this learning that influences participants' later responses could be associated with their experience of the first component or intervention; for example, participants who experience the side effects with the first intervention become sensitive and vigilant in monitoring and reporting minor discomfort with the second intervention.

The potential of carryover effects prevents the use of the crossover design in situations where the health problem is expected to exhibit no change (improvement or deterioration) over the trial period. The use of the crossover design is limited to the evaluation of interventions that work quickly, providing short-term relief that is not sustained over the trial period (Hui et al., 2015; Shadish et al., 2002).

### 14.3.1.3    Cluster Randomized Trial

A cluster is a discrete entity comprised of and serving groups of clients representing the target population. Examples of clusters include schools, clinics, in-patient units or wards, hospitals, community, or geographic locations. Some health interventions are designed to target and are delivered (in individual or group format) to individual clients within a cluster (e.g. behavioral therapy to promote physical activity given in group sessions), whereas others are designed to target and are implemented at the level of the cluster (e.g. professional development interventions to change health professionals' practices). In the first case, the conduct of an RCT within a cluster presents a few challenges: (1) the number of potentially eligible clients is limited; (2) the enrollment rate is slow and low; (3) the inclusion of a comparison group may not be acceptable; and (4) contamination or dissemination of the intervention to the comparison group is highly likely. To address these challenges, multiple clusters are selected and randomized to the experimental intervention or the comparison group (Choko et al., 2020; MRC, 2019; Verhaegher et al., 2012). However, the outcome analysis is done at the individual client level—a design referred to as multisite RCT or "cluster—individual trial" (Ford & Norrie, 2016). In the second case where the intervention is implemented at the cluster level, a large number of clusters is selected and randomized to the experimental intervention or the comparison group. Since the unit of analysis is the cluster, the outcome data, whether collected from individuals within each cluster (e.g. health professionals' practices, clients' engagement in physical activity) or from the cluster (e.g. prevalence of obesity), are aggregated and analyzed at the cluster level—a design called "cluster—cluster trial" (Ford & Norrie, 2016). In situations where: there is evidence supporting the benefits of the cluster level intervention; there is objection to withholding such an intervention from clusters randomized to the comparison group; there are practical issues in rolling out the intervention to all clusters simultaneously or within a short time frame; then the implementation of the intervention is staggered. The intervention is given sequentially to different clusters—a design known as "stepped wedge design" (Ford & Norrie, 2016; Hemming et al., 2015; MRC, 2019).

## Features

In general, the cluster randomized trial has features similar to those of the traditional RCT and the WLC group design, except that randomization is done at the level of the cluster. The design and conduct of the cluster randomized trial require specific considerations:

*Selection of clusters*: Ideally, and as is done in the traditional RCT, the selected clusters should be comparable in their characteristics in order to minimize potential confounding. These characteristics are identified in the intervention theory (Chapter 5) and pertain to the personal and health or clinical profiles of clients, the professional qualifications of health professionals, availability of human and material resources, and the physical and sociopolitical features of the context. In the absence of theory, main cluster characteristics that influence the implementation and the outcomes of the health intervention under evaluation are accounted for. Examples of clusters' characteristics are cluster size (i.e. number of clients), staff complement (i.e. number and mix of health professionals), and geographic location (reflecting socioeconomic status). In situations where the accessible clusters that agree to participate in the trial vary in their characteristics, it is highly recommended to collect relevant data from each site and conduct appropriate analysis to determine the contribution of the characteristics to the implementation and the outcomes of the intervention.

*Sample size*: In cluster–individual trials, the selected clusters are randomized to the intervention or the comparison group, but the unit of analysis is the client, that is, the analysis is done on the outcome data obtained from the individual participants. Therefore, the sample size calculation is done to determine the number of participants to include in each of the experimental intervention and the comparison treatment groups, regardless of the cluster in which they are housed. In cluster–cluster trials, the clusters are the units of randomization and of data analysis. As such, the sample size should include an adequate number of clusters to detect significant intervention effects, if the outcome data are collected at the cluster level, as well as an adequate number of clients within the clusters, if the outcome data are collected at the client level. The number of clients is balanced across clusters and is dependent on the expected level of within-cluster correlation. Overall, the sample size calculation takes into consideration the number of clusters, the number of clients, and the magnitude of the within-cluster correlation (for details, see Donner & Klar, 2004).

*Assignment to treatment groups*: In cluster—individual and cluster—trials, participating clusters are randomly assigned to the experimental intervention or the comparison treatment (treatment-as-usual being the most common). Randomization is expected to balance the clusters' characteristics between the two treatment groups and hence, control for their potential confounding. However, randomization increases the probability of a balanced distribution when the sample size (i.e. number of clusters) is large (Berger, 2018), and participating clusters have similar characteristics. Both requirements are not achievable in cluster trials for two reasons. First, the number of participating clusters is often limited due to constraints imposed by funding, trial time line and resources, or lack of readiness of some clusters. Second, the natural heterogeneity in the clusters' characteristics is the norm. With small and heterogeneous clusters, it is desirable to stratify or match the clusters on a few (i.e. less than the number of clusters) characteristics strongly associated with the outcomes, before randomization. Stratification or matching could generate challenges at the data analysis stage, particularly in the presence of differential attrition (Murray et al., 2004). In a stepped wedge design, an initial period is scheduled during which all participating clusters are not exposed to the intervention but are involved in outcome data collection. This initial period serves as a control condition. Subsequently, one cluster or a group of clusters is randomized to receive the intervention. Once post-treatment outcome data are obtained, another individual cluster or group of clusters is randomized to the intervention. This process is continued at regular time intervals until all clusters are exposed to the intervention (Ford & Norrie, 2016; Hemming et al., 2015; Mazzuca et al., 2018; MRC, 2019).

*Consent for participation*: Randomization of clusters to the experimental intervention and the comparison treatment groups has generated discussion regarding consent for participation in the trial. The specific questions raised are: Who should give consent? And what is the consent for? The answers to these questions may depend on the local contexts in which the trial is conducted and vary with local research ethics requirements. However, a few suggestions have been proposed. It is important to secure the approval of administrative or clinical decision-makers for the cluster's participation in the trial. In cluster trials involving collection of data from individual participants, some scholars argue for exempting participants' consent because the intervention targets the cluster and not individuals directly. Other scholars argue for obtaining consent from individual participants; however, during the consent process, participants are informed only of the treatment to which they will be exposed, which is determined by the cluster's allocation to either the experimental intervention or the comparison treatment. Participants are requested to consent for their involvement in outcome data collection. In cluster–cluster and stepped wedge design, obtaining consent from individual participants may be impractical, for instance, when the intervention involves a change in policy within a city or community. These ethical challenges have been explored, but not resolved (Anderson et al., 2015; Choko et al., 2020; Goldstein et al., 2019; Troxel et al., 2016).

*Outcome data analysis*: Cluster randomized trials in which outcome data are collected from individual participants present some challenges in the analysis. The challenges are related to the nesting of participants within clusters and the potential confounding effects of the clusters' characteristics. An additional challenge encountered in stepped wedge designs is the potential influence of calendar time (Arnup et al., 2017). Nesting of participants refers to the anticipated similarity of participants' characteristics and responses to treatment within a cluster. Within-cluster similarity may yield possible variability in characteristics and responses across clusters assigned to the same treatment group. Participants within a cluster share comparable socioeconomic, cultural, and health characteristics, particularly when the cluster is located in a specific geographical location (e.g. rural versus urban) or a unique community (e.g. defined by culture). Participants within a cluster are exposed to similar contextual factors (e.g. political, environmental, social norms) and the same health professionals; they also interact with each other and exchange health-related information. Comparable characteristics, contextual factors and experiences may influence, in the same way, their engagement and enactment of the allocated treatment and consequently, improvement in the outcomes.

The nesting of participants is quantified in the within-cluster correlation in the outcomes. A high correlation suggests that participants within clusters have responded to the allocated treatment in the same way, reflected in the same direction and amount of change in the outcomes, whereas a low correlation implies that participants' responses are independent (Lohr et al., 2014). When participants' outcome data are pooled across clusters to examine differences between the experimental intervention and the comparison treatment groups, and if across-cluster variability is not accounted for, the within-treatment group variability in outcomes is high, lowering the power to detect significant intervention effects. Consequently, the within-cluster variability should be tested and accounted for in outcome data analysis, using mixed-model or hierarchical linear models (Hox, 2010; Field & Wright, 2011; Raudenbush & Bryk, 2002). These models for outcome analysis can be extended to control for, or examine the extent to which cluster characteristics affect the outcomes (Jo et al., 2008). Calendar time at which different clusters are exposed to treatment is important to document in order to capture events or environmental changes that may occur at the time and affect the treatment implementation and outcome (Hemming et al., 2015). For instance, participants in a cluster exposed to a behavioral intervention to promote physical activity in the summer time may be able to engage in outdoor activities frequently and experience greater benefit than those receiving the intervention in the winter time, when engagement in such activities is limited due to weather conditions.

### Advantages/Strengths

The cluster–individual trial design has the advantages of (1) accruing the required sample size within a short time frame and (2) examining the influence of contextual factors on the implementation and outcomes of health interventions. The stepped wedge design in which clusters are exposed to both the comparison treatment and the experimental intervention has the advantage of controlling for potential confounding associated with the clusters' characteristics The control is achieved in the within-cluster comparison, where each cluster serves as its own control. This in turn, increases the power to detect significant changes in the outcomes following the delivery of the intervention (Hemming et al., 2015).

### Disadvantages/Limitations

Cluster randomized trials are susceptible to across-cluster variability in the contextual factors. The variability may necessitate modifications of the trial protocol (e.g. administering outcome measures by research assistants versus self-completing measures by participants; strategies for recruitment; timing of screening) to fit the resources available at each cluster. These modifications could introduce biases (e.g. application of some recruitment strategies may result in sample selection bias), weakening the validity of the trial's findings. Variability in contextual factors may also impact the delivery of health interventions with fidelity, and consequently the interventions' capacity to induce the hypothesized changes in outcomes. Ignoring the nesting of participants within clusters could result in biased estimates of the intervention effects.

### 14.3.1.4    Practical Clinical Trials

Embracing the pragmatic approach to intervention evaluation research, practical clinical trials (PCTs) (Tunis et al., 2003), also called pragmatic trials (Zwarestein & Treweek, 2009), are designed to determine the extent to which health interventions work, that is, produce the beneficial outcomes, when applied in real-world settings. The ultimate goal is to generate evidence on the intervention's effectiveness that is relevant, generalizable, and applicable to practice (Ford & Norrie, 2016; Taljaard et al., 2018). Accordingly, PCTs address questions that inform real-world treatment related decision-making. The questions include: What clients, presenting with what personal and health or clinical profiles, benefit from what health intervention, given by what health professionals, in what mode, at what dose? What risks and costs are associated with what intervention? To address these questions, PCTs are concerned with representing the real-world heterogeneity in clients, interventions, health professionals, and practice settings (Ford & Norrie, 2016; Patsopoulos, 2011; Zwarenstein, 2017). Nonetheless, PCTs still advocate randomization as the method for allocating clients to the treatments under evaluation (Taljaard et al., 2018; Troxel et al., 2016).

*Features*

The features of the PCTs are expected to mimic the circumstances characterizing real-world practice (Fernandez et al., 2015; Horwitz et al., 2017; Taljaard et al., 2018). However, the specific features could vary across trials. For instance, some PCTs are designed to enhance the representativeness of the sample, whereas other PCTs focus more on evaluating simple health interventions provided with flexibility as done in practice. PCTs have six main features.

*Selection of a broad representative sample.* The sample of clients participating in a PCT has to reflect the heterogeneity inherent in the client population seen in practice (Zwarenstein, 2017). This implies that the sample should represent the range of subgroups comprising the target client population. The subgroups are defined in terms of personal characteristics, health or clinical profile, and experience of the health problem. This broadly representative sample is essential for generating evidence on the profile of clients who benefit from the intervention.

The operationalization of this feature involves the specification of unrestrictive client eligibility criteria. The inclusion criteria are broad or general, geared toward ensuring the selection of clients typically seen in practice. A few exclusion criteria are applied to identify clients for whom the intervention is contraindicated (Fernandez et al., 2015; Horwitz et al., 2017; Troxel et al., 2016). The application of unrestrictive client eligibility criteria yields a sample of clients presenting with diverse personal and health or clinical profiles, health problem experiences, beliefs about the health problem and its treatment, and perceptions of the treatments under evaluation. This diversity influences participants' motivation, engagement and enactment of the intervention, and consequently achievement of beneficial outcomes. Thus, participants with different characteristics report varying levels of improvement in the outcomes. The variability in outcome achievement is naturally expected and therefore, should be examined. Examination of outcome variability, however, requires a large sample size to enable subgroup or moderator analysis (using hierarchical linear or mixed-models). The analysis aims to describe variability in the responses to treatment, determine the profile of clients who exhibit different responses (improvement, no change, worsening in outcomes), and identify those who benefit most (Ford & Norrie, 2016; Lowenstein & Castro, 2009).

*Selection of different practice settings.* Different practice settings are selected for participation in a PCT (Fernandez et al., 2015; Horwitz et al., 2017; Troxel et al., 2016). This feature enhances the accessibility of a large pool of clients who are representative of the target population, and the involvement of settings that vary in contextual factors with the potential to influence the implementation and the effectiveness of the intervention. Contextual factors are identified in the intervention theory and encompass the availability of material resources for implementing the intervention, the qualification and complement of health professionals entrusted the delivery of the intervention, and organizational culture reflected in general policies, vision and mission, and values that support the adoption of the intervention. Representing the diversity in settings and examining the influence (direct and indirect) of contextual factors (using multilevel or path analysis) on intervention implementation and outcomes enhance the generalizability and applicability of the findings to practice. The findings guide decisions regarding whether or not an intervention can be applied in a local setting and the modifications that can be safely made to the intervention and its delivery to fit with the characteristics of the client population, and with the human and material resources available within a local setting.

*Selection of different treatments.* The health intervention and the comparison treatment investigated in a PCT need to be relevant or meaningful to practice, in order to inform treatment-related decisions. This feature has two implications:

First, it is advisable to select health interventions that are feasible, inexpensive, and easy to implement with no specialized expertise and training of health professionals entrusted their delivery (Ford & Norrie, 2016; Taljaard et al., 2018). Therefore, the health intervention's protocol is rather simple to carry out by health professionals with different levels of expertise and easy to implement within the reality of day-to-day practice operations. The practice context is often described as having limited resources, high workload or caseload, and multiple competing demands. Having simple, clinically relevant interventions facilitate their scale up, that is, their uptake and integration in diverse practice settings (Troxel et al., 2016).

Second, health interventions are evaluated for their effectiveness relative to clinically relevant comparison treatments. A no-treatment control condition (unless it is a viable alternative, such as watchful waiting or monitoring for benign prostate cancer) and a placebo treatment (commonly used in RCTs) are not clinically meaningful treatments and thus, are not selected in PCTs. A range of alternative treatments are considered (see Chapter 15), with treatment-as-usual most commonly selected. The comparison of the intervention and the alternative treatment is done 'head-to-head" (Holtz, 2007) to determine the effectiveness, risk and cost of the intervention relative to the selected alternative treatment. The results of such a comparison are important in informing policy decision-makers in the process of approving the uptake of the intervention, and clinical decision-makers in the process of informing clients and prescribing treatments that are most appropriate and effective.

*Implementation of treatments.* The selected treatments (intervention and comparison) are implemented by health professionals employed in the practice settings participating in a PCT. The health professionals reflect the natural heterogeneity in personal characteristics and professional qualifications. Health professionals are trained in the intervention and the comparison treatment (if different from usual treatment). The training is often offered through continuing professional development workshops (Chapter 16). Further, the treatments are implemented with flexibility (Patsopoulos, 2011; Taljaard et al., 2018) to mimic real-world practice. Thus, health professionals may tailor, to varying extent, the treatments' components, mode of delivery and dose, to the characteristics and life circumstances of clients. In addition, clients differ in their level of treatment enactment. Variability in health professionals' implementation of the intervention and in clients' enactment of treatment is expected to yield variability in outcome achievement; this variability is examined at the stage of data analysis. To enable the latter analysis, the following methodological points are considered in the design and conduct of a PCT:

- Health professionals within and across participating settings are encouraged to provide all selected treatments. This crossing of health professionals and treatment is necessary to dismantle the influence of health professionals from the effects of treatment, on the outcomes. Data on health professionals' characteristics, including interpersonal style and working alliance, are collected and accounted for in the data analysis (see Chapter 8).
- The number of health professionals should be adequate and balanced across treatments. This is required to obtain significant and reliable estimates of their influence on outcomes. Similarly, the number of clients should be balanced across health professionals and treatments.
- Some scholars argue against close monitoring of treatment implementation and incorporating remedial strategies to improve fidelity of treatment delivery in the PCT (e.g. Taljaard et al., 2018). However, there is growing agreement to document variability in treatment delivery by health professionals and enactment of treatment by clients, as part of process evaluation as discussed in Chapter 13 (e.g. Ford & Norrie, 2016; MRC, 2019).
- The analysis of process and outcome data is done using advanced statistical tests (e.g. multilevel structural equation modeling) to determine: which treatments are well received and easily applied by health professionals and clients; what aspects of the treatments require what type of modification in what client subgroups; what health professionals' qualifications influence the delivery and outcome of treatments; and what client subgroups respond to what treatment and how. The findings are useful to refine the treatments' manual (e.g. revising or adding principles and methods for adapting the intervention) or to develop tailoring algorithms to inform treatment decision-making in practice (Sidani, 2015).

*Assessment of outcomes.* It is commonly advocated to investigate a range of outcomes over a long follow-up period, in order to determine the clinical utility of health interventions. The outcomes should be clinically meaningful; relevant to different stakeholder groups including clients, health professionals, and clinical and policy decision-makers (Sox et al., 2010); and simple to measure in practice or easy to obtain from available standard sources. The administration of relevant and simple outcome measures is important to reduce the burden of additional (i.e. not part of usual practice) and repeated data collection, for both health professionals (administering the measures) and clients (completing the measures) (Troxel et al., 2016).

Different categories of outcomes have been suggested: clinical end points related to the objective (e.g. biomarkers) and subjective (e.g. patient-oriented or patient-centered) indicators of the health problem; physical and psychosocial functioning; risks (adverse or side effects) associated with the treatments; and financial pertaining to the cost of implementing treatments and the cost incurred by clients enacting treatments. Recent emphasis has been on patient-centered outcomes (Taljaard et al., 2018; Zwarenstein, 2017). It is important to note that the outcomes should be selected to reflect the immediate, intermediate, and ultimate outcomes as hypothesized in the theory underpinning both the experimental intervention and the alternative comparison treatment evaluated in a PCT. Outcomes that are commonly anticipated for the selected treatments form the criteria for comparing their effectiveness and determining the most beneficial treatment. Furthermore, risks associated with treatments are monitored during and following treatment delivery.

The selected outcomes are assessed before providing the treatment, and at regularly scheduled time points after treatment delivery over an extended follow-up period. The time points for post-treatment outcome assessment are either specified based on the expected timing for change in the outcomes to take place (as proposed in the intervention theory) or on the usual follow-up encounters done in routine practice (Taljaard et al., 2018). The follow-up period is extended as long as needed to document the anticipated long term outcomes and feasible within funding constraints. The outcome analysis aims to determine not only statistical significance but most importantly clinical relevance (Page, 2014; Zwarenstein, 2017) of the treatments' direct effects on each outcomes, and to examine the extent to which the treatments induced the hypothesized mechanism of change using meditational analysis (Wiedermann & von Eye, 2015).

*Allocation to treatment.* Randomization is advocated as the method for treatment allocation in PCT, where necessary (i.e. exposure to treatment is likely to be associated with potentially confounding factors) and feasible (MRC, 2019). Randomization can be done at the practice site level (as is done in cluster randomized trials), the health professional level (e.g. professionals can be randomly allocated to treatments that they are expected to deliver), and the individual client level. However, randomization may not be acceptable nor feasible in practice. Other methods for treatment allocation can be used (see Chapter 15), with some capitalizing on procedures applied in day-to-day practice to select treatment.

### Advantages/Strengths

The advantages of PCT stem from its design to mimic real-world practice and to generate evidence that informs practice. By representing the natural heterogeneity of clients, health professionals, treatments, and practice settings; comparing the effects of different treatments that are delivered flexibly; and examining the complex interrelationships among contextual factors, implementation and outcomes, PCT results point to:

1. The profile of clients who benefit from the health intervention or the alternative (comparison) treatment under evaluation.
2. The reproducibility of the intervention's effects across settings with variable resources.
3. The robustness of the intervention's effects when delivered by a range of health professionals.
4. The intervention's components contributing most significantly to improvement in the short and long term outcomes.
5. The dose range that is optimal for producing beneficial outcomes and that is associated with potential risks.

It is important to mention that a subtype of PCT, referred to as hybrid designs (Curran et al., 2012; Eldh et al., 2017), has been proposed to evaluate, simultaneously, the health intervention and the techniques used to promote the implementation of the health intervention in practice. The PCT and hybrid designs have comparable features; however, in the hybrid design, the techniques applied to train health professionals (e.g. workshops) and support (e.g. supervision) their delivery of the health intervention, are also evaluated for their effectiveness in improving the quantity (e.g. number of health professionals using the health intervention in practice) and the quality (e.g. flexible fidelity) with which the health intervention is provided in practice (Chapter 16).

### Disadvantages/Limitations

The conduct of a PCT is demanding, requiring resources, efforts and time to: recruit practice settings, health professionals, and clients; negotiate support from administrative and clinical decision-makers to roll out the health intervention under evaluation; train health professionals in the implementation of the health intervention; gather information that tracks which client is given what treatment, in what mode, at what dose, by which health professional; and collect client outcome data, repeatedly, over time. Large samples of clients, health professionals, and settings are required to run the analysis. The analysis also accounts for the nesting of clients within treatment, health professionals and settings, for the influence of several factors operating at different levels on the treatment implementation and outcomes; and for the variability in treatment implementation—all of which is required to detect significant treatment effects.

### 14.3.1.5    Adaptive Designs

Adaptive designs represent an extension of the RCT used to evaluate adaptive health interventions. Adaptive interventions are individualized or tailored to address variability in participants' initial and changing characteristics and life circumstances or responses to treatment, over the course of the intervention delivery period (Lei et al., 2012). Adaptive interventions consist of protocolized sequences of treatment options. They are operationalized in clearly delineated algorithms that specify decision rules for modifying treatments at critical time points (Nahum-Shani et al., 2012). As explained in Chapter 5, the algorithms identify the set of tailoring variables, the procedure for measuring them, and the interpretation of scores. Also, the algorithms indicate which treatment is to be provided to participants presenting with different levels or scores on the tailoring variables. The tailoring algorithms inform the selection of an initial treatment option to address the personal and/or health or clinical characteristics with which participants present prior to exposure to the health intervention. In adaptive interventions, the algorithms are extended to critical time points over the intervention delivery period for further tailoring that is in alignment or responsive to participants' responses (i.e. level of improvement in the outcomes) to the initial treatment. The goal is to maximize improvement in the long-term outcomes (Lei et al., 2012; Nahum-Shani et al., 2012). The critical time points are specified on the basis of either the intervention theory (e.g. upon completion of each intervention component given sequentially) or clinical experience or judgment. At each critical time, participants' responses to treatment become the main tailoring variable informing the selection of the next treatment (Almirall et al., 2012). Other tailoring variables are also considered, such as participants' changing characteristics (e.g. life events resulting in increased stress) and adherence to treatment (Nahum-Shani et al., 2012). Participants' responses to treatment are quantified in their post-treatment scores on the immediate, intermediate, or ultimate outcomes. These scores are used to categorize participants as (1) responders, that is, they report the hypothesized improvement in the outcomes, or (2) nonresponders, that is, they report no changes in the outcomes. Responders to initial treatment are assigned the same treatment as needed. Nonresponders are assigned to an alternative treatment as delineated in the algorithms. Possible alternative treatments are: a conceptually different treatment (i.e. has different active ingredients) or modifications in the dose or mode of delivery of the same initial treatment (Nahum-Shani et al., 2020). The adaptive sequential multiple assignment randomized trial (SMART) has been used to evaluate adaptive interventions (Nahum-Shani et al., 2020).

## Features

The main feature of the SMART design is the multiple stages of randomization to sequential treatments. Each stage corresponds to a critical point at which a treatment decision is made, starting with allocation to initial treatment and continuing with allocation to alternative treatments at the prespecified time points. Each participant progresses through the stages and provides outcome data before and after exposure to each treatment. At each stage, participants are randomly assigned to one of several treatments selected either randomly or on the basis of the tailoring algorithms. It is believed that randomization allows inference regarding the causal effects of the different treatments included in the trial (Lei et al., 2012; Nahum-Shani et al., 2012). Mixed or multilevel or hierarchical linear models are used to analyze the outcomes within and across individual participants. These models enable examination of changes in the outcomes: (1) from pretest to posttest surrounding the delivery of each treatment and (2) cumulatively across all stages or time points (Nahum-Shani et al., 2020).

## Advantages/Strengths

The advantages of the SMART design stem from the flexibility inherent in the implementation and evaluation of adaptive treatments that are individualized to the initial and changing characteristics and life circumstances of participants as well as their responses to treatment (Hatfield et al., 2016). Accordingly, adaptive interventions are highly relevant to practice and the results of SMART studies are applicable to practice: they confirm the utility of the selected tailoring variables and of the algorithms in informing treatment decision-making; and they point to the specific treatment or the sequence of treatments that maximize the achievement of outcomes. In addition, since all participants receive treatment and the treatment is altered to meet their individual characteristics over time, the likelihood of attrition is reduced. Low attrition increases statistical power to detect significant treatment effects, and enhances the sample representativeness (Lei et al., 2012).

## Disadvantages/Limitations

The application of SMART requires: (1) the availability of well-delineated algorithms that clearly describe the decision rules for tailoring treatment; (2) careful monitoring of the fidelity with which the algorithms are followed and the treatments are delivered (Almirall et al., 2012); and (3) a rather large sample size to examine the effectiveness of different sequences of treatments and to reliably estimate their effects.

### 14.3.2   Quasi-Experimental or Nonrandomized Designs

With cumulating evidence demonstrating comparability (in direction and magnitude) of the estimated effects of health interventions reported in RCTs and nonrandomized studies (e.g. Finch et al., 2016; Soni et al., 2019), there is growing acceptance of quasi-experimental or nonrandomized designs as appropriate for outcome evaluation. These designs are used when randomization is not ethically acceptable, feasible, or possible. There are two categories of nonrandomized designs: between-subject and within-subject. Nonrandomized between-subject designs have the same features as those characterizing the RCT, except randomization. Other methods are used to allocate participants to treatment. Some treatment allocation methods are under the researcher's control as is the case in cohort and regression discontinuity designs, and others are not under the researcher's control as is the case in observational designs. Within-subject designs (e.g. single group with repeated measures) are used if forming a comparison group is not possible.

#### 14.3.2.1   Cohort Designs

The cohort design is also known as nonequivalent control group design (Shadish et al., 2002). It is used when randomization of participants to the experimental intervention and the comparison treatment is unethical or not feasible (Chavez-MacGregor & Giordano, 2016). Except for the method of treatment allocation, the cohort design has the same features as those of the RCT. Thus, when well planned and executed, cohort studies yield results that are comparable to those obtained in RCTs, as reported in recent meta-analyses (e.g. Mallard et al., 2016; Nelms & Castel, 2016; Rigato et al., 2017; Smeeing et al., 2017).

*Features*

Similar to the RCT, the cohort design is executed by the researcher. The researcher controls the selection of participants, the allocation of participants to treatment, the delivery of treatments, and the collection of outcome data at prespecified points in time. Participants are selected from a common pool, accessed on one or more practice settings that have comparable contextual factors, and using well-defined and clearly operationalized eligibility criteria. The criteria are preset to be less stringent than those specified for an RCT but enabling the control of potential confounding factors and the accrual of a sample that is representative of the target client population. Participants are allocated to the experimental intervention or the comparison treatment using nonrandom methods (see Chapter 5). The allocation is done by or under the control of the researcher, a feature that distinguishes cohort from observational designs. The comparison treatment may include a no-treatment control condition, placebo treatment, or any alternative treatment. The experimental intervention is delivered by well-trained interventionists, and the fidelity with which they deliver the intervention is closely monitored. The outcomes are measured before and after intervention delivery, with follow-up assessments done over an extended period required to detect changes in the long-term ultimate outcomes. The outcome analysis aims to determine the effects of the intervention, by comparing the mean outcome scores between the experimental intervention and the comparison treatment groups, while controlling statistically for between-group differences in personal and health profiles and outcomes assessed at pretest and known to confound the intervention effects (Hernán & Robins, 2016; Lobo et al., 2017). Statistical control of the confounding factors involves adjustment. Adjustment consists of partializing out the variance in the posttest outcomes that is directly associated with the confounding factors, prior to examining between-group differences in the posttest outcomes. Adjustment can be achieved with different statistical tests or techniques such as analysis of covariance (ANCOVA), subgroup analysis, and propensity scores (Johnson et al., 2018; Pan & Bai, 2018) and instrumental variables (Maciejewski & Brookhart, 2019; Werner et al., 2019; Yang et al., 2019). Each of these techniques has strengths and weaknesses, and there is no agreement on which is most appropriate. ANCOVA, propensity scores, and instrumental variables are statistical techniques that focus on the average effects of the intervention, whereas subgroup analysis is concerned with examining variability in outcome achievement relative to participants' baseline profile (Greenfield & Platt, 2012). The results of subgroup analysis are most informative to practice as they indicate which subgroups of participants, presenting with what profile, experience beneficial improvement in outcomes.

### Advantages/Strengths

The nonrandom method for treatment allocation in a cohort design is advantageous; it entices participants with unfavorable perceptions and reactions to randomization to enroll in the study. This in turn, facilitates the accrual of the required sample size within the study timeline, and in combination with less (than RCT) restrictive eligibility criteria, enhance the sample representativeness. Therefore, the generalizability of the findings is increased (Golfam et al., 2015).

### Disadvantages/Limitations

Traditionally, the main limitation of the cohort design has been attributed to the nonrandom method for treatment allocation. The nonrandom method is believed to result in selection bias and subsequent confounding that contributes to biased (often reported as over) estimates of the intervention effects. These beliefs have been dispelled by evidence showing that: (1) the treatment groups in RCTs differ on some baseline characteristics despite randomization because of the probabilistic nature of randomization (Rickles, 2009) as explained in Section 14.2.2; and (2) the estimates of the same intervention provided to the same client population are consistent across randomized and nonrandomized studies (Frieden, 2017). Further, statistical tests can be used to effectively control for confounding (Lobo et al., 2017), as mentioned previously.

### 14.3.2.2   Regression-Discontinuity Designs

The regression-discontinuity (RD) design, also known as cutoff experiment, has been used to evaluate interventions in economics, education, social welfare, and criminal justice (Cook, 2007). It has been recently advocated for the evaluation of health interventions in situations where randomization is not feasible or desirable. This can be the case when participants vary in their need for different treatments and a well-delineated algorithm is available to inform treatment assignment (Tomlison et al., 2015). The algorithm specifies the client characteristic (same as tailoring variable as mentioned in Section 14.3.1.5), called assignment variable (Shadish et al., 2002), the cutoff score, and the treatment that should be provided to participants with scores below or above the cutoff. The application of the algorithm by the researcher reflects the method for treatment allocation used in the RD design, which is a feature that distinguishes the RD design from the RCT and cohort designs, and makes the RD a form of adaptive design.

## Features

Just like the RCT and cohort designs, the RD design involves the prospective selection and allocation of participants to the experimental intervention and the comparison treatment. Also, both treatments are delivered by trained interventionists; and outcomes are assessed once before and once after treatment delivery. Although the comparison treatment may include no-treatment or treatment-as-usual, alternative active treatments are commonly used. The latter treatments are theoretically or clinically relevant, and if possible supported by empirical evidence of their appropriateness and effectiveness in subgroups of clients with different levels on the assignment variable. In general, the assignment variable cannot be caused by treatment; as such, client characteristics assessed at baseline, including personal, health, or clinical characteristics, as well as pretest outcomes, can be considered for selection as assignment variables (Glasgow et al., 2005; Shadish et al., 2002). The identification of a particular assignment variable is informed by the intervention theory, clinical knowledge, or empirical evidence of client subgroups likely to benefit from the treatments included in the RD study. The conceptual and operational definitions of the assignment variable guide the selection of its most appropriate measure. The measure should be valid and reliable, as well as have clear and if possible validated, cutoff scores.

The algorithm for allocating participants to treatment is developed to clearly delineate:

1. The assignment variable and its measure. In the example of insomnia, the assignment variable can be the perceived insomnia severity and measured by the Insomnia Severity Index (Morin et al., 2011).

2. The procedure for assessing the assignment variable and computing the total score, and for interpreting participants' scores relative to the cutoff score. For example, the Insomnia Severity Index is self-completed by participants at baseline and a total score is computed as the sum of the items' scores to quantify the level of insomnia severity. A total score equal or greater than 15 indicates highly severe insomnia.

3. The process for allocating participants with different levels on the assignment variable, to treatment. The process can be described in "If-Then" statements (as explained in Chapter 7). The statements specify the treatment to be given to participants with scores above or below the cutoff. For example, participants with a score $\geq 15$ on the Insomnia Severity Index are allocated to the behavioral therapy (e.g. stimulus control therapy) and those with a score $< 15$ are given sleep education and hygiene.

When the measure of the assignment variable yields a continuum of scores with no clear cutoff score, a complex computational formula can be used to generate the linkage between the assignment variable and the treatment to be allocated. This has been called "fuzzy" RD design (Imbens & Lemieux, 2008). It is also possible to have more than one assignment variable, which would require complex statistical techniques to generate a single cutoff score or a pattern of scores across the combination of assignment variables that would inform treatment allocation.

The outcome data analysis involves the comparison of the regression lines (intercepts and slopes) that quantify the relationship between the pretest and posttest outcomes, on either side of the cutoff score, between groups. This complex analysis is described in Shadish et al. (2002), Imbens and Lemieux (2008) and Henry et al. (2017).

### Advantages/Strengths

The method of treatment allocation is reflective of the treatment decision-making process applied in practice. It is attractive to participants with unfavorable views of randomization. This method of assignment has the potential of accruing the required sample size within the study time line and of enhancing the sample representativeness. The results may support the utility of the algorithm which is useful in guiding treatment decisions in practice. Furthermore, there is cumulating evidence indicating that the findings of RD designs are comparable to those reported in RCTs evaluating the same treatments (Chaplin et al., 2018; Henry et al., 2017; US Government Accountability Office, 2009).

### Disadvantages/Limitations

The RD design requires a large sample size. Cappelleri et al. (1994) estimated that the RD design requires 2.75 times the number of participants needed in an RCT. In addition, the selection and measurement of the assignment variable are critical for the validity of the RD design results. Selecting an inappropriate variable can lead to misassignment which, compounded by measurement error, increases the chance of committing type II error of inference. The complex analysis of outcome data requires a large sample size to increase the power to detect significant treatment effects at either end of the cutoff score.

### 14.3.2.3    Observational Designs

Observational designs are considered as natural experiments because the allocation to treatment and the provision of the experimental intervention and the comparison treatment follow a natural course. Observational designs are used to examine the impact of naturally occurring events (e.g. earthquake); to evaluate complex (e.g. implementation of best practice guidelines or public health programs) and simple (e.g. medication, behavioral therapy) interventions that target individual clients or communities and that are provided in real-world settings. As such, observational designs share many features of the PCT design; however, the assignment to treatment follows standard of practice and hence, is not under the researcher's control.

### Features

Observational designs involve the selection of a cohort of clients who meet pre-specified, less (than RCT) restrictive eligibility criteria and exposed to either the health intervention of interest or a comparison treatment which may include no-treatment. The designs also involve the prospective assessment of the outcomes, at least once before and repeatedly over time following implementation of the treatments (Lobo et al., 2017; Song & Chung, 2010). The allocation to the intervention or the comparison treatment is done according to the treatment decision-making process followed in practice. The process may be based on health professionals' clinical judgment or on clinical/administrative guidelines. Health professionals trained in the delivery of the health intervention (if not part of usual practice), are responsible for delivering the health intervention or the comparison treatment, to clients assigned to their care. Health professionals are also involved in assessing the outcomes and potential risks at different time points which usually coincide with regularly scheduled client visits. Data on clients' personal and health or clinical characteristics; the type, mode, and dose of treatment provided; and outcomes assessed at each time point are collected and documented in databases maintained by the researcher or by the participating practice settings (Stone & Pocock, 2010). Appropriate statistical tests are used to: (1) describe the characteristics of participants who received the different treatments, as well as the treatment type, mode, and dose that participants received; (2) comparing the baseline characteristics of participants exposed to the intervention and the comparison treatment in order to determine the need for statistical adjustment of their potentially confounding influence; (3) examining the change in outcomes, within each treatment group, over time; (4) exploring the experience of risks; and (5) determining the effectiveness of the intervention in achieving beneficial outcomes, while controlling for confounding variables and the nesting of participants within health professionals and settings, as needed.

### Advantages/Strengths

The advantage of observational designs relates to testing the effectiveness or comparative effectiveness of health interventions under the conditions of real-world practice, thereby enhancing the generalizability and the applicability of the findings to practice (Golfam et al., 2015). The findings indicate who would most benefit in the short and long term, from which treatment (experimental intervention or comparison treatment), provided in what mode and dose, and identify risks associated with each treatments. Accordingly, the findings inform the development of new or the refinement of guidelines for treatment decision-making.

### Disadvantages/Limitations

The main limitation of observational designs is selection bias that introduces possible confounding of the intervention effects, a belief dispelled by evidence presented previously (Section 14.3.2.1). Large samples are needed to conduct subgroup analyses aimed to determine participants that benefit from different treatments (Greenfield & Platt, 2012). Complete and accurate documentation of client characteristics, treatment delivery, and outcomes is essential for generating reliable estimates of treatment effects. However, completeness and accuracy of data can be jeopardized in practices characterized by high client volume, multiple demands imposed on health professionals, and limited resources to support data entry.

### 14.3.2.4    Single Group with Repeated Measure Designs

The single group with repeated measure design is appropriate for outcome evaluation in situations where it is difficult to find or form a comparison group representing the same client population targeted by the health intervention. These situations are encountered when the health intervention: (1) targets and is implemented to reach the whole population, in a large city, province or state, and a country, as is the case with public health campaigns or introduction of a new policy or law; (2) is designed to address the characteristics of a particular community or subgroup of the target client population, as is the case with culturally tailored interventions that are co-designed in collaboration with a particular community or subgroup; or (3) is designed to fit the resources available in a particular local context such as health interventions adapted for delivery to clients in geographically dispersed rural or remote areas. In addition, the single group with repeated measure design is used in situations where it is ethically and clinically unacceptable to withhold treatment.

In the single group with repeated measure design, the intervention is provided to all eligible participants and the outcomes are assessed repeatedly before and after the intervention delivery. The repeated outcome measurement before exposure to the intervention reflects the no-treatment condition, whereas the repeated outcome measurement after exposure reflects the intervention condition. Thus, this design operationalizes the counterfactual that forms the foundation for inferring causality. Also, in this design, participants serve as their own control.

## Features

The key feature of the single group with repeated measure design is the assessment of the outcomes at several time points before and after providing the intervention to the same participants. There are two subtypes of this design, characterized on the basis of the targeted participants and the number of outcome assessments conducted.

1. *Single group with repeated measure design*
   In this design, the health intervention targets either individual participants or a preexisting cluster (e.g. in-hospital unit or ward). However, the delivery of the intervention, the measurement of the outcomes, and the analysis of outcome data are done at the individual participant level. This design is illustrated with offering a professional development workshop to health professionals employed in an intensive care unit in a regional medical center; the workshop (i.e. intervention) is delivered to all health professionals who complete, individually, a self-report measure of the knowledge regarding the topic discussed; the outcomes are assessed, on the same group of health professionals exposed to the intervention, at prespecified time points before and after the intervention. Prior to intervention delivery, the outcomes are assessed at least twice, separated by a time period. The time period can be equivalent to the duration of the intervention (e.g. if the workshop is given over two weeks, then the time period in-between outcome assessments before the intervention would be two weeks); otherwise, it can be equivalent to a time period over which changes in the postintervention outcomes are expected to take place (e.g. improvement in health professionals' practices is anticipated to take place within three months of the workshop). The time period over which the outcomes are assessed before the intervention reflects the no-treatment condition. Once the second outcome assessment is completed, the intervention is delivered to all participants. Following completion of the intervention, the outcomes are assessed at least twice (e.g. immediately and three month follow-up). The outcome analysis, using repeated measure analysis of variance or mixed linear models, involves the comparison of outcomes within-group over time, with the expectation to detect no changes over the no-treatment time period and significant improvement in the outcomes after exposure to treatment.

2. *Interrupted time series design*

   In the interrupted time series design, the health intervention targets a cluster, such as the whole community as is usually the case with public health campaigns or the introduction of a new environmental policy (e.g. banning smoking in in-door public places). The outcomes are specified, assessed, and analyzed at the cluster level. Further, the outcomes are assessed at multiple prespecified time points before and after implementation of the intervention (Mazzuca et al., 2018). There is no clear agreement on the number of times for obtaining outcome data, but it is proposed to have 25–50 time points before and 25–50 time points after implementation of the intervention (Shadish et al., 2002). Collecting, prospectively, the outcome data across all time points may exceed the resources and time allocated for a particular study; however, it may be possible to obtain the required data from available large data sets maintained by the targeted cluster, such as clinical data maintained by a hospital and health indices (e.g. mortality rate) maintained by a public health agency. Obtaining outcome data from these databases requires that (1) the outcome of interest has been assessed with an instrument or measure that validly captures the outcome of interest; this implies that the content of the measure is in alignment with the theoretical and operational definitions of the outcome as specified in the intervention theory; and (2) the same instrument or measure has been used to assess the same outcome across all time points. The use of different instruments may introduce error of measurement and hence, fluctuation in the outcome scores over time. This fluctuation may lead to misinterpretation of the observed trends or patterns of change in the outcome over time. For instance, the change may mimic the hypothesized improvement in the outcome, yet the change may be associated with the characteristics of the newly administered measure. In interrupted time series design, the analysis focuses on examining the trend in the outcome scores before (which should be stable), the disruption or change following the intervention delivery, and gradual improvement reaching a plateau over the postintervention period. The analysis is done by (1) plotting the outcome scores against time and eyeball judgment of the observed trends and (2) using advanced statistical tests (e.g. autoregressive integrated moving average models, mixed linear models) to detect changes in the intercept or the slopes (reflecting the trend in the outcome scores before and after the intervention) around the time of intervention delivery (reflecting interruption or disruption in the levels of outcomes) (Henry et al., 2017).

## Advantages/Strengths

The main advantage of this type of design is the comparison on the outcome, for the same participants (individuals or clusters) subjected to no-treatment control condition and to the intervention. Thus, participants serve as their own control, a situation that (1) is consistent with the counterfactual posited as ideal for determining the causal effects of an intervention (Henry et al., 2017); (2) reduces the potential of confounding as the same participants with the same personal and health or clinical characteristics are exposed to both the control and the intervention conditions (Lawlor et al., 2004); and (3) decreases the number of individual participants needed to detect significant intervention effects in the single-group repeated measure design (Riley et al., 2013).

*Disadvantages/Limitations*

In the single group with repeated measure design targeting individual participants, there is potential for: (1) high attrition rates related to the burden of repeated assessments of outcomes, and (2) testing effects where participants' responses to outcome measures completed at later time points are influenced by their prior responses, their sensitization to the topic and their learning acquired through completing the measure. In interrupted time series design targeting clusters, the potential limitations are related to: (1) the validity, quality or accuracy, and completeness of the outcome data collected over time; (2) the occurrence of events or natural changes in the context or the environment (e.g. seasons) that could influence the outcomes and subsequently the estimation of the intervention effects; therefore, it is highly recommended to monitor, document, and account for these in the data analysis and the interpretation of findings; and (3) less-than-optimal number of time points, which contributes to unstable estimates of the intervention effects (Henry et al., 2017).

## 14.3.3   Mixed Designs

In general, mixed designs integrate elements of randomized and nonrandomized trials (Krauss, 2018) and/or qualitative research methods, into a study aimed to evaluate the effectiveness of health interventions. The proposed integration of different designs' elements or different research methods counterbalances the biases inherent in each and therefore, strengthens the validity of the inferences regarding the intervention's effects and the applicability of the findings to practice.

Novel mixed designs have been and continue to be developed (e.g. Golfam et al., 2015; Knox et al., 2019). Of these, three categories are commonly reported in intervention evaluation research: cohort multiple RCT, preference trial, and mixed quantitative and qualitative method design. These design categories address one or more limitations of the RCT, as discussed next.

### 14.3.3.1   Cohort Multiple RCT

The cohort multiple RCT is proposed to address the RCT limitations related to sample size and representativeness. By integrating elements of the RCT and of observation studies, this design is expected to examine the effectiveness of health interventions in large samples of participants representing the client population seen in practice. This is achieved with the method for identifying and assigning participants to the experimental intervention and the comparison treatment groups.

*Features*

The features of the cohort multiple RCT are similar to those of the RCT design in terms of having an experimental intervention group and a comparison treatment group, random allocation to treatment, and prospective assessment of the outcomes before and after treatment delivery. Health professionals are entrusted the delivery of all treatments included in the trial. However, the selection of participants and the random allocation method differ. Participants are selected on the basis of less (than RCT) restrictive eligibility criteria. Potentially eligible participants are identified from one or more practice settings to form a large cohort. A subsample of this cohort is randomly selected to receive the experimental intervention and is entered in the RCT arm of the study, whereas the remaining subsample of the cohort is not informed of the intervention or the study. The latter subsample continues to receive usual care and provide outcome data; it serves as the comparison treatment group (Golfam et al., 2015). Consent can be obtained only from the subsample randomly selected to receive the experimental intervention, which has been referred to as Zelen randomization. This method of randomization is considered unethical and found to be unacceptable to participants because they are not fully informed about the study (Velthuis et al., 2012). Alternatively, consent can be obtained from the large cohort; participants consent for randomization to treatment in the future (Candlish et al., 2017). In the cohort multiple RCT, the analysis focuses on comparing the posttest outcome between the subsamples that did and did not receive the intervention, to determine its effectiveness.

### Advantages/Strengths

The advantages of this design include improved efficiency of recruitment and enrollment, resulting in the accrual of a large sample that is representative of the target client population seen in practice. The sample representativeness enhances the generalizability of the study findings (Candlish et al., 2017; Golfam et al., 2015).

### Disadvantages/Limitations

This design has the potential for biases associated with: (1) low enrollment rates, which is highly likely among participants serving as comparison and having been not fully informed about the study aim (Velthuis et al., 2012); (2) high attrition in the comparison treatment group related to their disappointment with not being selected to receive the experimental intervention; and (3) contamination or enhanced usual care, whereby health professionals provide usual care that includes some components of the intervention and/or improve the quality of usual care to compensate and satisfy participants in the comparison group (Candlish et al., 2017).

### 14.3.3.2   Preference Trials

Preference trials address the limitations of the RCT associated with ignoring participants' perceptions of randomization and preferences for treatment (see Section 14.2.2 and Chapter 11). Briefly, participants with unfavorable perceptions of randomization and with preferences for a particular treatment (experimental intervention or comparison treatment) under evaluation are likely to decline enrollment in the RCT, or to withdraw from the study. The accrual of a small sample reduces the power to detect significant intervention effects. Alternatively, participants with unfavorable perceptions of randomization may enroll in the RCT but demonstrate less-than-optimal levels of engagement and enactment of treatment, as well as improvement in the outcomes. Accordingly, the RCT suffers from confounding by preference and potentially biased estimates of the intervention effects (Kowalski & Mrdjenovich, 2013; Marcus et al., 2012; Walter et al., 2017). Preference trials are advocated to account for participants' perceptions of randomization and preferences, thereby mitigating the influence of perceptions and preferences on participants' behaviors in a trial.

### Features

In general, preference trials share most features of the RCT except the type of comparison treatment and the method of allocation to treatment. In preference trials, the comparison treatment is an alternative treatment for managing the health problem targeted by the intervention under evaluation. The alternative treatment often has to be relevant to practice and to participating clients; it may consist of treatment-as-usual, another evidence-based health intervention, or a low dose or different mode for delivering the same health intervention under evaluation. A no-treatment condition may be included if it represents a meaningful alternative, such as watchful monitoring for benign prostate cancer. Two methods of assignment to treatment are used: random assignment and preference-based allocation. Randomization is done with procedures similar to the ones used in RCTs (see Chapter 15). Preference-based allocation involves assigning participants to the treatment (experimental or comparison) that they prefer. Accordingly, it is essential to assess participants' preferences. Although direct and indirect methods can be used to assess treatment preferences (see Chapter 11), the direct method is commonly used in preference trials because of its feasibility (simplicity and ease of administration) and its capacity to clearly identify the treatment of choice.

There are three types of preference trial: comprehensive cohort design, partially randomized preference trial, and two-stage randomized trial. All three designs yield four study groups representing participants allocated to the experimental intervention randomly (group 1) or by preference (group 2) and those assigned to the comparison treatment randomly (group 3) or by preference (group 4). However, they differ in the pattern of assignment to the experimental intervention and the comparison group.

1. *Comprehensive cohort design*: In this design, the initial plan is to randomize participants to treatment (same as the RCT). During the consent process, participants are informed of the treatments (intervention and comparison) under evaluation and of the randomization procedure. After providing baseline data, participants are reminded that they are to be randomly allocated to a treatment. At this stage, participants may either agree or decline randomization; the former group of participants are randomized to treatment as originally planned, whereas the latter group of participants are given the opportunity to choose treatment and are allocated to the treatment of choice (Donovan et al., 2018; He et al., 2016; Kowalski & Mrdjenovich, 2013; Kröz et al., 2017). Thus, the comprehensive cohort design addresses, directly, participants' perceptions of randomization and accounts for treatment preferences expressed by only participants who decline randomization.

2. *Partially randomized preferences trial (PRPT)*: The PRPT is very similar to the comprehensive cohort design (and in fact, the two terms have been used interchangeably) except for the pattern of assignment. In the PRPT, after providing baseline data, all participants are informed of the treatments (intervention and comparison) included in the trial and are asked to indicate whether or not they have a preference to any treatment. Participants expressing a preference are requested to identify and are allocated to the treatment of choice (Bradley-Gilbride & Bradley, 2010; Cao et al., 2014). Thus, the PRPT addresses, directly, participants' preferences. It is believed that the pattern of assignment to treatment used in the PRPT and the comprehensive cohort design contributes to selection bias associated with differences in the baseline characteristics of participants with and without preference, and subsequent confounding bias.

3. *Two-stage partially randomized trial*: This design, also called doubly randomized trial, has been developed to mitigate the selection and confounding biases introduced in the PRPT and comprehensive cohort design. As its name implies, assignment of participants to treatment is done in two stages. The first stage takes place upon participants' entry into the trial and consists of randomization to the random or the preference arm of the trial (Walter et al., 2017). The sec-

ond stage takes place at the time of treatment allocation within each trial arm. In the random arm, participants are informed that randomization is the method of assignment and are actually randomly assigned to treatment as is done in the traditional RCT. In the preference arm, participants are informed of the treatments and requested to indicate their preferences. Those with no preference are randomized, whereas those with a preference are allocated to the treatment of choice, as is done in the PRPT. It is believed that randomization at the first stage will maintain the comparability and a balanced number of participants allocated to the four groups described previously.

The analysis in preference trials aims to determine the effects of the intervention and of preference on the outcome. It involves comparison of the four groups generated with random and preference allocation to the intervention and comparison treatment on (1) the posttest outcomes (using analysis of variance), adjusted for baseline differences (using analysis of covariance); or (2) the change in outcomes from pretest to posttest (using mixed or hierarchical linear models). A significant treatment by method of allocation interaction effect and/or significant method of allocation main effect support the contribution of preference to outcome.

### Advantages/Strengths

Regardless of the specific type of preference trials, allocation of participants to the treatment of choice is advantageous. Preference-based allocation reflects, partially, the treatment decision-making process applied in practice. In practice, participants are informed of alternative treatments for managing the health problem and actively involved in treatment selection (Donovan et al., 2018). Involving participants in treatment selection and providing them the treatment of choice are beneficial: they induce favorable participants' reactions and behaviors throughout an outcome evaluation study. The advantages include:

1. Preference-based allocation is a design feature that is attractive to clients with unfavorable perceptions of randomization and strong preference. These clients participate in the trial, leading to increased enrollment rates and accrual of the required sample size within the study timeline. Higher enrollment rates have been consistently reported in individual studies and systematic reviews (Marcus et al., 2012; Mitchell-Jones et al., 2017; Wasmann et al., 2019).

2. Receiving the treatment of choice entices participants to engage, enact, and complete the allocated treatment (Sinclair et al., 2017). This advantage is supported by evidence generated in individual studies and/or synthesized in systematic reviews. The evidence shows increased attendance at the planned intervention sessions (Kwan et al., 2010; Raue et al., 2009); enhanced adherence to treatment recommendations (Kwan et al., 2010; Marcus et al., 2012; Raue et al., 2009); and low attrition rates (Lindheim et al., 2014; Prody et al., 2013; Swift et al., 2011, 2013; Wasmann et al., 2019) among participants allocated to their preferred treatment, as compared to those randomized.

3. Receiving the preferred treatment contributes to improved outcomes, either directly or indirectly through enhanced enactment of treatment. The evidence on the effects of exposure to the treatment of choice on outcomes is inconclusive: some individual studies and systematic reviews found no significant association (e.g. Franco et al., 2013; Kearney et al., 2011; Mitchell-Jones et al., 2017; Prody et al., 2013; Steidtmann et al., 2012; Winter and Barber 2013), whereas others reported a positive but small association between preference and

outcomes (e.g. Borradaile et al., 2012; Lindheim et al., 2014; Preference Collaborative Review Group, 2009; Swift et al., 2011). The inconsistent findings can be attributed to across-study variability in the treatments under evaluation, the target client population, the specific preference trial design used, and the method used to assess preferences (Franco et al., 2013). The inconsistent findings also suggest indirect effects of preferences on outcomes, mediated by enhanced enactment of treatment as found by Kwan et al.'s (2010).

### Disadvantages/Limitations

Two disadvantages have been identified for preference trials. First is the high probability of having disproportionate number of participants who decline randomization in a comprehensive cohort design and who have preferences for one of the treatments included in any type of preference trial. The unbalanced numbers of participants across the four groups limit meaningful between-group comparison, as illustrated in Coward's (2002) and Sidani et al.'s (2015) findings. Second is the selection, and subsequent confounding biases anticipated with preference-based allocation, resulting in biased (over) estimates of the intervention effects (Gemmell & Dunn, 2011). However, emerging evidence indicates either no (Donovan et al., 2018; Kearney et al., 2011; Mitchell-Jones et al., 2017) or minimal (i.e. on a small number of baseline characteristics, comparable to what is also reported in RCTs) (Hubacher et al., 2015; Prody et al., 2013; Wasmann et al., 2019) differences in the baseline profile of participants allocated to treatments by random or preference methods.

### 14.3.3.3   Mixed Methods Designs

Mixed or multiple method designs entail the use of quantitative and qualitative methods for data collection in an outcome evaluation study, regardless of its specific design (i.e. experimental, quasi-experimental, or mixed). Mixed quantitative and qualitative method designs are informed by a pragmatic approach to research. The pragmatic approach recognizes the strengths and limitations of the quantitative and the qualitative methods, and advocates the integration of both methods in a particular study so that the bias or limitation inherent in one method is counterbalanced by those associated with the other method (Fleming et al., 2008). The pragmatic approach values the equal and complementary contribution of quantitative and qualitative methods in enhancing the validity of the inferences regarding the effects of health interventions.

In intervention evaluation studies, generic qualitative methods, regardless of their underlying philosophical assumptions, are applied to complement and supplement the quantitative findings in generating an accurate and comprehensive understanding of what contributed to the observed intervention effects, how, why, and under what context (Kappen et al., 2016; Midgley et al., 2014). Therefore, mixed method designs are advocated to address the RCT limitations related to ignoring the influence of contextual factors and the mechanism of action responsible for the intervention's effects on the outcomes (Cheng & Metcalfe, 2018; Johnson & Schoonenboom, 2016). As described in the extant literature, mixed method designs incorporate qualitative methods for conducting a process evaluation within a randomized or nonrandomized trial (Belford et al., 2017; Moore et al., 2015; Nelson et al., 2015; O'Cathain et al., 2013; Wojewodka et al., 2017). However, the use of qualitative methods can be extended to collect data on a range of substantial and methodological factors that can potentially contribute to outcomes. The purposes for which qualitative methods can be used is presented in the first column of Table 14.2.

**TABLE 14.2**   Uses of qualitative research methods in outcome evaluation studies.

| Purpose/use | Method | Illustrative examples |
| --- | --- | --- |
| *Recruitment:* <br> To explore issues or concerns with recruitment strategies—to optimize strategies | Brief interview with recruiters (staff involved in active recruitment: health professionals or other agency personnel referring clients to study) <br> Brief interview with key informants representing the target client population | Capp et al. (2016), Drabble et al. (2014), Holm et al. (2017), Rengerink et al. (2015), Snowdon (2015), Verwey et al. (2016) |
| To identify reasons for clients' nonenrollment (barriers) and motivators for enrollment—to help generate solutions to enhance enrollment | Brief intervention with clients inquiring about the study | Buck et al. (2015), Horwood et al. (2016), O'Cathain et al. (2013), Rengerink et al. (2015) |
| *Reactions to randomization:* <br> To describe participants' perceptions and reactions to randomization (which affect their behaviors in a study and response to allocated treatment) | Brief interview with participants to explore (un)willingness to be randomized <br><br> Observation and documentation of participants' verbal and behavioral reactions to learning of the allocated treatment | Fleming et al. (2008), Meinich Petersen et al. (2014), Sidani et al. (2017) |
| *Attrition:* <br> To understand reasons or factors contributing to withdrawal from study—to inform generation of appropriate solutions to minimize attrition or improve retention | "Exit" semistructured interview with participants who withdraw at any time (question on general reasons for withdrawal, followed by questions focusing on the treatment and its delivery, and on the research methods) | Brueton et al. (2014), Drabble et al. (2014), Fleming et al. (2008), Johnson and Schoonenboom (2016) |
| *Process:* <br> A. Implementation of treatment by participant and interventionist <br> To explore issues/difficulties in implementation of treatment <br> To identify contextual factors (barriers or facilitators) to treatment implementation <br> To delineate variations in treatment implementation and factors contributing to the variations | Review documents recording occurrence of events at different levels <br><br> Unstructured observation of treatment delivery (to capture real time issues) <br><br> Individual or group interviews scheduled following treatment completion (questions on initiation, engagement, enactment of treatment; interfering factors; extent and reasons for variation in treatment implementation) <br><br> Open-ended questions (same as above) added to diary or posttest questionnaire | Cheng and Metcalfe (2018), Dixon et al. (2017), Drabble et al. (2014), Duberg et al. (2016), Johnson and Schoonenboom (2016), Kolltveit et al. (2017), Komatsu et al. (2016), Kozica et al. (2016), Lutge et al. (2014), Nelson et al. (2015), O'Cathain et al. (2013), Parsons et al. (2016), Omer et al. (2016), Schoultz et al. (2016), Storrar et al. (2015), van den Hurk et al. (2015), Verwey et al. (2016) |
| B. Perception of treatment (by participant and interventionist) | Individual or group interviews scheduled following treatment completion (questions on perceived/experienced usefulness of treatment or its components; components most or least valued, easy to carry out) | Duberg et al. (2016), Kikkenborg Berg et al. (2015), Komatsu et al. (2016), Moss et al. (2015), Schoultz et al. (2016), van den Hurk et al. (2015) |

**TABLE 14.2**   (Continued)

| Purpose/use | Method | Illustrative examples |
| --- | --- | --- |
| C. Mechanism of action (perspective of participant and interventionist) | | |
| To understand how treatment is experienced<br>To understand how treatment leads to (un)beneficial outcomes | Individual or group interviews scheduled following treatment completion (questions on perception of change/no change; component or any other aspect/element of treatment or its delivery that contribute to change/no change; how treatment works) | Cheng and Metcalfe (2018), Duberg et al. (2016), Johnson and Schoonenboom (2016), McArthur et al. (2016), Moss et al. (2015), Nelson et al. (2015), Omer et al. (2016), Saper et al. (2016), Ussher and Perz (2017) |
| *Outcomes* (as experienced by participant) | | |
| To explore individual variation in experience of improvement in outcomes | Individual interview scheduled following treatment completion (questions on experience of change in health problem and health functioning reflecting intended outcomes; and of change in other aspects of their condition or life) | Capp et al. (2016), Duberg et al. (2016), Johnson and Schoonenboom (2016); Midgley et al. (2014), Ussher and Perz (2017) |
| To detect unintended outcomes | Open-ended questions (on positive or negative impact of treatment on participants' general health condition) added to posttest questionnaire | |

*Features*

Mixed method designs are characterized by the integration in the outcome evaluation study, of: (1) unstructured or semistructured interviews with participants, interventionists, and research staff; (2) unstructured observation of treatment implementation by interventionists, and if feasible by participants; (3) adding open-ended questions to the questionnaire administered following treatment completion; and (4) review of documents recording the occurrence of events during the study period. These methods are used to collect pertinent qualitative data addressing the respective purposes, at different time points throughout the outcome evaluation study, as described in the second column of Table 4.1. Different strategies can be used to analyze the data (Miles et al., 2019), with thematic and content analyses (Lewin et al., 2009) being the most commonly applied in the analysis of short responses. The qualitative findings are integrated with the quantitative results to generate a comprehensive understanding of what exactly contributed to the observed outcomes, reflecting the effectiveness, or lack thereof, of the intervention. There is no agreement on the approach or strategy for integrating the quantitative and qualitative findings. Two have been proposed:

1. Mapping, which consists of considering one set of findings along another. This can be facilitated by creating a matrix where a particular quantitative result (e.g. correlation between a mediator and an outcome) is juxtaposed next to themes reflecting the same association (Rapport et al., 2013). This mapping exercise is extended in contribution analysis, to examine the inter-relationships among contextual factors, processes and outcomes, as delineated in the intervention theory and advocated in realist evaluation of interventions (e.g. Befani & Mayne, 2014; Budhwani & McDavis, 2017; Hansen & Jones, 2017).

2. Data transformation, which involves translating one data type into another prior to analyzing the whole data set. As suggested by Spillane et al. (2010), quantitizing techniques are used to transform qualitative data (e.g. a code) into numerical values (e.g. assign a value of "1" if a code is mentioned, "0" otherwise), whereas qualitizing techniques are used to transform quantitative data into descriptions.

### Advantages/Strengths

The incorporation of qualitative methods to collect process and outcome data in intervention evaluation studies is important for strengthening the validity of inferences on effectiveness. The qualitative methods integrated at different stages of the study, provide opportunities for elaboration and clarification of experiences and behaviors (Cooper et al., 2014; Kikkenborg Berg et al., 2015). The exploration of participants' and interventionists' perspectives on (1) recruitment, randomization, and attrition assists in understanding issues and in revising strategies to maximize recruitment and retention; (2) concerns or difficulties in applying the intervention provides evidence to refine its design and delivery to optimize its effectiveness; (3) the linkages among contextual factors, processes, mechanism of action, and outcomes (favorable or unfavorable) helps in validly attributing the outcomes to the intervention (issue of internal validity) and in determining the context or circumstances under which the intervention's effects are reproduced (issue of external validity) (Nelson et al., 2015; O'Cathain et al., 2013; White, 2013). The qualitative findings can corroborate the quantitative results (convergence) adding depth and real illustration of what exactly contributed to the intervention effects (Kikkenborg Berg et al., 2015; Rapport et al., 2013). The qualitative findings can also complement, supplement and clarify, by providing explanations to, the quantitative findings (Dixon et al., 2017; Kappen et al., 2016; Parsons et al., 2016) and answering questions related to what factors affected the outcomes, how and why.

### Disadvantages/Limitations

Collecting qualitative data from different sources (e.g. participants, interventionists), using different methods (e.g. observation, interviews), at different time points (e.g. during and after treatment), and analyzing the respective data is resource and time intensive. Completing both self-report questionnaires and interview is burdensome to participants (Midgley et al., 2014). Integrating quantitative and qualitative findings is challenging.

## 14.4   DESIGN SELECTION

For decades, the RCT was considered the most reliable, even the gold standard, for evaluating the effects of health interventions on outcomes. Recent critique presented in this chapter points to limitations of the RCT in accounting for the multiple factors that contribute to outcome achievement (i.e. notion of multicausality inherent in the real world) as delineated in the intervention theory, and in producing evidence that is generalizable, applicable, and useful in informing practice. Cumulating evidence, synthesized in systematic reviews cited in relevant sections of this chapter, supports the comparability of the intervention effects estimated in randomized and nonrandomized studies, raising questions about the superiority, or even the capacity, of randomization in reducing (let alone eliminating) selection and confounding bias. Therefore, the respective critique and evidence dispel the gold standard myth regarding the RCT (Concato et al., 2010) and refute the uncritical selection of the RCT for outcome evaluation (Krauss, 2018).

A range of experimental and quasi-experimental designs are proposed as alternatives for outcome evaluation. Each design, including the RCT, has inherent strengths and limitations (Frieden, 2017). Combining different designs and methods, as is done in mixed designs, is advocated to enhance the validity of inferences about the intervention's effects. Through this combination, different designs are integrated in the evaluation study, so that the strengths of one design complement those of the other design and simultaneously, the weaknesses of one are counterbalanced by those of the other (PCORI, 2019).

The selection of a research design and the specification of the methods to be used in an intervention evaluation study are carefully done in order to generate high-quality evidence that informs treatment decision-making in practice (Chavez-Mac-Gregor & Giordano, 2016). The selection of a design and respective methods should be informed by:

1. The question that the evaluation study is planned to address (Djurisic et al., 2017; Kowalski & Mrdjenovich, 2013; Lobo et al., 2017; MRC, 2019; Skivington et al., 2018). Some still advocate the RCT for evaluating the efficacy of simple and fixed treatments (e.g. Mohr et al., 2015) and nonrandomized (e.g. observational) studies, for evaluating the effectiveness of simple or complex, fixed or adaptive treatments (Anglemyer et al., 2014).

2. The theory underpinning the intervention, which identifies the range of factors contributing to the outcomes and proposes how to assess them, where and when (Marchal et al., 2013).

3. A critical review and analysis of the strengths and weaknesses of available designs and methods, with the possibility of using a mix to address the evaluation question and enhance validity.

4. Acceptability of the design and methods to stakeholder groups, including client population and clinical or policy decision-makers (Farquhar et al., 2011).

5. Feasibility, ethical and safety issues that could be encountered in implementing the intervention in the participating sites and in applying the research methods.

## REFERENCES

Almirall, D., Compton, S.N., Gunlicks-Stoessel, M., Duan, N., & Murphy, S.A. (2012) Designing a pilot sequential multiple assignment randomized trial for developing an adaptive treatment strategy. *Statistics in Medicine*, 31(17), 1887–1902.

Amaechi, A. & Counsell, S. (2013) Towards an approach for a conceptual system design. *Systems Research and Behavioral Science*, 30, 780–793.

Anderson, M.L., Califf, R.M., & Sugarman, J., for the participants in the NIH Health Care Systems Research Collaboratory Cluster Randomized Trial Workshop. (2015) Ethical and regulatory issues of pragmatic cluster randomized trials in contemporary health systems. *Clinical Trials*, 12(3), 276–286.

Anglemyer, A., Horvath, H.T., & Bero, L. (2014) Healthcare outcomes assessed with observational study designs compared with those assessed in randomized trials. *Cochrane Database of Systematic Reviews*, 4, MR000034.

Arnup, S.J., McKenzie, J.E., Hemming, K., Pilcher, D., & Forbes, A.B. (2017) Understanding the cluster randomized cross-over design: A graphical illustration of the components of variation and a sample size tutorial. *Trials*, 18, 381–395.

Baethge, C., Baethge, C., Assall, O.P., & Baldessarini, R.J. (2013) Systematic review of blinding assessment in randomized controlled trials in schizophrenia and affective disorders 2000-2010. *Psychotherapy and Psychosomatics*, 82, 152–160.

Befani, B. & Mayne, J. (2014) Process tracing and contribution analysis: A combined approach to generative causal inference for impact evaluation. *IDS Bulletin*, 45(6), 17–36.

Belford, M., Robertson, T., & Jepson, R. (2017) Using evaluability assessment to assess local community development health programmes: A Scottish case-study. *BMC Medical Research Methodology*, 17, 70–81.

Berger, V.W. (ed) (2018) *Randomization, Masking, and Allocation Concealment.* Chapman & Hall/CRC. Biostatistics Series. Taylor & Francis, New York.

Berry, C.C., Moore, P., & Dimsdale, J.E. (2006) Assessing the trade-offs between crossover and parallel group designs in sleep research. *Journal of Sleep Research*, 15, 348–357.

Beutler, L.E., Someah, K., Kimpara, S., & Miller, K. (2016) Selecting the most appropriate treatment for each patient. *International Journal of Clinical and Health Psychology*, 16, 99–108.

Blackwood, B., O'Halloran, P., & Porter, S. (2010) On the problems of mixing RCTs with qualitative research: The case of the MRC framework for the evaluation of complex healthcare interventions. *Journal of Research in Nursing*, 15(6), 511–521.

Bonell, C., Fletcher, A., Morton, M., Lorenc, T., & Moore, L. (2012) Realist randomised controlled trials: A new approach to evaluating complex public health interventions. *Social Science & Medicine*, 75, 2299–2306.

Borglin, G. & Richards, D.A. (2010) Bias in experimental nursing research: Strategies to improve the quality and explanatory power of nursing science. *International Journal of Nursing Studies*, 47, 123–128.

Borradaile, K.E., Helprn, S.D., Wyatt, H.R., et al. (2012) Relationship between treatment preference and weight loss in the context of a randomized controlled trial. *Obesity*, 20, 1218–1222.

Bothwell, L.E., Greene, J.A., Podolsky, S.H., et al. (2016) Assessing the gold standard— Lessons from the history of RCTs. *New England Journal of Medicine*, 374, 2175–81.

Boyer, B.E., Doove, L.L., Geurts, H.M., et al. (2016) Qualitative treatment-subgroup interactions in a randomized clinical trial of treatments for adolescents with ADHD: Exploring what cognitive-behavioral treatment works for whom. *PLoS One*, 11(3), e0150698.

Bradley, E.H., Curry, L.A., Ramanadhan, S., et al. (2009) Research in action: Using positive deviance to improve quality of health care. *Implementation Science*, 4, 25–35.

Bradley-Gilbride, J. & Bradley, C. (2010) Partially randomized preference trial design. In N.J. Salkind (Ed), *Encyclopedia of Research Design*, Vol 2. Sage, Thousand Oaks, CA.

Broadbent, H.J., van den Eynde, F., Guillaume, S., et al. (2011) Blinding success of rTMS applied to the dorsolateral prefrontal cortex in randomised controlled trials: A systematic review. *The World Journal of Biological Psychiatry*, 12(4), 240–248.

Brueton, V.C., Stevenson, F., Vale, C.L., et al. (2014) Use of strategies to improve retention in primary care randomized trials: A qualitative study with in-depth interviews. *BMJ Open*, 4, e003835.

Buck, D., Hogan, V., Powell, C.J., et al., on behalf of the SamExo (Surgery versus active-monitoring in intermittent exotropia) trial (2015) Surrounding control or nothing to lose: Parents' preferences about participation in a randomized trial of childhood strabismus surgery. *Clinical Trials*, 12(4), 384–393.

Budhwani, S. & McDavis, J.C. (2017) Contribution analysis: Theoretical and practical challenges and prospects for evaluators. *The Canadian Journal of Program Evaluation*, 32(1), 1–24.

Byrne, D. (2013) Evaluating complex social interventions in a complex world. *Evaluation*, 19(3), 217–228.

Campbell, R., Peters, T., Grant, C., Quilty, B., & Dieppe, P. (2005) Adapting the randomized consent (Zelen) design for trials of behavioural interventions for chronic disease: Feasibility study. *Journal of Health Sciences Research & Policy*, 10(4), 220–225.

Candlish, J., Pate, A., Sperrin, M., & van Staa, T., on behalf of GetReal Work Package 2 (2017) Evaluation of biases present in the cohort multiple randomized controlled trial design: A simulation study. *BMC Medical Research Methodology*, 17, 17–26.

Cao, H.-J., Liu, J.-P., Hu, H., & Wang, N.S. (2014) Using a partially randomized patient preference study design to evaluate the therapeutic effect of acupuncture and cupping therapy for fibromyalgia: Study protocol for a partially randomized controlled trial. *Trials*, 15, 280–286

Capp, R., Kelley, L., Ellis, P., et al. (2016) Reasons for frequent emergency department use by Medicaid enrollees: A qualitative study. *Academic Emergency Medicine*, 23, 476–481.

Cappelleri, J.C., Darlington, R.B., & Trochim, W.M. (1994) Power analysis of cutoff-based randomized clinical trials. *Evaluation Review*, 18(2), 141–152.

Cha, S., Erar, B., Niaura, R.S., & Graha, A.L. (2016) Baseline characteristics and generalizability of participants in internet smoking cessation randomized trial. *Annals of Behavioral Medicine*, 50(5), 751–761.

Chaplin, D.D., Cook, T.D., Zurovac, J., et al. (2018) The internal and external validity of the regression discontinuity design: A meta-analysis of 15 within-study comparisons. *Journal of Policy Analysis and Management*, 37, 403–429.

Chavez-MacGregor, M. & Giordano, S.H. (2016) Randomized clinical trials and observational studies: Is there a battle? *Journal of Clinical Oncology*, 34, 772–3.

Chemla, G. & Hennessy, C. (2016) *Bayesian Expectancy Invalidates Double-Blind Randomized Controlled Medical Trials*. CEPR Discussion Papers 11360, C.E.P.R. Discussion Papers

Cheng, K.K.F. & Metcalfe, A. (2018) Qualitative methods and process evaluation in clinical trials context: Where to head to? *International Journal of Qualitative Methods*, 17, 1–4.

Choko, A.T., Roshandel, G., Conserve, D.F., et al. (2020) Ethical issues in cluster randomized trials conducted in low- and middle-income countries: An analysis of two case studies. *Trials*, 21(Suppl 1), 314–322.

Concato, J., Peduzzi, P., Huang, G.D., et al. (2010) Comparative effectiveness research: What kind of studies do we need? *Journal of Investigative Medicine*, 58, 764–769.

Cook, T. D. (2007) Randomized experiments in education: Assessing the objections to doing them. *Economics of Innovation and New Technology*, 16(5), 331–355.

Cook, T. D. & Campbell, D. T. (1979) *Quasi-Experimentation: Design and Analysis Issues for Field Settings*. Houghton Mifflin, Boston, MA.

Cook, T.D., Scriven, M., Coryn, C.L.S., & Evergreen, S.D.H. (2010) Contemporary thinking about causation in evaluation: A dialogue with Tom Cook and Michael Scriven. *American Journal of Evaluation*, 31, 105–117.

Cooper, C., O'Cathain, A., Hind, D., et al. (2014) Conducting qualitative research within clinical trials units: Avoiding potential pitfalls. *Contemporary Clinical Trials*, 38, 338–343.

Coward, D.D. (2002) Partial randomization design in a support group intervention study. *Western Journal of Nursing Research*, 24, 406–421.

Cunningham, J.A., Kypri, K., & McCambridge, J. (2013) Exploratory randomize controlled trial evaluating the impact of a waiting list control design. *BMC Medical Research Methodology*, 13, 150–155.

Curran, G.M., Bauer, M., Mittman, B., Pyne, J.M., & Stetler, C. (2012) Effectiveness— Implementation hybrid designs: Combining elements of clinical effectiveness and implementation research to enhance public health impact. *Medical Care*, 50(3), 217–226.

D'Agostino, R.B. (2009) The delayed-start study design. *New England Journal of Medicine*, 361, 1304–1306.

Daniel, R.M., De Stavalo, B.L., & Vansteclandt, S. (2016) Commentary: The formal approach to quantitative causal inference in epidemiology: misguided or misrepresented? *International Journal of Epidemiology*, 45(6), 1817–1829.

Deaton, A. & Cartwright, N. (2018) Understanding and misunderstanding randomized controlled trials. *Social Science & Medicine*, 210, 2–21.

Diez-Roux, A.V. (2011) Complex system thinking and current impasses in health disparities research. *American Journal of Public Health*, 101(9), 1627–1634.

Dixon, B.E., Kasting, M.L., Wilson, S., et al. (2017) Health care providers' perceptions of use and influence of clinical decision support reminders: Qualitative study following a randomized trial to improve HPV vaccination rates. *BMC Medical Informatics and Decision Making*, 17, 119–129.

Djurisic, S., Rath, A., Gaber, S., et al. (2017) Barriers to the conduct of randomised clinical trials within all disease areas. *Trials*, 18, 360–369.

Donner, A. & Klar, N. (2004) Pitfalls of and controversies in cluster randomization trials. *American Journal of Public Health*, 94(3), 416–422.

Donovan, J.L., Young, G.J., Walsh, E.I., et al., ProtecT Study Group (2018) A prospective cohort and extended comprehensive-cohort design provided insights about the generalizability of a pragmatic trial: The ProtecT prostate cancer trial. *Journal of Clinical Epidemiology*, 96, 35–46.

Drabble, S.J., O'Cathain, A., Thomas, K.J., et al. (2014) Describing qualitative research undertaken with randomised controlled trials in grant proposals: A documentary analysis. *BMC Medical Research Methodology*, 14, 24–34.

Duberg, A., Möller, M., & Sunvisson, H. (2016) "I feel free": Experiences of a dance intervention for adolescent girls with internalizing problems. *International Journal of Qualitative Studies on Health and Well-Being*, 11, 31946–31960.

Eldh, A.C., Almost, J., DeCorby-Watson, K., et al. (2017) Clinical interventions, implementations and the potential greyness in between—A discussion paper. *BMC Health Services Research*, 17, 16–25.

Farquhar, M.C., Ewing, G., & Booth, S. (2011) Using mixed methods to develop and evaluate complex interventions in palliative care research. *Palliative Medicine*, 25(8), 748–757.

Fernandez, E., Salem, D., Swift, J.K., & Ramtahal, N. (2015) Meta-analysis of dropout from cognitive behavioral therapy: Magnitude, timing, and moderators. *Journal of Consulting and Clinical Psychology*, 86(6), 1108–1122.

Field, A.P. & Wright, D.B. (2011) A primer on using multilevel models in clinical and experimental psychopathology research. *Journal of Experimental Psychopathology*, 2(2), 271–293.

Finch, M., Jones, J., Yoong, S., Wiggers, J., & Wolfenden, L. (2016) Effectiveness of Centre-based childcare interventions in increasing child physical activity: A systematic review and meta-analysis for policymakers and practitioners. *Obesity Reviews*, 17(5), 412–428.

Fleming, K., Anderson, J., & Atkin, K. (2008) Improving the effectiveness of interventions in palliative care: The potential role of qualitative research in enhancing evidence from randomized controlled trials. *Palliative Medicine*, 22, 123–131.

Fletcher, A., Jamal, F., Moore, G., et al. (2016) Realist complex intervention science: Applying realist principles across all phases of the Medical Research Council framework for developing and evaluating complex intervention. *Evaluation*, 22(3), 286–303.

Ford, I. & Norrie, J. (2016) Pragmatic trials. *New England Journal of Medicine*, 375, 454–463.

Foster, N. (2012) Methodological issues in pragmatic trials of complex interventions in primary care. *British Journal of General Practice*, 62(594), 10–11.

Franco, M.R., Ferreira, M.L., Ferreira, P.H., et al. (2013) Methodological limitations prevent definitive conclusions on the effects of patients' preferences in randomized clinical trials evaluating musculoskeletal conditions. *Journal of Clinical Epidemiology*, 66, 586–598.

Frieden, T.R. (2017) Evidence for health decision making—Beyond randomized, controlled trials. *New England Journal of Medicine*, 377, 465–75.

Gemmell, I. & Dunn, G. (2011) The statistical pitfalls of the partially randomized preference design in non-blinded trials of psychological interventions. *International Journal of Methods in Psychiatric Research*, 20(1), 1–9.

Glasgow, R.E., Magid, D.J., Beck, A., Ritzwoller, D., & Estabrooks, P.A. (2005) Practical clinical trials for translating research to practice: Design and measurement recommendations. *Medical Care*, 43(6), 551–559.

Goldstein, C.E., Weijer, C., Taljaard, M., et al. (2019) Ethical issues in pragmatic cluster-randomized trials in dialysis facilities. *American Journal of Kidney Disease*, 74(5), 659–666.

Golfam, M., Beall, R., Brehaut J. et al. (2015) Comparing alternative design options for chronic disease prevention interventions. *European Journal of Clinical Investigation*, 45, 87–99.

Grapow, M.T.R., von Wattenwyl, R., Guller, U., Beyersdorf, F., & Zerkowski, H. R. (2006) Randomized controlled trials do not reflect reality: Real world analysis are critical for treatment guidelines. *The Journal of Theoretic and Cardio Surgery*, 132(1), 5–7.

Greenfield, S. & Platt, R. (2012) Can observational studies approximate RCTs? *Value in Health*, 15, 215–216.

Greenhalgh, T., Howick, J., & MasKreg, N., for the Evidence Based Medicine Renaissance Group (2014) Evidence based medicine: A movement in crisis? *BMJ*, 348, g3725.

Hansen, A.B.G. & Jones, A. (2017) Advancing "real world" trials that take account of social context and human volition. *Trials*, 18, 531–533.

Hansen, H.P. & Tjørnhøj-Thomsen, T. (2016) Meeting the challenges of intervention research in health science: An argument for a multimethod research approach. *Patient*, 9, 193–200.

Hatfield, I., Allison, A., Flight, L. et al. (2016) Adaptive designs undertaken in clinical research: A review of registered clinical trials. *Trials*, 17, 150–166.

He, Y., Gewirtz, A., Lee, S., Morrell, N., & August, G. (2016) A randomized preference trial to inform personalization of a parent training program implemented in community mental health clinics. *Translational Behavioral Medicine*, 6, 73–80.

Heinsman, D.T. & Shadish, W.R. (1996) Assignment methods in experimentation: When do nonrandomized experiments approximate answers from randomized experiments?. *Psychological Methods*, 1(2), 154–169.

Hemming, K., Haines, T.P., Chilton, P.J., Girling, A.J., & Lilford, R.J. (2015) The stepped wedge cluster randomised trial: Rationale, design, analysis, and reporting. *BMJ*, 350, h391.

Henry, D., Toaln, P., Gorman-Smith, D., & Schoeny, M. (2017) Alternatives to randomized control trial designs for community-based prevention evaluation. *Preventive Science*, 18, 671–680.

Hernán, M.A. (2018) The C-word: Scientific euphemisms do not improve causal inference from observational data. *American Journal of Public Health*, 108, 616–619.

Hernán, M.A. & Hernádez-Diaz, S. (2012) Beyond the intention-to-treat in comparative effectiveness research. *Clinical Trials*, 9, 48–55.

Hernán, M.A. & Robins, J.M. (2016) Using big data to emulate a target trial when a randomized trial is not available. *American Journal of Epidemiology*, 183(8), 758–764.

Hernán, M.A., Hernández-Diaz, S., & Robins, J.M. (2013) Randomized trials analyzed as observational studies. *Annals of Internal Medicine*, 159(8), 560–564.

Hershkop, E., Segal, L., Fainaru, O., & Kol, S. (2017) "Model" versus "everyday" patients: Can randomized controlled trial data really be applied to the clinic? *Reproductive Biomedicine Online*, 34, 274–279.

Holm, M., Alvariza, A., Fürst, C-J., et al. (2017) Recruiting participants in a randomized controlled trial testing an intervention in palliative cancer care—The perspectives of health care professionals. *European Journal of Oncology Nursing*, 31, 6–11.

Holtz, A. (2007) *Comparative effectiveness of health interventions: Strategies to change policy and practice*. Report from ECRI Institute's 15th Annual Conference. 1–8.

Horwitz, R.I., Hayes-Conroy, A., Coricchio, R., & Singer, B.H. (2017) Fromm evidence based medicine to medicine based evidence. *The American Journal of Medicine*, 130, 1246–1250.

Horwood, J., Johnson, E., & Gooberman-Hill, R. (2016) Understanding involvement in surgical orthopaedic randomized controlled trials: A qualitative study of patient and health professional views and experiences. *International Journal of Orthopaedic and Trauma Nursing*, 20, 3–12.

Hox, J.J. (2010) *Multilevel Analysis: Techniques and Applications* (2nd ed.). Routledge, Hove.

Hróbjartsson, A., Forgang, E., Haahr, M.T., Als-Neilson, B., & Brorsom, S. (2007) Blinded trials taken to the test: An analysis of randomized clinical trials that report tests for the success of blinding. *International Journal of Epidemiology*, 36, 654–663.

Hróbjartsson, A., Emanuelsson, F., Thomsen, A.S.S., Hilden, J., & Brorson, S. (2014) Bias due to lack of patient blinding in clinical trials. A systematic review of trials randomizing patients to blind and nonblind sub-studies. *International Journal of Epidemiology*, 43(4), 1272–128.

Hubacher, D., Spector, H., Monteith, C., Chen, P.-L., & Hart, C. (2015) Rationale and enrollment results for a partially randomized patient preference trial to compare continuation rates of short-acting and long-acting reversible contraception. *Contraception*, 91(3), 185–192.

Hui, D., Zhukovsky, D.S., & Bruera, E. (2015) Which treatment is better? Ascertaining patient preferences with crossover randomized controlled trials. *Journal of Pain and Symptom Management*, 49(3), 625–631.

Imbens, G. W. & Lemieux, T. (2008) Regression discontinuity designs: A guide to practice. *Journal of Econometrics*, 142(2), 615–635.

Jo, B., Muthen, B.O., Asparouhov, T., Ialongo, N.S., & Hendricks-Brown, C. (2008) Cluster randomized trials with treatment noncompliance. *Psychological Methods*, 13(1), 1–18.

Johnson, R.B. & Schoonenboom, J. (2016) Adding qualitative and mixed methods research to health intervention studies: Interacting with differences. *Qualitative Health Research*, 26(5), 587–602.

Johnson, S.R., Tomlinson, G.A., Hawker, G.A., Granton, J.T., & Feldman, B.M. (2018) Propensity score methods for bias reduction in observational studies of treatment effect. *Rheumatic Disease Clinics of North America*, 44, 203–213.

Kappen, T.H., van Loon, K., Kappen, M.A.M., et al. (2016) Barriers and facilitators perceived by physicians when using prediction models in practice. *Journal of Clinical Epidemiology*, 70, 136–145.

Kearney, R.S., Achten, J., Parsons, N.R., & Costa, M.L. (2011) The comprehensive cohort model in a pilot trial in orthopaedic trauma. *BMC Medical Research Methodology*, 11, 39.

Kikkenborg Berg, S., Moons, P., Christensen, A.V., et al. (2015) Clinical effects and implications of cardiac rehabilitation for implantable cardioverter defibrillator patients: A mixed methods approach embedding data from the Copenhagen outpatient programme E—Implantable Cardioverter defibrillator randomized clinical trial with qualitative data. *Journal of Cardiovascular Nursing*, 30(5), 420–427.

Knox, D., Yamamoto, T., Baum, M.A., & Berinsky, A.J. (2019) Design, identification, and sensitivity analysis for patient preference trials. *Journal of the American Statistical Association*, 114(528), 1532–1546.

Kolltveit, B-C.H., Thorne, S., Graue, M., et al. (2017) Telemedicine follow-up facilitates more comprehensive diabetes foot ulcer care: A qualitative study in home-based and specialist health care. *Journal of Clinical Nursing*, 27, e1134–e1145.

Komatsu, H., Yagaski, K., & Yamaguchi, T. (2016) Effects of a nurse-led medication self-management programme in cancer patients: Protocol of a mixed-method randomized controlled trials. *BMC Nursing*, 15, 9–18.

Kowalski, C.J. & Mrdjenovich, A.J. (2013) Patient preference clinical trials: Why and when they will sometimes be preferred. *Perspectives in Biology and Medicine*, 56(1), 18–35.

Kozica, S.L., Teede, H.J., Harrison, C.L., Klein, R., & Lombard, C.B. (2016) Optimizing implementation of obesity prevention programs: A qualitative investigation within a large-scale randomized controlled trials. *The Journal of Rural Health*, 32, 72–81.

Krauss, A. (2018) Why all randomized controlled trials produce biased results. *Annals of Medicine*, 50(4), 312–322.

Kröz, M., Reif, M., Glinz, A., et al., and on Behalf of the CRF-2 Study Group (2017). Impact of a combined multimodal aerobic and multimodal intervention compared to standard aerobic treatment in breast cancer survivors with chronic cancer-related fatigue—Results of a three-armed pragmatic trial in a comprehensive cohort design. *BMC Cancer*, 17, 166–178.

Kwan, B.M., Dimidjian, S., & Rizvi, S.L. (2010) Treatment preferences, engagement, and clinical improvement in pharmacotherapy versus psychotherapy for depression. *Behavior Research and Therapy*, 48, 799–804.

Lawlor, D.A., Smith, G.D., Bruckdorfer, K.R., Kundu, D., & Ebrahim, S. (2004) Those confounded vitamins: What can we learn from the differences between observational versus randomized trial evidence? *The Lancet*, 363, 1924–27.

Lei, H., Nahmu-Shani, I., Lynch, K., Oslin, D., & Murphy, S.A. (2012) A "SMART" design for building individual treatment sequences. *Annual Review of Clinical Psychology*, 8, 21–48.

Leviton, L.C. (2017) Generalizing about public health intervention: A mixed-methods approach to external validity. *Annual Review of Public Health*, 38, 371–391.

Lewin, S., Glenton, C., & Oxman, A. (2009) Use of qualitative methods alongside randomised controlled trials in complex health case interventions: Methodological study. *BMJ*, 339, b3496.

Lindheim, O., Bennett, O., Trentacosta, C.J., & McLear, C. (2014) Client preferences affect treatment satisfaction, completion and clinical outcome: A meta-analysis. *Clinical Psychology Review*, 34, 506–517.

Ling, T. (2012) Evaluating complex and unfolding intervention in real time. *Evaluation*, 18(1), 79–91.

Liu, Q. & Maxwell, S.E. (2020) Multiplicative treatment effects in randomized pretest-posttest experimental designs. *Psychological Methods*, 25 (1), 71–87.

Lobo, M.A., Kagan, S.H., & Corrigan, J.D. (2017) Research design options for intervention studies. *Pediatric Physical Therapy*, 29 (Suppl 3), S57–63.

Lohr, S., Schochet, P.Z., & Sanders, E. (2014) *Partially Nested Randomized Controlled Trials in Education Research: A Guide to Design and Analysis.* US Department of Education—National Center for Education Research, Washington, DC.

Lowenstein, P.R. & Castro, M.G. (2009) Uncertainty in the translation of preclinical experiments to clinical trials: Why do most Phase III clinical trials fail? *Current Gene Therapy*, 9(5), 368–374.

Lutge, E., Lewin, S., & Volmink, J. (2014) Economic support to improve tuberculosis treatment outcomes in South Africa: A qualitative process evaluation of a cluster randomized controlled trial. *Trials*, 15, 236–247.

Maciejewski, M.L. & Brookhart, M.A. (2019) Using instrumental variables to address bias from unobserved confounders. *Journal of the American Medical Association*, 321(21), 2124–2125.

Mallard, S.R., Howe, A., & Houghton, L.A. (2016) Vitamin D status and weight loss: A systematic review and meta-analysis of randomized and nonrandomized controlled weight-loss trials. *American Journal of Clinical Nutrition*, 104, 1151–1159.

Marchal, B., van Belle, S., De Brouwere, V., & Witter, S. (2013) Studying complex interventions: Reflections from the FEMHealth project on evaluating fee exemption policies in West Africa and Morocco. *BMC Health Services*, 13, 469–477.

Marcus, S.M., Stuart, E.A., Wang, P., Shadish, W.R., & Steiner, P.M. (2012) Estimating the causal effect of randomization versus treatment preference in a doubly randomized preference trial. *Psychological Methods*, 17(2), 244–254.

Mazzuca, S., Tabak, R.G., Pilar, M., et al. (2018) Variation in research designs to test the effectiveness of dissemination and implementation strategies: A review. *Frontiers in Public Health*, 6, 32.

McArthur, K., Cooper, M., & Berdondini, L. (2016) Change processes in school-based humanistic counseling. *Counseling and Psychotherapy Research*, 16(2), 88–99.

McCurry, S.M., Shortreed, S.M., Von Korff, M, et al. (2014) Who benefits from CBT for insomnia in primary care? Important patient selection and trial lessons from longitudinal results of the lifestyle trial. *Sleep*, 37(2), 299–308.

Medical Research Council [MRC] (2019) *Developing and evaluating complex interventions: Following considerable development in the field since 2006.* The authors. Available on: https://mrc.ukri.org/documents/pdf/complex-interventions-guidance (accessed in May 13, 2019).

Meinich Petersen, S., Zoffman, V., Kjærgaard, J., Steensballe, L.G., & Greisen, G. (2014) Disappointment and adherence among parents of newborns allocated to the control group: A qualitative study of a randomized clinical trial. *Trials*, 15, 126–136.

Midgley, N., Ansaldo, F., & Target, M. (2014) The meaningful assessment of therapy outcomes: Incorporating a qualitative study into a randomized controlled trial evaluating the treatment of adolescent depressions. *Psychotherapy*, 51(1), 128–137.

Miles, M.B., Huberman, A.M., & Saldana, J. (2019) *Qualitative Data Analysis. A Methods Sourcebook* (4th ed.). Sage Publications, Inc., Thousand Oaks, CA

Mitchell-Jones, N., Farren, J.A., Tobias, A., Bourne, T., & Bottomley, C. (2017) Ambulatory versus inpatient management of severe nausea and vomiting of pregnancy: A randomised control trial with patient preference arm. *BMJ Open*, 7, e017566.

Mohr, D.C., Schueller, S.M., Riley, W.T., et al. (2015. Trials of intervention principles: Evaluation methods for evolving behavioral intervention technologies. *Journal of Medical Internet Research*, 17(7), e166.

Moore, G.F., Audrey, S., Barker, M., et al. (2015) Process evaluation of complex interventions: Medical Research Council guidance. *BMJ*, 350, h1258.

Morin, C.M., Belleville, G., Bélanger, L., & Ivers, H. (2011) The insomnia severity index: Psychometric indicators to detect insomnia cases and evaluate treatment response. *Sleep*, 34(5), 601–608.

Moss, A.S., Reibel, D.K., Greeson, J.M., et al. (2015) An adapted mindfulness-based stress reduction program for elders in a continuing care retirement community: Quantitative and qualitative results from a pilot randomized controlled trial. *Journal of Applied Gerontology*, 34(4), 518–538.

Mulder, R., Singh, A.B., Hamilton, A., et al. (2018) The limitations of using randomised controlled trials as a basis for developing treatment guidelines. *Evidence-Based Mental Health*, 21(1), 4–6.

Murray, D.M., Varnell, S.P., & Blitstein, J. L. (2004) Design and analysis of group randomized trials: A review of recent methodological developments. *American Journal of Public Health*, 94(3), 423–432.

Mustafa, F.A. (2015) Non-consent bias in OCTET. *The Lancet*, 2, 233–234.

Nahum-Shani, I., Qian, M., Almirall, D., et al. (2012) Experimental design and primary data analysis methods for comparing adaptive interventions. *Psychological Methods*, 17(4), 457–477.

Nahum-Shani, I., Almirall, D., Yap, J.R.T., et al. (2020) SMART longitudinal analysis: A tutorial for using repeated outcome measures from SMART studies to compare adaptive interventions. *Psychological Methods*, 25(1), 1–29.

Nelms, J.A. & Castel, L. (2016) A systematic review and meta-analysis of randomized and nonrandomized trials of clinical emotional freedom techniques (EFI) for the treatment of depression. *Explorer*, 12, 416–426.

Nelson, G., Mcnaughton, E., & Goering, P. (2015) What qualitative research can contribute to a randomized controlled trial of a complex community intervention. *Contemporary Clinical Trials*, 45, 377–384.

O'Cathain, A., Thomas, K.J., Drabble, S.J., et al. (2013) What can qualitative research do for randomised controlled trials? A systematic mapping review. *BMJ Open*, 3, e002889.

Omer, S., Golden, E., & Priebe, S. (2016) Exploring the mechanisms of a patient-centered assessment with a solution focused approach (DIALOG+) in the community of patients with psychosis: A process evaluation within a cluster-randomised controlled trial. *PLoS One*, 11(2), e0148415.

Page, P. (2014) Beyond statistical significance: Clinical interpretation of rehabilitation research literature. *The International Journal of Sports Physical Therapy*, 9(5), 726–736.

Page, M.J., Higgins, J.P.T., Clayton, G., et al. (2016) Empirical evidence of study design biases in randomized trials: Systematic review of meta-epidemiological studies. *PLoS One*, 11, e0159267.

Pan, W. & Bai, H. (2018) Propensity score methods for causal inference: An overview. *Behaviormetrike*, 45, 317–334.

Parsons, J.A., Yu, C.H.Y., Baker, N.A., et al. (2016) Practice doesn't always make perfect: A qualitative study explaining why a trial of an educational toolkit did not improve quality of care. *PLoS One*, 11(2), e0167878.

Patsopoulos, N.A. (2011) A pragmatic view on pragmatic trials. *Dialogues in Clinical Neuroscience*, 13, 217–224.

PCORI (2012) Methodological standards and patient-centredness in comparative effectiveness research. The PCORI perspective. *Journal of the American Medical Association*, 307(15), 1636–1640.

PCORI (2019) *Patient-Centered Outcomes Research Institute (PCORI) Methodology Committee. The PCORI Methodology Report.* PCORI is solely responsible for the final content of this report.

Preference Collaborative Research Group (2009) Patients' preferences within randomized trials: Systematic review and patient level meta-analysis. *British Medical Journal*, 338, a1864.

Probst, P., Zaschke, S., Heger, P., et al. (2019) Evidence-based recommendations for blinding in surgical trials. *Archives of Surgery*, 404, 273–284.

Prody, S.L., Burch, J., Crouch, S., & MacPherson, H. (2013) Insufficient evidence to determine the impact of patient preferences on clinical outcomes in acupuncture trials: A systematic review. *Journal of Clinical Epidemiology*, 66, 308–318.

Ranganathan, P., Pramesh, C.S., & Aggarwal, E. (2016) Common pitfalls in statistical analysis: Intention-to-treat versus per-protocol analysis. *Perspectives in Clinical Research*, 7(3), 144–146.

Rapport, F., Storey, M., Porter, A., et al. (2013) Qualitative research within trials: Developing a standard operating procedure for a clinical trials unit. *Trials*, 14, 54–61.

Raudenbush, S.W. & Bryk, A.S. (2002) *Hierarchical Linear Models: Applications and Data Analysis Methods.* Sage, Thousand Oaks, CA.

Raue, P.J., Schulberg, H.C., Heo, M., Klimstra, S., & Bruce, M.L. (2009) Patients' depression treatment preferences and initiation, adherence, and outcome: A randomized primary care study. *Psychiatric Services*, 60, 337–343.

Rengerink, K.O., Logtenberg, S., Hooft, L., Bossuyt, P.M., & Mol, B.W. (2015) Pregnant women's concerns when invited to a randomized trial: A qualitative case control study. *BMC Pregnancy and Childbirth*, 15, 207–217.

Renjith, V. (2017) Blinding in randomized controlled trials: What researchers need to know? *Journal of Nursing and Health Sciences*, 3(1), 45–50.

Reynolds, J., DiLiberto, J., Mangham-Jefferies, L., et al. (2014) The practice of 'doing' evaluation: Lessons learned from nine complex intervention trials in action. *Implementation Science*, 9, 75–86.

Rickles, D. (2009) Causality in complex interventions. *Medical Health Care and Philosophy*, 12, 77–90.

Rigato, M., Monami, M., & Fadini, G.P. (2017) Autologous cell therapy for peripheral arterial disease. Systematic review and meta-analysis of randomized, nonrandomized, and noncontrolled studies. *Circulation Research*, 120, 1326–1340.

Riley, W.T., Glasgow, R.E., Etheredge, L., & Abernethy, A.P. (2013) Rapid, responsive, relevant (R3) research: A call for a rapid learning health research enterprise. *Clinical and Translational Medicine*, 2, 10–14.

Robins, J.M. & Weissman, M.B. (2016) Commentary: Counterfactual causation and street lamps: What is to be done? *International Journal of Epidemiology*, 45(6), 1830–1835.

Saltaji, H., Armijo-Olivo, S., Cummings, G.G., et al. (2018) Influence of blinding on treatment effect size estimate in randomized controlled trials of oral health interventions. *BMC Medical Research Methodology*, 18, 42–58.

Saper, R.B., Lemaster, C.M., Elwy, A.R., et al. (2016) Yoga versus education for veterans with chronic low back pain: Study protocol of a randomized controlled trial. *Trials*, 17, 224–241.

Schoultz, M., Macaden, L., & Hubbard, G. (2016) Participants' perspectives on mindfulness-based cognitive therapy for inflammatory bowel disease: A qualitative study nested within a pilot randomised controlled trial. *Pilot and Feasibility Studies*, 2, 3–16.

Shadish, W.R., Cook, T.D., & Campbell, D.T. (2002) *Experimental and Quasi-Experimental Design for Generalized Causal Inference.* Houghton-Mifflin, Boston, MA.

Shean, G. (2014) Limitations of randomized control designs in psychotherapy research. *Advances in Psychiatry*, 2014, 561452.

Sidani, S. (2006) Random assignment: A systematic review. In: R. R. Bootzin & P. E. McKnight (eds) *Strengthening Research Methodology. Psychological Measurement and Evaluation.* American Psychological Association Books, Washington, DC.

Sidani, S. (2015) *Health Intervention Research: Advances in Research Design and Methods.* Sage, London, UK.

Sidani, S., Bootzin, R.R., Epstein, D.R., Miranda, J., & Cousins, J. (2015) Attrition in randomized and preference trials of behavioral treatments for insomnia. *Canadian Journal of Nursing Research*, 47(1), 17–34.

Sidani, S., Fox, M., & Esptein, D.R. (2017) Contribution of treatment acceptability to acceptance of randomization: An exploration. *Journal of Evaluation in Clinical Practice*, 23(1), 14–20.

Sil, A., Kumar, P., Kumar, R., & Das, N.K. (2019) Selection of control, randomization, blinding, and allocation concealment. *Indian Dermatology Online Journal*, 10(5), 601–605.

Sinclair, C., Auret, K.A., Evans, S.F., et al. (2017) Advance care planning uptake among patients with severe lung disease: A randomised patient preference trial of a nurse-led, facilitated advance care planning intervention. *BMJ Open*, 7, e013415.

Skivington, K., Matthews, L., Craig, P., Simpson, S., & Moore, L. (2018) Developing and evaluating complex interventions: Updating Medical Research Council guidance to take account of new methodological and theoretical approaches. *Lancet*, 392, S2.

Smeeing, D.P.J., van der Ven, D.J.C., Hietbrink, F., et al. (2017) Surgical versus nonsurgical treatment for midshaft clavicle fractures in patients aged 16 years and older. A systematic review, meta-analysis, and comparison of randomized controlled trials and observational studies. *The American Journal of Sports Medicine*, 45(8), 1937–1945.

Snowdon, C. (2015) Qualitative and mixed methods research in trials. *Trials*, 16, 558–560.

Song, J.W. & Chung, K.C. (2010) Observational studies: Cohort and case-control studies. *Plastic & Reconstruction Surgery*, 126(6), 2234–2242.

Soni, P.D., Hartman, H.E., Dess, R.T., et al. (2019) Comparison of population-based observational studies with randomized trials in oncology. *Journal of Clinical Oncology*, 37(14), 1209–1216.

Sox, H.C., Helfand, M., Grimshaw, J., Dickerson, K., The PLoS Medicine, Torvey, D., et al. (2010) Comparative effectiveness research: Challenges for medical journals. *Trials*, 7(4), 45.

Spillane, J.P., Pareja, A.S., Dorner, L., et al. (2010) Mixing methods in randomized controlled trials (RCTs): Validation, contextualization, triangulation and control. *Educational Assessment, Evaluation and Accountability*, 22, 5–28.

Steidtmann, D., Manber, R., Arnow, B.A., et al. (2012) Patient treatment preference as a predictor of response and attrition in treatment for chronic depression. *Depression and Anxiety*, 29, 896–905.

Stone, G.W. & Pocock, S.J. (2010) Randomized trials, statistics, and clinical inference. *Journal of the American College of Cardiology*, 55(5), 428–431.

Storrar, W., Dewey, A., Chauhan, A., et al. (2015) Early qualitative analysis to enhance trial process. *Trials*, 16(Suppl 2), 73.

Streiner, D.L. & Sidani, S. (eds) (2015) *When Research Goes off the Rails. Why It Happens and What you Can Do About It*. The Guilford Press, New York.

Swift. J.K., Callahan. J.L., & Vollmer, B.M. (2011) Preferences. *Journal of Clinical Psychology*, 67(2), 155–65.

Swift, J.K., Callahan, J.L., Ivanovic, L.M., & Kominiak, N. (2013). Further examination of the psychotherapy preference effect: A meta-regression analysis. *Journal of Psychotherapy Integration*, 23(2), 134–145.

Taljaard, M., Weijer, C., Grimshaw, J.M., et al. (2018) Developing a framework for the ethical design and conduct of pragmatic trials in healthcare: A mixed methods research protocol. *Trials*, 19, 525–537.

Tang, W., Xu, Q., Hong, G., et al. (2016) Comparative efficacy of anti-diabetic agents on nonalcoholic fatty liver disease in patients with type 2 diabetes mellitus: A systematic review and meta-analysis of randomized and non-randomized studies. *Diabetes/Metabolism Research and Reviews*, 32, 200–216.

Tarquinio, C., Kivits, J., Minary, L., Coste, J., & Alla, F. (2015) Evaluating complex interventions: Perspective and issues for health behavior change interventions. *Psychology and Health*, 30(1), 35–51.

TenHave, T.R., Normand, S-L.T., Marcus, S.M., et al. (2008) Intent-to-treat vs non-intent-to-treat analyses under treatment non-adherence in mental health randomized trials. *Psychiatry Annals*, 38(12), 772–783.

Tomlison, M., Ward, C.L., & Marlow, M. (2015) The strengths and limitations of randomized controlled trials. *SA Crime Quarterly*, 51, 43–52.

Troxel, A.B., Asch, D.A., & Volpp, K.G. (2016) Statistical issues in pragmatic trials of behavioral economic interventions. *Clinical Trials*, 13(5), 578–483.

Tunis, S.R., Stryer, D.B., & Clancy, C. M. (2003) Practical clinical trials: Increasing the value of clinical research for decision making in clinical and health policy. *Journal of the American Medical Association*, 290(12), 1624–1632.

United States Government Accountability Office (2009) *Program Evaluation: A variety of rigorous methods can help identify effective interventions*. Available on: `http://www.gao.gov/products/GAO-10-30\` (accessed in May 2019).

Ussher, J.M. & Perz, J. (2017) Evaluation of the relative efficacy of a couple cognitive-behaviour therapy (CBT) for premenstrual disorders (PMDs), in comparison to one-to-one CBT and a wait list control: Randomized controlled trial. *PLoS One*, 12(4), e0175068.

Van Belle, S., Wong, G., Westrop, G. et al. (2016) Can "realist" randomised controlled trials be genuinely realist? *BMC Trials*, 17, 313–320.

Van den Hurk, D.G.M., Schellekens, M.P.J., Molema, J., Speckens, A.E.M., & van der Drift, M.A. (2015) Mindfulness-based stress reduction for lung cancer patients and their partners: Results of a mixed methods pilot study. *Palliative Medicine*, 29(7), 652–660.

VanderWeele, T. (2016) Commentary: On causes, casual inference, and potential outcomes. *International Journal of Epidemiology*, 45(6), 1809–1816.

Velthuis, M.J., May, A.M., Monninkhof, E.M., van der Wall, E., & Peeters, P.H.M. (2012) Alternatives for randomization in lifestyle intervention studies in cancer patients were not better than conventional randomization. *Journal of Clinical Epidemiology*, 65, 288–292.

Verhaegher, N., De Maeseneer, J., Maes, L., et al. (2012) Health promotion intervention in mental health care: Design and baseline findings of a cluster preference randomized controlled trial. *BMC Public Health*, 12, 431–441.

Verwey, R., van der Weegen, S., Spreeuwenberg, M., et al. (2016) Process evaluation of physical activity counseling with and without the use of mobile technology: A mixed methods study. *International Journal of Nursing Studies*, 53, 3–16.

Villeval, M., Bidault, E., Shoveller, J., et al. (2016) Enabling the transferability of complex interventions: Exploring the combination of an intervention's key functions and implementation. *International Journal of Public Health*, 61, 1031–1038.

Walter, S.D., Turner, R.M., Macaskill, P., McCaffery, K.J., & Irwig, L. (2017) Estimation of treatment preference effects in clinical trials when some participants are indifferent to treatment choice. *BMC Medical Research Methodology*, 17, 29–38.

WanderWeele, T.J., Hernán, M.A., Techtgan, E.J., & Robins, J.M. (2016) Letters to the editor—Re: Causality and casual inference in epidemiology: The need for a pluralistic approach. *International Journal of Epidemiology*, 45(6), 2199–2200.

Wartolowska, K., Beard, D., & Carr, A. (2018) Blinding in trials of interventional procedures is possible and worthwhile. *F1000Research*, 6, 1663.

Wasmann, K., Wijsman, P., van Dieren, S., Bemelman, W., & Buskens, C. (2019) Influence of patients' preference in randomised controlled trials. *Journal of Crohn's and Colitis*, 13(Suppl 1), S517–S518.

Wellek, S. & Blettner, M. (2012) On the proper use of the crossover design in clinical trials: Part 18 of a series on evaluation of scientific publication. *Deutsches Ärzteblatt International*, 109(15), 276–281.

Werner, R.M., Coe, N.B., Qi, M., & Konetzka, R.T. (2019) Patient outcomes after hospital discharge to home with home healthcare vs to a skilled nursing facility. *JAMA Internal Medicine*, 179(5), 617–623.

West, S.G. & Thoemmes, F. (2010) Campbell's and Rubin's perspectives on causal inference. *Psychological Methods*, 15(1): 18–37.

White, H. (2013) The use of mixed methods in randomized control trials. In: D.M. Mestens & S. Hesse-Biber (eds) *Mixed Methods and Credibility of Evidence in Evaluation: New Directions for Evaluation, Number 138*. Jossey-Bass, San Francisco, CA

Wiedermann, W. & von Eye, A. (2015) Direction of effects in mediation analysis. *Psychological Methods*, 20(2), 221–244.

Winter, S. E. & Barber, J.P. (2013) Should treatment for depression be based more on patient preference? *Patient Preference and Adherence*, 7, 1047–1057.

Winter, A.C. & Colditz, G.A. (2014) Clinical trial design in the era of comparative effectiveness research. *Open Access Journal of Clinical Trials*, 6, 101–110.

Wojewodka, G., Hurley, S., Taylor, S.J.C., et al. (2017) Implementation fidelity of a self-management cause of epilepsy: Method and assessment. *BMC Medical Research Methodology*, 17, 100–109.

Woodman, R.W. (2014) The role of internal validity in evaluation research on organizational change interventions. *The Journal of Applied Behavioral Science*, 50(1), 40–49.

Yang, R., Carter, B.L., Gums, T.H., et al. (2017) Selection bias and subject refusal in a cluster-randomized controlled trial. *BMC Medical Research Methodology*, 17, 94–103.

Yang, J.Y., Webster-Clark, M., Lund, J.L., et al. (2019) Propensity score methods to control for confounding in observational cohort studies: A statistical primer and application to endoscopy research. *Gastrointestinal Endoscopy*, 90(3), 360–369.

Younge, J.O., Kouwenhoven-Pasmooij, T.A., Freak-Poli, R., Koos-Hesselink, J.W., & Hunink, M.G.M. (2015) Randomized study designs for lifestyle interventions: A tutorial. *International Journal of Epidemiology*, 44(6), 2006–2019.

Zeilstra, D., Younes, J.A., Brummer, R.J., & Kleerebezem, M. (2018) Perspective: Fundamental limitations of the randomized controlled trial methods in nutritional research: The example of probiotics. *Advances in Nutrition*, 9, 561–571.

Zwarenstein, M. (2017) "Pragmatic" and "explanatory" attitudes to randomised trials. *Journal of the Royal Society of Medicine*, 110(5), 208–218.

Zwarestein, M. & Treweek, S. (2009) What kind of randomized trials do we need?. *Canadian Medical Association Journal*, 180(10), 998–1000.

# CHAPTER 15

# Outcome Evaluation: Methods

The selection of a design is the first step in devising the plan for a study aimed to evaluate the outcomes of health interventions. A design specifies the overall schema of the study, pointing to the treatment groups to be included, the way in which participants are to be assigned to these groups, the timing for outcome assessment relative to treatment delivery, and whether or not a process evaluation is to be embedded within the outcome evaluation study. More information is required to guide the conduct of the study. It is essential to delineate the type of comparison treatment, as well as the methods for sampling participants, allocating participants to the health intervention under evaluation and the comparison treatment, collecting outcome (and process, if planned) data, and analyzing the data to determine the effectiveness of the intervention. If not carefully selected and applied, these methods can introduce biases that threaten the validity of inferences regarding the intervention's effects. The selection of methods and procedures is based on their relevance to the study question and designs, on a critical appraisal of their strengths and limitations, and most importantly, on their acceptability to stakeholder groups including the target client population and their feasibility.

In this chapter, the range of comparison treatments (alluded to in Chapter 14) is presented, and their advantages and disadvantages are discussed. Methods and procedures for sampling, treatment allocation, and outcome data collection and analysis are described, and their importance in maintaining validity is reviewed. Where available, evidence supporting the usefulness of particular methods or procedures is presented.

## 15.1 COMPARISON TREATMENT

### 15.1.1 Importance

As mentioned in Chapters 10 and 14, a comparison treatment is included in outcome evaluation studies to make valid inferences in attributing changes in posttest outcomes to the health intervention under evaluation. A valid attribution is supported by empirical evidence showing: (1) no significant differences in the baseline characteristics of

*Nursing and Health Interventions: Design, Evaluation, and Implementation*, Second Edition.
Souraya Sidani and Carrie Jo Braden.
© 2021 John Wiley & Sons Ltd. Published 2021 by John Wiley & Sons Ltd.

participants assigned to the intervention group and to the comparison group; (2) significant improvement in the outcomes in the intervention group from pretest to posttest, maintained at follow-up; (3) no significant changes in the outcomes in the comparison treatment group from pretest to posttest; and (4) significant differences between the two groups in the outcomes measured following treatment completion.

It is possible that participants in the comparison group report changes in the post-test outcomes. The changes may reflect worsening or improvement (to varying degree) in the outcomes over time. The changes may be related to life events (history), naturally expected changes in their condition (maturation or spontaneous recovery), learning that occurs with repeated completion of the outcome measures (testing), as well as participants' perceptions and reactions, favorable or unfavorable, to the allocated comparison treatment (as explained in Chapter 11). Alternatively, the changes could reflect the effects of the comparison treatment. The pattern of change, operationalized in the direction (i.e. improvement, no change, worsening) and magnitude (size or extent), in the outcomes reported for participants in the comparison group affects the estimates of the intervention effects. Participants exposed to no-treatment at all may experience worsening (of any magnitude) of outcomes. The worsening (quantified in posttest outcome scores of a direction opposite to hypothesized) yields large between-group differences in the posttest outcomes which result in overestimated intervention effects. Participants receiving a comparison treatment that incorporates some components (content, activities) of the experimental intervention may experience minimal change, in the hypothesized direction, in the posttest outcomes; this change translates into small between-group differences in the posttest outcomes. The small between-group differences potentially lead to underestimated intervention effects. Participants exposed to an alternative active treatment may experience moderate-to-large improvement in the outcomes. Large improvement results in no significant between-group differences in the posttest outcomes. The interpretation of nonsignificant between-group differences differs with the purpose of the study: in efficacy and effectiveness studies, they weaken the confidence in attributing the outcomes to the intervention, whereas in comparative effectiveness studies, they indicate that the intervention is as beneficial as the comparison treatment.

The influence of the type of comparison treatment on the estimates of the intervention effects is illustrated in the findings of a recent systematic review. Frost et al. (2018) reviewed the results of studies that evaluated motivational interviewing. They reported significant effects where motivational interviewing was compared to no-treatment and no beneficial effects where it was compared to alternative active treatments, that is, treatments with active components that differ from those comprising the experimental intervention.

The selection of a comparison treatment therefore, is informed by the overall study purpose and an understanding of the different types of comparison treatment. In general, studies aimed to examine the efficacy of health interventions include a no-treatment condition, placebo treatment, or treatment-as-usual. Studies concerned with demonstrating the effectiveness of interventions consider comparison treatments that are relevant to practice, such as usual care or treatment-as-usual. Studies focusing on comparative effectiveness select alternative active treatments.

The different types of comparison treatments that are commonly used in the evaluation of health interventions are described next; their strengths and limitations are highlighted to assist in deciding which one to select. There are two general points to consider regarding comparison treatments:

1. It is widely acknowledged that the comparison treatment should not incorporate the components reflecting the active ingredients of the health intervention

under evaluation. With overlap in components (content, activities, and/or treatment recommendations), participants exposed to the comparison treatment may experience improvement in the outcomes similar to the improvement reported by participants receiving the health intervention. Comparable levels of improvement are quantified in posttest outcome scores that do not differ much between the experimental intervention and the comparison treatment groups. Small between-group differences reduce the size of the intervention effects and increase the probability of type II error in efficacy and effectiveness studies. The intervention is claimed ineffective when it is successful in initiating the mechanism of action and in inducing the hypothesized improvement in the ultimate outcomes.

2. It is important to develop a manual to guide the delivery of the selected comparison treatment and to monitor the fidelity with which the comparison treatment is provided, as part of the process evaluation embedded in the outcome evaluation study (Chapter 13). Adherence to the manual and assessment of fidelity help in preventing overlap and in determining the extent of variations in providing the comparison treatment; these variations could have led, intentionally or unintentionally, to the integration of some intervention components into the comparison treatment which, as explained previously, reduces the size of the health intervention's effects. Therefore, fidelity data are useful in the interpretation of findings, especially when no significant between-group differences in the posttest outcomes are observed.

## 15.1.2   No-Treatment Control Condition

In a no-treatment control condition, participants do not receive any treatment for the health problem, as part of the evaluation study. Participants who may be taking treatment are requested to withhold it or to maintain its dose constant for the duration of the study.

The advantage of a no-treatment control condition is that it creates a situation that generates the evidence for demonstrating the criterion of covariation for inferring causality (Chapter 10). The evidence shows no change in the outcomes at posttest in participants assigned to the no-treatment control condition and improvement in the outcomes in participants assigned to the intervention.

There are disadvantages to the no-treatment control condition:

1. It presents an ethical dilemma because treatment is withheld for participants who may have a pressing need for treatment, potentially jeopardizing their health.

2. It generates unfavorable reactions among participants assigned to the no treatment control condition. These participants demand an explanation for withholding treatment to which they are entitled. They lose motivation and withdraw from the study to seek treatment elsewhere (De Moat et al., 2007). Those who complete the study may experience worsening of the health problem over the study duration.

3. Participants' reactions introduce biases. Differential attrition is highly likely when a larger number of participants in the no treatment control group than in the intervention group withdraw. Differential attrition is a major threat to internal (i.e. confounding) and statistical (i.e. low power) validity (Chapter 10). Participants who seek treatment outside the trial (concurrent treatment) and

complete the evaluation study may report improvement in the outcomes, which may reduce the size of the between-group differences in the posttest outcomes and increase the chance of type II error.

### 15.1.3   Placebo Treatment

Placebo refers to an inert, innocuous treatment that has no inherent power or capacity to induce changes in the health problem. To be included in intervention evaluation studies, placebo treatments have to be credible (Foster, 2012) so that they appear meaningful to participants. Accordingly, placebo treatments should be comparable to the health intervention under evaluation in all respects except the active ingredients that characterize the experimental intervention. Thus, placebo treatments are designed to be structurally equivalent to the experimental intervention.

Structural equivalence means that the placebo treatment has the same nonspecific components as those planned for the delivery of the experimental intervention. Therefore, placebo treatments are delivered by trained interventionists, in the same mode (e.g. individual or group, face-to-face sessions), dose (e.g. number of sessions) and setting (e.g. facility and room). The sessions or modules are provided in a similar format as planned for the experimental intervention. Participants are (1) informed of the treatment rationale at the beginning of treatment; the rationale maintains credibility of the placebo treatment and avoids disappointment associated with the receipt of a less desirable treatment; (2) provided information about general health or topics that are not directly related to the health problem and its management; this is done to minimize overlap with the content covered in the experimental intervention; and (3) are encouraged to engage in a discussion of health-related topics and to carry out homework such as problem solving. Interventionists providing placebo treatment are also encouraged to develop a working alliance with participants, as is also anticipated with the delivery of the experimental intervention.

The advantage of using a placebo treatment in an outcome evaluation study is the "control" for the nonspecific components of treatment delivery on the outcomes. A well-designed placebo treatment that is structurally equivalent to the experimental intervention incorporates the same nonspecific components as those comprising the intervention. It is believed that participants exposed to the same nonspecific components respond to these components in the same way, whether assigned to the placebo treatment or the intervention. The same responses are reflected in the same pattern (direction and magnitude) of changes in the outcomes observed at posttest. When participants exposed to placebo treatment and to the intervention exhibit the same responses to the nonspecific components, then differences between the two groups in the posttest outcomes are attributable solely and uniquely to the intervention's active ingredients, thereby enhancing the validity of the causal inferences (van Die et al., 2009).

The disadvantages of the placebo treatment are associated with the placebo response (also called placebo effects) it induces. Although placebo treatments are theoretically expected to be inert, they have been found to produce favorable outcomes such as improvement in the experience of the health problem, or unfavorable outcomes such as the development of side effects. Several mechanisms have been proposed to explain the placebo response: (1) the natural fluctuation in the experience or the natural resolution of the health problem over the evaluation study period; (2) participants' motivation to apply the homework or placebo treatment recommendations; the motivation results from the perceptions of good rapport and/or working alliance with the interventionist; (3) expectancy of improvement associated with the belief that the placebo treatment is credible and useful; (4) classical conditioning, where improvement is anticipated with the mere fact of receiving a treatment; and (5) neurobiological mechanisms reflected in endogenous opioids (Autret et al., 2012; Finnis et al., 2010; van Die et al., 2009).

Developing a placebo treatment that is structurally equivalent to health interventions presents challenges. Placebo treatments addressing general health topics that are not directly or obviously related to the health problem targeted by the intervention may not be perceived favorably. Participants become aware of the experimental intervention and the placebo treatment during recruitment and the consent process; research ethics may require informing participants of the risks involved in assignment to placebo treatment (Wandile, 2018). Therefore, participants may view the placebo treatment as less credible and less desirable; they may be unwilling to be randomized and withdraw from the study, leading to differential attrition. Participants who enroll in the study and are exposed to the placebo treatment may not experience improvement in the health problem. Some withdraw from the study and others may attempt to please the researchers by reporting socially desirable responses, resulting in response bias (Younge et al., 2015).

In general, placebo responses affect the size of differences in the posttest outcomes between the placebo treatment and the intervention groups, yielding biased (under or over) estimates of the intervention effects as indicated in the results of meta-analyses. A few meta-analytic studies reported no or weak placebo effects (Finnis et al., 2010; Kaptchuk et al., 2010), whereas others found a high prevalence of the placebo response and a high magnitude of the placebo effects. Large placebo effects were reported for subjective outcomes (e.g. symptoms), placebo treatments that were not structurally equivalent to the experimental intervention, and placebo treatments involving frequent encounters with empathetic and supportive interventionists (Autret et al., 2012; Baskin et al., 2000; Finnis et al., 2010; Kaptchuk et al., 2010; van Die et al., 2009).

### 15.1.4 Treatment-as-Usual

In treatment-as-usual, also called usual care or usual treatment, participants continue to receive the treatment that is prescribed by their healthcare providers, for the management of the health problem addressed by the experimental intervention. In some evaluation studies, participants allocated to the comparison group only are asked to continue with treatment-as-usual and those in the experimental intervention group are not offered or are requested to stop the application of usual treatment. In this situation, between-group differences in the posttest outcomes are assumed to reflect the unique effects of the experimental intervention. In other evaluation studies, participants in both the comparison treatment group and the experimental intervention group continue with treatment-as-usual. In this situation, the experimental intervention is provided along with usual care; between-group differences in the posttest outcomes indicate the contribution of the experimental intervention above and beyond treatment-as-usual.

Treatment-as-usual is commonly resorted to in situations where it is unethical and unacceptable to stakeholder groups (participants, health professionals, researchers, decision-makers) to withhold usual care. However, the use of treatment-as-usual as a comparison treatment generates methodological challenges that should be carefully addressed during the conduct of the study in order to enhance validity. The challenges stem from the variability in the definition and delivery of treatment-as-usual across participants recruited from the same or different practice settings, over the study duration. Whether informed by best practice guidelines adopted in some but not all participating practice settings, or by individual health professionals' judgment, usual care is often individualized. Accordingly, participants assigned to the experimental intervention or the comparison treatment, receive different types of usual treatments. Usual treatments are given in different modes and doses that are responsive to participants' initial experience of the health problem, characteristics, preferences and life circumstances, and adapted to progress in their experience of the health problem and overall health condition, over time. It is possible that usual treatments contain the specific components reflecting the active ingredients of the experimental intervention and/or its nonspecific components. The variability in the types and delivery of the treatment-as-usual, and the possible overlap of its components with those of the experimental intervention, increases the within-group variance in the responses (levels of improvement or scores in the posttest outcomes) to the allocated treatment. High within-group variance decreases the power to detect significant experimental intervention effects (Younge et al., 2015).

It, therefore, is important to address the methodological challenges associated with the use of treatment-as-usual in an outcome evaluation study. This can be achieved by: (1) selecting into the study, practice settings that provide standardized usual care; standardized usual care adheres to clearly defined best practice guidelines; (2) obtaining agreement from health professionals and decision-makers at the selected practice settings, to maintain treatment-as-usual (as much as ethically and clinically appropriate) consistent across participants and constant over the study duration; and (3) monitoring the fidelity with which treatment-as-usual is delivered. Alternatively, provision of "devised care" has been suggested to address the challenges with treatment-as-usual. Devised care involves the development of treatment-as-usual from available best practice guidelines; it is delivered consistently by interventionists hired for the evaluation study (Barkauskas et al., 2005). An additional strategy to address the methodological challenges is to collect data on what treatment-as-usual is given to what participant. Analysis of these data is helpful in clarifying the distinction between the experimental intervention and the comparison treatment in an evaluation study, and in interpreting the findings.

### 15.1.5   Active Treatment

Alternative active treatments include theory-informed or evidence-based interventions designed to manage the health problem addressed by the health intervention under evaluation. Different types of active treatments are available and can be used in an outcome evaluation study.

Active treatments can comprise *selected components operationalizing some active ingredients of a complex health intervention*. This type of active treatment is often used in dismantling studies. These studies focus on determining the contribution of each component or a combination of components relative to that of the complex intervention as-a-whole (e.g. Epstein et al., 2012). In other words, the goals are to identify which components are most and least effective, and to refine the design of the complex intervention so that it includes only the combination of components found most beneficial. This revision of the complex intervention is believed to optimize its effectiveness and efficiency.

Despite its utility, this type of active treatment may generate challenges in the interpretation of the outcome evaluation study's findings. With an active treatment that contains selected components of the same intervention, there is an overlap in the components comprising the experimental intervention and those comprising the comparison treatment. If the components comprising the comparison treatment are beneficial, then participants in both groups experience comparable levels of improvement in the outcomes. As explained previously, comparable levels of improvement reduce the magnitude of the between-group differences in the posttest outcomes, and decrease the likelihood of detecting significant intervention effects (i.e. type II error of inference). It is also possible that the components included in the comparison treatment interact with each other. The components may weaken each other's effects, resulting in worsening or no change in the outcomes; this yields large between-group differences in the posttest outcomes. Alternatively, the components may strengthen or enhance each other's effects, resulting in large improvement in the posttest outcomes; this leads to small between-group differences, or findings that support the superiority of the comparison treatment relative to the experimental intervention.

Active treatments may consist of the *experimental intervention given at a low dose or in a different mode or format*. This type of active treatment is perceived favorably by participants as they are given a credible, acceptable, and potentially effective treatment that addresses their pressing need to manage the presenting health problem. This favorable perception has the potential to enhance participants' enrollment, willingness to be randomized, as well as engagement, enactment, and completion of treatment. Participants' perceptions and behaviors yield improvement in the outcomes that is comparable to that reported for the experimental intervention, thereby obscuring the intervention's effects.

Alternative treatments may consist of *interventions or therapies with active ingredients* that differ from those characterizing the experimental intervention. These treatments induce different mechanisms of action responsible for the effective management of the health problem. Alternative treatments are commonly used in comparative effectiveness research. The experimental intervention's effects are compared relative to those of the alternative treatment. The goal is to determine that the experimental intervention is as effective (i.e. non-inferiority trial) or more beneficial (i.e. superiority trial) as the comparison treatment.

The inclusion of an active treatment in an outcome evaluation study is advantageous. It has the potential of enhancing recruitment, enrollment, and retention of participants. Comparing the effectiveness of the experimental health intervention to alternative active treatments provides evidence to guide treatment decision-making in practice.

## 15.2  SAMPLING

### 15.2.1  Importance

Sampling involves the application of methods for accruing an adequate number of participants who are representative of the target client population, excluding client subgroups with characteristics known to confound the intervention's effects. The methods are applied to recruit clients, screen for eligibility, determine the required sample size, and prevent attrition or retain participants in the study. The choice and application of these methods is critical for maintaining or enhancing the validity of inferences regarding the effects of the health intervention under evaluation.

Recruitment and screening contribute to the composition of the sample in an evaluation study. The sample should represent the target client population in order to enhance the generalizability of the study findings (issue of external validity).

Therefore, participants should experience the health problem addressed by the experimental intervention and have the personal and health or clinical characteristics that are comparable to those defining the target client population. Recruitment is expanded to reach the various subgroups (defined in terms of personal and health characteristics) comprising the target client population and avoid, intentionally or unintentionally, the exclusion of a specific subgroup (Fayler et al., 2007). Exclusion of client subgroups may yield sampling selection bias which limits the applicability of the evaluation study findings to the subgroups of the target population represented in the sample. Simultaneously, the sample should exclude participants with personal and health characteristics that are known, based on the intervention theory, empirical evidence, and clinical observation, to influence their capacity and ability to engage and enact treatment, to confound the intervention effects, or to increase the risk of untoward consequences. Therefore, screening for eligibility is done to generate a representative sample (and hence, maintain external validity) and to minimize the potential for confounding bias (and hence, maintain internal validity).

Determination of the required sample size indicates the number of eligible participants to enroll in the outcome evaluation study. The sample size is a determinant of the study's statistical power to detect significant intervention effects (issue of statistical conclusion validity). The sample size should be adequate, that is, not too large and not too small. With large samples, there is a general tendency to find "statistically" significant differences in the posttest outcomes between the experimental intervention and the comparison treatment groups, potentially leading to type I error (claiming that the intervention is effective when it is not). With small samples, there is a tendency to observe "statistically" nonsignificant differences, potentially leading to type II error (claiming that the intervention is ineffective when it is) (Lipsey, 1990). Therefore, the sample size required for an evaluation study is best determined on the basis of power analysis (Cohen, 1988).

Retention is critical to maintain the composition and the size of the study sample, and to minimize the potential for confounding. If a large number of participants assigned to the intervention and the comparison treatment groups withdraw from the study, then the sample size is decreased, which jeopardizes the power to detect significant intervention effects and increases the chance of type II error. If a larger number of participants assigned to one group drop out, then the groups' sizes, and the within-group variances in the outcomes are unbalanced. This imbalance affects the estimates of the intervention's effects when it is not accounted for in the statistical analysis (issue of statistical conclusion validity). Differential attrition can also be encountered when participants who withdraw from one group differ in their personal and health characteristic than those who drop out of another group. Differential attrition introduces confounding (issue of internal validity). Thus, the findings are based on the subgroups of the target client population that completed the study; they may not be applicable and replicated across different subgroups of the target client population (Sidani, 2015).

There are general points to consider in planning for screening, recruitment, and determination of the sample size for an outcome evaluation study. These are:

1. Screening assesses for the prespecified eligibility (inclusion and exclusion) criteria, using relevant validated measures. It is done in the early stages of an evaluation study, with clients' oral/verbal agreement and/or written consent, based on the level of intrusiveness/invasiveness of the screening tests, and the requirements of the research ethics boards at participating settings. Early screening reduces the burden of extensive assessment for clients who do not

meet the general eligibility criteria (such as language or experience of the health problem).

2. Multiple recruitment strategies are planned to reach various subgroups of the target client population. It is useful to consult key informants or representatives of the target client population regarding the most appropriate and acceptable recruitment strategies. Recruitment is done at the start of the evaluation study and at regularly scheduled intervals over the study period to coincide with the planned waves for delivering the intervention. Monitoring the effectiveness of the recruitment strategies helps in optimizing recruitment within available resources.

3. Determination of the sample size has to account for the accessibility and size of the sampling pool (i.e. number of potentially eligible clients at the participating practice settings, geographic or catchment area, or community) and the anticipated (based on previous research involving the same target client population) enrollment and attrition rates. The goal is to accrue a final sample (i.e. participants who complete the study) of the size required to detect significant intervention effects.

4. Multiple retention strategies are incorporated in a study. The strategies need to be relevant and attractive to the target client population, and not perceived as coercive. The strategies can be provided at different time points throughout participants' involvement in the evaluation study.

5. The relevance, feasibility, and effectiveness of the methods for recruitment, screening and retention are examined in pilot studies (Chapter 12) and optimized prior to use in the large-scale outcome evaluation study. But, be cognizant of Murphy's law and prepare for it by having multiple methods and alternative ways or procedures for applying the methods (Streiner & Sidani, 2010).

## 15.2.2   Screening

Screening aims to determine if clients referred to the outcome evaluation study meet the eligibility criteria. It is informed by the prespecified inclusion and exclusion criteria and conducted with relevant measures that can be administered by health professionals or service providers involved in client referral, and by the research personnel, at the time of enrollment. The eligibility criteria are specified on the basis of (1) the intervention theory: the theory clarifies the nature of the health problem, describes its indicators, and identifies its determinants as well as aspects of the problem addressed by the intervention (forming inclusion criteria). The theory also highlights client characteristics that may influence engagement, enactment, and response to the intervention (forming exclusion criteria); (2) available empirical evidence and clinical observations: these point to subgroups of clients who do not benefit from the intervention or are at risk of developing discomfort or side effects associated with the health intervention. Evidence and observation may highlight possible interaction between the intervention and the treatment-as-usual prescribed to clients (forming exclusion criteria).

It is worth reiterating that the prespecification of restrictive or stringent criteria limits the number of potentially eligible clients (sampling pool). A limited sampling pool, in combination with the number of clients who do not consent (for any reason), decrease enrollment rate and thus, the accrued sample size. The end result is reduced statistical power to detect significant intervention effects and limited applicability of the findings to the range of clients seen in practice (see Chapter 14).

Well-specified eligibility criteria are foundational for the selection of practice settings for recruitment and measures for screening. Recruitment settings (e.g. hospital, clinic, community centers, online, or social media) that have large pools of potentially eligible clients are selected. Information on the size of the sampling pool is gathered from clinical or administrative managers, relevant community leaders, available public health records, or other databases; the information point to the number, within the respective settings, of clients experiencing the health problem addressed by the intervention under evaluation, and the personal profile of clients. A review of this information indicates not only the sampling pool available at each setting, but also if the available pool is restricted to a particular subgroup of the target population (e.g. defined by ethnicity, economic affluence). The information gives direction for determining the number and diversity of settings to be selected in order to recruit a representative sample of adequate size.

The eligibility criteria are clearly delineated to inform the selection of respective measures for screening. Each criterion is defined at the conceptual (what it is) level and operational (what are its indicators) level. The operational definition guides the selection of a measure: the measure should be content valid and capture all indicators of the criterion. Whether containing one question (e.g. How old are you?) or multiple items (e.g. Mini-Mental State Exam [MMSE] assessing cognitive status), the measure should have validated cutoff scores as well as excellent sensitivity and specificity to correctly identify eligible clients. Failure of screening measures could lead to the inclusion of participants who present with potentially confounding characteristics or who may not benefit from the intervention. Inclusion of these participants results in high variability in their response to the allocated treatment and biased estimates of the intervention effects.

It is useful to develop a protocol that delineates the screening procedures. The protocol provides an overview of the eligibility criteria, the rationale for the specified inclusion and exclusion criteria, the conceptual and operational definitions of each criterion, the measure to be used in the assessment of each criterion, and relevant cutoff scores. The protocol describes:

1. The equipment or material (e.g. sphygmomanometer to assess blood pressure) and supplies (e.g. paper on which the command "close your eyes" is written in large font for administering an item of the MMSE) needed to administer the screening measures.

2. The instructions and script for obtaining oral agreement to administer the measures assessing general nonintrusive eligibility criteria such as age or language proficiency.

3. Instructions for securing written consent to administer the measures assessing specific, possibly intrusive eligibility criteria such as cognitive status or ethnicity.

4. The logistics for administering the screening measures, including: the personnel responsible and the appropriate time for conducting the screening. For instance, the general eligibility criteria, including medical diagnosis, can be determined by health professionals at the recruitment settings who are involved in referring clients to the evaluation study. Alternatively, the general eligibility criteria can be assessed via telephone conferencing by research personnel involved in recruitment.

5. Clients meeting the general eligibility criteria are then referred to trained research personnel responsible for obtaining written consent and administering measures of additional, potentially intrusive, or invasive eligibility criteria under conditions that ensure privacy and confidentiality.

6. The step-by-step procedures for administering the measures, appropriately. The sequence for administering the screening measures is specified. Details are provided for computing the total scores for multi-item measures; and for interpreting the participants' responses or total scores correctly, relative to the cutoff score, and hence, for accurately determining whether or not a participant is eligible to enroll in the study.

7. The script to be followed in informing clients of their eligibility.

After training the research personnel in the screening protocol, it is important to monitor their performance of the screening procedures and provide remedial strategies as needed. It is equally important to periodically review the results of screening to assist in identifying the number of eligible participants. A low number suggests the need to extend recruitment to additional settings. Review of the screening results helps in delineating the exclusion criteria most frequently reported; these criteria may be revised to increase the sampling pool and the accrual of the required sample size. McDonald et al. (2006) reported that fewer than expected number of clients met their eligibility criteria, a phenomenon they called as the "Lasagna Law." Refer to Streiner and Sidani (2010) for real-life examples of this phenomenon.

## 15.2.3   Recruitment

Recruitment involves the application of strategies to disseminate information on the outcome evaluation study to the accessible client population (i.e. available at participating settings). The goal is to invite potentially eligible clients to enroll in the study. There are two broad categories of recruitment strategies: active and passive (Cooley et al., 2003). Within each category, there are different specific recruitment strategies that are appropriate to use with, and effective in enrolling different subgroups of the client population in different contexts. Because of these differences, it is useful to select and use multiple strategies in an evaluation study.

### 15.2.3.1   Active Recruitment Strategies

Active, also called proactive, strategies consist of direct contacts between the recruiters and potentially eligible clients. Recruiters include research staff, and health professionals, or community leaders involved in referring clients to the study. In the direct contact, the recruiters introduce the study's purpose; briefly describe the health intervention and the comparison treatment that address the health problem of interest; provide an overview of the research activities in which clients will engage; and mention the potential benefits and risks of participation in the study, and the incentives offered. The direct contact can take the form of:

1. face-to-face meeting, scheduled during regular clients' visits, with individual clients receiving usual services at the participating practice settings, which is often used by health professionals or service providers involved in recruitment;

2. face-to-face meeting with individual clients attending a clinic or hospitalized, which is often used by research personnel responsible for recruitment; in this situation, the meeting should be held privately; and

3. presentation, given by research staff, to individual or group of clients attending a health (e.g. health fair) or social (e.g. community gathering) event.

The advantages of active recruitment strategies are related to the interactions that take place between recruiters and clients. The interactions offer opportunities to provide detailed information about the study; clarify any misperception of the treatments under evaluation and the planned research activities; discuss the benefits and risks of participation; and address any other concern that clients may have. Clarification of information promotes clients' understanding of the study and development of realistic expectations of their participation in the study, which are necessary to support their enrollment decision. Through these interactions, clients become familiar with the research staff and begin to develop trust and good rapport. Trust and rapport are important in promoting enrollment in a study, in particular for clients of different ethnic or cultural backgrounds (Timraz et al., 2017). Integrating recruitment closely with client care (Mattingly et al., 2015) and using direct contact (Bower et al., 2014) are reported as effective recruitment strategies.

The active recruitment strategies have limitations. They are time consuming and resource intensive. The recruiters need to be trained. They are required to arrange for the planned contact at the settings' and clients' convenience, travel to the settings, and be present throughout the health or social event serving as the context for recruitment. Despite extensive efforts, a rather small percentage of clients can be reached, confined to those available at the event. Further, the available clients may represent a select subgroup of the target client population; for example, those who attend a health fair are likely to be health-conscious persons. Thus, there is the potential for limited representativeness of the accrued sample. Active strategies can be complemented by passive strategies to reach a wider range of clients.

### 15.2.3.2  Passive Recruitment Strategies

Passive, also called reactive, strategies involve the use of different media to disseminate information on the study to clients. The information identifies the overall purpose of the study and the general eligibility criteria; highlights the nature of the treatments (experimental intervention and comparison treatment) under evaluation; and instructs interested clients to contact the research staff to learn more about the study. The content is presented in simple, easy to understand terms; using short sentences or phrases written in an attractive, interactive and uncluttered format. The interactive format is illustrated with the statement of a question such as: Who can take part in the study. The question is followed by answers given in point format such as: people who are: (1) 18 years of age or older; (2) have difficulty falling asleep, that is, it takes more than 20 minutes to fall asleep. The amount of information to cover depends on the medium to be used. For example, flyers can afford short key messages or points whereas brochures can expand on the main message. The funding agency and affiliation of the research team are added to the recruitment materials, which contributes to the perceived credibility of the study.

The information is available in printed material (brochures, flyers, advertisement) or in verbal script (announcement, short video). It can be disseminated through a wide range of media, including:

1. distributing brochures or pamphlets in areas within the participating settings that are frequently visited by potentially eligible clients (e.g. waiting area in outpatient clinics or community health centers);
2. posting flyers in strategic locations in the participating settings (e.g. bulletin board) or other locations frequented by the target population (e.g. ethnic food stores, sites of worship);

3. placing advertisements in newspapers, newsletters (distributed door-to-door in local communities) or magazines with wide distribution or in those targeting the client population of interest (such as newsletters for specific immigrant or ethnic groups printed in their respective language, or magazines focusing on topics of relevance to older persons), or in social media such as freely and commonly accessed websites for the general public (e.g. Kijjiji) or those maintained by relevant associations or organizations (e.g. Sleep Society or Alzheimer's Society);

4. making announcements on television or radio; these are aired in stations and at time slots carefully selected to reach the target population (e.g. classical music radio station to reach older people) at the most opportune time (e.g. lunch time);

5. sending an electronic message to clients belonging to an association (through the association's listserv) such as an association for the caregivers of persons with Alzheimer' disease;

6. uploading written material or short recruitment video on the website created for the study, or other online recruitment strategies (e.g. Juraschek et al., 2018).

7. snowballing, where health professionals, service providers, community leaders, and participants "spread the word" about the study (Williams et al., 2017).

The advantages of passive recruitment strategies relate to the wide dissemination of the information about the study, which increases the likelihood of reaching a large number of diverse subgroups of the target client population. This wide reach has the potential to accrue the required sample size within the study time line and to enhance the representativeness of the sample. Compared to active strategies, the use of passive strategies reduces research staff time incurred with recruitment. However, passive strategies may increase the need and cost of other resources associated with printing of materials, travel to distribute and replenish these materials, and placing advertisements in newspapers (e.g. the cost of a business-card size advertisement is $400, at the least) or announcement in media (e.g. cost is $800, at least). Additional expenses are associated with research staff time spent in responding to a large number of inquiries and explaining the study to clients, who may end up being ineligible.

### 15.2.3.3 Recruitment Process

Developing a recruitment plan is useful in directing the selection and application of the recruitment strategies at different time intervals throughout the evaluation study. The selection of strategies is guided by evidence on their effectiveness in combination with "knowledge" of the target client population and/or input from key informants or representatives of the population. Effectiveness of a recruitment strategy is indicated by the number of clients informed of the study and showing interest in learning more about it (Sidani, 2015). It is assessed by the number of clients who contact the research staff. Results of systematic reviews were inconsistent in identifying the most promising strategies. For instance, Leach (2003) reported face-to-face, referral by health professionals, and use of media as most effective. McDonald et al. (2006) found advertisement in newspapers, mail shots sent to clients or to their healthcare providers, and having dedicated research staff spearheading recruitment as most effective. Ibrahim and Sidani (2013) concluded that active strategies are more successful than passive ones in recruiting clients of diverse ethno-cultural background. Caldwell et al. (2010) found that strategies to increase potential participants' awareness of the health problem are useful in enhancing recruitment, whereas Tre-week et al. (2018) reported the use of open-label trials and telephone reminders as most useful.

The inconsistency in results suggests that different recruitment strategies may be effective for different client populations, and that multiple strategies may be used in an evaluation study to reach a large number of clients. Accordingly, it is important to "know" the target population not only in terms of the general characteristics but also the location (Williams et al., 2017) of clients; the health, social, and recreational services they frequently use; the media they commonly access; and possible variation in their ability or motivation to participate in the health intervention. The importance of "knowing" the population is illustrated with these findings: a slightly larger number of smokers entered a study evaluating a web-based smoking cessation program around the new year (resolution) period than in the summer or fall period (Graham et al., 2013). Such information, gathered in formal or informal consultation with representatives of the target client population, assists in selecting the most appropriate strategy and timing for recruitment. For example, if the target client population such as persons with insomnia, is widely dispersed, then passive strategies would reach a large proportion of the population. Also awareness that older persons with insomnia read the hard copy (more so than electronic copy) of the daily newspapers and avoid going out in the winter time (because of fear of slipping on icy sidewalks and breaking their hips) assists in selecting the newspapers for advertisement and in planning to intensify recruitment efforts in the fall, spring, and summer. In contrast, it may be more appropriate to use social media to recruit young persons with insomnia. This example highlights the importance of selecting multiple strategies to recruit various subgroups of the target client population.

Spacing the implementation of the selected recruitment strategies, where they are applied at different time intervals throughout the study duration serves two purposes. First and foremost is that this scheduling provides the opportunity to evaluate the effectiveness of each recruitment strategy. This requires documentation of the specific recruitment strategy used (e.g. advertisement in a particular newspaper or presentation at an event), the date it was carried out, and the number of clients contacting the research staff to inquire about the study, within a prespecified time interval (e.g. one week) following the implementation of the strategy. The number of inquiries indicates the effectiveness of the strategy. The recruitment data are discussed at regularly scheduled research team meetings. The discussion involves the identification of: possible challenges with the use of a particular recruitment strategy (e.g. recruiters share their perceptions of what may have or have not worked; Williams et al., 2017); the need to modify any aspect of the strategy's implementation (e.g. timing of an advertisement to maximize its reach); and ways to increase the efficiency of the recruitment plan, within available resources (e.g. discontinuing ineffective strategies).

The second purpose for spacing the implementation of recruitment strategies has to do with the practicality of responding to inquiries promptly, within the constraints of available human resources. For instance, it is important to contact interested clients within 24–48 hours of their inquiry (i.e. leaving a voice mail message or sending an electronic message) as a means of showing respect and appreciation, and of developing a good rapport with them. This prompt response may demand the availability of an adequate number of research staff who are responsible to contact clients, at a convenient time; explain the study; address their concerns; and invite them to participate; all of which take time and must not be rushed. Interactions that demonstrate respect and patience are essential for developing a good rapport, which is a recommended strategy to promote enrollment.

The importance of developing a good rapport underscores the necessity to prepare a recruitment protocol that details the steps in responding to clients' inquiries. The protocol specifies the timing of contact, ways to ascertain convenience of the time, the description of the study and of techniques to inquire about clients' concerns. It is also necessary to train all personnel responsible for recruitment in the skills and procedures delineated in the protocol, to monitor their performance and to give feedback as needed, to promote the development of a good rapport with clients.

In the extant literature, enrollment is discussed alongside recruitment because the ultimate goal of recruitment is to enroll clients in the study. Multiple recruitment strategies have been increasingly used in outcome evaluation studies. However, the enrollment rates (i.e. percentage of clients recruited that consent to participate in the study) have been and still are consistently low. Low enrollment rates result in smaller (than required) sample size, and a in sample that is not representative of all subgroups of the target population, thereby jeopardizing statistical conclusion and external validity, respectively (Bower et al., 2014; Horwood et al., 2016; Thoma et al., 2010). Cumulative evidence shows that less than half of the funded RCTs achieve the required sample size (Butler et al., 2015; Califf et al., 2012; Hughes-Morley et al., 2015; Treweek et al., 2013). To understand what contributes to low enrollment, despite extensive and effective recruitment, assessment of reasons for declining entry into an intervention evaluation study has been (and should be done in any study) integrated as part of the recruitment or the consent process. The assessment involves inquiring about the clients' willingness to enroll in the study and if not, the reasons for declining. The questions eliciting reasons for nonenrollment can be generic or general (e.g. what were the reasons or what led you to not wanting to take part in the study). Additional more specific questions are used to ask about reasons for nonenrollment. The questions inquire about factors known to affect enrollment. The factors are usually related to: personal life circumstances (e.g. Is it for personal reasons like lack of time or transportation issues?); the health intervention and the comparison treatment (e.g. Does your decision have to do with the type of treatments or with the way the treatments are given?); and the research methods (e.g. Is there any particular aspect of the study, such as invasiveness of the test, that led you to not take part in the study?).

Participants' responses are content analyzed to identify frequent barriers to enrollment. Awareness of the barriers informs necessary modifications in the following:

1. the recruitment message: for example, adding points that may address some reasons for nonenrollment such as "you will receive an incentive" or "transportation costs will be covered";
2. the study methods: for example, the design of the study can be revised from a traditional RCT to a comprehensive cohort design, which is increasingly being reported as a means to enhance enrollment; and
3. the mode of intervention delivery: for instance, later intervention sessions can be offered by telephone instead of face-to-face individual format, to address transportation barriers.

Results of several evaluation studies suggest that, in addition to personal client characteristics such as older age, general health status, perceptions of randomization and of the treatments under evaluation including possible side effects are frequently mentioned reasons for nonenrollment (Costenbader et al., 2007; Moorcraft et al., 2016;

Murphy et al., 2012; Thoma et al., 2010). Modifications in the study design and methods are made to address client-reported barriers to enrollment such as using an open-label design (Treweek et al., 2018) where blinding participants could not be applied or is not well received, and allowing flexibility in research methods. The effectiveness of these strategies in enhancing recruitment and enrollment was examined. Results of systematic reviews identified promising strategies in improving enrollment. The strategies were: applying active recruitment strategies (i.e. direct contact with clients); providing incentives to recruiters (i.e. health professionals or service providers) and to participants; using open-label design; planning the study methods in a way that reduces burden on participants and that maintains flexibility; and building and maintaining good rapport between research personnel and participants (Bower et al., 2014).

## 15.2.4 Determination of Sample Size

Determination of sample size involves calculations of the number of participants to include in the evaluation study, in order to detect significant intervention effects. The sample size should be adequate to reach valid conclusions regarding the intervention's effects, while minimizing the chance of type I error (i.e. false conclusion that the intervention is effective) and type II error (i.e. false conclusion that the intervention is ineffective). Thus, the calculations are done to optimize the sample size so that it is not too small to the point it is unable to detect existing effects, and not large to the point it is able detect any effect even if not theoretically and/or clinically meaningful (Noordzij et al., 2010).

Sample size calculations are based on power analysis. Power analysis consists of applying formulae that take into consideration three components and that vary with the design planned for the outcome evaluation study. The components are:

*Alpha ($\alpha$) level*: The alpha level represents the rate of type I error. It is commonly set at 0.05, which implies a desire for less than 5% chance of drawing a false conclusion that the intervention is effective. Conventionally, a more liberal alpha level (e.g. 0.10) can be set for pilot studies aimed to explore the effects of a new intervention or the effect of an evidence-based intervention in a new client population in a new context. A more conservative alpha level (e.g. 0.01) can be set for full scale studies aimed to confirm the efficacy, effectiveness and safety of the intervention.

*Beta ($\beta$) level and Power*: The beta ($\beta$) level reflects the rate of type II error. It is usually set at 0.20, which implies a desire for less than 20% chance of drawing a false conclusion that the intervention is ineffective. Power reflects the ability to detect intervention effects that are present in the client population, based on the sample's estimates of these effects. Power is the complement of $\beta$ and is computed as $1 - \beta$. It is conventionally set at 0.80 or 80%, which represents the probability of avoiding type II error (Noordzij et al., 2010).

*Magnitude of the intervention effect*: The magnitude of the intervention effect is the anticipated size of the difference in the primary outcome. The effect size represents the magnitude of the difference between the intervention and the comparison treatment groups, in the primary outcome measured at posttest in a between-subject design. The effect size can also quantify the difference between the pretest and the posttest outcome scores, within the intervention group, in a within-subject design. The size of the difference is quantified in either of two ways. The first is the minimal, clinically relevant, difference that is anticipated to be detected. The difference is estimated from previous research (Noordzij et al., 2010); it can be meaningfully estimated for outcomes with established metrics (e.g. blood pressure) on the basis of clinical judgment, or derived from available evidence that validated what constitutes a minimal clinically important difference for self-reported patient-oriented outcomes (e.g. pain rating scale). The second way is the standardized mean difference or effect size (e.g. Cohen's d). The effect size can be estimated on the basis of theoretical expectations (proposed in the intervention theory) or available empirical evidence.

There are a few points to clarify in estimating the magnitude of the intervention effects:

- The terms "primary" outcome has been frequently used but not explicitly defined in the literature. However, it appears to reflect the outcome of most interest to the researchers or stakeholder groups such as policy makers. Accordingly, the primary outcome considered in sample size determination often represents an ultimate outcome such as mortality or quality of life. This could be potentially problematic, as the intervention theory hypothesizes an indirect effect of the health intervention on the ultimate outcomes, mediated by immediate and intermediate outcome. Therefore, the direct impact of the intervention is expected to be large on the immediate outcomes, moderate on the intermediate outcomes and small on the ultimate outcome. Large samples are needed to detect small effect sizes. In full mediation, the direct effect of the intervention on the selected (for power analysis) ultimate outcome is anticipated to be nonsignificant (Wiedermann & von Eye, 2015), presenting challenges in determining the required sample size.

- Conventionally, it has been advised to conduct a pilot study in order to estimate the magnitude of the intervention effect on the primary outcome. The effect size, computed on the basis of a pilot study's data, is then used in the power analysis to determine the sample size required for the large-scale or full evaluation study. This practice is no longer recommended because the effect sizes estimated in a pilot study involving a small number of participants are unreliable, unstable and imprecise. They give inaccurate directions in determining the sample size required for the large-scale evaluation study (Leon et al., 2011). Instead, it is recommended to estimate the magnitude of the intervention effect from previous research where available, or informed by the intervention theory or clinical judgment.

Different formulae are available to determine the sample size required for different between-subject, individual or cluster level, randomized and nonrandomized designs, and within-subject designs. The formulae are well covered in other sources (Cohen, 1988; Chow et al., 2008; Rutterford et al., 2015). The formulae are applied to determine either the total sample size or the number of participants needed for each treatment group. Many statistical packages are available for power analysis (e.g. G-power). It is worth noting the importance of carefully specifying the values of the three components of power analysis, as these affect the adequacy of the sample size calculations. The general trend is that, with a low alpha level (e.g. 0.01), a high power (e.g. 0.90), and an anticipated small magnitude of the intervention effect, a very large sample is required (Noordzij et al., 2010). Accruing a large sample may not be logistically possible within the evaluation study time line and resources; it demands the availability of a large sampling pool across a large number of practice settings to account for nonenrollment and attrition.

The sample size, determined with power analysis, should be inflated as a means for addressing nonenrollment and attrition. Nonenrollment and attrition rates can be computed from previous research that evaluated the same health intervention or similar interventions, in the same or comparable target client population. The obtained nonenrollment rates are then used to specify the number of participants to recruit. For example, the rate of nonenrollment in studies evaluating behavioral therapies for insomnia is estimated at 45%; if power analysis indicates that the required sample size is 100, then 145 persons should be recruited. The attrition rates estimated from previous research indicate the additional (to required) number of participants to accrue in order to account for attrition. For example, attrition rates in studies evaluating behavioral therapies for insomnia are estimated at 50%; thus, 50 additional persons must be enrolled to end up with 100 persons completing the study.

## 15.2.5   Retention

Obtaining the required number of clients who consent and enroll in the outcome evaluation study is important. It, however, is highly likely (if not certain) that some participants withdraw from the study. Withdrawal or attrition jeopardizes the validity of inferences regarding the effectiveness of the health intervention. Therefore, it is advisable to document the number of participants who withdraw from the outcome evaluation study, to inquire about the reasons for withdrawal, to incorporate retention strategies, and to examine the impact of attrition on sample representativeness and on estimates of the intervention effects (discussed in Section 15.5).

### 15.2.5.1   Attrition

Attrition, also called mortality, dropout, or loss to follow-up, refers to the withdrawal of consenting participants from the evaluation study. The withdrawal occurs at any time following consent, surrounding the delivery of the intervention: before exposure to the allocated treatment (called pre-inclusion attrition), during and/or following exposure to treatment (called post-inclusion).

Withdrawal is initiated by the participants or the researchers. Participants with various personal and health characteristics drop out of the study for reasons related to personal life circumstances, to their perceptions and expectations of the allocated treatment and to their views of the research methods and procedures (see section 15.2.5.2). Researchers exclude participants from the study on the basis of prespecified criteria. Common criteria include: nonadherence to the allocated treatment (e.g. nonattendance at treatment sessions, poor enactment of the treatment recommendations); failure to carry out key aspects of the study protocol (e.g. noncompletion of daily diary related to the experience of the health problem, which is necessary to tailor treatment); worsening of the health problem or of general health (e.g. not sleeping for one week); or experience of discomforts or severe side effects.

The pattern of attrition varies in different evaluation studies. It impacts the validity of inferences regarding the effectiveness of the intervention. Pattern has to do with the number and characteristics of participants who withdraw:

1. When the total number of participants who withdraw from any evaluation study, in particular those using a within-subject design, is large (>50%), then the sample available for outcome data analysis is small. Small samples reduce the power to detect significant intervention effects (issue of statistical conclusion validity).

2. When participants who withdraw differ in personal and health characteristics from those who complete the study, then the sample available for outcome data analysis is not representative of the target client population. Rather, the sample comprises select subgroups of the population, who may respond to the allocated treatment in a unique way. Therefore, the estimated intervention effects are not generalizable or applicable to the subgroups of the population not represented in the study (issue of external validity).

3. When the number as well as the personal and health characteristics of participants who withdraw are comparable for the experimental intervention and comparison treatment groups (a situation called equal attrition), then the sample available for analysis and the statistical power are reduced (issue of statistical conclusion validity). The comparability of the two groups on baseline profiles is maintained, which enhances internal validity.

4. When the number as well as the personal and health characteristics of participants who withdraw differ between the intervention and the comparison group (a situation called differential attrition), then the risk of selection bias and subsequent confounding bias is increased (issue of internal validity).

Monitoring and documenting attrition are essential in an intervention evaluation study. Monitoring attrition is facilitated by: (1) clarifying, upfront (i.e. during the consent process) and throughout involvement in the study (where applicable), to participants their right of self-determination, including withdrawal from the study at any time, and requesting their cooperation in informing research staff of their decision to withdraw; (2) close surveillance of participants' behavior (verbal and nonverbal) that may be indicative of the potential for attrition, such as expression of discomfort with the allocated treatment or with completion of the outcome measures. The surveillance is done by interventionists and research staff, throughout the study participation period; (3) contacting participants who miss a treatment session or a planned data collection session, to inquire about the reasons (e.g. due to unexpected event or to decision to withdraw). To document attrition, a participant log is developed. The log lists, sequentially, the research activities in which participants should engage, starting with inquiring about the study and agreement to enroll, through consenting, completing baseline data collection measures, completing treatment, and ending with completing posttest and follow-up measures. Participants' completion of each activity is documented as well as the time and reasons for withdrawal are identified and documented.

### 15.2.5.2  Reasons for Attrition

Attrition is pervasive in intervention evaluation research. The median attrition rate was 7% for studies of medical treatments (Dumville et al., 2006) but reached 40% for cognitive behavioral therapy for insomnia (Ellis & Barclay, 2014) and 50% for smoking cessation programs (Young et al., 2006). Attrition has been found to be associated with a range of factors. The evidence of this association was derived from three sources: the quantitative results of individual studies where participants who withdrew were compared to those who completed the study on personal and health characteristics assessed at baseline; and qualitative results pertaining to reasons for withdrawal provided by participants who dropped out of the study at any time; and results of systematic reviews that synthesized the results of studies. The factors are categorized into:

**TABLE 15.1**  Participant characteristics associated with attrition.

| Category | Characteristics | References |
| --- | --- | --- |
| Personal (i.e. sociodemographic) | Age | Warden et al. (2009) and Wasmann et al. (2019) |
| | Gender | Gucciardi (2008) |
| | Level of education | Ahern and Le Brocque (2005) |
| | Marital status | Graham et al. (2013) |
| | Employment status or socioeconomic status | Graham et al. (2013) |
| | Race, ethnicity, or culture | Gucciardi (2008) |
| | Transportation issues | Coday et al. (2005) |
| | Multiple competing demands (e.g. family obligations) | Keller et al. (2005) |
| Health | Presence of comorbid mental health problems (e.g. depression) or physical health problems (e.g. functional limitations) | Hebert et al. (2010), Warden et al. (2009) |
| | Poor general health | Adams et al. (2013) |
| | Cognitive ability | Ahern and LeBrocque (2005) |
| | Severity of the health problem | Gucciardi (2008), Hebert et al. (2010) |
| Psychological or behavioral | Experience of life stress | Glombiewski et al. (2010) |
| | Experience of loneliness | Ahern and LeBrocque (2005) |
| | Motivation, perceived susceptibility to the health problem, perceived benefit from enrollment in the study | Grave et al. (2005) |

*Characteristics of participants*: Several sociodemographic, health, behavioral, and psychological characteristics were reported to predict attrition. The set of predictors varied across primary studies and systematic reviews that examined different types of health interventions addressing different health problems in different client populations. Table 15.1 lists factors found to be associated with attrition. The direction of the associations is often inconsistent. For example, high attrition rates were found to be related to younger age in some and to older age in other studies and reviews.

*Characteristics of treatments*: Participants' perceptions and experiences with the allocated treatment contribute to attrition, as discussed in Chapter 11. In general, participants who view the allocated treatment as unacceptable or undesirable; complex or demanding that is, requiring changes in different aspects of life and the application of multiple treatment recommendations, which are cumbersome and difficult to enact; inflexible in that it does not account for their individual needs and life circumstances; potentially ineffective that is, participants have low expectation that the treatment will successfully manage the health problem; and harmful that is, associated with side effects considered as intolerable, are likely to withdraw from treatment and the study (Gucciardi et al., 2009; Sidani, 2015; Warden et al., 2009). In their systematic review, Akl et al. (2012) found higher attrition rates in RCTs evaluating nonmedical (versus medical) treatments, which reflect the complexity of nonmedical therapies. Further, higher attrition rates were reported for the comparison treatment group, specifically the no-treatment control and placebo treatments in studies that evaluated pharmacological or nonpharmacological therapies (Karras-Jean Gilles et al., 2019; Kemmler et al., 2005). In other studies, higher attrition rates were observed in the experimental intervention group as compared to the placebo treatment group (e.g. Maneeton et al., 2012); these researchers attributed high attrition to the concern or experience of the medications' side effects. Participants' experience, whether positive or negative, with the allocated treatment contributes to attrition. Some participants may drop out once they experience improvement in the health problem. Others withdraw if they are dissatisfied with the allocated treatment (Glombiewski et al., 2010), experience no changes in the health problem, or report discomfort or side effects (Warden et al., 2009).

*Characteristics of the study*: The study's methods and procedures have been reported to contribute to withdrawal. Overall, high attrition rates were observed: (1) in delayed treatment group within a waiting-list design, which was attributed to the loss of interest in the study, or the spontaneous recovery experienced over a long waiting period; (2) in randomized trials or randomized arms of trials, which was related to the mismatch between the allocated and the preferred treatment (see Chapters 11 and 14); (3) in studies involving burdensome data collection procedures (e.g. completion of a daily diary and long questionnaires), invasive procedures (e.g. taking blood samples), frequent administration of measures within short time intervals, incentives perceived as inappropriate by participants, inflexibility in carrying out the treatments and research activities (e.g. location and schedule of data collection sessions that may be convenient to participants) (Sidani, 2015), as well as long time intervals between research activities during which no contact with participants is initiated (Akl et al., 2012; Karras-Jean Gilles et al., 2019).

### 15.2.5.3   Strategies to Identify Factors Associated with Attrition

There are two general strategies to identify factors that contribute to attrition in an outcome evaluation study. The first strategy involves the conduct of an "exit" interview with participants who withdraw. The interview is done after obtaining participants' verbal agreement or written consent, in a face-to-face or telephone format. The interview aims to explore reasons for withdrawal. It can be semistructured, beginning with a "grand tour" open-ended question (e.g. What led the participant to quit the study?), followed by focused questions inquiring about each categories of factors known to contribute to attrition. Examples of focused questions are: Are the reasons for quitting related to personal issues or life condition (participant characteristics); to the type of treatment received (treatment characteristics); and to the way the study is done (study characteristics). If participants find the interview inconvenient, then they can be invited to respond to the questions in writing. Participants' responses are content analyzed to identify the most common factors contributing to attrition, from the participants' perspective.

The second strategy is applied at the stage of data analysis. It consists of determining factors that are associated with attrition. In a particular study, the factors can include: participants' characteristics (e.g. severity of the health problem) assessed at baseline; perceptions (acceptability, credibility, satisfaction) of treatments;

match–mismatch between the allocated and the preferred treatment; response to treatment (i.e. level of improvement in the outcomes); and experience of side effects. The associations between these factors and attrition are examined with logistic regression analysis. Understanding the factors and how they operate guides the development and incorporation of strategies to minimize attrition and maximize retention.

### 15.2.5.4   Retention Strategies

Numerous strategies have been proposed to promote retention in outcome evaluation studies. However, there is limited evidence supporting their effectiveness in reducing attrition. The strategies are, to some extent, designed to address specific factors commonly reported as associated with attrition and to make involvement in the study attractive and convenient to participants. Therefore, it is recommended to select and integrate multiple retention strategies in a study in order to mitigate the potential influence of several predictors of attrition that may be operating in different subgroups of participants. The strategies can be categorized into those addressing (i.e. enhancing or reducing) the following aspects of a study:

*Convenience of participation.* Making involvement in the study convenient to participants is commonly advised to promote retention (Leach, 2003; Lindsay Davis et al., 2002; Lyons et al., 2004). Convenience is maintained by allowing some flexibility in the performance of the research activities to accommodate participants' life circumstances and to overcome barriers to sustained engagement in the study, while maintaining study integrity (Sidani, 2015). Strategies to promote convenience include:

- Initiating recruitment at locations that are frequented or salient to participants, and where they feel comfortable (Baucom et al., 2018; Karras-Jean Gilles et al., 2019).
- Offering the intervention and holding the data collection sessions, in a face-to-face format, at a place that is convenient to participants. The location must be trusted, accessible to participants with varying levels of physical functioning, and within reasonable travel distance. Covering transportation or parking costs is suggested to assist participants with limited resources overcome this barrier to sustained engagement in the evaluation study (Baucom et al., 2018; Michelet et al., 2014).
- Scheduling the delivery of the intervention and the data collection sessions, in face-to-face or distance format, at a time that is convenient to individual or subgroups of participants. The time can be determined in consultation with participants to minimize potential conflict with their usual activities such as work and childcare. Providing childcare support overcome this barrier, which is commonly reported by working participants of low socioeconomic status and of diverse ethno-cultural backgrounds (Baucom et al., 2018).
- Allowing flexibility in the mode of intervention delivery (e.g. switching face-to-face to telephone format for providing individual sessions focused on reinforcing treatment recommendations); and in the completion of data collection measures such as using the format (hard or electronic) of preference to participants.
- Accommodating diversity of languages spoken by participants of different ethno-cultural backgrounds. This involves hiring and training bilingual, and if possible bicultural, interventionists and research staff, translating intervention materials and data collection measures to the preferred language, and offering the intervention and the measures in the language of preference.

*Communication.* Communication is foundational to initiating and maintaining a good rapport between research staff and participants throughout the study. Good rapport enhances retention. Demonstrating flexibility (as discussed in the previous section) contributes to the initiation of a good rapport, which is reinforced with the following strategies:

- Employing interventionists with appropriate personal qualities, including interactional style (Chapter 8), and research staff with good communication skills.

- Training research staff in skills required for demonstrating genuineness, caring, respect, and acceptance; and recognizing or praising strengths in staff's interactions with participants, especially those of diverse ethno-cultural backgrounds (Baucom et al., 2018).

- Providing thorough information about the study that is easily understood by participants of different literacy levels (Michelet et al., 2014). The information should be comprehensive, clear and unbiased, and relayed in simple lay terms (i.e. avoid medical or research jargon), at the fourth grade reading level. It covers the purpose of the study, the types of treatments, the target population, the sequence and timing of all planned research activities, the discomfort or side effects as well as the effectiveness of the intervention. The benefits of participation are also presented. The information is relayed at initial encounters with participants such as recruitment and consent processes; the information is clarified and reinforced, as needed, throughout the study (Sidani, 2015). This strategy ensures that participants have a clear understanding of the study and realistic expectations of their involvement; this in turn, prevents misperceptions and potential disappointment with the allocated treatment or with the study methods that contribute to withdrawal.

- Following up with participants who miss a treatment or a data collection session. Research staff contact these participants to inquire about their general status and the reasons for nonattendance, and to discuss their interest in continued involvement in the study. The contact conveys a sense of genuine interest in the participants' well-being, respect for the persons, and valuing their involvement. The contact provides an opportunity to identify possible barriers and to apply relevant strategies to overcome the barriers. The contact also allows to reschedule the missed session at the participants' convenience.

- Maintaining contacts with participants over the course of the study. The contacts are scheduled at different points in time before and after the intervention delivery to remind participants of upcoming research activities and of the importance of completing the activities in a timely manner. The contacts, also called reminders, are planned around: (1) one week or a few days before the intervention, to remind participants of the place, date, and time of the first session or module; (2) one week or a few days before an in-person (face-to-face) data collection session to remind participants of the place, date, and time of the session; if a participant misses the session, then a contact is made within one to two days, to inquire about the participants' status and continued interest in the study, and to reschedule the session if possible; (3) one week after sending (in hard or electronic copy) the data collection questionnaire to determine if the questionnaire has been received, remind participants to complete and return the completed questionnaire, or inquire about participants' continued interest in the study; (4) the mid-point of the time interval between planned research activities (e.g. 1.5 month within a 3-month period between posttest and follow-up data collection); this contact is useful to remind participants of their involvement in the study and of the upcoming research activity, as well as to request an update on their contact information if it has changed. The contacts may involve a telephone call, an email or a text message, letters, or postcards (Baucom et al., 2018; Michelet et al., 2014). The contacts have been reported as useful in improving completion of questionnaires (Brueton et al., 2017).

- Creating a study identity that reflects the essence of what the study is about. The identity is in the form of an acronym or logo. It is added to: envelopes for mailing study-related materials; hard and electronic copies of the questionnaires to be completed by participants; and reminder letters and postcards. The appearance of the acronym or logo on all correspondence materials helps participants remember that they are enrolled in the study and recognize the materials and hence, attend to it (Brueton et al., 2017; Michelet et al., 2014). Generating a study newsletter reporting on the progress made and presenting general information of relevance to the target client population, and distributing it to participants and recruitment settings, have the potential to maintain participants' and recruiters' interest in the study.

- Acknowledging participants' contribution. The acknowledgement can be done by expressing gratitude for participants' involvement in the study. Expression of gratitude can take different forms. The interventionists can verbally thank participants for attending an intervention session. A communication can be automatically sent for completing a web-based module or the words "THANK YOU" can be added at the end of self-reported measures. A card can be mailed to thank participants for completing the questionnaire. Such acknowledgement promotes participants' sense of being respected and valued, which contributes to their sustained involvement in the study.

*Incentives.* Offering incentives to participants is a commonly used retention strategy. There are two categories of incentives: monetary and nonmonetary. Monetary incentives consist of direct payment to participants. The payment often aims to reward participants and to offset costs they incur with their involvement in the study such as transportation and childcare costs. The amount and timing for giving the monetary incentives vary with the funding agency policy (i.e. some agencies put a cap on the amount that can be offered), the local research ethics board (i.e. the board may have guidance on what is considered coercive) and the needs of the target client population. For example, monetary incentives may be useful to overcome barriers to participants in under-resourced or low-income communities but are discouraged in studies involving substance abusers. The monetary incentives can be offered (1) as a lump sum provided upon completion of the study, which is believed to improve full participation in the study but is considered coercive; or (2) in smaller amounts provided upon completion of the measures at pretest, posttest and follow-up, which is viewed as another means of acknowledging participants' contribution in a timely manner (Baucom et al., 2018). Brueton et al. (2017) reported that the effectiveness of monetary incentives depended on participants' age, socioeconomic status, education, and medical condition, and that the overall benefit is small.

Nonmonetary incentives include items, other than direct payment, that are provided to participants at different points over the course of the study. The items can be creative but need to be of relevance (or attractive) to the target client population. A wide range of items has been used such as running shoes (to facilitate engagement in physical activity by low income women), movie pass (which is motivating to adolescents), gift card at local grocery store or coffee shop or bookstore (which may be attractive to students), and T-shirts, pens, or mugs with the study logo. Brueton et al. (2017) reported that nonmonetary incentives are useful to acknowledge participants' contribution but are of limited benefit in improving retention. Offering the intervention free-of-charge is considered an incentive that is highly valued by low-income, under-resourced communities in countries with no universal healthcare coverage.

*Burden*. Strategies that minimize the burden, demands, and efforts of involvement in the evaluation study have the potential to enhance retention. The strategies most commonly used, and reported by Brueton et al. (2017) as useful, relate to data collection. It is advisable to collect data pertaining only to the conceptual variables of relevance to the study and meaningful to the target client population, and to obtain the relevant data at the most significant time points that are defined by the intervention theory as those at which changes in the immediate and ultimate outcomes are expected to occur. This schedule for collecting data on relevant variables is expected to reduce participants' response burden and to maintain their interest and willingness to complete the measures. Another strategy to reduce burden consists of selecting measures that are most accurate in operationalizing the variables of interest; this decreases the number of measures to complete by participants, without jeopardizing construct validity. Lastly, the use, where available, of validated short versions of the measures and/or measures containing clearly written and easy to understand and complete items would decrease the time required for participants to complete the measures and minimize response fatigue.

*Treatments*. Designing health interventions in a way that is meaningful and attractive to participants has the potential of promoting enthusiasm for, engagement in, and satisfaction with treatment, and consequently enhancing retention. Strategies for designing attractive intervention are presented in Chapters 4 and 5. Few points are reiterated. It is important to convey the content in simple terms; present the content and activities in a logical sequence; select the most appropriate mode and dose of delivery; specify how the content, activities, and treatment recommendations can be adapted to fit the participants' experiences of the health problem, concerns, and life circumstances; and integrate approaches to support participants' engagement and enactment of treatment. Allowing flexibility in scheduling the intervention sessions is equally useful in promoting retention. In addition, the comparison treatment can be carefully selected to provide meaningful comparison; yet it should be perceived favorably by participants, as discussed in Section 15.1.

*Other study characteristics*. The method of assignment to treatment is a study characteristic that can be modified to promote retention. Allowing participants who refuse randomization to choose treatment, as is done in a comprehensive cohort or preference trial, is a strategy found effective in reducing attrition (see Chapter 14 for evidence of this strategy's effectiveness). Brueton et al. (2017) reported that open-label RCTs (where participants are not blinded and are aware of treatment allocation) improve retention, whereas use of motivational strategies or case-management were not beneficial in preventing attrition.

There is limited evidence supporting the effectiveness of most retention strategies because some strategies like showing respect, may not be amenable to measurement or quantification. In light of limited evidence on effectiveness and of the possibility that different strategies may be appropriate and potentially beneficial for different subgroups of participants, it is highly recommended to include multiple retention strategies in an outcome evaluation study. This recommendation is widely endorsed and supported by the results of Coday et al. (2005). The latter investigators interviewed research staff to gain their perspective on the most useful retention strategies. The staff advocated a combination of strategies: being flexible in scheduling research activities with participants' input, offering incentives and emphasizing the benefits to participants of their involvement in the study.

## 15.3    TREATMENT ALLOCATION

### 15.3.1    Importance

Eligible consenting participants are allocated to the experimental intervention or to the comparison treatment. Since all participants meet the same set of inclusion and exclusion criteria, participants in both groups are expected to have comparable characteristics at baseline and to differ only in their exposure to the experimental intervention. Differences in the outcomes assessed following treatment completion represent the evidence supporting the efficacy or effectiveness of the experimental intervention. Two general approaches can be used to allocate participants to treatment: random and nonrandom.

### 15.3.2    Random Allocation

Random allocation, also referred to as random assignment or randomization, rests on chance in the process of placing participants in the experimental intervention or the comparison treatment groups (Berger, 2018). The randomization process gives participants (individuals or clusters) an equal chance of receiving the experimental intervention. Randomization is believed to maintain the comparability on baseline characteristics of participants allocated to the experimental intervention and the comparison treatment groups, and to balance the number of participants in both groups (Henry et al., 2017). Thus, randomization is considered as a "practical tool" to reduce confounding (Bonell et al., 2016). To ensure that allocation to treatment group is based on chance only, devoid of human (researchers, research personnel, health professionals, or participants) interference, the randomization process is applied in two phases: (1) the generation of the allocation sequence using appropriate randomization procedures and schemes; and (2) concealment of the allocation sequence, that is, not disclosing the sequence to those involved in the treatment allocation process.

#### 15.3.2.1    Randomization Procedures

Different randomization procedures are available. The selection of a procedure is informed by a careful consideration of its strengths and limitations, and of accessibility to resources required for its implementation.

*Flip of a coin.* This procedure consists of having a research staff member toss a coin and follow a preset rule in determining the treatment group to which a participant is allocated. The rule specifies the treatment group for participants' assignment if the toss yields Heads (e.g. in this case, participants are allocated to the experimental intervention) or Tails (e.g. in this case, participants are allocated to the comparison treatment). Although easy to apply, the flip of a coin has limitations. It is not appropriate or feasible in studies including more than two treatment groups. It has the potential to result in unbalanced number of participants assigned to two groups, due to pure chance in the toss yields; for example, the toss may yield Heads more frequently than Tails. Concealment is not maintained with this procedure; the procedure is highly subject to tampering by the research staff who can repeat the toss until the treatment that the staff deems suitable or the participant desires, is allocated. This procedure is rarely used nowadays (with the advent of computerized randomization programs) but it may be the only accessible procedure in a few situations.

*Table of random numbers.* This procedure consists of having a research staff member randomly select a number listed in a table (usually appended to research or statistical textbooks, or available electronically). The research staff follow a preset guideline in determining treatment allocation. The guideline delineates the linkages of treatments (e.g. experimental intervention) with particular numbers (e.g. odd numbers or numbers less than a specific value such as 5). For details on how to apply this procedure, refer to Sidani (2015). The procedure has the same strengths and limitations as those identified for flip of a coin, and is also rarely used nowadays.

*Sealed opaque envelopes.* This procedure consists of preparing envelopes containing a paper on which the name of a treatment included in the outcome evaluation study is written. The envelopes are sealed and put in a box accessible to research staff. The research staff or if possible, the participant, pick up an envelope to identify the treatment group to which the participant is allocated. The type (i.e. experimental intervention or comparison treatment) or the name (e.g. stimulus control therapy or sleep education and hygiene) is written on the paper. The paper is folded prior to placing it in an opaque envelope, as a means to maintain concealment. The selection of the treatment, which name is written on the paper, can be done by: (1) following the table of random numbers (as described previously) or (2) preparing a number of envelopes that is consistent with the total sample size required for the study (e.g. 100) and equally divided across the study treatments (e.g. 50 for experimental intervention and 50 for the comparison treatment). The strengths of this procedure include: (1) it is simple and easy to implement; (2) it maintains chance allocation and balanced numbers of participants assigned to the treatment groups; and (3) it increases the likelihood of concealment, though instances of tampering have been reported (see Streiner & Sidani, 2010). The practicality or logistics of carrying out this procedure in evaluation studies with large sample and number of participating sites is a potential limitation.

*Computer-generated allocation.* Computer-generated allocation is considered the standard randomization procedure. This procedure involves the use of computer software or programs to generate the list of random numbers for allocating participants to treatment groups. The list is usually generated by central randomization services or the statistical consultant, using widely and freely accessible programs through websites such as Random.org 2017 (Berger, 2018). The list is kept under lock. Research staff connect with the randomization services or the consultant to learn about the treatment to which each participant is to be assigned. The strengths of this procedure are the ability to maintain chance-based allocation, concealment, and balanced numbers of participants across groups. As well, the procedure is convenient in applying various allocation schemes (discussed in Section 15.3.2.2). Its limitations relate to the accessibility of the randomization services and the logistics of prompt communication and coordination between the research staff and the randomization services.

*Zelen randomization.* This procedure for treatment allocation has been proposed by Zelen (1979) to overcome the nonconsent bias and the low enrollment rate. These biases are associated with participants' unfavorable perceptions of randomization and sense of discontentment and demoralization expressed by participants assigned to the comparison treatment group, in RCTs evaluating the effectiveness of health interventions in the practice setting. The Zelen randomization procedure involves four steps. First is the identification of the pool of eligible clients seen in the practice setting. Second is the generation of a list of clients and corresponding identification code numbers (e.g. health record number). The third step consists of randomly sampling or selecting (e.g. using table of random numbers) a cohort of clients. The fourth step entails inviting and obtaining consent only from the cohort selected to receive the experimental intervention. The remaining clients (i.e. those comprising the initial pool but not selected) continue to receive treatment-as-usual, and serve as the comparison group. The application of the Zelen randomization procedure has raised ethical and practice concerns. From an ethical perspective, clients in the comparison group are not informed of the study and do not provide consent to collect data on their treatment and health outcomes; this violates their fundamental rights of respect and self-determination. From a practical or scientific perspective, no additional data of relevance to the evaluation study can be gathered from clients in the comparison group. Accordingly, the Zelen randomization procedure is not recommended.

*Pseudo or quasi-randomization.* This procedure entails the generation of an allocation sequence that alternates assignment to the experimental intervention and the comparison treatment by any of the following four ways. First, the allocation is done by participant, such as allocating the first participant to the experimental intervention group, the second participant to the comparison treatment group, and so on. Second, the assignment is done by day or week, such as participants attending a health clinic on a particular day or week are assigned to the intervention group and those attending the clinic on the next day or week are assigned to the comparison treatment group. Third, the allocation is done by time period, such as assigning participants to the experimental intervention until the number of participants required for this group is attained, and allocating the remaining participants to the comparison treatment group. Fourth, the assignment is done on the basis of a select number (e.g. month or year of participants' birth, hospital identification number), such that participants with an odd number are assigned to the experimental intervention and an even number to the comparison treatment. The strengths of this procedure relate to its simplicity and feasibility. Although based on chance, the sequence of allocation is known to the researchers (Berger, 2018), limiting concealment. Further, the procedure may introduce selection bias if different subgroups of participants are available at different points in time (Sidani, 2015).

### 15.3.2.2   Randomization Schemes

The randomization procedures have the potential to yield an unbalanced number and composition or characteristics of participants allocated to the experimental intervention and the comparison treatment groups, by chance, especially when the sample size is small (Berger, 2018). Randomization schemes are embedded in the randomization procedures in order to reduce the potential for imbalances in the number and/or characteristics of participants in the experimental intervention and the comparison treatment groups. The most common schemes (for detail, refer to Sidani, 2015), include:

*Block randomization.* With this scheme, a random sequence of blocks is generated. Each block reflects a pattern of assignment to the treatment groups for a prespecified number of participants. The prespecified number is a multiple of the number of treatment groups. When the prespecified number of consenting participants is reached, individual participants are allocated to the group as delineated for the respective block. For instance, in a study including one experimental intervention group and one comparison treatment group, the block size can be specified as 2 groups $\times$ 2 (i.e. multiple of the group) = 4; the pattern of allocation to groups can be: experimental, comparison, comparison, experimental; thus, the first 4 participants are assigned to the respective groups delineated in the pattern. Block randomization is used to maintain a balanced number of participants assigned to the experimental intervention and the comparison treatment groups, should the study end early (for whatever reason).

*Stratified randomization.* In this scheme, participants are first stratified on a baseline (personal or health) characteristic known to be associated with the outcome (i.e. a confounder) and second, randomized to the experimental intervention and the comparison treatment groups within each stratum (i.e. subgroup of participants with similar levels on the confounding characteristic). Stratified randomization is advocated to "ensure" or enhance the comparability of participants assigned to the experimental intervention and the comparison treatment in a particular study, where the sample size is small. Its application, however, is challenging: it may be difficult to quantify similarity on the confounding characteristic, especially if it is measured on a continuous (versus categorical) scale; it also is challenging to find an adequate number of participants who are similar on the selected characteristic.

*Minimization.* Conceptually, minimization is similar to stratified randomization, aiming to maintain between-group comparability, but differs in its application. With advances in technology (computer programming), minimization has the capacity to account for several, categorical and continuous, confounding characteristics in assigning participants to the experimental intervention and the comparison treatment groups. The assignment process consists of: (1) randomizing the first 10 participants to the intervention and the comparison groups; (2) examining the distribution of the confounding characteristics in each group (e.g. two women in the intervention group and eight men in the comparison group); (3) assessing the status on the confounding characteristics of the next set of participants prior to randomization; (4) assigning the latter participants to the respective group on the basis of their status on the confounding characteristics (e.g. more women are assigned to the intervention group). The goal is to maintain the groups' comparability on the confounding characteristics. The use of minimization demands accessibility to central randomization services and close collaboration and prompt communication between these services and the research personnel.

*Adaptive (Urn) randomization.* In this scheme, the assignment process involves: (1) randomizing the first set of participants to the experimental intervention and the comparison groups; (2) assessing their responses to the allocated treatment; and (3) using the information on the type of responses (success or improvement versus failure or no change/worsening) reported in each treatment group as the basis for allocating subsequent participants. For instance, if a large number of participants assigned to the intervention group show improvement in the outcomes, then the next participant is allocated to the intervention group. The goal is to expose a large number of participants to the successful treatment and hence, to address the ethical concerns of denying participants in the comparison group a useful intervention or of providing participants in the intervention group a harmful intervention. The application of adaptive randomization requires that changes in the outcomes are clearly specified (i.e. what constitutes success or failure is accurately defined) and take place in a short time period (to inform subsequent assignments). The potential of having the majority of participants in one group is a limitation of this scheme.

### 15.3.3    Concealment of Allocation

Concealment implies not disclosing the randomization sequence to research staff or health professionals involved in recruitment, enrollment, and assignment to treatment. Concealment is considered important in ensuring that allocation is done on the basis of chance alone, with no interference by these persons. Concealment can be maintained by: (1) folding the paper on which the treatment is written and enclosing it in an opaque envelope; (2) hiding the computer-generated sequence of allocation and communicating with the central randomization services at the point in time when participants are to be informed of the allocated treatment; and (3) not disclosing the alternating pattern of assignment characterizing pseudo-randomization. Results of systematic reviews were inconsistent in determining the contribution of concealment to the validity of the intervention effects' estimates: some reviews' findings indicated that lack of adequate concealment led to overestimated effects (Savovíc et al., 2011), whereas others showed no association between concealment and the estimated effects (Hyde, 2004; Lindsay, 2004). Incidences of tampering with randomization procedures and concealment have been reported (Schulz & Grimes, 2002; Streiner & Sidani, 2010), leading to the conclusion that concealment cannot be ensured (Berger, 2018).

### 15.3.4    Nonrandom Allocation

The two procedures for nonrandom allocation illustrate those commonly applied in real world treatment decision-making. The first involves others' selection of treatment and the second entails participants' self-selection of treatment.

*Others' selection of treatment.* In this procedure, someone other than participants determines the treatment to which participants are assigned. The person selecting the treatment may be: the researcher as done in the cohort and regression-discontinuity designs and in studies evaluating tailored interventions, or the health professional responsible for the participants' care as done in observational studies and some pragmatic trials. Treatment selection can be informed by: (1) well-delineated algorithms developed for the evaluation study. The algorithms are based on propositions of the intervention theory combined with relevant empirical or clinical evidence; the algorithms detail the protocol for assessing the tailoring variables and interpreting the participants' scores on the respective measures, as well as the decision rules for treatment selection (as explained in Chapter 5); (2) clinical guidelines in use in the practice setting where the study is conducted; the guidelines recommend specific treatments (included in the evaluation study) for participants presenting with varying personal and health characteristics, or demonstrating varying responses to treatments (as explained for adaptive designs in Chapter 13); (3) clinical judgment that is based on health professionals' expert knowledge. The similarity of this procedure to that for treatment selection used in practice, makes others' selection a feature of evaluation studies that is acceptable and valued by participants, contributing to enhanced enrollment. The vulnerability of this and the next (self-selection) procedures to selection and subsequent confounding bias is disputed, as cumulative evidence (presented in Chapter 13) supports the comparability of intervention effects estimated in randomized and nonrandomized studies.

*Participants' self-selection of treatment.* In this procedure, participants are allocated to the treatment (experimental intervention or comparison treatment) of their choice, as advocated in preference trials. As explained in Chapter 11, participants should be provided with information on both treatments and appraise the treatments relative to appropriateness, effectiveness, severity of discomfort or side effects, and convenience, before expressing their preferences. This procedure for treatment allocation is attractive to participants and has been found to enhance enrollment, retention, and intervention effectiveness. However, it has the potential to yield unbalanced groups' sizes if the majority of participants prefer one treatment over the other.

## 15.4  OUTCOME DATA COLLECTION

### 15.4.1  Importance

Outcomes are the criteria for determining the effectiveness, benefits, or success of health interventions. Accordingly, they have been of primary concern in intervention evaluation research. Traditionally, the focus has been on evaluating the effects of health interventions on the primary outcomes, often represented in clinical end points covering objective and subjective indicators of the disease or general health. Recently, attention has shifted to the investigation of the mechanism of action through which the intervention contributes to the ultimate outcomes. The mechanism is represented in the interrelationships among the immediate, intermediate, and ultimate outcomes. Furthermore, there is growing interest in exploring unintended outcomes (beneficial or harmful) associated with health interventions.

The centrality of outcomes in determining the success (or failure) of health interventions requires careful considerations in their selection and assessment in an outcome evaluation study. First and foremost, the outcomes should be carefully selected to represent those expected to be impacted by the experimental intervention. The common practice of including a wide range of outcomes that may not be sensitive to the intervention increases: (1) the likelihood of observing no significant improvement in these outcomes and consequently, inferring that the intervention is not effective; (2) the burden on participants who have to provide data on a large number of outcomes, resulting in response fatigue that negatively affects the quality of the data; and (3) the probability of type I error associated with repeated testing to examine the effect of the intervention on each outcome.

Second, the outcomes should be assessed with valid and reliable measures. *Valid measures* are essential to accurately reflect the selected outcomes, quantify the participants' levels on the outcomes, and capture the anticipated changes in the outcomes in participants exposed to the intervention and no changes in those exposed to the comparison treatment (issue of construct validity).

*Reliable measures* have the capacity to assess the outcomes with consistency, precision and minimal error (issue of statistical conclusion validity). Measurement error increases variability in the posttest outcome scores that is not attributable to the intervention. Therefore, it reduces the power to detect significant intervention effects. Measurement error represents variability in participants' scores on an outcome that is associated with the use of the measure itself and not with the participants' actual level on the outcome being measured. The error can be random or systematic. *Random error* is introduced by chance, through factors such as: (1) the content of the measure, exemplified by misspelled words that change their meaning or by unclear directions for completing the measure; (2) the application of the measure, illustrated with improper functioning of the equipment (e.g. pedometer); and (3) conditions or circumstances under which the measure is completed such as participants' fatigue or improper storage of specimens. *Systematic error* is introduced by factors that interfere with or influence participants' responses to all items in a measure. The factors are related to misunderstanding the instructions on how to complete the measure, difficulty in grasping the items' content due to low literacy level, cultural or language barriers, social desirability, and acquiescence (i.e. tendency to select the same response option for all items).

Outcomes should be assessed at the appropriate points in time surrounding treatment delivery. The time points are carefully specified in order to detect the pattern (direction and magnitude) of change in the outcomes that are attributable to the intervention. The pattern of change in the immediate, intermediate, and ultimate outcomes is specified in the intervention theory (Chapter 5).

### 15.4.2    Selection of Outcomes

Conventionally, the focus in intervention evaluation research has been on what is considered "primary" outcomes. These are outcomes of interest to researchers as well as clinical and policy decision-makers. Most primary outcomes usually reflect (1) clinical end points, covering objective and subjective indicators of the health problem addressed by the intervention and of disease or general health (e.g. mortality, complications, biomarkers, health-related quality of life); and (2) financial outcomes related to the use of healthcare resources or services and the cost-efficacy or cost-effectiveness of the intervention. Recently, attention has shifted to outcomes of relevance to clients, referred to as patient-centered or patient-oriented outcomes. These outcomes encompass symptoms commonly experienced by various client populations (e.g. fatigue, insomnia); physical functioning (e.g. performance of activities of daily living like bathing and cooking; engagement in physical activity like walking); social functioning (e.g. visits with family and friends); health-related behaviors (e.g. smoking); and psychological well-being (e.g. low anxiety). Thus, there is a wide range of outcomes that can be investigated to determine the success of health interventions.

Including a combination of clinical end points, patient-centered, and financial outcomes in health intervention evaluation studies, is common practice. This practice has some advantages. It enables the assessment of the intervention's impact on different domains of health valued by different stakeholder groups (clients, health professionals, policy makers); the comparative effectiveness and cost-effectiveness of alternative health interventions addressing the same health problem, using the same set of criteria for effectiveness (i.e. the same set of outcomes); and the identification of intended (i.e. hypothesized) and unintended (i.e. not anticipated) outcomes (Sidani, 2015). The limitations of including a wide range of outcomes are related to the investigation of outcomes that are not sensitive to the intervention; this in turn, increases the potential for incorrect inferences regarding the effects of the intervention (mentioned in Section 15.4.1). Furthermore, the findings quantifying the direct impact of the intervention on multiple outcomes are prone to misinterpretation. It may be difficult to discern if the significant beneficial outcomes are solely attributable to the intervention, or if they reflect happenstance. Also, it may be hard to determine if the nonsignificant changes in the ultimate outcomes are related to their nonsensitivity to the intervention, to measurement error, or if they reflect the intervention's indirect effects on the ultimate outcomes (expected to be small or nonsignificant, as explained by Wiedermann & von Eye, 2015). The practice of combining outcomes, without attendance to the propositions of the intervention theory, resembles a fishing expedition, yielding results that may not be accurate, robust or replicable, and clearly interpreted.

Outcome selection should be explicitly informed by the intervention theory, which is advantageous. As explained in Chapter 5, the theory:

1. identifies the ultimate outcomes expected of the intervention, and the mechanism of action. The latter is represented by the interrelationships among the immediate, intermediate, and ultimate outcomes;

2. provides conceptual and operational definitions of each outcome; these definitions give clear directions for selecting the instrument for validly measuring the outcomes;

3. specifies the time points at which changes in the outcomes are anticipated, which indicates when exactly the outcomes are assessed surrounding (before, during, and after) the delivery of the intervention;

4. describes the pattern of change expected for immediate, intermediate, and ultimate outcomes; the pattern of change is important for the correct specification of the mathematical function that quantifies change over time in the outcome data analysis and for the correct interpretation of the findings; for instance, no to minimal improvement in the ultimate outcomes is expected at posttest, that is, immediately following completion of the intervention; and

5. delineates the interrelationships among exposure to the intervention, and the immediate, intermediate, and ultimate outcomes. The proposed interrelationships guide the outcome data analysis. The analysis aims to determine the direct and indirect (or mediated) effects of the intervention. Evidence on the interrelationships assists in figuring out the extent to which the intervention is successful in initiating the mechanism of action and hence, in understanding how or why the intervention works or does not work in improving the ultimate outcomes.

The limitation of the theory-informed selection of outcomes is the inability to examine quantitatively, possible unintended outcomes. However, these could be explored with qualitative methods for data collection.

### 15.4.3 Selection of Measures

After identifying relevant outcomes, the search begins for appropriate measures. In intervention research, there is a tendency to choose measures simply because they are widely used or because their names suggest that they capture the outcome of interest. This approach for selecting outcome measures may lead to results that are hard to interpret, even meaningless. Instead, the process for selecting an outcome measure is systematic, involving:

1. *A thorough review of the conceptual and operational definitions of an outcome.* The conceptual definition specifies the attributes that characterize the outcome and distinguish it from others. For example, chronic insomnia is generally defined as a disturbance in the quantity and quality of sleep, experienced over three months or more. The operational definition delineates the indicators of each attribute. The indicators can be directly measured. The operational definition also specifies the dimension (e.g. severity, frequency, duration) of the outcome to be assessed. For instance, the attribute of quantity of sleep is indicated by: (1) self-reported difficulty falling asleep and staying asleep (i.e. perceived severity); (2) the time it takes to fall asleep or time spent

awake, and the total sleep time during a night; the number of nights within a week (frequency); and (3) the number of months (duration) over which the difficulty is experienced. The attribute of sleep quality is operationalized in subjectively reported satisfaction with sleep and impact of the sleep disturbance on daily functioning.

2. *A search for available measures of the outcome*

The search for available measures of outcomes is completed in two types of databases. The first type includes general health-related databases. The search is for studies that report on the development and evaluation of the psychometric properties of instruments measuring the selected outcome, and for intervention evaluation studies that examined the effects of health interventions on the selected outcome. The second type consists of instrument-specific databases (e.g. Health and Psychosocial Instruments [HaPI]) that list or publish a copy of instruments measuring the selected outcome. A review of relevant studies assists in generating a list of available instruments measuring the same outcome. In addition, the review should identify the conceptual and operational definitions of the outcome underpinning the development of each measure, a description of the domains and dimensions of the outcome captured by each measure, and evidence of validity and reliability.

3. *Careful appraisal of the measures*

The content captured in the items comprising each measure is carefully appraised to determine its congruence with the operational definition of the outcome advanced in the intervention theory. The appraisal involves two steps. The first step focuses on clarifying the attributes of the outcome that are measured in each instrument. The attributes are reflected in respective indicators, and the indicators are assessed in the items. All items measuring one attribute are lumped into a subscale. Thus, in the first step of the appraisal, the outcome attributes and relevant indicators are delineated for each measure. The second step involves judging the correspondence or alignment of the outcome attributes, and the respective indicators, as represented in each measure. A matrix can be generated to document the results of this exercise applied on each available outcome measure. The first column of the matrix specifies the attributes and respective indicators of the outcome as proposed in the intervention theory. The remaining columns represent the attributes and indicators captured in measures reviewed. The cells of the matrix are populated with check marks indicating the attributes and indicators of the outcome as specified in the intervention theory (and presented in the first column of the matrix) captured in each measure. Items assessing additional indicators of the outcome that are inconsistent with those proposed in its operational definition, are identified and listed in an additional row in the matrix. These additional indicators are scrutinized to determine if they reflect (1) indicators of other related outcomes (e.g. measures of depressive symptomatology often include items assessing insomnia): overlap in content of instruments measuring conceptually distinct outcomes has the potential to confound the effects of the intervention on the outcomes; therefore, the overlap in content should be minimized (by selecting measures that show nonoverlap in content or by excluding overlapping items); or (2) indicators of the same outcome concept as experienced by a particular client population: items assessing these indicators are kept if applicable to the client population targeted in the evaluation study. For instance, items capturing somatic indicators of depression are included in measures of depression when the target client population consists of ethno-cultural groups known to express depression somatically, even though the operational definition of depression presented in the intervention theory focuses on the cognitive or emotional expression of this outcome. The point is that the operational definition and the content of the measure should be relevant to various subgroups of the target client population.

The appraisal of outcome measures' content is relevant to self-report and observational measures and should also be considered in the selection of objective measures. Some objective indicators (e.g. blood pressure) can equally reflect distinct outcomes (e.g. anxiety and pain). Some objective measures (e.g. actigraphy) claimed to accurately assess an outcome (e.g. sleep) may indeed capture a different concept (e.g. inactivity rather that sleep).

4. *Choice of a measure*

   A thorough review of the matrix data assists in determining the measure to be selected for assessing the outcome. The measure is the one with items that comprehensively operationalize all attributes and respective indicators of the outcome.

There are additional points to consider before finalizing the selection of an outcome measure. The points relate to the psychometric properties and clinical utility of the measure.

*Evidence of construct validity.* Validity refers to the accuracy with which an instrument measures the concept it purports to measure. There are several approaches and methods for assessing construct validity (see Streiner et al., 2015). Of most relevance to the selection of an outcome measure are those that assess its capacity to distinguish different levels on the outcome for participants exposed and not exposed to the intervention (sometimes called responsiveness), and to detect true changes in the outcome in participants exposed to the intervention, over time (sometimes called sensitivity to change).

Capacity to distinguish different levels on the outcome is assessed with the contrasted group approach. In this approach, participants belonging to naturally occurring (e.g. men and women) or experimentally generated (e.g. intervention and comparison treatment) groups and known (based on theoretical or clinical predictions) to differ on the outcomes, complete the outcome measure. Differences in their responses or scores on the measure support the measure's capacity to distinguish among levels on the outcome. The measure's capacity to detect true changes in the outcome is inferred from evidence showing: (1) significant changes, in the anticipated direction and magnitude, in participants exposed to an intervention of known efficacy, and/or (2) concordance or congruence between the level of change in the outcome captured by the measure, and the level of change in the same outcome detected by a criterion instrument. The criterion instrument could be another subjective or objective measure completed by participants, their healthcare providers, or interventionists delivering the intervention. Statistical formulae for estimating true change are available (see Liang, 2000). Outcome measures that are suspected or have demonstrated floor or ceiling effects are not useful for assessing outcomes, as these measures have limited capacity to register further changes in the outcomes.

*Evidence of reliability.* Reliability refers to the consistency with which an instrument measures the concept of interest. There are different approaches and methods for examining reliability (see Streiner et al., 2015) of: (1) biophysiological and physical measures: evidence of the measure's precision can be obtained from the laboratory conducting the test or from the manufacturer of the equipment; (2) behavioral measures completed by observers: interrater reliability is assessed to reflect the level of agreement in the observers' ratings of the same behavior exhibited by the same participants; and (3) self-report measures completed by participants.

Two approaches for evaluating the reliability of self-report measures can be used. The first is internal consistency reliability. It reflects consistency in the responses to the items contained in the outcome measure and obtained at one point in time. The second is test–retest reliability or stability. It reflects consistency in responses to the same items by the same participants, over time. In intervention evaluation research, the internal consistency reliability, quantified in the Cronbach's alpha coefficient, is of relevance; however, estimates of reliability, based on the total sample (i.e. participants in both the intervention and comparison treatment groups) are anticipated to be low (less than the cutoff value of 0.80 for established measures and 0.70 for new measures) at pretest because the sample is homogenous relative to their experience of the outcomes. Homogeneity of experience is manifested in low variability in participants' responses or scores on the outcome measure. In contrast, the Cronbach's alpha coefficient is expected to be high at posttest, reflecting heterogeneity in responses or scores on the outcome measures. Heterogeneity is generated by results indicating that participants in the experimental intervention group show improvement (e.g. high scores) and those in the comparison treatment group report no change (e.g. low scores). Outcome measures demonstrating high (>0.80) stability are not appropriate because they may not have the capacity to register or detect changes.

*Suitability to the target client population.* Suitability has to do with the relevance of the outcome measure to clients. Relevant measures have items with content that taps onto all indicators of the outcome as experienced by clients. In addition, the content is presented in simple, easy to understand, lay terms, preferably written at the fourth or sixth grade level. The response options represent meaningful nuances in the outcome's experience. For example, an 11-point Likert type scale offers fine gradations that are not easy to discern by many clients.

*Clinical utility.* Clinical utility relates to the convenience of administering the measure, computing the scores and interpreting the scores (Streiner et al., 2015) in intervention evaluation research.

*Convenience of administering the measure*: it would be ideal to select measures that capture all relevant indicators of the outcome, with a small number of items. Long, multiple item measures take time to complete, potentially leading to response burden. Response burden is heightened when a large number of outcome measures are administered repeatedly. Response burden lowers the quality of responses (e.g. acquiescence or careless responses) and contribute to high amount of missing data. Both quality and missingness affect the accuracy of the estimates of the intervention's effects.

Two solutions are proposed to reduce response burden. Firstly, short versions of the measure could be selected if available. Secondly, transition or perceived change scales are promising alternative measures of outcomes. They consist of single items, administered at posttest and requesting participants to indicate the extent of change (from pretest to posttest) they experienced or perceived in each outcome. The response options represent different levels of change (e.g. much better, better, no change, worse, much worse). Transition scales are simple to complete, familiar to many clients (as they are often used in practice), and provide a direct and efficient quantification of change in the overall outcome experience. However, the use of single transition items limits the ability to examine change in specific attributes of the outcome. Transition scales have been validated and found capable of detecting clinically important changes in different outcomes and in different client populations (Kamper et al., 2009).

*Ease of scoring and interpreting scores*: Outcome measures with validated cutoff scores are useful in determining the clinical relevance or significance of the evaluation study's results. In addition to quantifying the size of the intervention's effects, cutoff scores assist in identifying the number of participants in remission (i.e. no longer meet the diagnostic criteria of the health problem).

*Measures for detecting unintended outcomes.* Open-ended questions are most useful to identify unintended outcomes as experienced by participants. Examples of questions are: How did this treatment affect you, in a positive or negative way? What impact did this treatment have on you, your health, your life? The questions are added to the questionnaire for self-completion by participants, or are asked in an interview with participants, at posttest. The responses are content analyzed to determine the type and frequently experienced unintended, beneficial, or nonbeneficial outcomes.

### 15.4.4   Specification of Outcome Assessment Times

The times for assessing the outcomes are carefully specified to enable the detection of the anticipated level and pattern of change in the immediate, intermediate, and ultimate outcomes. The specification of the time points is informed by the intervention theory, as detailed in Chapter 5. At a minimum, the outcomes should be assessed once before and once after the intervention delivery. Additional time points are included in between-subject and within-subject designs, as described in Chapter 14. The time interval separating the outcome assessments are also guided by theoretical expectation of change.

## 15.5   OUTCOME DATA ANALYSIS

### 15.5.1   Importance

The analysis of outcome data aims to determine the extent to which the health intervention is successful in producing the hypothesized outcomes. Success is inferred from the results of comparisons between the experimental intervention and the comparison treatment groups on the outcomes measured at different points in time surrounding treatment delivery. Valid inferences rest on having unbiased estimates that accurately quantify the intervention's effects. Whereas the analysis cannot rectify all design-related biases, it can be planned to assess and address some biases, such as those associated with confounding and attrition. Points to consider in planning the outcome analysis of an intervention evaluation study, along with recent advances in the field, are presented next. The plan usually involves preliminary steps and main analysis steps.

### 15.5.2   Preliminary Steps

The preliminary steps are undertaken to assess the quality of the data and the suitability of the data for the main analysis. The preliminary steps include:

*Data cleaning.* Data cleaning focuses on determining the accuracy of the data entered. When participants complete hard copies of the measures, this step involves having two research staff check the values (i.e. numbers assigned to the responses to the items comprising all measures administered to all participants at all points in time) entered in the computerized database, against the responses reported in the questionnaire. Alternatively, two research staff enter the same data set separately and use existing software or program to examine the consistency in the values they entered separately. Discrepancies are resolved by checking the values entered in the databases to the values reported in the questionnaire completed by the participants. In addition, data cleaning entails initial descriptive statistics. Descriptive statistics (frequency distribution) are applied for each item to identify possible out-of-range values; these are checked for accuracy against those reported by participants in the questionnaire.

Data cleaning may be skipped when participants complete the measures online. Regardless of how data are collected, this step also involves computation of the total score to quantify participants' level on each outcome variable at each time point. The calculation follows the instructions provided by the measure developer, where the total score is calculated as either the sum or mean of the items' values.

*Knowing the data.* The purpose of this step is to "get to know" or "have a good sense" of the data. It involves running descriptive statistics, including frequency distribution, histogram, and measures of central tendency and of dispersion. The purpose of this descriptive analysis is to explore the extent of missing data and the pattern of missing data on specific items and variables (where variables are quantified in the total scores on respective multi-item measures). This analysis is critical to determine whether or not the data are missing at random and hence, to select the most appropriate strategy for handling missing data (for details, see McKnight et al., 2007). The descriptive analysis also aims to examine the shape of the distribution of the scores quantifying each outcome variable; the analysis assists in identifying participants with extreme values on the outcome and in inquiring about the reasons underlying extreme values. The results of this analysis inform the decision on the strategy to handle these cases. For example, extreme values may represent a distinct subgroup of the target client population that may respond differently to the intervention, which is best handled in a planned subgroup analysis. The descriptive analysis determines the level of variance in the outcome scores within and across treatment groups, interventionists, and settings or sites. The level of variance has implication for selecting statistical tests most appropriate to handle the nesting of participants within this hierarchy of treatment, interventionist, and site (Bell & Rabe, 2020).

Additional analyses are performed in this step. The reliability of outcome measures is assessed. Testing the internal consistency of multi-item outcome measures is highly recommended in an evaluation study because the reliability estimates are sample dependent (i.e. they vary from one sample to another) and affect the power to detect significant intervention effects. Also in this step, the comparability of participants assigned to the experimental intervention and the comparison treatment groups on personal and health characteristics, the health problem and other outcomes assessed at baseline or pretest, is examined. This analysis is important to identify potential confounding variables and to devise the most appropriate strategies to address them. Confounding variables are those showing between-group differences at baseline and known or found (in previous research or current study) to be associated with the outcomes measured at posttest. Statistical strategies to address confounding variables include adjustment of the confounding variables' correlation with the posttest outcomes (e.g. analysis of covariance) and determination of the intervention's effects in subgroups of participants with varying levels on the confounding variables (e.g. factorial analysis of variance or multilevel or hierarchical linear models). Lastly, the pattern of change in each outcome is examined in the total sample and in each treatment group. It is examined using change or difference scores for outcomes assessed at two time points only, or individual regression coefficient for outcomes assessed at more than two time points. Awareness of the pattern of change in the outcomes has implications for selecting pertinent analytic strategies in the analysis of outcome data. For instance, differences in the pattern of change observed within the experimental intervention group suggests the need for subgroup analysis or exploration of the influence of treatment, interventionist, setting, and/or client characteristics on the level of improvement in the outcomes (Engel et al., 2013).

*Understanding the sample.* In this step, participants who did and did not enroll, and those who did and did not complete the study, are compared on their characteristics. Where data are available (either collected from individuals or from participating settings), clients who refuse enrollment are compared to enrollees on personal and health characteristics to determine the representativeness of the enrollees of various subgroups of the client population. The results are useful in delineating the generalizability or applicability of the intervention's effects reported in the evaluation study. Similar comparisons are done on baseline characteristics between participants who complete the study and those who withdraw. These comparisons determine the presence of differential attrition and resulting confounding, which should be addressed when estimating the intervention's effects.

*Addressing attrition.* In RCTs, the intention-to-treat or intent-to-treat (ITT) principle is used to handle three possible biases: attrition, violations of study protocol (i.e. participants crossing over to nonassigned treatment; nonadherence to treatment recommendations; exposure to concurrent treatment available outside the trial); and confounding that can be introduced with attrition. In the ITT analysis, participants are analyzed in the treatment group to which they are randomized, regardless of their subsequent behaviors such as dropping out, over the course of the trial. The ITT analysis is done to maintain both the balance in the number of participants and the comparability on baseline characteristics of the experimental intervention and the comparison treatment groups, which are achieved through randomization; therefore, the ITT analysis eliminates potential confounding bias (Ragonathan et al., 2016). For participants who drop out of the trial, their missing outcome data are imputed with different strategies, with the last observation carried forward commonly advocated. The last observation carried forward is based on the assumption that participants' responses or scores on the outcomes remain the same after withdrawal. Thus, the last outcome score recorded prior to withdrawal is imputed for the remaining time points.

The ITT analysis has been criticized on conceptual and empirical grounds. Conceptually, IIT estimates the effects of "treatment assignment", and not the effects of the treatment that participants engage in and enact. The ITT analysis has been found to dilute the actual treatment effects, represented in underestimated (low) effects (Shrier et al., 2017). To enhance the validity of inferences, it is now recommended to conduct per-protocol analysis, to supplement the results of ITT. In per-protocol analysis, the outcome data are analyzed for participants who adhered to the allocated treatment, after adjusting for possible confounding (Hernán & Robins, 2017). Recent statistical analytic strategies (i.e. multilevel or hierarchical linear models) have the capacity to efficiently handle missing outcome data (Bell & Rabe, 2020; Chakraborty & Gu, 2009) and are highly recommended.

### 15.5.3   Main Analysis Steps

The main analytic steps consist of applying appropriate tests to determine the significance of the estimated intervention effects. Traditionally, statistical significance was emphasized. However, the main outcome analysis should also address clinical significance. Most statistical tests are devised to determine whether or not the null hypothesis (i.e. participants in the experimental intervention and the comparison treatment groups belong to the same population and therefore, do not differ in the posttest outcomes). The $p$-value and power are preset at criterion or cutoff levels to reduce the chance of committing error in making inferences regarding accepting or rejecting the null hypothesis (Page, 2014). This prevalent practice and reliance on statistical significance is of limited scientific (Wasserstein et al., 2019) and clinical / practical / substantive relevance (Page, 2014; Pek & Flora, 2018). Statistically significant results indicate that the outcomes differ between the treatment groups, but fail to quantify the magnitude of the treatment effects (Kelly & Preacher, 2012); yet, it is the magnitude of the effects that is meaningful in informing practice.

*Statistical tests.* A range of statistical tests are available to examine the effects of the experimental intervention on the outcomes. These include tests to:

1.  examine between-group differences in each outcome (e.g. independent sample $t$-test or one way analysis of variance) or all outcomes (e.g. multivariate analysis of variance or discriminant analysis) measured at each time point following delivery of the intervention, and where required, adjusting for confounding variables (e.g. analysis of covariance or regression analysis);
2.  examine within-group differences in each outcome measured at two points in time (e.g. dependent or paired $t$-test) or multiple time points before and after treatment delivery (e.g. repeated measure analysis of variance);
3.  examine between-group differences in each outcome measured at multiple time points (e.g. repeated measure analysis of variance including treatment as a between-subject factor); and
4.  conduct subgroup analyses in which the variable representing the subgroup (e.g. gender or concurrent treatment) is added as a between-subject factor in the analytic model (e.g. regression or analysis of variance).

Although widely used, the abovementioned tests focus on the average direct effects of the intervention on the outcomes. The focus on the average effects ignores the interindividual variability in participants' responses to treatment. Yet, interindividual variability in responses to treatment is important for two reasons. First, if large, the variability reduces the likelihood of detecting between-group differences, yielding type II error. Second, the variability in responses to treatment across subgroups of clients is of importance to practice, addressing the question of: Who would most benefit from the intervention? Subgroups analysis is a useful approach for providing answers to this question.

The outcome analysis should also test the extent to which the intervention initiated its mechanism of action, which is represented in the interrelationships among exposure to the intervention, and immediate, intermediate and ultimate outcomes. Path analysis or structural equation modeling is the statistical approach for examining the indirect intervention effects on the ultimate outcomes, mediated through the immediate and intermediate outcomes (Wiedermann & von Eye, 2015).

There are some limitations to widely used statistical tests. The results of widely used tests such as repeated measure analysis of variance with a between-subject factor representing treatment received, indicate whether or not there are differences over time (time effect), between groups (group effect) and between groups over time (interaction effect). Post hoc comparisons are conducted to determine where exactly the differences occurred, which has the potential of increasing type I error rate. Carefully planning the post hoc comparisons (informed by theory) is the strategy to minimize type I error. Only a few variables can be examined in widely used statistical tests; also, these tests do not account for the nesting or clustering of participants within interventionists, treatment, and setting. Ignoring the possible interaction among variables and the nesting of participants impacts the estimated intervention effects. Multilevel, hierarchical, or mixed models are recommended to account for the multilevel nesting of the outcome data and for multiple variables that are theoretically hypothesized to influence the outcomes. In these models, the pattern (direction and magnitude) of change in an outcome is estimated for each participant and a range of (continuous or categorical, time-invariant or time-variant) predictors occurring at different levels are included in the analytic model to investigate their influence on the outcome. These models have been extended to enable analysis of mediated effects (Bell & Rabe, 2020; Engel et al., 2013; Field & Wright, 2011; Hox, 2010; Twisk et al., 2017).

*Clinical significance.* Different approaches can be used to quantify the magnitude of health intervention effects. The common approaches include:

1. the size of the difference in the mean of the experimental intervention and the comparison treatment groups. The difference is used for an outcome assessed with a measure that has a standard, well recognized and clearly interpretable metric such as blood pressure or weight;

2. the standardized mean difference (Cohen's d). The standardized difference is used for an outcome assessed with a measure with nonstandard metric. The standardized difference is useful in comparing the magnitude of the intervention's effects on different outcomes. However, the interpretation of its value is done with caution as what is considered small, moderate, or large effect sizes varies across outcomes or fields;

3. comparing the mean or the standardized mean difference to minimal clinically important differences validated as important or worthwhile or meaningful in practice (Kelly & Preacher, 2012; Page, 2014; Pek & Flora, 2018); and

4. the rate of remission in the experimental intervention (versus the comparison treatment) group; remission is the percentage of participants considered as no longer experiencing the health problem, based on well-established criteria.

## REFERENCES

Adams, K.F., Sperl-Hillen, J.M., Davis, H., et al. (2013) Factors influencing patient completion of diabetes self-management education. *Diabetes Spectrum: A Publication of the American Diabetes Association*, 26(1), 40–47.

Ahern, K. & Le Brocque, R. (2005) Methodological issues in the affects of attrition: Simple solutions for social scientists. *Field Methods*, 17, 53–69.

Akl, E.A., Briel, M., Yov, J.J., et al. (2012) Potential impact on estimated treatment effects of information lost to follow-up in randomised controlled trials (LOST-IT): Systematic review. *BMJ*, 344, e2809.

Autret, A., Valade, D., & Debiais, S. (2012) Placebo and other psychological interactions in headache treatment. *Journal of Headache and Pain*, 13, 191–198.

Barkauskas, V.H., Lusk, S.L., & Eakin, B.L. (2005) Intervention research: Selecting control interventions for clinical outcome studies. *Western Journal of Nursing Research*, 27, 346–363.

Baskin, T.W., Tierney, S.C., Minami, T., & Wampold, B.E. (2000) Establishing specificity in psychotherapy: A meta-analysis of structural equivalence of placebo controls. *Journal of Consulting and Clinical Psychology*, 71(6), 973–979.

Baucom, K.J.W., Chen, X.S., Perry, N.S., et al. (2018) Recruitment and retention of low-SES ethnic minority couples in intervention research at the transition to parenthood. *Family Process*, 57(2), 308–323.

Bell, M.L. & Rabe, B.A. (2020) The mixed model for repeated measures for cluster randomized trials: A simulation study investigating bias and type I error with missing continuous data. *Trials*, 21, 148–158.

Berger, V.W. (ed) (2018) *Randomization, Masking, and Allocation Concealment*. Chapman & Hall/CRC. Biostatistics Series, Taylor & Francis, New York.

Bonell, C., Warren, E., Fletcher, A., & Viner, R. (2016) Realist trials and the testing of context-mechanism-outcome configurations: A response to van belle et al. *Trials*, 17, 478–482.

Bower, P., Brueton, V., Gamble, C., et al. (2014) Interventions to improve recruitment and retention in clinical trials: A survey and workshop to assess current practice and future priorities. *Trials*, 15, 399–407.

Brueton, V., Stenning, S.P., Stevenson, F., Tierney, J., & Rait, G. (2017) Best practice guidance for the use of strategies to improve retention in randomized trials developed from two consensus workshops. *Journal of Clinical Epidemiology*, 88, 122–132.

Butler, J., Tahhan, A.S., Georgiopoulou, K.A., et al. (2015) Trends in characteristics of cardiovascular clinical trials 2001-2012. *American Heart Journal*, 170, 263–272.

Caldwell, P.H.Y., Hamilton, S., Tan, A., & Craig, J.C. (2010) Strategies for increasing recruitment to randomised controlled trials: Systematic review. *PLoS Medicine*, 7(11), e1000368.

Califf, R.M., Zarin, D.A., Kramer, J.M., et al. (2012) Characteristics of clinical trials registered in ClinicalTrials.gov, 2007-2010. *Journal of the American Medical Association*, 307(17), 1838–1847.

Chakraborty, H. & Gu, H. (2009) *A Mixed Model Approach for Intent-to-Treat Analysis in Longitudinal Clinical Trials with Missing Values*. RTI Press publication No. MR-0009-0903. Research Triangle Park, NC: RTI International. Available on: http://www.rti.org/rtipress (accessed in June 2020).

Chow, S.-C., Shao, J., & Wang, H. (2008) *Sample Size Calculations in Clinical Research* (2nd Ed). Chapman and Hall/CRC, Boca Raton.

Coday, M., Boutin-Foster, C., Goldman Sher, T., et al. (2005) Strategies for retaining study participants in behavioural intervention trials: Retention experiences of the NIH behaviour change consortium. *The Society of Behavioural Medicine*, 29(suppl), 55–65.

Cohen, J. (1988) *Statistical Power Analysis for the Social Sciences* (2nd ed.). Lawrence Erlbaum, Hillsdale, NJ.

Cooley, M.E., Sarna, L., Brown, J.K., et al. (2003) Challenges of recruitment and retention in multisite clinical research. *Cancer Nursing*, 26(5), 376–386.

Costenbader, K.H., Brome, D., Blanch, D., et al. (2007) Factors determining participation in prevention trials among systematic lupus erythematosus patients: A qualitative study. *Arthritis Care & Research*, 57, 49–55.

De Moat, S., Dekker, J., Schoevers, R., & de Jonghe, F. (2007) The effectiveness of long term psychotherapy: Methodological research issues. *Psychotherapy Research*, 17(1), 59–65.

Dumville, J. C., Torgerson, D. J., & Hewitt, C. E. (2006) Reporting attrition in randomized controlled trials. *British Medical Journal*, 332(22), 969–971.

Ellis, J.G. & Barclay, N.L. (2014) Cognitive behavior therapy for insomnia: State of the science or a stated science? *Sleep Medicine*, 15, 849–850.

Engel, C., Meisner, C., Wittorf, A., et al. (2013) Longitudinal data analysis of symptom score trajectories using linear mixed models in a clinical trial. *International Journal of Statistics in Medical Research*, 2, 305–315.

Epstein, D.R., Sidani, S. Bootzin, R.R., & Belyea, M.J. (2012) Dismantling multi-component behavioral treatment for insomnia in older adults: A randomized controlled trial. *Sleep*, 35(6), 797–805.

Fayler, D., McDaid, C., & Eastwood, A. (2007) A systematic review highlights threats to validity in studies of barriers to cancer trial participation. *Journal of Clinical Epidemiology*, 60, 990–1001.

Field, A.P. & Wright, D.B. (2011) A primer on using multilevel models in clinical and experimental psychopathology research. *Journal of Experimental Psychopathology*, 2(2), 271–293.

Finnis, D.G., Kaptchuk, T.J., Miller, F., & Benedetti, F. (2010) Biological, clinical, and ethical advances of placebo effects. *Lancet*, 375, 686–695.

Foster, N. (2012) Methodological issues in pragmatic trials of complex interventions in primary care. *British Journal of General Practice*, 62(594), 10–11.

Frost, H., Campbell, P., Maxwell, M., et al. (2018) Effectiveness of motivational interviewing on adult behavior change in health and social care settings: A systematic review of reviews. *PLoS One*, 13 (10), e0204890.

Glombiewski, J.A., Hartwich-Tersek, J., & Rief, W. (2010) Two psychological interventions are effective in severely disabled, chronic back pain patients: A randomised controlled trial. *International Journal of Behavioural Medicine*, 17(2), 97–107.

Graham, A.L., Cha, S., Cobb, N.K., et al. (2013) Impact of seasonality on recruitment, retention, adherence, and outcomes in a web-based smoking cessation intervention: Randomized controlled trial. *Journal of Medical Internet Research*, 15(11), e249.

Grave, R.D., Calugi, S., Molinari, E., et al. and the QUOVADIS Study group (2005) Weight loss expectations in obese patients and treatment attrition: An observational multi center study. *Obesity Research*, 13(11), 1961–1969.

Gucciardi, E. (2008) A systematic review of attrition from diabetes and education services: Strategies to improve attrition and retention research. *Canadian Journal of Diabetes*, 32(1), 53–65.

Gucciardi, E., DeMelo, M., Booth, G., Tomlinson, G., & Stweart, D.E. (2009) Individual and contextual factors associated with follow-up use of diabetes self-management education programmes: A multisite prospective analysis. *Diabetic Medicine*, 26, 510–517.

Hebert, E.A., Vincent, N., Lewycky, S., & Walsh, K. (2010) Attrition and adherence in the online treatment of chronic insomnia. *Behavioral Sleep Medicine*, 8(3), 141–150.

Henry, D., Toaln, P., Gorman-Smith, D., & Schoeny, M. (2017) Alternatives to randomized control trial designs for community-based prevention evaluation. *Preventive Science*, 18, 671–680.

Hernán, M.A. & Robins, J.M. (2017) Per-protocol analyses of pragmatic trials. *New England Journal of Medicine*, 377(14), 1391–1398.

Horwood, J., Johnson, E., & Gooberman-Hill, R. (2016). Understanding involvement in surgical orthopaedic randomized controlled trials: A qualitative study of patient and health professional views and experiences. *International Journal of Orthopaedic and Trauma Nursing*, 20, 3–12.

Hox, J.J. (2010) *Multilevel Analysis: Techniques and Applications* (2nd ed.) Routledge, Hove.

Hughes-Morley, A., Young, B., Waheed, W., Small, N., & Bower P. (2015) Factors affecting recruitment into depression trials: Systematic review, meta-synthesis and conceptual framework. *Journal of Affective Disorders*, 172, 274–290.

Hyde, P. (2004) Fool's gold: Examining the use of gold standards in the production of research evidence. *British Journal of Occupational Therapy*, 67(2), 89–94.

Ibrahim, S. & Sidani, S. (2013) Strategies to recruit minority persons: A systematic review. *Journal of Immigrant and Minority Health*, 16(5), 882–8.

Juraschek, S.P., Plante, T.B., & Charleston, J. (2018) Use of online recruitment strategies in a randomized trial of cancer survivors. *Clinical Trials*, 15(2), 130–138.

Kamper, S.J., Maher, C.G., & Mackay, G. (2009) Global rating of change scales: A review of strengths and weaknesses and considerations for design. *The Journal of Manual & Manipulative Therapy*, 17(3), 163–170.

Kaptchuk, T.J., Friedlander, E., Kelley, J.M., et al. (2010) Placebos without deception: A randomized controlled trial in irritable bowel syndrome. *Public Library of Science One*, 5(12), 1–7.

Karras-Jean Gilles, J., Astuto, J., Gjicali, K., & LaRue, A. (2019) Sample retention in an urban context: Exploring influential factors within a longitudinal randomized evaluation. *American Journal of Evaluation*, 40(2), 268–290.

Keller, C.S., Gonzales, A., & Fleuriet, K.J. (2005) Retention of minority participants in clinical research studies. *Western Journal of Nursing*, 27(3), 292–306.

Kelly, K. & Preacher, K.J. (2012) On effect size. *Psychological Methods*, 17(2), 137–152.

Kemmler, G., Hummer, M., Widschwendter, C, et al (2005) Dropout rates in placebo-controlled and active-control clinical trials of antipsychotic drugs—A meta-analysis. *Archives of General Psychiatry*, 62, 1305–12.

Leach, M.J. (2003) Barriers to conducting randomized controlled trials: Lessons learnt from the Horsechestnut & Venous Leg Ulcer Trial (HAVLUT). *Contemporary Nurse*, 15, 37–47.

Leon, A.C., Davis, L.L., & Kraemer, H.C. (2011) The role and interpretation of pilot studies in clinical research. *Journal of Psychiatric Research*, 45(5), 626–629.

Liang, M.H. (2000) Longitudinal construct validity. Establishment of clinical meaning in patient evaluative instruments. *Medical Care*, 38(9, Suppl II), 84–90.

Lindsay, B. (2004) Randomized controlled trials of socially complex nursing interventions: Creating bias and unreliability? *Journal of Advanced Nursing*, 45(1), 84–94.

Lindsay Davis, L., Broome, M.E., & Cox, R.P. (2002) Maximizing retention in community-based clinical trials. *Journal of Nursing Scholarship*, 34, 47–53.

Lipsey, M.W. (1990) *Design Sensitivity. Statistical Power for Experimental Research*. Sage, Thousand Oaks, CA.

Lyons, K.S., Carter, J.H., Carter, E.H., et al. (2004) Locating and retaining research participants for follow-up studies. *Research in Nursing & Health*, 27, 63–68.

Maneeton, N., Maneeton, B., Srisurapanont, M., et al. (2012) Quetiapine monotherapy in acute phase for major depressive disorder: A meta-analysis of randomized, placebo-controlled trials. *BMC Psychiatry*, 12, 160.

Mattingly, W.A., Kelley, R.R., Wiemken, T.L., et al. (2015) Real-time enrollment dashboard for multisite clinical trials. *Contemporary Clinical Trials Communications*, 1, 17–21.

McDonald, A.M., Knight, R.M., Campbell, M.K., et al. (2006) What influences recruitment to randomized controlled trials? A review of trials funded by two UK funding agencies. *Trials*, 7, 9.

McKnight, P.E., McKnight, K.M., Sidani, S., & Figueredo, A.J. (2007) *Missing Data: A Gentle Introduction*. Guilford Publications, Inc., New York, NY

Michelet, M., Lund, A., & Sveen, U. (2014) Strategies to recruit and retain older adults in intervention studies: A qualitative comparative study. *Archives of Gerontology and Geriatrics*, 59(1), 25–31.

Moorcraft, S.Y., Marriott, C., Peckitt, C. et al. (2016) Patients' willingness to participate in clinical trials and their views on aspects of cancer research: Results of a prospective patient survey. *Trials*, 17, 17–26.

Murphy, V., Awatagiri, K.R., Tike, P.K., et al. (2012) Prospective analysis of reasons for non-enrollment in a phase III randomized controlled trial. *Journal of Cancer Research and Therapeutics*, 8, S94–S99.

Noordzij, M., Tripepi, G., Dekker, F.W., et al. (2010) Sample size calculations: Basic principles and common pitfalls. *Nephrology, Dialysis, Transplantation*, 25, 1388–1393.

Page, P. (2014) Beyond statistical significance: Clinical interpretation of rehabilitation research literature. *The International Journal of Sports Physical Therapy*, 9(5), 726–736.

Pek, J. & Flora, D.B. (2018) Reporting effect sizes in original psychological research: A discussion and tutorial. *Psychological Methods*, 23(2), 208–225.

Ragonathan, P., Pramesh, C.S., & Aggrawal, R. (2016) Common pitfalls in statistical analysis: Intention-to-treat versus per-protocol analysis. *Perspectives in Clinical Research*, 7(3), 144–146.

Rutterford, C., Copas, A., & Eldridge, S. (2015) Methods for sample size determination in cluster randomized trials. *International Journal of Epidemiology*, 44(3), 1052–1067.

Savovíc J., Jones, H.E., Altman, D.G., et al. (2011) Influence of reported study design characteristics on intervention effect estimates from randomized, controlled trials. *Annals of Internal Medicine*, 157, 429–438.

Schulz, K.F. & Grimes, D.A. (2002) Allocation concealment in randomised trials: Defending against deciphering. *The Lancet*, 359, 614–618.

Shrier, I., Verhagen, E., & Stovitz, S.D. (2017) The intention-to-treat analysis is not always the conservative approach. *The American Journal of Medicine*, 130(7), 867–871.

Sidani, S. (2015) *Health Intervention Research: Advances in Research Design and Methods*. Sage, London, UK.

Streiner, D.L. & Sidani, S. (eds) (2010) *When Research Goes Off the Rails. Why It Happens and What you Can Do About It*. The Guilford Press, New York

Streiner, D.L., Norman, G.R., & Cairney, J. (2015) *Health Measurement Scales: A Practical Guide to Their Development and Use* (5th ed). Oxford University Press, Oxford, UK.

Thoma, A., Farrokhyar, F., McKnight, L., & Bhandari, M. (2010) Practical tips for surgical research: How to optimize patient recruitment. *Canadian Journal of Surgery. Journal canadien de chirurgie*, 53(3), 205–210.

Timraz, S.M., Alhasanat, D.I., Albdour, M.M., et al. (2017) Challenges and strategies for conducting sensitive research with an Arab American population. *Applied Nursing Research*, 33, 1–4.

Treweek, S., Lockhart, P., Pitkethly, M., et al. (2013) Methods to improve recruitment to randomised controlled trials: Cochrane systematic review and meta-analysis. *BMJ Open*, 3, e002360.

Treweek S., Pitkethly, M., Cook, J. et al. (2018) Strategies to improve recruitment to randomised trials. *Cochrane Database of Systematic Reviews*, 22(2): MR000013. doi: `10.1002/14651858.MR000013.pub6`.

Twisk, J.W.R., de Vente, W., Apeldoorn, A.T., & de Boer, M.R. (2017) Should we use logistic mixed model analysis for the effect estimation in a longitudinal RCT with a dichotomous outcome variable? *Epidemiology, Biostatistics and Public Health*, 14(3), e12613-1.

van Die, D.M., Bone, K.M., Burger, H.G., & Teede, H. J. (2009) Are we drawing the right conclusions from randomized placebo-controlled trials? A post-hoc analysis of data from a randomized controlled trial. *BioMed Central Medical Research Methodology*, 9, 41–47.

Wandile, P.M. (2018) Placebos in clinical trials. *Clinical Research*, 32(10). Accessed on: `https://acrpnet.org/2018/12/06/ethical-deliberations-on-using-placebos-in-clinical-trials` (accessed in July 2020).

Warden, D., Trivedi, M.H., Wisniewski, S.R., et al. (2009) Identifying risk for attrition during treatment for depression. *Psychotherapy and Psychosomatics*, 78, 372–379.

Wasmann, K., Wijsman, P., van Dieren, S., Bemelman, W., & Buskens, C. (2019) Influence of patients' preference in randomised controlled trials. *Journal of Crohn's and Colitis*, 13(Suppl 1), S517–S518. doi: `10.1093/ecco-jcc/jjy222.915`.

Wasserstein, R.L., Schirm, A.L., & Lazar, N.A. (2019) Moving to a world beyond "p < 0.05". *The American Statistician*, 73(Sup1), 1–19.

Wiedermann, W. & von Eye, A. (2015) Directions of effects in mediation analysis. *Psychological Methods*, 20(2), 221–244.

Williams, A., Duggleby, W., Ploeg, J., et al. (2017) Overcoming recruitment challenges for securing a survey of caregivers of community-dwelling older adults with multiple chronic conditions. *Journal of Human Health Research*, 1(1), 16–24.

Young, B., Beidel, D., Turner, S., et al. (2006) Pretreatment attrition and childhood social phobia. *Anxiety Disorders*, 20, 1133–1147.

Younge, J.O., Kouwenhoven-Pasmooij, T.A., Freak-Poli, R., Koos-Hesselink, J.W., & Hunink. M.G.M. (2015) Randomized study designs for lifestyle interventions: A tutorial. *International Journal of Epidemiology*, 44(6), 2006–2019.

Zelen, M. (1979) A new design for randomized clinical trials. *The New England Journal of Medicine*, 300, 1242–1245.

# IMPLEMENTING INTERVENTIONS

# CHAPTER 16

# Frameworks and Methods for Implementing Interventions

Health interventions that demonstrate effectiveness (also called evidence-based interventions) have to be integrated in practice in order to benefit clients experiencing the health problem. Implementation is the actively planned and deliberately initiated effort to promote the uptake or adoption and use of evidence-based interventions in real-world practice (Pfadenhaver et al., 2017). Implementation must be carefully planned and well executed to facilitate health professionals' adoption and delivery of evidence-based interventions, and consequently clients' engagement and enactment of treatment; the ultimate goal is improvement in clients' experience of the health problem, general health, and well-being. To this end, the implementation plan should account for a range of factors that are inherent in the real world and that influence the actual use of evidence-based interventions in practice. Knowledge of the most influential factors informs the selection of strategies to disseminate evidence-based interventions to health professionals and to support them in the delivery of these interventions to clients. The implementation plan is executed in a multistage process that actively involves different stakeholder groups, including clients, health professionals, and decision-makers. The success of the implementation initiative is evaluated with designs that enable collection of data, with different methods, from multiple sources, on the factors that affect the use of the evidence-based interventions, on the fidelity with which the interventions are delivered and on the outcomes achieved within practice. Implementation initiatives are informed by frameworks that provide a useful structure for planning, executing, and evaluating them.

In this chapter, implementation frameworks are briefly reviewed. Practical guidance for applying the implementation process is provided. Research designs for evaluating the success of the implementation initiatives are highlighted.

## 16.1 IMPLEMENTATION FRAMEWORKS

Recognizing the importance of theory in guiding implementation initiatives, a large number of implementation frameworks have been, and still are being, developed. Examples of frameworks include: Practical Robust Implementation and Sustainability Model (PRISM), Consolidated Framework for Implementation Research,

Normalization Process Theory, General Theory of Implementation, Diffusion of Innovation Theory, the Ottawa Model, Behavior Change Model, and Promoting Action on Research Implementation in Health Services. Recent reviews of implementation frameworks (Harris et al., 2017; Moullin et al., 2015; Nilsen, 2015) classified the frameworks into three main categories: determinants, process, and evaluation. Each category consists of frameworks that emphasize one aspect of implementation more so than the remaining aspects.

## 16.1.1   Determinants Frameworks

Determinants frameworks identify the range of factors, operating at different levels within the healthcare system, that may influence the adoption and implementation of evidence-based interventions, as well as the effectiveness of these interventions in practice (Damschroder, 2020). The factors represent a set of characteristics, inherent in the context of implementation, that enable (i.e. facilitators) or hinder (i.e. barriers) the use of evidence-based interventions in practice. The factors manifest at the levels of:

*Clients*: Clients are the recipients or end users of the evidence-based interventions. Multiple client characteristics affect their uptake, engagement and enactment of evidence-based health interventions as detailed in Chapters 5, 9, 12, and 13. Of relevance are practical problems associated with access to the evidence-based interventions in practice (e.g. transportation, time at which the intervention is offered); clients' experience of the health problem and general health condition (e.g. level of severity at which the problem is experienced, presence of comorbid conditions); clients' motivation to seek treatment; and clients' beliefs about the health problem and its treatment that may shape their acceptability of the evidence-based interventions (Harvey & Gumport, 2015; Nilsen & Bernhardsson, 2019; Pfadenhaver et al., 2017).

Clients seen in practice may experience the health problem and present with sociodemographic and health characteristics in a way that differs, to various extent, from those reported for clients who participated in research studies that demonstrated the effectiveness of the interventions. The differences in the experience of the health problem and characteristics between the two cohorts of clients raise concerns about the applicability of the evidence, generated in research, to practice (as mentioned in Chapter 14). The limited relevance of evidence to practice can potentially influence the adoption of the evidence-based intervention in practice.

Clients seen in practice may be aware of the evidence-based intervention and its benefits. Therefore, they demand or seek it, which motivates the implementation initiatives aimed to make the evidence-based intervention available and accessible in the local practice. Alternatively, clients may perceive an evidence-based intervention as unacceptable, and consequently decline its uptake when offered in the local practice setting.

*Health professionals*: Health professionals are the users of evidence-based interventions. Personal attributes and professional qualifications, mentioned in Chapters 5, 8, 9, and 13, affect the adoption and delivery of evidence-based interventions in practice. Health professionals vary in their underlying philosophy of care and attitudes toward change in practice, which shape their perceptions of evidence-based interventions. In general, health professionals value a client-centered approach to care, characterized by flexibility and individualization of treatment. In health professionals' opinion, these features are not afforded in evidence-based interventions, limiting their acceptability and adoption of the interventions. In addition, health professionals may not have the theoretical knowledge underlying the evidence-based interventions and the competence or sense of self-efficacy to deliver the evidence-based interventions, which reduce their enthusiasm for adopting the interventions (Harvey & Gumport, 2015; Lau et al., 2016).

*Evidence-based interventions*: The features of the evidence-based interventions and the evidence supporting their effectiveness, influence their adoption, implementation, and effectiveness in practice. The specific features of interventions of concern include their complexity, applicability, and relevance to the local practice context; clarity and practicality of its protocol; customization; and cost (Lau et al., 2016). Evidence-based interventions that are complex, involving multiple components that are delivered by interprofessional team members, following a standardized or fixed protocol that contains limited practical guidance, are difficult and expensive to carry out. Furthermore, the supportive evidence of many health interventions indicates that, although the interventions had statistically significant effects, the observed effects are often of a small size and not maintained over time. The effects are estimated and thus applicable to clients who experience the health problem, but do not have comorbid conditions, limiting the relevance of the evidence-based intervention to all subgroups of clients seen in practice (Hartveit et al., 2019; Harvey & Gumport, 2015). Evidence-based interventions that are complex, costly, and provide benefits comparable to those achieved with usual care may not be adopted.

*Context*: The context in which the evidence-based intervention is implemented is influential. The contextual factors operate at different levels, including the local practice setting (e.g. clinic, hospital, community center), the organization or the community, and the healthcare system or society at large. The factors may directly or interactively affect the adoption, implementation, and effectiveness of evidence-based interventions as discussed in Chapters 5, 9, and 13. Contextual factors that are commonly identified include: communication and collaboration among health professionals; peer relationships or pressure; availability of human and material resources, in an adequate amount required to implement an intervention; culture prevalent in the practice setting, organization, community, or society (e.g. presence of commonly held values and beliefs); readiness for change, that is, decision-makers and health professionals' collective confidence to implement change and commitment to pursue a course of action leading to successful change (Teal et al., 2012); and practice setting or organization climate, that is, the perception shared among health professionals of the extent to which implementation of the evidence-based intervention is supported and expected (DiMartino et al., 2018; Harvey & Gumport, 2015; Lau et al., 2016; Nilsen & Bernhardsson, 2019; Pfadenhaver et al., 2017).

*Strategies*: Strategies used to facilitate the implementation of evidence-based interventions can influence their adoption and delivery. In addition to the specific strategies used to disseminate an intervention (see Section 16.1.2), the material or instrumental (e.g. increasing availability and access to resources), social (e.g. strong leadership making necessary changes in policies and practice guidelines), and financial support influence the success of the implementation initiatives (DiMartino et al., 2018; Lau et al., 2016; Nilsen, 2015; Pfadenhaver et al., 2017).

## 16.1.2   Process Frameworks

Process frameworks specify the phases or stages and steps to plan and execute the implementation initiatives (Damschroder, 2020; Nilsen, 2015). The process aims to facilitate change in practice (i.e. adoption and use of evidence-based interventions) at the individual (i.e. health professionals) and the collective (i.e. healthcare team members, support staff, decision-makers) levels (Hartveit et al., 2019). Despite some variability in its description, the implementation process comprises two main stages: pre-implementation and implementation (Moullin et al., 2015). Recent emphasis on the importance of accounting for the features of the local context in which the evidence-based intervention is implemented, contributed to the embracement of a collaborative process. In a collaborative process, stakeholder groups encompassing clients, health professionals, and decision-makers are engaged in preparing for and monitoring the implementation of evidence-based interventions (Aarons et al., 2017; Glandon et al., 2017; Pfadenhaver et al., 2017; Wandersman et al., 2016). The steps of this collaborative approach are reviewed next, and practice guidance for carrying them out is presented in Section 16.2.

### 16.1.2.1   Stage 1—Pre-implementation

The pre-implementation phase focuses on the preparation for the implementation of an evidence-based intervention. The preparation involves steps that (1) explore the local practice need for change in practice and local stakeholder groups' views on the evidence-based intervention; (2) determine the need for adapting the evidence-based intervention to the local practice context, and engage stakeholder groups in the adaptation of the evidence-based intervention; (3) assess for facilitators and barriers to implementation; and (4) engage local stakeholder groups in the selection of strategies or techniques to facilitate implementation.

Adaptation of the evidence-based intervention is advocated to improve its relevance and applicability to the local practice context. The adaptation promotes favorable perceptions and buy-in of the evidence-based intervention by local stakeholder groups, which enhances the adoption of the intervention (Aarons et al., 2017; Bach-Mortensen et al., 2018; Harvey & Gumport, 2015). Choosing training and support strategies that meet health professionals' learning needs and style is expected to build their personal competence in implementing the evidence-based intervention. Selecting techniques that address the specific (to the local context) facilitators and barriers are anticipated to promote collective implementation of the intervention. The end result is implementation of the evidence-based intervention with flexible fidelity (see Chapter 9).

### 16.1.2.2   Stage 2—Implementation

The implementation stage involves the actual roll-out of the plan. This entails: providing the training and support to health professionals responsible for implementing the evidence-based intervention; carrying out other implementation strategies (e.g. changes in policy); and monitoring the delivery of the evidence-based intervention in practice (Nilsen, 2015; Pfadenhaver et al., 2017). A process evaluation is conducted to monitor the delivery of the evidence-based intervention and identify challenges in implementation, which should be appropriately and promptly addressed.

### 16.1.3   Evaluation Frameworks

Evaluation frameworks delineate the outcomes expected of the implementation initiatives. The outcomes form the basis for designing research studies to evaluate the success of the implementation initiatives (Damschroder, 2020; Nilsen, 2015). Generally, two sets of outcomes are specified.

The first set entails outcomes expected as a result of the implementation strategies aimed to promote the adoption of the evidence-based intervention in practice. These outcomes manifest as changes in health professionals' perceptions (e.g. acceptability) of the evidence-based intervention, knowledge, and competence in providing the intervention, adoption (i.e. actual use of the intervention in practice), and appropriate delivery (i.e. with fidelity) of the intervention in daily practice. Changes in these outcomes take place and are assessed at the health professionals' individual level and at the collective level. The collective level is often represented in the number or percentage of health professionals implementing the evidence-based intervention within the local practice setting.

The second set of outcomes reflects the benefits, to clients, anticipated of the evidence-based intervention. They include improvement in the clients' experience of the health problem, general health, and well-being. These outcomes are assessed at the individual client level and may be reported at the practice level as the percentage of clients exhibiting improvement (Fixsen et al., 2019a; Procter et al., 2011).

### 16.1.4   Selection of a Framework

Although implementation frameworks are categorized as focusing on determinants, processes, or outcomes, there is overlap in the categories; that is, some frameworks cover combinations of determinants, processes and outcomes. Selecting one particular framework may not provide a full or comprehensive understanding of the complexity of implementation, thereby limiting the careful planning, conduct and evaluation of the implementation initiatives (Nilsen, 2015). Therefore, it is advisable to develop, in collaboration with stakeholder groups, a logic model that specifies the determinants, processes and outcomes of relevance to the local practice context of implementation. As suggested by Smith et al. (2020), the implementation logic model identifies:

1. Determinants of implementation: These include the facilitators and barriers to implementation operating in the local practice setting.
2. Implementation strategies: These are the activities selected to address the locally experienced determinants, and applied to facilitate the adoption of the evidence-based intervention.
3. Mechanisms of action: These reflect the series of events or processes responsible for the success of the implementation strategies in enhancing adoption of the evidence-based intervention in practice. The processes represent changes in the determinants or in immediate outcomes induced by the strategies; examples are increased health professionals' knowledge and competence in delivering the evidence-based intervention.
4. Outcomes: The outcomes usually operationalize the ultimate outcomes of the implementation strategies. These are illustrated with the adoption of the evidence-based intervention in practice.

The implementation logic model focuses on the implementation strategies. It should be supplemented with the logic model of the evidence-based intervention to comprehensively evaluate the success of the implementation initiatives in improving clients' experiences. The intervention's logic model operationalizes the theory underlying the intervention as described in Chapter 5. The logic model guides the specification of client outcomes (i.e. second set of outcomes as mentioned in

Section 16.1.3) to be assessed in the implementation evaluation initiatives. The logic model also informs the design and conduct of the process and outcome evaluation of the evidence-based intervention, which are embedded within the implementation evaluation project, forming a hybrid or dual evaluation of the implementation strategies and of the evidence-based intervention.

## 16.2   GUIDANCE FOR APPLYING THE IMPLEMENTATION PROCESS

The success of the implementation process rests on a collaborative approach in applying the pre-implementation and the implementation stages. The collaborative approach entails engaging local stakeholder groups in the process. The stakeholder groups include: (1) decision-makers (administrative or clinical) who play a key role in supporting the implementation initiative; (2) health professionals (i.e. users of the intervention) who are expected to adopt and deliver the evidence-based intervention; and (3) clients (i.e. end users of the intervention) who receive the evidence-based intervention and carry out its treatment recommendations. Stakeholder groups' engagement in the process contributes to favorable perceptions of the evidence-based intervention and heightens the stakeholder groups' enthusiasm, motivation, and willingness to adopt the intervention and to collectively participate in resolving challenges that may be encountered throughout the process (Aarons et al., 2017; Glandon et al., 2017). Strategies for engaging stakeholder groups in pertinent steps of the pre-implementation (Sections 16.2.1–16.2.4, and the implementation (Section 16.2.5) stages are described next.

### 16.2.1   Exploration of Stakeholder Groups' Views of the Evidence-Based Intervention

The implementation of the evidence-based intervention is frequently challenged by problems of acceptability that limit adoption and proper implementation of the intervention, and undermine the intervention's effectiveness in practice (Aarons et al., 2017; Cabassa et al., 2014; Procter et al., 2011; Sekhon et al., 2017). It is helpful to explore clients', health professionals', and decision-makers' perception of the acceptability of the evidence-based intervention to be implemented in the local practice setting. Different designs and methods for assessing acceptability of health interventions are presented in Chapter 11. A mixed, quantitative and qualitative, method is useful and efficient in gathering relevant data from each stakeholder group. It involves individual or group sessions (Fox et al., 2019; Sidani et al., 2016; Yamada et al., 2020), during which the facilitator:

- Describes the evidence-based intervention. The description clarifies the intervention's goals, components (i.e. content, activities, and treatment recommendations), mechanism of action (i.e. immediate and intermediate outcomes) underlying its effects on the ultimate outcomes. In addition, resources needed for implementing the evidence-based intervention by health professionals and clients are identified, and evidence of benefits and risks (synthesized from the scientific literature) is presented. The description is informed by the intervention's logic model. A copy of the evidence-based intervention logic model (in the form of a figure, table, or infographic) is shared with participants to help them follow through the description and visualize what the intervention entails.

- Requests participants to individually rate the acceptability of the evidence-based intervention that was described. Validated measures of acceptability (see Chapter 11) are administered. Having two versions of the same measure would be helpful in comparing clients' and health professionals' perceived acceptability of the evidence-based intervention. Results of the comparison indicate convergence and divergence of their views, and guides attempts at resolving discrepancies. For example, two versions, one for clients and one for health professionals, of the Treatment Perception and Preference scale have been generated and validated (Fox et al., 2019; Sidani et al., 2018).
- Engages participants in a discussion of the evidence-based intervention. The discussion is focused on generating an understanding of participants' views or ratings of the overall acceptability of the evidence-based intervention and aspects (e.g. specific content, activity, mode, and dose of delivery) of the intervention that are viewed favorably (i.e. considered suitable, appropriate, useful, convenient) and unfavorably, and why.

The quantitative and qualitative findings are analyzed descriptively to identify aspects of the evidence-based intervention that are acceptable and those that are unacceptable. Acceptable aspects of the intervention are maintained, whereas unacceptable aspects are adapted in collaboration with the stakeholder groups. Assessment of the evidence-based intervention's acceptability can be done independently (as described previously) or can be integrated as the first step in the adaption of the intervention (as described next).

## 16.2.2   Adaptation of the Evidence-Based Intervention

As mentioned in Chapters 4, 5, and 13, and emphasized in the extant literature (Aarons et al., 2017; Bach-Mortensen et al., 2018; Cabassa et al., 2014), the evidence-based intervention has to be adapted in order to enhance its fit within the local practice setting. The adaptation enhances its adoption and reduces the potential of deviations or drifts in its implementation and subsequently, its effectiveness (Harvey & Gumport, 2015). The adaptation, however, should be carefully done in a way that improves its fit to the local practice context but maintains its active ingredients that are operationalized in the specific components. The need for drastic modifications in the evidence-based intervention's active ingredients indicates lack of fit, acceptability and utility of the intervention in a particular context, and calls for exploration of other evidence-based interventions.

The adaptation involves modifications in the wording of the information or content to be relayed, in nonspecific components and respective activities, as well as the mode (including format such as switching from standardized to tailored format) and dose of delivery. The modifications are justifiable to make the evidence-based intervention desirable and feasible within the resources available to clients and health professionals in the local practice setting. Accordingly, engagement of stakeholder groups in the adaptation is highly recommended.

Qualitative methods are appropriate to elicit the stakeholder groups' perspectives on the aspects of the evidence-based interventions to modify and how. These consist of individual, but preferably group sessions (to reach common or collective agreement). The sessions are held separately or integrated as the next step of the session focusing on assessing acceptability (described in Section 16.2.1). The session facilitator (Fox et al., 2019; Sidani et al., 2016) proceeds as follows:

- Describes the evidence-based intervention (i.e. its goals, components, mode, and dose of delivery), its mechanism of action, and the human and material resources required for its implementation, as delineated in the intervention's logic model.

- Identifies the active ingredients and the respective specific components (including content, activities and treatment recommendations) of the evidence-based intervention and explains the centrality of these components in activating the mechanism responsible for the intervention's effects on the ultimate outcomes.

- Reminds participants that the active ingredients are not to be modified in order to maintain the effectiveness of the evidence-based intervention when implemented in practice.

- Engage participants in a thorough discussion of the acceptability and feasibility of the evidence-based intervention, and of possible modifications that could be made to promote its implementation. The discussion of acceptability is the same as that described in Section 16.2.1. The discussion of feasibility focuses on: the capacity or ability of health professionals and clients to carry out the intervention; content or information that may not be relevant to the target client population; activities that may be challenging to perform within the constraints or resources available in the local context; aspects of the mode and dose of the intervention's delivery that may be challenging or convenient.

- Once potentially unacceptable and inconvenient aspects of the intervention and its delivery are identified, the facilitator invites participants in a problem-solving exercise aimed to delineate ways or changes to be made in each aspect that would render the evidence-based intervention acceptable, feasible, or convenient to provide by health professionals, and to engage in and enact by clients. The changes encompass not only modifications of the evidence-based intervention but also alterations in the context (e.g. introduction of new policies, hiring additional staff, or renovation of the physical environment) that facilitate the implementation of the evidence-based intervention in the local practice setting.

Participants' responses are content analyzed to clarify what aspects of the evidence-based intervention are to be adapted and how. The proposed modifications, agreeable to all stakeholder groups, are clearly delineated and integrated in the intervention's theory, logic model, and manual, which are used for training of, and as references for, health professionals involved in its implementation in practice.

## 16.2.3   Assessment of Facilitators and Barriers

As explained in Section 16.1.1, there is a myriad of factors that enable or hinder the adoption and implementation of evidence-based interventions in practice. The factors operate at different levels. Acceptability and feasibility are characteristics of the evidence-based intervention that influence its adoption, and are handled with appropriate adaptation as described in Sections 16.2.1 and 16.2.2. Identification of other facilitators and barriers, operating within the local practice setting, is important for the selection of the most appropriate and relevant implementation techniques that are designed to support health professionals' adoption of the intervention and practices related to the provision of the intervention (Lau et al., 2015; Powell et al., 2017). Different methods can be used to assess facilitators and barriers to implementation. The assessment has commonly involved health professionals and decision-makers who are responsible for making the evidence-based intervention available or accessible to clients. The methods for assessing facilitators and barriers include:

- Quantitative, survey-type, studies. The design of these studies is informed by determinants frameworks that identify factors affecting adoption and implementation of the evidence-based intervention. Single or multiple item measures assessing each factor are collated in a questionnaire that can be administered in hard or electronic format. Examples of measures are provided by Hartveit et al. (2019) and Smith and Hasan (2020). All health professionals and decision-makers in the local practice setting are requested to complete the questionnaire. Descriptive analysis of the data indicates the most relevant (e.g. commonly reported or highly rated) facilitators and barriers. Alternatively, the questionnaire can be developed to directly assess the importance of the influential factors. In this case, the questionnaire consists of a list of factors, a brief description of each factor, and a rating scale to determine respondents' perceptions of the most important factors in the local practice, or to prioritize (i.e. rank order) the factors as reported by Craig et al. (2017).
- Qualitative interviews. The interviews are held with a representative sample of health professionals and decision-makers. The interviews are held with individuals or groups, using a semistructured approach to elicit participants' perspectives on what factors may influence adoption and implementation of the evidence-based intervention and how the factors exert their influence (Damschroder, 2020; Hamilton & Finley, 2019). Content or thematic analysis of responses highlights the most influential factors and delineates the pathways through which they influence adoption and implementation.
- Mixed, quantitative and qualitative methods. Health professionals and decision-makers participate in an individual or group data collection session; self-complete relevant measures; and engage in a discussion focusing on identifying the most influential factors and elucidating the mechanism underlying their influence, as illustrated in Bell et al.'s (2014) study.
- Concept mapping. This is a structured exercise inviting participants to brainstorm to identify barriers and facilitators; to sort them into categories; and to rate them relative to their importance, feasibility, and changeability (for details, refer to Powell et al., 2017). Data analysis focuses on determining the most important yet changeable factors.

Assessment of facilitators and barriers identifies influential factors that should be addressed with relevant strategies in order to enhance adoption and implementation of the evidence-based intervention. The assessment can be done independently (as described previously), or in conjunction with methods for selecting implementation strategies (as explained in the next section).

## 16.2.4 Selection of Implementation Strategies

A wide array of implementation strategies have been used and evaluated for their success in promoting the adoption and implementation of evidence-based interventions in practice. Frequently mentioned strategies are: distribution of educational materials, educational meetings, local consensus processes, educational outreach visits, involvement of local opinion leaders, patient-mediated techniques, audit and feedback, reminders, marketing, mass media, and publishing performance data (Gagliardi, 2011). Systematic reviews of the empirical literature resulted in different categorization of the strategies. For example, Johnson and May (2015) identified four general types of strategies or techniques to change the behavior or practices of health professionals and synthesized evidence of their effectiveness. The four types included:

1. Persuasive techniques: These techniques focus on persuading local stakeholder groups to adopt the evidence-based intervention. They involve diffusion strategies such as marketing or mass media, or direct strategies such as building consensus or exploiting local opinion leaders to inform and convince local stakeholder groups of the importance of adopting the intervention. Persuasive techniques were found to have inconsistent and ambiguous effects in promoting adoption and implementation.

2. Educational and informational strategies: These are concerned with relaying knowledge related to the evidence-based intervention, through different media such as presentation and dissemination of written materials. Educational and informational techniques are somewhat successful in changing health professionals' practices but had unclear effects on client outcomes.

3. Action and monitoring techniques: These techniques consist of continuous monitoring and reinforcing (including provision of incentives) desired health professionals' behaviors reflective of change in practice. They produced some benefits.

4. Guideline implementation strategies: These entail multiple strategies that seek to restructure stakeholder groups, norms, and expectations of practice. They were useful in changing practice.

On the other hand, Lau et al. (2015) synthesized evidence derived from systematic reviews and categorized implementation strategies into those targeting health professionals (e.g. distribution of printed materials, educational outreach visits or meetings, audit, and feedback) and the organization (e.g. introduction of new roles), providing incentives, and changing policy. There was limited evidence on the utility of strategies targeting the organization, whereas those targeting health professionals, whether comprised of single or multiple components, were effective.

Michie et al. (2007, 2011, 2014) developed the Behavioural Change Wheel Model. The model identifies behavioral change strategies that can be used to address factors influencing health professionals' adoption and implementation of evidence-based interventions. Informed by relevant behavioral theories, they delineated three categories of factors that enable or hinder health professionals' change of practice (i.e. adoption and implementation of evidence-based interventions). The categories are: (1) capability, reflecting individuals' psychological and physical capacity to engage in an activity or behavior; (2) motivation, including habitual processes, emotional responding, and decision-making; and (3) opportunity, representing factors that lie outside the individual and that affect performance of the behavior. Nine categories of strategies were generated to address the factors. These were: education, persuasion, incentivization, coercion, training, restriction, environmental restructuring, modeling, and enablement (for details, refer to Michie et al., 2014).

Additional strategies that can be used in training health professionals in the evidence-based intervention are presented in Chapter 8.

The selection of implementation strategies is based on the facilitators and barriers operating in the local practice setting, and on input from the stakeholder groups (Wensig et al., 2010). The goal is to maintain consistency between the nature of the influential factors and the nature of the strategies' active ingredients, as suggested by Michie and colleagues and explained for the design of health interventions (Chapter 4). Further, stakeholder groups are engaged in the selection and operationalization of the strategies, with the goal of choosing the ones that are locally acceptable and feasible, which increases the likelihood of their effectiveness and efficiency. To this end, stakeholder groups are engaged in a group model building or intervention mapping exercise as described by Powell et al. (2017). Basically, this involves holding individual or group sessions during which participants are: (1) informed of the task at hand; (2) identify most influential factors, using a mix of quantitative and qualitative methods described in Section 16.2.3; (3) prioritize the factors; and either (4) generate ideas for strategies to address each prioritized factor (as is done in group model building described by Powell et al., 2017) and reach an agreement on the most appropriate, feasible and potentially useful ones; or (5) are informed of techniques derived from pertinent literature and found beneficial, asked to rate the acceptability of each technique, discuss the relevance and feasibility of the techniques to the local practice setting, and adapt the technique as necessary using the method described in Section 16.2.3. For each selected strategy, a protocol is developed to identify resources for its application are acquired prior and to guide its actual use in the implementation stage.

## 16.2.5   Implementation

All stakeholder groups are actively involved in the implementation stage, with the support of decision-makers. The selected implementation strategies are provided, whereby clients are informed of the evidence-based intervention and encouraged to demand it of health professionals, health professionals are trained in the theory underpinning the intervention and the skills for its delivery in practice (using techniques mentioned in Chapter 4 and in Section 16.2.4), and decision-makers revise policies and practices to ensure availability and accessibility of the required human and material resources, and offer instrumental support and reinforcement for all those involved in the adoption and implementation of the evidence-based intervention.

A comprehensive and in-depth process evaluation is conducted in the initial (e.g. 3–6 months) implementation stage in order to identify challenges in providing the intervention. Mixed quantitative (e.g. survey, observation) and qualitative (e.g. interviews with all stakeholder groups) methods are used to gain a thorough understanding of what did and did not work, why, and under what circumstances or context. The results of process evaluation inform necessary revisions or refinement of the implementation strategies (e.g. plan for more intensive or extensive training) and/or the evidence-based intervention logic model and manual, in preparation for evaluating the success of the implementation efforts.

## 16.3   RESEARCH DESIGNS FOR EVALUATING IMPLEMENTATION INITIATIVES

Implementation initiatives are often considered complex. They involve two sets of interventions comprised of single or multiple components and targeting change in health professionals' behavior or practices (implementation strategies) and in clients' experience of the health problem (evidence-based intervention). The complex interventions, combining implementation strategies and the evidence-based intervention, activate different mechanisms responsible for their effects on two sets of outcomes taking place at the level of health professionals and clients, respectively. Furthermore, the interventions are implemented in the real world, where various factors, operating at different levels, influence the health professionals' adoption and implementation of the evidence-based intervention; health professionals' practices, along with clients' experience of the health problem, beliefs, and life circumstances, affect the clients' perceptions of the evidence-based intervention and subsequently clients' engagement, enactment, and adherence to treatment recommendations, and ultimately the effectiveness of the evidence-based intervention.

A thorough and valid evaluation of the implementation initiatives should account for this complexity. Accordingly, the evaluation is guided by relevant intervention theory (Chapter 5) or implementation frameworks (Section 16.1.4). The logic model guides the overall plan of the study evaluating the implementation initiative; the logic model points to the concepts or variables to be measured at different levels and from different sources, to the most opportune time for assessing the variables, and to interrelationships among them that should be examined. The examination aims to determine (1) the success of the implementation strategies in promoting adoption of the evidence-based intervention; (2) the fidelity with which the evidence-based intervention is provided by health professionals; (3) the uptake, engagement and enactment of the evidence-based intervention by clients; (4) the capacity of the evidence-based intervention in inducing its mechanism of action responsible for its effectiveness on the ultimate outcomes; and (5) contextual factors that influenced implementation and effectiveness of the evidence-based intervention.

A pragmatic approach and respective designs, described in Chapter 14, are most appropriate and feasible for evaluating implementation initiatives. The evaluation focuses on process and outcome, while accounting for context, embedded within a mix of designs and methods. A range of designs are considered for implementation initiatives carried out at the group (e.g. in-patient unit), organization (e.g. long-term care facility), or community levels. In these designs, the experimental group consists of these entities that receive the implementation strategies and the evidence-based intervention, and the comparison group consists of comparable entities that are not exposed to the strategies and intervention. Designs advocated for implementation evaluation include: (1) experimental (i.e. cluster randomized trial, stepped-wedge design, or practical clinical trials); (2) quasi-experiment, involving nonrandomized trials with experimental and comparison groups (e.g. cohort and observation designs) or single-group with repeated measures or time series; and (3) mixed design, specifically the hybrid design and mixed quantitative and qualitative methods designs (Fixsen et al., 2019b; Smith & Hasan, 2020). These designs are detailed in Chapter 14 and are briefly described by Hwang et al. (2020).

Actively engaging stakeholder groups in the process of designing and conducting the implementation evaluation project, in the role of either consultants or collaborators or partners (with equal status in decision-making) is important to enhance the feasibility of the evaluation. In addition, the stakeholder groups provide informative input in the interpretation of the implementation evaluation study's findings. They offer useful insight regarding what actually may have happened, on the ground, that contributed to the success (or failure) of the implementation efforts.

# REFERENCES

Aarons, G.A., Sklar, M., Mustanski, B., Benbow, N., & Brown, H. (2017. "Scaling-out" evidence-based interventions to new populations or new health care delivery system. *Implementation Science*, 12, 111–123. doi:10.1186/s13012-017-0640-6

Bach-Mortensen, A.M., Lange, B.C.L., & Montgomery, P. (2018. Barriers and facilitators to implementing evidence-based interventions among third sector organization: A systematic review. *Implementation Science*, 13, 103–121. doi; 10.1186/s13012-018-0789-7

Bell, J.J., Rossi, T., Bauer, J.D., & Capra, S. (2014) Developing and evaluating interventions that are applicable and relevant to inpatients and those who care for them; A multiphase, pragmatic action research approach. *BMC Medical Research Methodology*, 14, 98–107.

Cabassa, L.J., Gomes, A.P., Meyreles, Q., et al. (2014) Using the collaborative intervention planning framework to adapt a health-care manager intervention to a new population and provider group to improve the health of people with serious mental illness. *Implementation Science*, 9(178), 1–11.

Craig, L., Churilov, L., Olenko, L., et al. (2017) Testing a systematic approach to identify and prioritise barriers to successful implementation of a complex healthcare intervention. *BMC Medical Research Methodology*, 17, 24–37. doi:10.1186/s12874-017-0298-4

Damschroder, L.J. (2020. Clarity out of chaos: Use of theory in implementation research. *Psychiatry Research*, 283, 112461. doi:10.1016/j.psychres.2019.06.036

DiMartino, L.D., Birken, S.A., Hanson, L.C., et al. (2018) The Influence of formal and informal policies and practices on healthcare innovation implementation: A mixed-methods analysis. *Health Care Manage Review*, 43(3), 249–260. doi:10.1097/HMR.0000000000000019

Fixsen, D.L., Van Dyke, M., & Blase, K.A. (2019a) *Implementation Science: Fidelity Predictions and Outcomes*. Active Implementation Research Network, Chapel Hill, NC. www.activeimplementation.org/resources

Fixsen, D.L., Van Dyke, M.K., & Blase, K.A. (2019b) *Implementation Methods and Measures*. Active Implementation Research Network, Chapel Hill, NC. www.activeimplementation.org/resources

Fox, M.T., Sidani, S., Butler, J.I., Skinner, M.W., & Alzghoul, M.M. (2019. Protocol of a multimethod descriptive study: Adapting hospital-to-home transitional care interventions to the rural healthcare context in Ontario, Canada. *BMJ Open*, 9:e028050. doi:10.1136/bmjopen-2018-028050

Glandon, D., Paina, L., Alonge, O., Peters, D.H., & Bennett, S. (2017) 10 Best resources for community engagement in implementation research. *Health Policy and Planning*, 32, 1457–1465. doi:10.1093/heapol/czx123

Gagliardi, A.R. (2011) Tailoring interventions: Examining the evidence and identifying gaps. *Journal of Continuing Education in Health Professions*, 31(4), 276–282.

Hamilton, A.B. & Finley, E.P. (2019) Qualitative methods in implementation research: An introduction. *Psychiatry Research*, 280, 112516. doi:10.1016/j.psychres.2019.112516

Harris, M., Lawn, S.J., Morello, A., et al. (2017) Practice change in chronic conditions care: An appraisal of theories. *BMC Health Services Research*, 17, 170–179. doi:10.1186/s12913-017-2012-x

Hartveit, M., Hovlid, E., Nordin, M.H.A., et al. (2019) Measuring implementation: development of the implementation process assessment tool (IPAT). *BMC Health Services Research*, 19, 721–731. doi:10.1186/s12913-019-4496-0

Harvey, A.G. & Gumport, N.B. (2015) Evidence-based psychological treatments for mental disorders: Modifiable barriers to access and possible solutions. *Behavior Research and Therapy*, 68, 1–12. doi:10.1016/j.brat.2015.02.004

Hwang, S., Birken, S.A., Melvin, C.L., Rohweder, C.L., & Smith, J.D. (2020) Designs and methods for implementation research: Advancing the mission of the CTSA program. *Journal of Clinical and Translational Science*, 4, 159–167. doi:10.1017/cts.2020.16

Johnson, M.J. & May, C.R. (2015) Promoting professional behaviour change in healthcare: What interventions work and why? A Theory-led overview of systematic reviews. *BMJ Open*, 5, e008592. doi:10.1136/bmjopen-2015-008592.

Lau, R., Stevenson, F., Ong, B.N., et al. (2016) Achieving change in primary care – causes of the evidence to practice gap: Systematic reviews of reviews. *Implementation Science*, 11, 40–78. doi:10.1186/s13012-016-0396-4

Lau, R., Stevenson, F., Ong, B.N., et al. (2015) Achieving change in primary care – effectiveness of strategies for improving implementation of complex interventions: Systematic reviews of reviews. *BMJ Open*, 5, e009993. doi:10.1136/bmjopen-2015-00993.

Michie, S., Atkins, L., & West, R. (2014) *The Behavioural Change Wheel. A Guide to Designing Interventions*, 1st edn. Silverback Publishing, Great Britain, pp. 1003–1010.

Michie, S., Pilling, S., Garety, P., et al. (2007) Difficulties implementing a mental health guideline: An exploratory investigation using psychological theory. *Implementation Science*, 2, 8–15. doi:10.1186/1748-5908-2-8.

Michie, S., van Stralen, M.M., & West, R. (2011) The behaviour change wheel: A new method for characterizing and designing bahaviour change interventions. *Implementation Science*, 6, 42–52. http://www.implementation.com/content/6/1/42

Moullin, J.C., Sabater-Hernández, D., Fernandez-Llimos, F., & Benrimoj, S.I. (2015) A systematic review of implementation frameworks of innovations in healthcare and resulting generic implementation framework. *Health Research Policy and Systems*, 13, 16–26. doi:10.1186/s12961-015-0005-z

Nilsen, P. (2015) Making sense of implementation theories, models and frameworks. *Implementation Science*, 10, 53–65. doi:10.1186/s13012-015-0242-0

Nilsen, P. & Bernhardsson, S. (2019) Context matters in implementation science: A scoping review of determinant frameworks that describe contextual determinants for implementation outcomes. *BMC Health Services Research*, 19, 189–200. doi:10.1186/s12913-019-4015-3

Pfadenhaver, L.M., Gerhardus, A., Mozygemba, K., et al. (2017) Making sense of complexity in content and implementation: The Context and Implementation of Complex Interventions (CICI) framework. *Implementation Science*, 12, 21–37.

Powell, B.J., Beidas, R.S., Lewis, C.C., et al. (2017) Methods to improve the selection and tailoring of implementation strategies. *Journal of Behavioral Health Services Research*, 44(2), 177–194. doi:10.1007/s11414-015-9475-6

Procter, E., Silmere, H., Raghavan, R., et al. (2011) Outcomes for implementation research: Conceptual distinctions, measurement challenges and research agenda. *Administration & Policy in Mental Health*, 38, 65–76. doi:10.1007/s10488-010-0319-7

Sekhon, M., Cartwright, M., & Francis, J.J. (2017) Acceptability of healthcare interventions: An overview of reviews and development of a theoretical framework. *BMC Health Services Research*, 17, 88–100. doi:10.1186/s12913-017-2031-8

Sidani, S., Manojlovich, M., Doran, D., et al. (2016) Nurses' perception of interventions for the management of patient-oriented outcomes: An exploration. *Worldviews on Evidence-Based Nursing*, 13(1), 66–74.

Sidani, S., Epstein, D.R., Miranda, J., & Fox, M. (2018) Psychometric properties of the Treatment Perception and Preferences scale. *Clinical Nursing Research*, 27(6), 743–761. doi:10.1177/1054773816654137

Smith, J.D., Li, D., & Rafferty, M.R. (2020) The implementation research logic model: A method for planning, executing, reporting, and synthesizing implementation projects. *BMJ medRxiv* 2020.04.05.20054379. doi:10.1101/2020.04.05.20054379

Smith, J.D. & Hasan, M. (2020) Quantitative approaches for the evaluation of implementation research studies. *Psychiatry Research*, 283, 112521. doi:10.1016/j.psychres.2019.112521

Teal, R., Bergmire, D.M., Johnston, M., & Weiner, B.J. (2012) Implementing community-based provider participation in research: An empirical study. *Implementation Science*, 7, 41–55.

Wandersman, A., Alia, K., Cook, B.S., Hsu, L.L., & Ramaswamy, R. (2016) Evidence-based interventions are necessary but not sufficient for achieving outcomes in each setting in a complex world: Empowerment evaluation, getting to outcomes and demonstrating accountability. *American Journal of evaluation*, 37(4), 544–561. doi:10.1177/1098214016660613

Wensig, M., Bosch, M., & Grol, R. (2010) Developing and selecting interventions for translating knowledge to action. *Canadian Medical Association Journal*, 182(2), E85–E88. doi:10.1503/cmaj.081233

Yamada, J., Ballantyne, M., Kron, A., & Sidani, S. (2020). Parents' perceptions of evidence-based interventions to support transition to rehabilitation services. *Canadian Journal of Nursing Research*. doi:10.1177/0844562120931661

# Index

## A

Acceptability, intervention
  assessment of
    confirmation of desirability,
        230–31, 231t
    development of interven-
        tion, 229–30
    examining acceptability in descriptive
        studies, 231
    examining acceptability in evaluative
        studies, 232
  examination of
    conceptualization, 226–27
    measure acceptability, 227–29
  formulation of
    awareness of treatment, 220
    beliefs about health problem,
        219–20
    evaluation study, 220–21
    personal and health profiles, 219
  significant contribution of, 218–19
  treatment perceptions
    and attrition, 223–25
    and enrollment, 223
    and implementation, 225–26
    and outcomes, 222–23
Active ingredients, 24
Adaptation debate, 125–26
Adaptive designs, 324–25
Adaptive interventions, 87–88
Adaptive (Urn) randomization, 383
Adherence, 172–73
  client report on adherence, 184–84
  instruments measuring adherence,
      179–80

intervention delivery, 181–83
interventionist self-report on
    adherence, 183–84
Armstrong, T.S., 180
Assessing fidelity, 122–24
Attitudes and Expectations
    Questionnaire, 236
Audition-style interviews, 156

## B

Baethge, C., 306
Bartholomew, L.K., 56, 72
Beasly, M.J., 236
Behavior Change Model, 404
Behavior health, 21
Bellg, A.J., 171
Bishop, D.B., 32
Block randomization, 382–83
Borkovec, T.D., 235
Broadbent, H.J., 306

## C

Carter, S.L., 227
Categorization of health problems, 33
Causative factors, 35
Chavalarias, D., 199
Client-centered care, 4, 7–8
Client responsiveness, 174
  enactment, 287–88
  engagement
    interventionist report, 285–86
    observation, 284–85
    participant report, 286–87
  exposure, 283–84
Client Satisfaction Questionnaire, 237